Soft Biological Shells in Bioengineering

IPEM–IOP Series in Physics and Engineering in Medicine and Biology

About the Series

Series in Physics and Engineering in Medicine and Biology will allow IPEM to enhance its mission to 'advance physics and engineering applied to medicine and biology for the public good.'

Focusing on key areas including, but not limited to:

- clinical engineering
- diagnostic radiology
- informatics and computing
- magnetic resonance imaging
- nuclear medicine
- physiological measurement
- radiation protection
- radiotherapy
- rehabilitation engineering
- ultrasound and non-ionising radiation.

A number of IPEM–IOP titles are published as part of the EUTEMPE Network Series for Medical Physics Experts.

Soft Biological Shells in Bioengineering

Roustem N Miftahof
Technische Universität Hamburg, Institut für Kontinuums - und Werkstoffmechanik, Germany

Nariman R Akhmadeev
Kazan State Medical University, Republican Clinical Hospital of Ministry of Health, Republic of Tatarstan, Russia

IOP Publishing, Bristol, UK

ISBN 978-0-7503-2195-2 (ebook)
ISBN 978-0-7503-2193-8 (print)
ISBN 978-0-7503-2194-5 (mobi)

DOI 10.1088/2053-2563/ab1a9e

Version: 20190701

IOP Expanding Physics
ISSN 2053-2563 (online)
ISSN 2054-7315 (print)

British Library Cataloguing-in-Publication Data: A catalogue record for this book is available from the British Library.

Published by IOP Publishing, wholly owned by The Institute of Physics, London

IOP Publishing, Temple Circus, Temple Way, Bristol, BS1 6HG, UK

US Office: IOP Publishing, Inc., 190 North Independence Mall West, Suite 601, Philadelphia, PA 19106, USA

Contents

Preface

Publications dedicated to the modeling of soft visceral organs, including the eyeball, esophagus, stomach, small intestine, colon, gallbladder, uterus, ureter, and urinary bladder, remain sparse. The novelty and strength of this book lies in the holistic modeling of these organs as soft biological active shells, an approach never previously achieved. Here, the precise study of mathematics has been combined with the descriptive science of biology and medicine to form a coherent structure that accurately represents the organs' function.

This book serves three functions: (i) introducing the general principles of the construction of multiscale models of organs by integrating existing experimental data at different structural levels; (ii) providing an understanding of the intricacies of physiological processes through numerical simulations; and (iii) giving a perspective to current knowledge. It is intended as a textbook for courses in computational systems biology for advanced undergraduate and/or first year graduate students, as well as researchers and instructors of applied mathematics, biomedical engineering, and computational biology, alongside mathematically savvy medical doctors.

The book is divided into two parts. In part I, the general theory of shells introduces the basic concepts of: the theory of surfaces; the parameterization of shells of complex geometry; the nonlinear theory of thin elastic and soft shells; boundary conditions; the modeling of biological tissues; the neurochemical processes of signal transduction in neuronal networks; and pharmacological modulations. Although the material provided is sufficient to understand the fundamentals used in the applications described in the book (see part II), the reader is advised, in addition, to consult special texts for fuller details.

Part II is dedicated to modeling the stomach, small intestine, uterus, and urinary bladder. Their functions are studied under both normal and pathological conditions using an approach based on the combined reduction of integrated systems biology approach. In such an approach, the first consideration is always to understand the biological essentials that support the principles involved in the construction of a model; a summary of these is provided at the start of each chapter. This is followed by a formulation of the one-dimensional model and an investigation of a functional unit of the organ. Each chapter concludes with the modeling of the organ as a soft biological shell.

At the time of writing, publications dedicated to the modeling of soft visceral organs remain sparse. Instead of providing a comprehensive reference list on different aspects of the topics covered in each chapter, a suggested list of further reading is given at the end of that chapter. The intention is to indicate the original research papers of importance in the area concerned in the hope of assisting and motivating the more diligent reader to study in depth some of the more complex areas of the material presented here.

The book has depended on the assistance, advice, and encouragement of many people. We are indebted to all who have contributed both directly and indirectly to this book. We are particularly grateful to Ms Wendy Pearson for thoroughly reviewing the manuscript, providing valuable comments on its content, and editing the text. Our gratitude extends to our families for their continuous support and, finally, we are grateful to the publisher, the Institute of Physics Publishing LLC, Bristol, UK, who supported the project and made its successful publication possible.

Professor Dr Roustem N Miftahof
Dr Nariman R Akhmadeev

Author biographies

Roustem N Miftahof

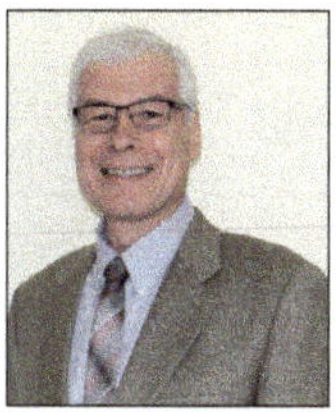

Roustem N Miftahof is a Professor, Dr of Medicine and Applied Mathematics. Internationally acclaimed as a leading scientist in the field of systems computational biology and medicine, Professor Miftahof has authored and co-authored six previous books on these subjects.

Nariman R Akhmadeev

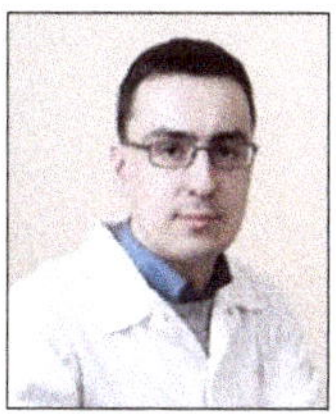

Nariman R Akhmadeev works as an Assistant Professor at the Department of Obstetrics and Gynecology at Kazan State Medical University, Russia. With an MD/MBBS degree and PhD, he combines a career as an academician and physician with a specific research interest in the application of mathematical and computational methods in his area.

Notations

$\overset{0}{S}, S, \overset{*}{S}$	cut, undeformed and deformed (*) middle surface of a shell
S_z	surface co-planar to S such that $S_z \parallel S$
S^r	middle surface of a net
$\Sigma, \overset{*}{\Sigma}$	boundary faces of an undeformed and deformed shell
$d\Sigma, d\overset{*}{\Sigma}$	differential line elements on $\Sigma, \overset{*}{\Sigma}$
h	thickness
x_1, x_2, x_3	rectangular coordinates
$\{\bar{i}_1, \bar{i}_2, \bar{i}_3\}$	orthonormal base of $\{x_1, x_2, x_3\}$
$\{\bar{k}_1, \bar{k}_2, \bar{k}_3\}$	orthonormal base of $\{r, \varphi, z\}$
(α_1, α_2), $(\overset{*}{\alpha}_1, \overset{*}{\alpha}_2)$	coordinates of the undeformed and deformed shell
$\bar{m}, \overset{*}{\bar{m}}$	vectors normal to S and $\overset{*}{S}$
$\bar{\tau}, \bar{\tau}^z, \overset{*}{\bar{\tau}}$	tangential vectors to a line on S, S_z, $\overset{*}{S}$ or their boundaries
$\bar{n}, \bar{n}^z, \overset{*}{\bar{n}}$	normal vectors to a line on the boundary of S, S_z, and $\overset{*}{S}$
$\bar{r}, \bar{\rho}, \overset{*}{\bar{\rho}}$	position vectors of points $M \in S$, $M_z \in S_z$, and $\overset{*}{M}_z \in \overset{*}{S}_z$, respectively
$\bar{r}_i, \bar{\rho}_i$	tangential vectors to coordinate lines on S and S_z
$\{\bar{r}_1, \bar{r}_2, \bar{m}\}$, $\{\bar{r}^1, \bar{r}^2, \bar{m}\}$	covariant and contravariant bases at point $M \in S$
$\{\bar{\rho}_1, \bar{\rho}_2, \bar{\rho}_3\}$	covariant base at point $M_z \in S_z$
$\{\bar{n}, \bar{\tau}, \bar{m}\}$, $\{\overset{*}{\bar{n}}, \overset{*}{\bar{\tau}}, \overset{*}{\bar{m}}\}$	orthogonal bases on Σ and $\overset{*}{\Sigma}$, respectively
$\chi, \chi^z, \overset{*}{\chi}$	angles between coordinate lines defined on S, S_z, $\overset{*}{S}$
γ	shear angle
$A_i, \overset{*}{A}_i, H_i$	Lamé coefficients on S, $\overset{*}{S}$, and S_z
a_{ik}	components of the metric tensor
$a, \overset{*}{a}$	determinants of the metric tensor
b_{ik}	components of the second fundamental form
$\bar{e}_i, \bar{e}_i^z, \overset{*}{\bar{e}}_i, \overset{*}{\bar{e}}_i^z$	unit base vectors on S, S_z, and $\overset{*}{S}$
$ds, ds_z, d\overset{*}{s}$	lengths of line elements on S, S_z, and $\overset{*}{S}$
ds_Δ	surface area of a differential element of S
$\Gamma_{ik,j}, \Gamma_{ik}^j$	Christoffel symbols of the first and second kind
A_{ik}^j	deviator of the Christoffel symbols
$\bar{v}(\alpha_1, \alpha_2)$	displacement vector
u_1, u_2, ω	projections of the displacement vector on x_1, x_2, x_3 axes

$\varepsilon_{ik}, \varepsilon_{ik}^{z}$	components of the tensor of planar deformation through points $M \in S$ and $M_z \in S_z$
$\tilde{\varepsilon}_{ik}, \overset{*}{\tilde{\varepsilon}}_{ik}$	physical components of the tensor deformation in undeformed and deformed configurations of a shell
$\varepsilon_1, \varepsilon_2$	principal physical components of the tensor of deformation
$\varsigma_{ij}, \Delta_{ij}$	elastic and viscous parts of deformation
$\varepsilon_n, \varepsilon_\tau\ \varepsilon_{n\tau}$	components of deformation of the boundary of a shell in $\bar{n}$, $\bar{\tau}$ directions
$\underline{\varepsilon}_{ik}, \underline{æ}_{ik}$	components of the tensor of tangent and bending fictitious deformations
$\lambda_i, \lambda_{c,l}$	stretch ratios (subscripts c and l refer to the circular and longitudinal directions of a bioshell)
$\mathbf{\Lambda}_1, \mathbf{\Lambda}_2$	principal stretch ratios
$I_1^{(\mathbf{E})}, I_2^{(\mathbf{E})}$	invariants of the tensor of deformation
$æ_n, æ_\tau, æ_{n\tau}$	components of bending deformation and twist of the boundary of a shell in $\bar{n}$, $\bar{\tau}$ directions
$e_{nn}, e_{n\tau}, e_{n\tau}$, $e_{\tau n}, \omega_n, \omega_\tau$	rotation parameters
$e_{\alpha 1}, e_{\alpha 2}$	elongations in directions α_1, α_2, respectively
$\underline{e}_i^{k}, \underline{e}_{ki}, \underline{\omega}_i$	rotation parameters in fictitious deformation
$k_{ii}, \overset{*}{k}_{ii}$	normal curvatures of S and $\overset{*}{S}$
$k_{ik}, \overset{*}{k}_{ik}$	twists of S and $\overset{*}{S}$
$k_n, k_\tau, k_n^*, k_\tau^*$	normal curvatures in $\bar{n}$, $\bar{\tau}$, $\overset{*}{\bar{n}}$, $\overset{*}{\bar{\tau}}$ directions
$k_{n\tau}, k_{n\tau}^*$	twists of the contours Σ and $\overset{*}{\Sigma}$
$1/R_{1,2}, 1/R_{1,2}{}^*$	principal curvatures of S and $\overset{*}{S}$
K, K_0	Gaussian curvatures of S and $\overset{*}{S}$
$L'_j(\varepsilon_{ik}), L_i(T_{ik})$	differential operators
$\bar{p}_i$	stress vector
$\bar{R}_i$	resultant of force vector
$\bar{p}_{(+)}, \bar{p}_{(-)}$	external forces applied over the free surface area of a shell
$\overset{*}{\bar{p}}{}_n^{z}$	normal stress vector on $\overset{*}{\Sigma}$
$\bar{F}$	vector of mass forces per unit volume of the deformed element of a shell
$\bar{X}$	resultant external force vector on $\overset{*}{S}$
$\bar{M}$	resultant external moment of external forces on $\overset{*}{S}$
$\overset{*}{T}_{ii}, \overset{*}{T}_{ik}, \overset{*}{N}_i$	normal, shear, and lateral forces per unit length
$T_{c,l}$	total force per unit length
$T_{c,l}^{\mathrm{p}}, T_{c,l}^{\mathrm{a}}$	passive and active components of the total forces per unit length
T_1^r, T_2^r	forces per unit length of reinforced fibers
T_1, T_2	principal stresses

$I_1^{(\mathbf{T})}$, $I_2^{(\mathbf{T})}$	invariants of the stress tensor
$\overset{*}{M}_{ii}$, $\overset{*}{M}_{ik}$	bending and twisting moments per unit length of a shell perpendicular to α_1, α_2 directions on $\overset{*}{S}$
$\overset{*}{M}_i$	projections of the moment vector on $\overset{*}{\bar{e}}_1$, $\overset{*}{\bar{e}}_2$, $\overset{*}{\overline{m}}$
$\overset{*}{X}_i$	projections of the external force vector on $\overset{*}{\bar{e}}_1$, $\overset{*}{\bar{e}}_2$, $\overset{*}{\overline{m}}$
$\bar{R}_n^*$	resultant force vector per unit length acting on $d\overset{*}{\Sigma}_z$ in the $\overset{*}{\bar{n}}$ direction
$\bar{M}_n^*$	resultant moment vector per unit length acting on $d\overset{*}{\Sigma}_z$ in the $\overset{*}{\bar{n}}$ direction
$\overset{*}{G}$, $\overset{*}{H}$	bending and twisting moments in a boundary of a shell
$\bar{G}_i$, $\bar{M}_p$, $\bar{M}_q$	resultant moment vectors per unit length of a soft shell
σ_{ij}	stresses in a shell
σ_{ij}^{α}	stresses in the α phase of a biomaterial
c_i	material constants
d_m, d_f	diameter of smooth muscle fiber and nerve terminal, respectively
L, L^s, L_0^s	length of bioshell/muscle fiber, axon, and nerve terminal, respectively
ρ, $\overset{*}{\rho}$	densities of undeformed and deformed material of a shell
ρ_ζ^α	partial density of the ζth substrate in the α phase of a biomaterial
m_ζ^α	mass of the ζth substrate in the α phase of a biomaterial
υ, υ^α	total and elementary volumes of a biomaterial
c_ζ^α	mass concentration of the ζth substrate in the α phase of a biomaterial
η	porosity of the phase α
Q_ζ^e, Q_ζ	influxes of the ζth substrate into the α phase; external sources and exchange flux between phases
$\nu_{\zeta j}$	stoichiometric coefficient in the jth chemical reaction.
$U^{(\alpha)}$	free energy
$s^{(\alpha)}$, S_ζ^1	entropy of the α phase and partial entropy of the entire biomaterial
μ_ζ^α	chemical potential of the ζth substrate in the α phase of a biomaterial
$\bar{q}$	heat flux vector
$\boldsymbol{R}$	dissipative function
Λ_j	affinity constant of the jth chemical reaction
$\bar{J}_i$, $\bar{J}_o$	intra- (i) and extracellular (o) ion currents
I_{m1}, I_{m2}	transmembrane ion currents
I_{Appl}	applied external membrane current
I_{ion}	total ion current

$\tilde{I}^s_{Ca}$, $\tilde{I}^f_{Ca}$, $\tilde{I}_{Ca-K}$, $\tilde{I}_K$, $\tilde{I}_{Cl}$, I_{Ca}, I_{Ca-K}, I_{Na}, I_K, I_{Cl}, $\tilde{I}_{Na}$, I_{Cl}	ion currents
Ψ_i, Ψ_o	electrical potentials
V, V^s_n, V^e, V^d, V^s_l, V^s_c, V_i, $\overset{0}{V}$	transmembrane potentials
$\overset{(\sim)}{V}_{Ca}$, $\overset{(\sim)}{V}_{Ca-K}$, $\overset{(\sim)}{V}_{Na}$, $\overset{(\sim)}{V}_K$, $\overset{(\sim)}{V}_{Cl}$	reversal membrane potentials for respective ion currents
$V^{(+,-)}_{syn}$, $V_{syn,0}$	actual excitatory (+)/inhibitory (−) and resting synaptic membrane potentials
C_m, C^s_n, C_p, C^f_a, C_d	membrane capacitances of smooth muscle, synapse, postsynaptic structures, axon, and the free nerve endings, respectively
$R^{ms}_{i(0)}$	membrane resistance
R_s, R_v, R^f_a	specific membrane resistances of a myofiber, synapse and axon, respectively
$\hat{g}_{ij}$, $\hat{g}_{oj}$	intra- (i) and extracellular (o) conductivities
$\hat{g}^*_{i(0)}$	maximal intra- (i) and extracellular (o) conductivities
$g_{Ca(i)}$, $g_{Ca-K(i)}$, $g_{Na(i)}$, $g_{K(i)}$, $g_{Cl(i)}$, $\tilde{g}^f_{Ca}$, $\tilde{g}^s_{Ca}$, $\tilde{g}_K$, $\tilde{g}_{Ca-K}$, $\tilde{g}_{Cl}$, $\tilde{g}_{Na}$, g^f_{Na}, g^f_K, g^f_{Cl}	maximal conductances of respective ion channels
$\tilde{m}$, $\tilde{h}$, $\tilde{n}$, h_{Na}, n_K, z_{Ca}, ρ_∞, $\tilde{x}_{Ca}$	dynamic variables of respective ion currents
m_f, n_f, h_f	dynamic variables of ion channels at the synapse
$\tilde{\alpha}_y \tilde{\beta}_y$	activation and deactivation parameters of ion channels
f_{aD}, f_{aS}	normalized activity functions for the detrusor (D) and urethral sphincter (S)
ω^D_e, ω^D_i, ω_s	normalized excitatory (subscript e), inhibitory (i), and excitatory somatic (s) neural inputs
$Z^{(*)}_{mn}$	'biofactor'
$[Ca^{2+}_i]$	intracellular concentration of free Ca^{2+} ions
ϑ_{Ca}	parameter of calcium inhibition
λ, $\hbar$, $\wp_{Ca}$, τ_{Ca}, τ_m	electrical numerical parameters and constants

$\overset{0}{\breve{V}}, \breve{V}$	initial and current volumes
p_0, p	initial and current pressures
$\dot{p}$	rate of pressure change
$k_{(\pm)i}$	rate constants of chemical reactions
$\bar{v}_u(u_u, v_u, w_u)$	velocity vector of urine
μ_u, μ_w	dynamic viscosity of urine and water, respectively
ν_u	kinematic viscosity of urine
$\chi_1, \cdots, \chi_n$	physicochemical parameters
$\mathbf{A}$, $\mathbf{B}$, $\mathbf{C}$, $\mathbf{D}$	matrices of rate coefficients
$\mathbf{X}(X_i)^T$, $\mathbf{C_0}(C_i)^T$	vectors of reacting substrates

Acronyms

AC	adenylyl cyclase
ACh	acetylcholine
AChE	acetylcholinesterase
ACh–R	acetylcholine–receptor complex
AD	adrenaline
AHP	after-hyperpolarization
AP(s)	action potential(s)
ATP	adenosine-5′-triphosphate
BK_{Ca}	large conductance Ca^{2+} activated K^+ channel
cAMP	cyclic adenosine monophosphate
COX-1/2	cyclooxygenase 1 and 2
DAG	diacylglycerol
DMV	dorsal motor nucleus of the vagus
DP	dominant pacemaker
ECM	extracellular matrix
ENS	enteric nervous system
$EP_{1,2,3A,D}$	prostaglandin $E_{1,2,3A,D}$ receptors
EPSP	excitatory postsynaptic potential
hCG	human chorionic gonadotrophin
GDP/DTP	guanosine diphosphate/guanosine triphosphate
ICs	interstitial cells
ICC (MY, IM)	interstitial cells of Cajal (myenteric, intramuscular)
IGLE	intraganglionic laminar ending
IL	interleukin
IMA	intramuscular array
IP_3	inositol-1,4,5-triphosphate
IPSP	inhibitory postsynaptic potential
K_{ATP}	ATP sensitive K^+ channel
K_V	voltage-gated K^+ channel
MAPK	mitogen-activated protein kinase
MLCK	myosin light chain kinase
(f)MRI	(functional) magnetic resonance imaging
MP	myenteric nervous (Auerbach's) plexus
NA	noradrenaline
NCSCs	neural crest multipotent stem cells
NO	nitric oxide
nNOS	neuronal nitric oxide synthase
NTS	nucleus tractus solitaries
OT	oxytocin
P2X	purine type 2X receptors
PDE	phosphodiesterase
$PDGFR\alpha^+$	platelet-derived growth factor receptor α
PAG	periaqudactal gray
$PGF_{2\alpha}$	prostaglandin $F_{2\alpha}$
PGN	preganglionic neuron
PIP_2	inositide-4,5-biphosphate

PKA	protein kinase A
PKC	protein kinase C
PLC	phospholipase C
PMC	pontine micturition center
PR	progesterone
*m*PR, *n*PR	membrane and nuclear progesterone receptors
SIP	smooth muscle-interstitial cells of Cajal-syncytium
SM(C)	smooth muscle (cell)
SP	substance P
SR	sarcoplasmic reticulum
TTX	tetrodotoxin
VIP	vasoactive intestinal peptide
5-HT	5-hydroxytryptamine/serotonin

Part I

Fundamentals of soft biological shells

IOP Publishing

Soft Biological Shells in Bioengineering

Roustem N Miftahof and Nariman R Akhmadeev

Chapter 1

Geometry of the surface

A shell is a body bounded by two closely spaced curved boundary surfaces separated at a given distance (thickness). The shell is classified as thin or thick based on the ratio of the thickness to the radii of the curvature of the shell; if the ratio $\leqslant 0.05$ the shell is considered to be thin, otherwise it is regarded as thick. In this chapter, the classical results of the theory of surfaces in general curvilinear coordinates are introduced, followed by an analysis of the deformed surface under the assumption of finite deformations and displacements. The equations of continuity of deformations are derived.

1.1 Intrinsic geometry

Consider a smooth surface S in three-dimensional Euclidean space. It is referred to using a right-handed global orthogonal Cartesian system x_1, x_2, x_3. Let S also be associated with a set of independent parameters α_1 and α_2 (figure 1.1), such that

$$x_1 = f_1(\alpha_1, \alpha_2), \quad x_2 = f_2(\alpha_1, \alpha_2), \quad x_3 = f_3(\alpha_1, \alpha_2), \tag{1.1}$$

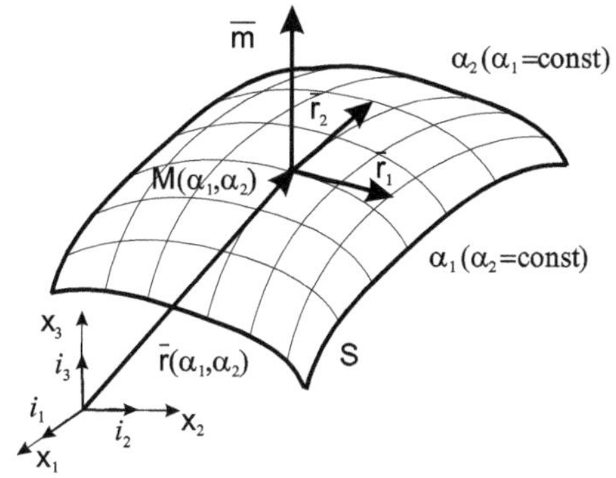

Figure 1.1. Intrinsic parameterization of the surface.

doi:10.1088/2053-2563/ab1a9ech1

where f_j (j = 1, 2, 3) are single-valued functions that possess derivatives up to any required order. Putting α_1 = const and varying the parameter α_2 in $f_j(c, \alpha_2)$, a curve is obtained that lies entirely on S. Successively giving α_1 a series of constant values, a family of curves is obtained along which only the parameter α_2 varies. These curves are called the α_2-coordinate lines. Similarly, setting α_2 = const the α_1-coordinate lines of S are obtained. It is assumed that only one curve of the family passes through a point of the given surface. Thus, any point M on S can be treated as a cross-intersection of the α_1 and α_2 curvilinear coordinate lines.

The position of a point M with respect to the origin O of the reference system is defined by the position vector $\bar{r}$:

$$\bar{r} = \bar{i}_1 x_1 + \bar{i}_2 x_2 + \bar{i}_3 x_3 = \sum_{i=1}^{3} \bar{i}_i x_i,$$

where $\{\bar{i}_1, \bar{i}_2, \bar{i}_3\}$ is the orthonormal triad of unit vectors associated with $\{x_1, x_2, x_3\}$. By the virtue of equations (1.1) it can be written in the form

$$\bar{r} = \bar{i}_1 f_1(\alpha_1, \alpha_2) + \bar{i}_2 f_2(\alpha_1, \alpha_2) + \bar{i}_3 f_3(\alpha_1, \alpha_2). \tag{1.2}$$

Equation (1.2) is the vector equation of a surface. Differentiating $\bar{r}$ with respect to α_i (i = 1, 2), the vectors tangent to the α_1- and α_2-coordinate lines are found to be

$$\bar{r}_1 = \frac{\partial \bar{r}}{\partial \alpha_1}, \quad \bar{r}_2 = \frac{\partial \bar{r}}{\partial \alpha_2}. \tag{1.3}$$

Modules and the scalar product of $\bar{r}_i$ (i = 1, 2) are defined by

$$\begin{aligned} |\bar{r}_1| &= \bar{r}_1 \bar{r}_1 = A_1 = \sqrt{a_{11}}, \\ |\bar{r}_2| &= \bar{r}_2 \bar{r}_2 = A_2 = \sqrt{a_{22}}, \\ \bar{r}_1 \bar{r}_2 &= A_1 A_2 \cos\chi = \sqrt{a_{12}}, \end{aligned} \tag{1.4}$$

where χ is the angle between coordinate lines, A_i are the Lamé parameters, and a_{ik} are the coefficients of the metric tensor $\mathbf{A}$ on S. Using equation (1.4) we introduce the unit vectors $\bar{e}_i$ in the direction of $\bar{r}_i$ which are described by

$$\bar{e}_1 = \frac{\bar{r}_1}{|\bar{r}_1|} = \frac{\bar{r}_1}{A_1}, \qquad \bar{e}_2 = \frac{\bar{r}_2}{|\bar{r}_2|} = \frac{\bar{r}_2}{A_2}. \tag{1.5}$$

The vector $\bar{m}$ normal to $\bar{r}_1$ and $\bar{r}_2$ is found from

$$\bar{m} = \bar{r}_1 \times \bar{r}_2 \quad \text{and} \quad \bar{m}\bar{r}_1 = 0, \quad \bar{m}\bar{r}_2 = 0, \tag{1.6}$$

where $\bar{r}_1 \times \bar{r}_2$ is the vector product. The vectors $\bar{r}_1$, $\bar{r}_2$, and $\bar{m}$ are linearly independent and comprise a covariant base $\{\bar{r}_1, \bar{r}_2, \bar{m}\}$ on S. The reciprocal base $\{\bar{r}^1, \bar{r}^2, \bar{m}\}$ is defined by

$$\bar{r}^1 = \frac{\bar{r}_2 \times \bar{m}}{\bar{r}_1(\bar{r}_2 \times \bar{m})}, \quad \bar{r}^2 = \frac{\bar{m} \times \bar{r}_1}{\bar{r}_2(\bar{m} \times \bar{r}_1)}, \tag{1.7}$$

where $\bar{r}_i(\bar{m} \times \bar{r}_j)$ is the scalar triple product. Evidently, the vectors $\bar{r}^k$ and $\bar{r}_i$ are mutually orthogonal, i.e.

$$\bar{r}^k \bar{r}_i = \delta_i^k, \quad \bar{r}^k \bar{m} = 0.$$

Here δ_i^k is the Kronecker delta such that $\delta_i^k = 1$ if $i = k$ and $\delta_i^k = 0$ if $i \neq k$.

Let $\bar{m}(\bar{r}_i \times \bar{r}_k) = c_{ik}$ and $\bar{m}(\bar{r}^i \times \bar{r}^k) = c^{ik}$. Hence,

$$\begin{aligned} c_{ik}\bar{m} &= \bar{r}_i \times \bar{r}_k, & c^{ik}\bar{m} &= \bar{r}^i \times \bar{r}^k, \\ c_{ik}\bar{r}^k &= \bar{m} \times \bar{r}_i, & c^{ik}\bar{r}_i &= \bar{m} \times \bar{r}^i. \end{aligned} \tag{1.8}$$

It follows that

$$\begin{aligned} c^{ii} &= 0, \quad c^{12} = -c^{12} = 1/\sqrt{a}, \quad a = (A_1 A_2 \sin\chi)^2 \\ c_{ii} &= 0, \quad c_{12} = -c_{12} = \sqrt{a}, \end{aligned} \tag{1.9}$$

$$c_{ik}c^{km} = \delta^m{}_i, \quad c_{ik}c^{ki} = \delta^i{}_i = 2, \ (i, k = 1, 2). \tag{1.10}$$

The length of a line element between two infinitely close points $M(x_1, x_2, x_3)$ and $N(x_1 + dx_1, x_2 + dx_2, x_3 + dx_3)$ (figure 1.2) is given by

$$ds^2 = dx_1{}^2 + dx_2{}^2 + dx_3{}^2 = |d\bar{r}|^2 = |\bar{r}_i d\alpha_i|^2.$$

Using equation (1.4) in the above we have

$$ds^2 = A_1^2 d\alpha_1^2 + 2A_1A_2 \cos\chi d\alpha_1 d\alpha_2 + A_2^2 d\alpha_2^2 = a_{ik} d\alpha_i d\alpha_k. \tag{1.11}$$

The quadratic form (equation (1.11)) is called the first fundamental form of the surface. It allows the calculation of the length of line elements, the angle between coordinate curves and the surface area

$$ds_\Delta = |\bar{r}_1 \times \bar{r}_2| d\alpha_1 d\alpha_2 = \sqrt{a}\, d\alpha_1 d\alpha_2, \tag{1.12}$$

and therefore, it fully describes the intrinsic geometry of S.

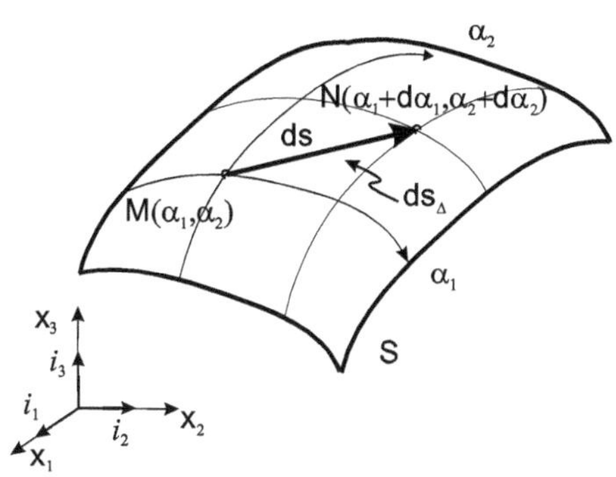

Figure 1.2. First fundamental form of the surface.

1.2 Extrinsic geometry

Let Γ be a non-singular curve on S (figure 1.3)

$$\bar{r} = \bar{r}(s) = \bar{r}(\alpha_1(s), \alpha_2(s)).$$

Differentiating $\bar{r}(s)$ with respect to s the unit vector $\bar{\tau}$ the tangent to Γ is found to be

$$\bar{\tau} = \frac{d\bar{r}}{ds} = \bar{r}_1\frac{d\alpha_1}{ds} + \bar{r}_2\frac{d\alpha_2}{ds}. \tag{1.13}$$

Applying the Frenet–Serret formula, for the derivative of $\bar{\tau}$ with respect to s we obtain

$$\frac{d\bar{\tau}}{ds} = \frac{\bar{n}}{R_c}, \tag{1.14}$$

where $1/R_c$ is the curvature and $\bar{n}$ is the vector normal to Γ. Substituting equation (1.7) into (1.8) we obtain

$$\bar{n} = \sum_{i=1}^{2}\sum_{k=1}^{2}\bar{r}_{ik}\frac{d\alpha_i}{ds}\frac{d\alpha_k}{ds} + \bar{r}_1\frac{d\alpha_1^2}{ds} + \bar{r}_2\frac{d\alpha_2^2}{ds}, \tag{1.15}$$

where

$$\bar{r}_{ik} = \frac{\partial^2\bar{r}}{\partial\alpha_i\partial\alpha_k} = \frac{\partial^2\bar{r}}{\partial\alpha_k\partial\alpha_i}, \quad \bar{r}_{ik} = \bar{r}_{ki}.$$

Let φ be the angle between the vectors $\bar{m}$ and $\bar{n}$ such that $\bar{m}\bar{n} = \cos\varphi$. Then the scalar product of equation (1.15) by $\bar{m}$ yields

$$\frac{\cos\varphi}{R_c} = \frac{b_{11}d\alpha_1^2 + 2b_{12}d\alpha_1 d\alpha_2 + b_{22}d\alpha_2^2}{ds^2}, \tag{1.16}$$

where

$$b_{11} = \bar{m}\bar{r}_{11}, \quad b_{12} = \bar{m}\bar{r}_{12} = \bar{m}\bar{r}_{21}, \quad b_{22} = \bar{m}\bar{r}_{22}. \tag{1.17}$$

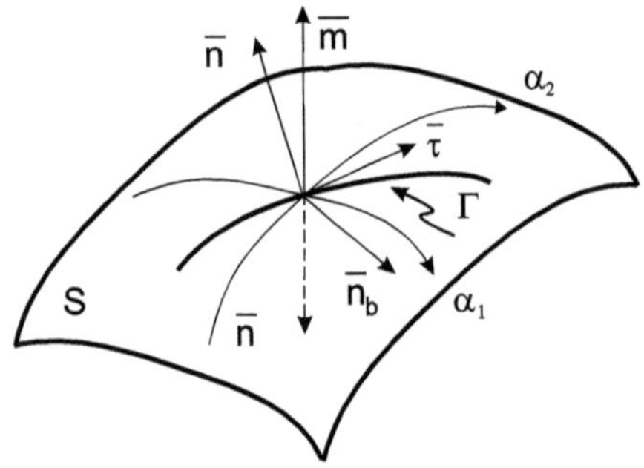

Figure 1.3. Extrinsic geometry of the surface and a local base $\{\bar{n}, \bar{n}_b, \bar{\tau}\}$ associated with a curve Γ.

The quadratic form

$$b_{11}d\alpha_1^2 + 2b_{12}d\alpha_1 d\alpha_2 + b_{22}d\alpha_2^2$$

is called the second fundamental form of the surface. Differentiating equation (1.6) with respect to α_i we find

$$b_{ik} = -\bar{m}_i\,\bar{r}_k = -\bar{m}_i\,\bar{r}_i, \tag{1.18}$$

here

$$\bar{m}_i = \frac{\partial \bar{m}}{\partial \alpha_i}. \tag{1.19}$$

A normal section at $\forall\, M(\alpha_1, \alpha_2) \in S$ is the section by some plane that contains the vector $\bar{m} \perp S$. Assuming $\varphi = \pi$, which implies that $\bar{m}$ and $\bar{n}$ are oriented in opposite directions, from equation (1.10) for the curvature of the normal section $1/R_n$, we obtain

$$-\frac{1}{R_n} = \frac{b_{11}d\alpha_1^2 + 2b_{12}d\alpha_1 d\alpha_2 + b_{22}d\alpha_2^2}{A_1^2 d\alpha_1^2 + 2A_1A_2 d\alpha_1 d\alpha_2 + A_2^2 d\alpha_2^2}. \tag{1.20}$$

Henceforth, it is assumed that the coordinate lines are arranged in such a way that $\bar{m}$ is positive when pointing from the concave to the convex side of the surface. Putting $\alpha_2 = \text{const}$ and $\alpha_1 = \text{const}$ in equation (1.20), for the curvatures k_{11}, k_{22} of the normal sections in the direction of α_1, α_2 we find

$$\frac{1}{R_{\alpha 1}} := k_{11} = -\frac{b_{11}}{A_1^2}, \quad \frac{1}{R_{\alpha 2}} := k_{22} = -\frac{b_{22}}{A_2^2}, \tag{1.21a}$$

and the twist k_{12} of the surface

$$\frac{1}{R_{\alpha 1 \alpha 2}} := k_{12} = -\frac{b_{12}}{A_1 A_2}. \tag{1.21b}$$

It becomes evident from the above considerations that the second fundamental form describes the intrinsic geometry of the surface.

At any point $M(\alpha_1, \alpha_2) \in S$ there exist two normal sections where $1/R_n$ assumes extreme values called principal sections. Two perpendicular directions at M belonging to the corresponding tangent plane are called the principal directions and the principal curvatures $(1/R)_{\max} = 1/R_1$, and $(1/R)_{\min} = 1/R_2$ (figure 1.4). Thus, there is at least one set of principal directions at any point on S. A curve on the surface such that the tangent at any point to it is collinear with the principal direction is called the line of curvature. Thus, two lines of curvature intersect at right-angles and pass through each point of S. It is assumed that the coordinate lines α_1, α_2 are the lines of curvature ($\chi = \pi/2$, $b_{12} = 0$). Such coordinates have an advantage over other coordinate systems since the governing equations in them have a relatively simple form.

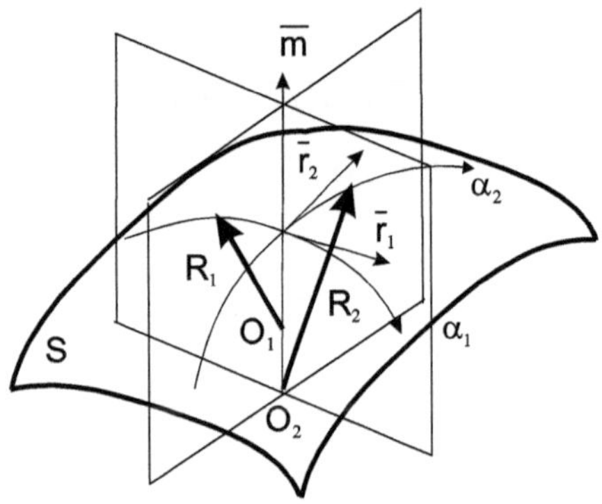

Figure 1.4. Normal curvatures R_1, R_2 of the surface.

Let $\bar{r}_{ik}$ be second derivatives of the position vector with respect to $\alpha_{i(k)}$ $(i, k = 1, 2)$. Decomposing $\bar{r}_{ik}$ with respect to the covariant base $\{\bar{r}_1, \bar{r}_2, \bar{m}\}$ we obtain

$$\bar{r}_{ik} = \Gamma^1_{ik}\bar{r}_1 + \Gamma^2_{ik}\bar{r}_2 + \bar{m}b_{ik}. \tag{1.22}$$

Here Γ^j_{ik} $(\Gamma^j_{ik} = \bar{r}^j\bar{r}_{ik})$ are the Christoffel symbols of the second kind. Multiplying subsequently both sides of equation (1.22) by $\bar{r}_1$ and $\bar{r}_2$, and making use of equations (1.4) and (1.6) we find

$$\bar{r}_1\,\bar{r}_{ik} = \Gamma^1{}_{ik}A_1^2 + \Gamma^2{}_{ik}A_1A_2\cos\chi$$
$$\bar{r}_2\,\bar{r}_{ik} = \Gamma^1{}_{ik}A_1A_2\cos\chi + \Gamma^2{}_{ik}A_2^2.$$

Solving the system with respect to Γ^j_{ik} we obtain

$$\begin{aligned} a\Gamma^1_{ik} &= A_2^2(\bar{r}_1\,\bar{r}_{ik}) - A_1A_2\cos\chi(\bar{r}_2\,\bar{r}_{ik}) \\ a\Gamma^2_{ik} &= A_1^2(\bar{r}_2\,\bar{r}_{ik}) - A_1A_2\cos\chi(\bar{r}_1\,\bar{r}_{ik}). \end{aligned} \tag{1.22a}$$

Differentiating $\bar{r}_1^2 = A_1^2, \bar{r}_2^2 = A_2^2$, and $\bar{r}_1\,\bar{r}_2 = A_1A_2\cos\chi$ with respect to α_1 and α_2, we find

$$\bar{r}_i\,\bar{r}_{ii} = A_i\frac{\partial A_i}{\partial\alpha_1}, \quad \bar{r}_1\,\bar{r}_{12} = A_1\frac{\partial A_1}{\partial\alpha_2}, \quad \bar{r}_2\,\bar{r}_{12} = A_2\frac{\partial A_2}{\partial\alpha_1} \tag{1.22b}$$

$$\bar{r}_2\,\bar{r}_{11} + \bar{r}_1\,\bar{r}_{12} = \frac{\partial a_{12}}{\partial\alpha_1} = a_{12,1} \tag{1.22c}$$

$$\bar{r}_2\,\bar{r}_{12} + \bar{r}_1\,\bar{r}_{22} = \frac{\partial a_{12}}{\partial\alpha_2} = a_{12,2}, \tag{1.22d}$$

where $a_{12} = a_{21} = A_1 A_2 \cos\chi$, $a_{12,i} = \frac{\partial a_{12}}{\partial \alpha_i}$. From (1.22*b*) and (1.22*c*) we have

$$\begin{aligned} \bar{r}_2\,\bar{r}_{11} &= \frac{\partial a_{12}}{\partial \alpha_1} - A_1 \frac{\partial A_1}{\partial \alpha_2}, \\ \bar{r}_1\,\bar{r}_{12} &= \frac{\partial a_{12}}{\partial \alpha_2} - A_2 \frac{\partial A_2}{\partial \alpha_1}. \end{aligned} \tag{1.22e}$$

Substituting expressions (1.22*b*) and (1.22*d*) into (1.22*a*) we obtain

$$\begin{aligned} a\Gamma^1_{11} &= A_1 A_2^2 \frac{\partial A_1}{\partial \alpha_1} - a_{12}\left(\frac{\partial a_{12}}{\partial \alpha_1} - A_1 \frac{\partial A_1}{\partial \alpha_2}\right) \\ a\Gamma^1_{12} &= A_1 A_2^2 \frac{\partial A_1}{\partial \alpha_2} - A_2 a_{12} \frac{\partial A_2}{\partial \alpha_1} \\ a\Gamma^1_{22} &= A_2^2 \frac{\partial a_{12}}{\partial \alpha_2} - A_2^3 \frac{\partial A_2}{\partial \alpha_1} - A_2 a_{12} \frac{\partial A_2}{\partial \alpha_2} \\ a\Gamma^2_{22} &= A_2 A_1^2 \frac{\partial A_2}{\partial \alpha_2} - a_{12}\left(\frac{\partial a_{12}}{\partial \alpha_2} - A_2 \frac{\partial A_2}{\partial \alpha_1}\right) \\ a\Gamma^2_{12} &= A_2 A_1^2 \frac{\partial A_2}{\partial \alpha_1} - A_1 a_{12} \frac{\partial A_1}{\partial \alpha_2} \\ a\Gamma^2_{11} &= A_1^2 \frac{\partial a_{12}}{\partial \alpha_1} - A_1^3 \frac{\partial A_1}{\partial \alpha_2} - A_1 a_{12} \frac{\partial A_1}{\partial \alpha_1}. \end{aligned} \tag{1.23}$$

Derivatives of the normal vector $\bar{m}$ with respect to α_i, lie in the tangent plane $(\bar{r}_1, \bar{r}_2)$ of S. Decomposing $\bar{m}_i$ $(i = 1, 2)$ along $\bar{r}_i$ we obtain

$$\bar{m}_i = -b_i^1 \bar{r}_1 - b_i^2 \bar{r}_2, \tag{1.24}$$

where b_i^1, b_i^2 are the mixed coefficients of the second fundamental form. The scalar product of equation (1.24) by $\bar{r}_1$ and $\bar{r}_2$, respectively, yields

$$\begin{aligned} \bar{m}_i\,\bar{r}_1 &= -\,b_i^1 \bar{r}_1^2 - b_i^2 \bar{r}_2\,\bar{r}_1, \\ \bar{m}_i\,\bar{r}_2 &= -\,b_i^1 \bar{r}_1\,\bar{r}_2 - b_i^2 \bar{r}_2^2. \end{aligned}$$

Using equations (1.4) and (1.18), b_{1i}, b_{2i} are found to be

$$\begin{aligned} b_{1i} &= A_1^2 b_i^1 + a_{12} b_i^2, \\ b_{2i} &= A_2^2 b_i^2 + a_{12} b_i^1. \end{aligned} \tag{1.25}$$

It is easy to show that

$$\begin{aligned} b_i^1 &= \frac{1}{A_1 \sin^2\chi}\left(\frac{b_{i1}}{A_1} - \frac{b_{i2}}{A_2}\cos\chi\right) \\ b_i^2 &= \frac{1}{A_2 \sin^2\chi}\left(\frac{b_{i2}}{A_2} - \frac{b_{i1}}{A_1}\cos\chi\right). \end{aligned} \tag{1.26}$$

Assuming that the surface is referred to orthogonal coordinates $\chi = \pi/2$, $a_{12} = a_{12} = 0$, $a = (A_1A_2)^2$, equations (1.23) take the form

$$\Gamma_{11}^1 = \frac{1}{A_1}\frac{\partial A_1}{\partial \alpha_1}, \quad \Gamma_{12}^1 = \frac{1}{A_1}\frac{\partial A_1}{\partial \alpha_2}, \quad \Gamma_{22}^1 = -\frac{A_2}{A_1^2}\frac{\partial A_2}{\partial \alpha_1},$$
$$\Gamma_{22}^2 = \frac{1}{A_2}\frac{\partial A_2}{\partial \alpha_2} \quad \Gamma_{12}^2 = \frac{1}{A_2}\frac{\partial A_2}{\partial \alpha_1}, \quad \Gamma_{11}^2 = -\frac{A_1}{A_2^2}\frac{\partial A_1}{\partial \alpha_2}. \tag{1.27}$$

Substituting equation (1.27) into equation (1.22) and making use of equations (1.5), (1.22*a*), (1.22*b*), the formulas for the derivatives of unit vectors $\bar{e}_1$ and $\bar{e}_2$ are found to be

$$\frac{\partial \bar{e}_1}{\partial \alpha_1} = -\frac{\bar{e}_2}{A_2}\frac{\partial A_1}{\partial \alpha_2} - A_1k_{11}\overline{m}, \quad \frac{\partial \bar{e}_1}{\partial \alpha_2} = -\frac{\bar{e}_2}{A_1}\frac{\partial A_2}{\partial \alpha_1} - A_2k_{12}\overline{m}$$
$$\frac{\partial \bar{e}_2}{\partial \alpha_1} = -\frac{\bar{e}_1}{A_2}\frac{\partial A_1}{\partial \alpha_2} - A_1k_{12}\overline{m}, \quad \frac{\partial \bar{e}_2}{\partial \alpha_2} = -\frac{\bar{e}_1}{A_1}\frac{\partial A_2}{\partial \alpha_1} - A_2k_{22}\overline{m}. \tag{1.28}$$

From equation (1.24) we have

$$A_1^2b_i^1 = b_{1i}, \quad A_2^2b_i^1 = b_{i2},$$

from whence, using equation (1.18), we obtain

$$A_1b_i^1 = -A_ik_{1i}, \quad A_2b_i^1 = -A_ik_{2i}.$$

Substituting the above into equation (1.24), and using equation (1.5), we obtain

$$\overline{m}_i = A_i(k_{1i}\bar{e}_i + k_{2i}\bar{e}_i). \tag{1.29}$$

If the coordinate lines are the lines of principal curvature ($k_{12} = 0$, $k_{ii} = 1/R_i$), equations (1.28) and (1.29) can be simplified to take the form

$$\frac{\partial \bar{e}_1}{\partial \alpha_1} = -\frac{\bar{e}_2}{A_2}\frac{\partial A_1}{\partial \alpha_2} - \overline{m}\frac{A_1}{R_1}, \quad \frac{\partial \bar{e}_1}{\partial \alpha_2} = \frac{\bar{e}_2}{A_1}\frac{\partial A_2}{\partial \alpha_1},$$
$$\frac{\partial \bar{e}_2}{\partial \alpha_1} = \frac{\bar{e}_1}{A_1}\frac{\partial A_1}{\partial \alpha_2}, \quad \frac{\partial \bar{e}_2}{\partial \alpha_2} = -\frac{\bar{e}}{A_1}\frac{\partial A_2}{\partial \alpha_1} - \overline{m}\frac{A_2}{R_2}.$$
$$R_i\overline{m}_i = A_i\bar{e}_i. \tag{1.30}$$

1.3 Equations of Gauss and Codazzi

Coefficients of the first and second fundamental forms are interdependent and satisfy the three differential Gauss–Codazzi equations. The Gauss formula defines the Gaussian curvature K of the surface

$$K = \frac{1}{R_1 R_2} = \frac{b_{11} - b_{12}^2}{a} = \frac{A_1 A_2 (k_{11} k_{22} - k_{12}^2)}{a}. \tag{1.31}$$

With the help of equations (1.21a), (1.21b), (1.26) it can be written in the form

$$\begin{aligned} \frac{b_{11} - b_{12}^2}{A_1 A_2 \sin\chi} &= \frac{\partial^2 \chi}{\partial\alpha_1 \partial\alpha_2} + \frac{\partial}{\partial\alpha_1} \frac{\frac{\partial A_2}{\partial\alpha_1} - \cos\chi \frac{\partial A_1}{\partial\alpha_2}}{A_1 \sin\chi} \\ &+ \frac{\partial}{\partial\alpha_2} \frac{\frac{\partial A_1}{\partial\alpha_2} - \cos\chi \frac{\partial A_2}{\partial\alpha_1}}{A_2 \sin\chi}. \end{aligned} \tag{1.32}$$

To derive the Codazzi equations we proceed from

$$\frac{\partial b_{11}}{\partial\alpha_2} - \frac{\partial b_{12}}{\partial\alpha_1} = -\frac{\partial \bar{r}_1 \bar{m}_1}{\partial\alpha_2} + \frac{\partial \bar{r}_2 \bar{m}_2}{\partial\alpha_1} = -\bar{m}_1 \bar{r}_{12} + \bar{m}_2 \bar{r}_{22}.$$

Substituting $\bar{r}_{ik}$ given by equation (1.22) the first Codazzi equation is found to be

$$\begin{aligned} \frac{\partial b_{11}}{\partial\alpha_2} - \frac{\partial b_{12}}{\partial\alpha_1} &= -\bar{m}_1(\Gamma_{12}^1 \bar{r}_1 + \Gamma_{12}^2 \bar{r}_2) + \bar{m}_2(\Gamma_{11}^1 \bar{r}_1 + \Gamma_{11}^2 \bar{r}_2) \\ &= \Gamma_{12}^1 b_{11} + (\Gamma_{12}^2 - \Gamma_{11}^2) b_{12} - \Gamma_{11}^2 b_{22}. \end{aligned} \tag{1.33}$$

Here use is made of equation (1.18) and the fact that $\bar{m}_i \bar{m} = 0$.

Similarly, proceeding from the difference $\frac{\partial b_{22}}{\partial\alpha_1} - \frac{\partial b_{12}}{\partial\alpha_2}$ and repeating the steps as above, we obtain the second Codazzi equation

$$\frac{\partial b_{22}}{\partial\alpha_1} - \frac{\partial b_{12}}{\partial\alpha_2} = \Gamma_{12}^1 b_{22} + (\Gamma_{12}^1 - \Gamma_{22}^2) b_{12} - \Gamma_{22}^1 b_{11}. \tag{1.34}$$

The Christoffel symbols Γ_{ik}^j in equation (1.26) satisfy equation (1.17).

Substituting equations (1.21*a*), (1.21*b*) into the left-hand side of equation (1.34), we obtain

$$\begin{aligned} \frac{\partial b_{11}}{\partial\alpha_2} - \frac{\partial b_{12}}{\partial\alpha_1} &= A_1\left(\frac{\partial A_1 k_{12}}{\partial\alpha_1} - \frac{\partial A_1 k_{11}}{\partial\alpha_2}\right) \\ &+ A_2 k_{12} \frac{\partial A_1}{\partial\alpha_1} - A_1 k_{11} \frac{\partial A_1}{\partial\alpha_2}. \end{aligned} \tag{1.35}$$

On using equation (1.35) in (1.33) and dividing the resultant equation by $-A_1$ and $-A_2$, respectively, we obtain

$$
\begin{aligned}
&\frac{\partial A_1 k_{11}}{\partial \alpha_2} - \frac{\partial A_2 k_{12}}{\partial \alpha_1} + k_{11}\left(\frac{\partial A_1}{\partial \alpha_2} - A_1 \Gamma_{12}^1\right) \\
&\qquad - A_2 k_{12}\left(\frac{1}{A_1}\frac{\partial A_1}{\partial \alpha_1} - \Gamma_{11}^1 + \Gamma_{12}^2\right) - \frac{A_2^2 k_{22} \Gamma_{11}^1}{A_1} = 0,\ A_2^2 = (A_2)^2. \\
&\frac{\partial A_2 k_{22}}{\partial \alpha_1} - \frac{\partial A_1 k_{12}}{\partial \alpha_2} + k_{22}\left(\frac{\partial A_2}{\partial \alpha_1} - A_2 \Gamma_{12}^2\right) \\
&\qquad - A_1 k_{12}\left(\frac{1}{A_2}\frac{\partial A_2}{\partial \alpha_2} - \Gamma_{22}^2 + \Gamma_{12}^1\right) - \frac{A_1^2 k_{11} \Gamma_{22}^2}{A_2} = 0.
\end{aligned}
\tag{1.36}
$$

In the case of orthogonal coordinates, equations (1.32) and (1.36) can be written in the form

$$
\begin{aligned}
&\frac{\partial}{\partial \alpha_1}\left(\frac{1}{A_1}\frac{\partial A_2}{\partial \alpha_1}\right) + \frac{\partial}{\partial \alpha_2}\left(\frac{1}{A_2}\frac{\partial A_1}{\partial \alpha_2}\right) \\
&\qquad = A_1 A_2 (k_{12}^2 - k_{11} k_{22}) = -\frac{A_1 A_2}{R_1 R_2}, \\
&\frac{\partial A_1 k_{11}}{\partial \alpha_2} - \frac{\partial A_2 k_{12}}{\partial \alpha_1} - k_{12}\frac{\partial A_2}{\partial \alpha_1} - k_{22}\frac{\partial A_1}{\partial \alpha_2} = 0, \\
&\frac{\partial A_2 k_{22}}{\partial \alpha_1} - \frac{\partial A_1 k_{12}}{\partial \alpha_2} - k_{12}\frac{\partial A_1}{\partial \alpha_2} - k_{11}\frac{\partial A_2}{\partial \alpha_1} = 0.
\end{aligned}
\tag{1.37}
$$

Here use is made of equation (1.27) for the Christoffel symbols Γ_{ik}^j.

If the coordinate lines are the lines of curvature ($k_{12} = 0$, $k_{ii} = 1/R_i$), then equation (1.37) takes the simplest form

$$
\begin{aligned}
&\frac{\partial}{\partial \alpha_1}\left(\frac{1}{A_1}\frac{\partial A_2}{\partial \alpha_1}\right) + \frac{\partial}{\partial \alpha_2}\left(\frac{1}{A_2}\frac{\partial A_1}{\partial \alpha_2}\right) = -\frac{A_1 A_2}{R_1 R_2} \\
&\frac{\partial}{\partial \alpha_2}\left(\frac{A_1}{R_1}\right) = \frac{1}{R_2}\left(\frac{\partial A_1}{\partial \alpha_1}\right),\quad \frac{\partial}{\partial \alpha_1}\left(\frac{A_2}{R_2}\right) = \frac{1}{R_1}\left(\frac{\partial A_2}{\partial \alpha_1}\right).
\end{aligned}
\tag{1.38}
$$

1.4 General curvilinear coordinates

Consider a non-singular surface S_z that is located at a distance z to S and $S_z \parallel S$. Let $\bar{\rho}$ be the position vector of a point $M_z \in S_z$ (figure 1.5)

$$
\bar{\rho}(\alpha_1, \alpha_2) = \bar{r}(\alpha_1, \alpha_2) + z\bar{m}(\alpha_1, \alpha_2). \tag{1.39}
$$

Here z is the normal distance measured from the point $M \in S$ and to M_z. Differentiating equation (1.39) with respect to α_i and z, we find

$$
\bar{\rho}_i = \frac{\partial \bar{\rho}}{\partial \alpha_i} = \bar{r}_i + \bar{m}_i z,\quad \bar{\rho}_3 = \frac{\partial \bar{\rho}}{\partial z} = \bar{m}_i. \tag{1.40}
$$

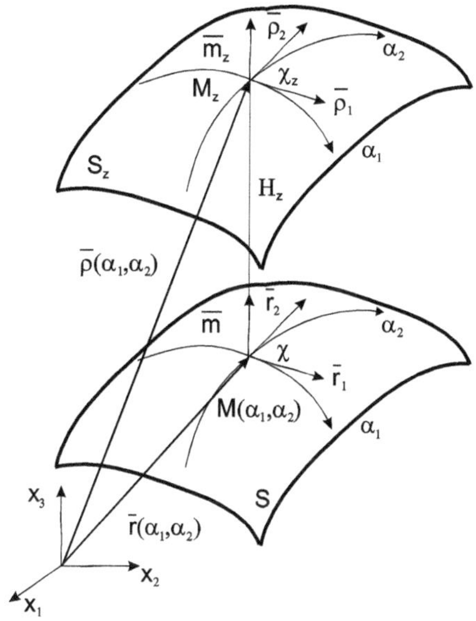

Figure 1.5. Parameterization of the equidistant surface S_z.

The vectors $\bar{\rho}_1, \bar{\rho}_2$ are tangent to the α_1, α_2-coordinate lines and are linearly independent. Thus, together with $\bar{\rho}_3$, they comprise a local base $\{\bar{\rho}_1, \bar{\rho}_2, \bar{\rho}_3\}$ at M_z.

Substituting $\bar{m}_i$ given by equation (1.24) into (1.40), we obtain

$$\begin{aligned} \bar{\rho}_1 &= \bar{r}_1(1 - zb_1^1) - \bar{r}_1 zb_1^2, \\ \bar{\rho}_2 &= \bar{r}_2(1 - zb_2^2) - \bar{r}_1 zb_1^1, \quad \bar{\rho}_3 = \bar{m}. \end{aligned} \tag{1.41}$$

If the coordinate system is orthogonal then using equation (1.29) for $\bar{m}_i$ we obtain

$$\bar{\rho}_i = A_i\bar{e}_i + (A_i k_{1i}\bar{e}_1 + k_{2i}\bar{e}_2)z, \quad \bar{\rho}_3 = \bar{m}. \tag{1.42}$$

Further, if the coordinate lines are the lines of curvature, equation (1.42) becomes

$$\bar{\rho}_i = A_i\bar{e}_i + (1 + z/R_i), \quad \bar{\rho}_3 = \bar{m}. \tag{1.43}$$

The scalar product of equations (1.41) and (1.42) by $\bar{m}$, yields

$$\bar{\rho}_i\bar{m} = 0. \tag{1.44}$$

Let g_{ik} and H_i be the scalar product of $\bar{\rho}_i$ and $\bar{\rho}_k$ in general and orthogonal curvilinear coordinates, respectively,

$$g_{ik} = \bar{\rho}_i\bar{\rho}_k \quad (i, k = 1, 2) \tag{1.45}$$

$$H_i = |\bar{\rho}_i|, \tag{1.46}$$

H_i are the Lamé coefficients of S_z. The unit vectors $\bar{e}_i^z \in S_z$ are given by

$$\bar{e}_i^z = \frac{\bar{\rho}_i}{H_i}. \tag{1.47}$$

Making use of equation (1.42) in (1.47), for $\bar{e}_1^z$, $\bar{e}_2^z$ we find

$$\begin{aligned} \bar{e}_1^z &= \frac{A_1}{H_1}(\bar{e}_1 + \bar{e}_1 k_{11} z + \bar{e}_2 k_{12} z), \\ \bar{e}_2^z &= \frac{A_2}{H_2}(\bar{e}_2 + \bar{e}_2 k_{22} z + \bar{e}_1 k_{12} z). \end{aligned} \tag{1.48}$$

Using equations (1.42) and (1.47) in (1.48), after simple algebra, we obtain

$$\begin{aligned} H_1 &= A_1\sqrt{(1 + k_{11}z)^2 + k_{12}z^2} = A_1(1 + k_{11}z + \cdots) \\ H_2 &= A_2\sqrt{(1 + k_{22}z)^2 + k_{12}z^2} = A_2(1 + k_{22}z + \cdots). \end{aligned} \tag{1.49}$$

In equation (1.49) we neglected terms $O(z^2)$. Such an approximation is proven to be satisfactory for z being sufficiently small when compared to the degree of accuracy required in practical applications. If the coordinate lines are the lines of curvature, $k_{12} = 0$, the formulas (1.49) become accurate

$$H_i = A_i(1 + k_{ii}z) = A_i(1 + k_{11}z/R_{ii}). \tag{1.50}$$

Also, the unit vectors $\bar{e}_i^z \in S_z$ and $\bar{e}_i \in S$ become identical if the chosen coordinate lines are the lines of curvature. Indeed, by setting $k_{12} = 0$ in equation (1.48) and using formula (1.50), we obtain

$$\bar{e}_1^z = \bar{e}_1, \quad \bar{e}_2^z = \bar{e}_2. \tag{1.51}$$

The length of a line element on S_z is given by

$$\begin{aligned} (ds^z)^2 &= |d\bar{\rho}|^2 = |\bar{\rho}_1 d\alpha_1 + \bar{\rho}_2 d\alpha_2 + \bar{m} dz|^2 \\ &= g_{11} d\alpha_1^2 + 2g_{12} d\alpha_1 d\alpha_2 + dz^2. \end{aligned} \tag{1.52}$$

Substituting equation (1.39) into equation (1.45), we obtain

$$g_{ik} = \bar{r}_i \bar{r}_k + 2\bar{m}_i \bar{r}_k z + \bar{m}_i \bar{m}_k z^2.$$

Further, with the help of equations (1.4) and (1.24), we obtain

$$\begin{aligned} g_{ik} &= A_i(1 + 2k_{ii}z) + (\bar{m}_i z)^2, \\ g_{12} &= A_1 A_2(\cos\chi + 2k_{12}z) + \bar{m}_1 \bar{m}_2 z^2. \end{aligned} \tag{1.53}$$

Neglecting higher-order terms $O(z^2)$, we find

$$\begin{aligned} g_{ik} &= A_i(1 + 2k_{ii}z), \\ g_{12} &= A_1 A_2(\cos\chi + 2k_{12}z). \end{aligned} \tag{1.54}$$

Assume the coordinate system is orthogonal $g_{12} = \bar{\rho}_1\bar{\rho}_2 = 0$. Hence from equation (1.54) we have $k_{12}z \approx 0$. Note, that the condition (1.51) remains valid in orthogonal coordinates even if the coordinate lines are not the lines of curvature.

Let χ^z be the angle between coordinate lines on S_z. Since

$$g_{12} = \bar{\rho}_1\bar{\rho}_2 = |\bar{\rho}_1| \cdot |\bar{\rho}_2| \cos\chi^z,$$

then

$$\cos\chi^z = \frac{g_{12}}{|\bar{\rho}_1| \cdot |\bar{\rho}_2|} = \frac{g_{12}}{\sqrt{g_{11}g_{12}}}.$$

Using equation (1.54), we obtain

$$\cos\chi^z = \frac{\cos\chi + 2k_{12}z}{\sqrt{(1 + 2k_{11}z)(1 + 2k_{22}z)}}. \tag{1.55}$$

We conclude this section with some useful formulas for the cross product of vectors

$$\begin{gathered} H_2(\bar{\rho}_1 \times \bar{m}) = -\bar{\rho}_2 H_1, \quad H_1(\bar{\rho}_2 \times \bar{m}) = \bar{\rho}_1 H_2, \\ H_1H_2(\bar{\rho}_1 \times \bar{\rho}_2) = \bar{m}, \quad A_2(\bar{r}_1 \times \bar{m}) = -A_1\bar{r}_2, \\ A_1(\bar{r}_2 \times \bar{m}) = A_2\bar{r}_1, \quad A_1A_2(\bar{r}_1 \times \bar{r}_2) = \bar{m}, \end{gathered} \tag{1.56}$$

$$(\bar{e}_1 \times \bar{m}) = \bar{e}_2, \quad (\bar{e}_2 \times \bar{m}) = \bar{e}_1, \quad (\bar{e}_1 \times \bar{e}_2) = \bar{m}. \tag{1.57}$$

1.5 Deformation of the surface

As a result of deformation the surface S changes into a new surface $\overset{*}{S}$ with a point $M \in S$ sent into the point $\overset{*}{M} \in \overset{*}{S}$. Henceforth, all quantities that refer to the deformed configuration will be designated by an asterisk (*) unless otherwise specified. Let $\bar{v}(\alpha_1, \alpha_2)$ be the vector of displacement of point M. Then the position of $\overset{*}{M}$ after deformation (figure 1.6) is described by

$$\overset{*}{\bar{r}}(\alpha_1, \alpha_2) = \bar{r}(\alpha_1, \alpha_2) + \bar{v}(\alpha_1, \alpha_2). \tag{1.58}$$

Projections of $\bar{v}$ onto the base $\{\bar{e}_1, \bar{e}_2, \bar{m}\}$ are given by

$$u_1 = \bar{v}\bar{e}_1 = \bar{v}\bar{r}_1/A_1, \quad u_2 = \bar{v}\bar{e}_2 = \bar{v}\bar{r}_2/A_2, \quad \omega = \bar{v}\bar{m}. \tag{1.59}$$

Hence

$$\bar{v} = u_1\bar{e}_1 + u_2\bar{e}_2 + \omega\bar{m}, \tag{1.60}$$

where u_1, u_2 are the tangent, and ω is the normal displacement (deflection), respectively.

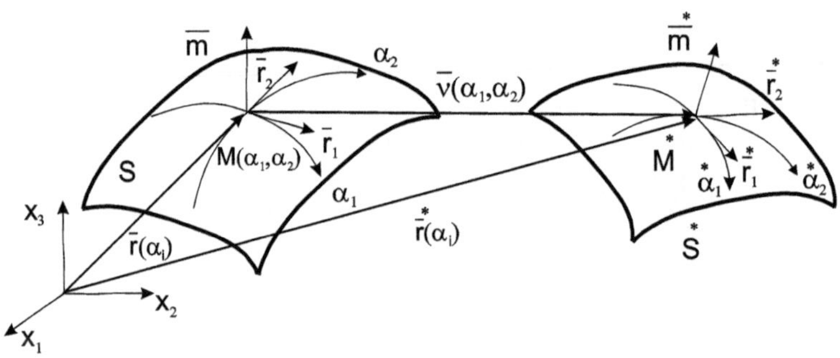

Figure 1.6. Deformation of the surface.

Differentiating equation (1.58) with respect to α_i and using equations (1.28) and (1.29), we find

$$\overset{*}{\bar{r}}_1 = A_1\{(1 + e_{11})\bar{e}_1 + e_{12}\bar{e}_2 + \bar{m}\varpi_1\},$$
$$\overset{*}{\bar{r}}_2 = A_2\{e_{21}\bar{e}_1 + (1 + e_{22})\bar{e}_2 + \bar{m}\varpi_2\}, \tag{1.61}$$

where

$$\begin{aligned}
e_{11} &= \frac{1}{A_1}\frac{\partial u_1}{\partial \alpha_1} + \frac{u_2}{A_1A_2}\frac{\partial A_1}{\partial \alpha_2} + k_{11}\omega,\\
e_{22} &= \frac{1}{A_2}\frac{\partial u_2}{\partial \alpha_2} + \frac{u_1}{A_1A_2}\frac{\partial A_2}{\partial \alpha_1} + k_{22}\omega,\\
e_{12} &= \frac{1}{A_1}\frac{\partial u_2}{\partial \alpha_1} - \frac{u_1}{A_1A_2}\frac{\partial A_1}{\partial \alpha_2} + k_{12}\omega,\\
e_{21} &= \frac{1}{A_2}\frac{\partial u_1}{\partial \alpha_2} - \frac{u_1}{A_1A_2}\frac{\partial A_2}{\partial \alpha_2} + k_{21}\omega,\\
\varpi_1 &= \frac{1}{A_1}\frac{\partial \omega}{\partial \alpha_1} - k_{11}u_1 - k_{12}u_2,\\
\varpi_2 &= \frac{1}{A_2}\frac{\partial \omega}{\partial \alpha_2} - k_{22}u_1 - k_{21}u_1.
\end{aligned} \tag{1.62}$$

The length of a line element on the deformed surface $\overset{*}{S}$ is defined by

$$(d\overset{*}{s})^2 = (\overset{*}{A}_1)^2 d\alpha_1^2 + 2\overset{*}{A}_1\overset{*}{A}_2 d\alpha_1 d\alpha_2 + (\overset{*}{A}_2)^2 d\alpha_2^2 = \overset{*}{a}_{ij} d\alpha_i d\alpha_j, \tag{1.63}$$

where

$$\overset{*}{A}_1 = |\overset{*}{\bar{r}}_1|, \quad \overset{*}{A}_2 = |\overset{*}{\bar{r}}_2|, \quad \overset{*}{a}_{12} = \overset{*}{\bar{r}}_1 \overset{*}{\bar{r}}_2 = \overset{*}{A}_1\overset{*}{A}_2 \cos\overset{*}{\chi}, \tag{1.64}$$

$\overset{*}{\chi}$ is the angle between coordinate lines on $\overset{*}{S}$. Substituting equation (1.61) into (1.64) we find

$$(\overset{*}{A}_1)^2 = A_1^2(1 + 2\varepsilon_{11}), \quad (\overset{*}{A}_2)^2 = A_2^2(1 + 2\varepsilon_{22}), \tag{1.65}$$

$$\cos\overset{*}{\chi} = \frac{2\varepsilon_{12}}{\sqrt{(1 + 2\varepsilon_{11})(1 + 2\varepsilon_{22})}}, \tag{1.66}$$

where

$$\begin{aligned} 2\varepsilon_{11} &= 2e_{11} + e_{11}^2 + e_{12}^2 + \varpi_1^2, \\ 2\varepsilon_{22} &= 2e_{22} + e_{22}^2 + e_{21}^2 + \varpi_2^2, \\ 2\varepsilon_{12} &= (1 + e_{11})e_{21} + (1 + e_{22})e_{12} + \varpi_1\varpi_2. \end{aligned} \tag{1.67}$$

To provide a physically appealing explanation for ε_{ik} $(i, k = 1, 2)$, consider the lengths of the same line element before $(ds)_i$ and after deformation $(\overset{*}{ds})_i$

$$\begin{aligned} (ds)_1 &= A_1\partial\alpha_1, \quad (ds)_2 = A_2\partial\alpha_2, \\ (\overset{*}{ds})_1 &= \overset{*}{A}_1\partial\alpha_1, \quad (\overset{*}{ds})_2 = \overset{*}{A}_2\partial\alpha_2. \end{aligned}$$

Relative elongations $e_{\alpha 1}$, $e_{\alpha 2}$, along the α_1, α_2 lines and the shear angle γ between them, are found to be

$$e_{\alpha i} = \frac{\overset{*}{ds}_i - ds_i}{ds_i} = \sqrt{1 + 2\varepsilon_{ii}} - 1 \quad (i = 1, 2) \tag{1.68}$$

$$\cos\overset{*}{\chi} = \cos\left(\frac{\pi}{2} - \gamma\right) = \sin\gamma = \frac{2\varepsilon_{12}}{\sqrt{(1 + 2\varepsilon_{11})(1 + 2\varepsilon_{22})}}. \tag{1.69}$$

It follows from equations (1.68) and (1.69) that ε_{11} and ε_{22} describe tangent deformations along the coordinate lines and ε_{12} is the shear deformation that characterizes the change in γ.

Changes in curvatures, $æ_{ii}$, and the twist, $æ_{12}$, of the surface are described by

$$\begin{aligned} æ_{11} &= \frac{1}{\overset{*}{R}_1} - \frac{1}{R_1} = \overset{*}{k}_{11} - k_{11} \\ æ_{22} &= \frac{1}{\overset{*}{R}_2} - \frac{1}{R_2} = \overset{*}{k}_{22} - k_{22} \\ æ_{12} &= æ_{21} = \overset{*}{k}_{12} - k_{12} = \overset{*}{k}_{21} - k_{21}. \end{aligned} \tag{1.70}$$

Here $\frac{1}{R_i}$ and $\frac{1}{\overset{*}{R_i}}$ are curvatures of coordinate lines before and after deformation, and $\overset{*}{k}_{ij} = -\overset{*}{b}_{ij}/\overset{*}{A}_i\overset{*}{A}_j$ $(i, j = 1, 2)$.

To express $\overset{*}{\bar{m}}$ in terms of the middle surface displacements we proceed from the formula

$$\overset{*}{\bar{m}} = (\overset{*}{\bar{r}}_1 \times \overset{*}{\bar{r}}_2)/\overset{*}{A}_1\overset{*}{A}_2 \sin \overset{*}{\chi}.$$

Substituting $\overset{*}{A}_i$ and $\sin \overset{*}{\chi}$ given by equations (1.65) and (1.66) into the above, we find

$$\overset{*}{\bar{m}} = (\overset{*}{\bar{r}}_1 \times \overset{*}{\bar{r}}_2)/A_1A_2\sqrt{\mathfrak{A}}, \quad \overset{*}{A}_1\overset{*}{A}_2 \sin \overset{*}{\chi} = A_1A_2\sqrt{\mathfrak{A}}. \tag{1.71}$$

Here

$$\mathfrak{A} = 1 + 2(\varepsilon_{11} + \varepsilon_{22}) + (\varepsilon_{11}\varepsilon_{22} - \varepsilon_{12}^2). \tag{1.72}$$

Substituting $\overset{*}{\bar{r}}_i$ given by equations (1.61) and (1.57) into (1.71), we find

$$\overset{*}{\bar{m}} = (\bar{e}_1\mathbb{S}_1 + \bar{e}_2\mathbb{S}_2 + \bar{m}\mathbb{S}_3)/\sqrt{\mathfrak{A}}, \tag{1.73}$$

where

$$\begin{aligned} \mathbb{S}_1 &= e_{12}\varpi_2 - (1 + e_{22})\varpi_1, \\ \mathbb{S}_2 &= e_{21}\varpi_1 - (1 + e_{11})\varpi_2, \\ \mathbb{S}_3 &= (1 + e_{11})(1 + e_{22}) - e_{12}e_{21}. \end{aligned} \tag{1.74}$$

The scalar product of equations (1.61) and (1.73) by $\bar{e}_i$ and $\bar{m}$, yields

$$\begin{aligned} \cos(\overset{*}{\bar{r}}_i, \bar{e}_k) &= (\delta_{ik} + e_{ik})/\sqrt{1 + 2\varepsilon_{ii}}, \\ \cos(\overset{*}{\bar{r}}_i, \bar{m}) &= \varpi_i/\sqrt{1 + 2\varepsilon_{ii}}, \\ \cos(\overset{*}{\bar{m}}, \bar{e}_k) &= \mathbb{S}_k/\sqrt{\mathfrak{A}}, \\ \cos(\overset{*}{\bar{m}}, \bar{m}) &= \mathbb{S}_3/\sqrt{\mathfrak{A}}. \end{aligned}$$

The quantities e_{ik}, ϖ_i, $\mathbb{S}_i$, $\mathbb{S}_3$ describe the rotations of tangent and normal vectors during deformation.

Differentiating equation (1.73) with respect to α_i and making use of equations (1.28) and (1.29), we find

$$\sqrt{\mathfrak{A}}\overset{*}{\bar{m}}_i = A_i(\bar{e}_1\mathfrak{M}_{i1} + \bar{e}_2\mathfrak{M}_{i2} + \bar{m}\mathfrak{M}_{i3}) - \overset{*}{\bar{m}}\frac{\partial\sqrt{\mathfrak{A}}}{\partial\alpha_i}, \tag{1.75}$$

where

$$
\begin{aligned}
\mathfrak{M}_{11} &= \frac{1}{A_1}\frac{\partial \mathbb{S}_1}{\partial \alpha_1} + \frac{\mathbb{S}_2}{A_1 A_2}\frac{\partial A_1}{\partial \alpha_2} + k_{11}\mathbb{S}_3,\\
\mathfrak{M}_{21} &= \frac{1}{A_2}\frac{\partial \mathbb{S}_2}{\partial \alpha_2} + \frac{\mathbb{S}_1}{A_2 A_1}\frac{\partial A_2}{\partial \alpha_1} + k_{22}\mathbb{S}_3,\\
\mathfrak{M}_{12} &= \frac{1}{A_1}\frac{\partial \mathbb{S}_2}{\partial \alpha_1} - \frac{\mathbb{S}_1}{A_1 A_2}\frac{\partial A_1}{\partial \alpha_2} + k_{12}\mathbb{S}_3,\\
\mathfrak{M}_{22} &= \frac{1}{A_2}\frac{\partial \mathbb{S}_1}{\partial \alpha_2} - \frac{\mathbb{S}_2}{A_1 A_2}\frac{\partial A_2}{\partial \alpha_1} + k_{12}\mathbb{S}_3,\\
\mathfrak{M}_{13} &= \frac{1}{A_1}\frac{\partial \mathbb{S}_3}{\partial \alpha_1} - k_{11}\mathbb{S}_1 - k_{12}\mathbb{S}_2,\\
\mathfrak{M}_{23} &= \frac{1}{A_2}\frac{\partial \mathbb{S}_3}{\partial \alpha_2} - k_{22}\mathbb{S}_2 - k_{12}\mathbb{S}_1.
\end{aligned}
\tag{1.76}
$$

Substituting equation (1.60) into (1.75), and using the fact that $\overset{*}{\bar{m}}\overset{*}{\bar{r}}_j = 0$, $A_i A_1 \overset{*}{k}_{i1} = \overset{*}{\bar{m}}_i \overset{*}{\bar{r}}_1$, $A_i A_2 \overset{*}{k}_{i2} = \overset{*}{\bar{m}}_i \overset{*}{\bar{r}}_2$, we obtain

$$
\begin{aligned}
\sqrt{\mathfrak{A}}\,\overset{*}{k}_{i1} &= (1 + e_{11})\mathfrak{M}_{i1} + e_{12}\mathfrak{M}_{i2} + \varpi_1\mathfrak{M}_{i3},\\
\sqrt{\mathfrak{A}}\,\overset{*}{k}_{i2} &= e_{21}\mathfrak{M}_{i1} + (1 + e_{22})\mathfrak{M}_{i2} + \varpi_2\mathfrak{M}_{i3}
\end{aligned}
\tag{1.77}
$$

e_{ik}, ϖ_i, $\mathbb{S}_i$, $\mathbb{S}_3$ satisfy the following algebraic equalities

$$
\begin{aligned}
\mathbb{S}_1(1 + e_{11}) + e_{12}\mathbb{S}_2 + \mathbb{S}_3\varpi_1 &= 0,\\
\mathbb{S}_2(1 + e_{22}) + e_{21}\mathbb{S}_1 + \mathbb{S}_3\varpi_2 &= 0.
\end{aligned}
\tag{1.78}
$$

Equation (1.78) can be verified by substituting $\overset{*}{\bar{r}}_j$ and $\overset{*}{\bar{m}}$ given by equations (1.61) and (1.73) into equality $\overset{*}{\bar{m}}\overset{*}{\bar{r}}_j = 0$. The following is also true:

$$
\begin{aligned}
\mathbb{S}_1 e_{12} - \mathbb{S}_2(1 + e_{11}) &= (1 + 2\varepsilon_{11}) - 2\varepsilon_{12}\varpi_1 = f_{12}\\
\mathbb{S}_3(1 + e_{11}) - \mathbb{S}_1\varpi_1 &= (1 + e_{22})(1 + 2\varepsilon_{11}) - 2\varepsilon_{12}e_{12} = g_{12} \quad 1 \overset{\leftrightarrow}{,} 2\\
\mathbb{S}_3 e_{12} - \mathbb{S}_2\varpi_1 &= (1 + e_{22})2\varepsilon_{11} - (1 + 2\varepsilon_{11})e_{12} = h_{12}.
\end{aligned}
\tag{1.79}
$$

The result can be confirmed by substituting $\mathbb{S}_i$, $\mathbb{S}_3$ given by equation (1.74) and making use of equation (1.67).

Substituting equation (1.76) into equation (1.78), we find

$$\begin{aligned}
\sqrt{\mathfrak{A}}\overset{*}{k}_{11} &= \frac{1}{A_1}\left[(1+e_{11})\frac{\partial \mathbb{S}_1}{\partial \alpha_1} + e_{12}\frac{\partial \mathbb{S}_2}{\partial \alpha_1} + \varpi_1\frac{\partial \mathbb{S}_3}{\partial \alpha_1}\right] \\
&\quad - \frac{f_{12}}{A_1A_2}\frac{\partial A_1}{\partial \alpha_2} + k_{11}g_{12} + k_{12}h_{12} \\
\sqrt{\mathfrak{A}}\overset{*}{k}_{22} &= \frac{1}{A_1}\left[e_{21}\frac{\partial \mathbb{S}_1}{\partial \alpha_1} + (1+e_{22})\frac{\partial \mathbb{S}_2}{\partial \alpha_1} + \varpi_2\frac{\partial \mathbb{S}_3}{\partial \alpha_1}\right] \\
&\quad + \frac{f_{12}}{A_1A_2}\frac{\partial A_1}{\partial \alpha_2} - k_{11}h_{12} - k_{12}g_{12}.
\end{aligned} \tag{1.80}$$

Differentiating equation (1.80) with respect to α_1, we obtain

$$\begin{aligned}
(1+e_{11})\frac{\partial \mathbb{S}_1}{\partial \alpha_1} + e_{12}\frac{\partial \mathbb{S}_2}{\partial \alpha_1} + \varpi_1\frac{\partial \mathbb{S}_3}{\partial \alpha_1} &= -\mathbb{S}_1\frac{\partial e_{11}}{\partial \alpha_1} - \mathbb{S}_2\frac{\partial e_{12}}{\partial \alpha_1} - \mathbb{S}_3\frac{\partial \varpi_1}{\partial \alpha_1}, \\
(1+e_{22})\frac{\partial \mathbb{S}_2}{\partial \alpha_1} + e_{21}\frac{\partial \mathbb{S}_1}{\partial \alpha_1} + \varpi_2\frac{\partial \mathbb{S}_3}{\partial \alpha_1} &= -\mathbb{S}_2\frac{\partial e_{22}}{\partial \alpha_1} - \mathbb{S}_1\frac{\partial e_{21}}{\partial \alpha_1} - \mathbb{S}_3\frac{\partial \varpi_2}{\partial \alpha_1}.
\end{aligned} \tag{1.81}$$

Substituting the right-hand sides of equation (1.81) into (3.22), the final formulas for the curvatures $\overset{*}{k}_{11}$, $\overset{*}{k}_{22}$ are found to be

$$\begin{aligned}
\sqrt{\mathfrak{A}}\overset{*}{k}_{11} &= -\frac{1}{A_1}\left(\mathbb{S}_1\frac{\partial e_{11}}{\partial \alpha_1} + \mathbb{S}_2\frac{\partial e_{12}}{\partial \alpha_1} + \mathbb{S}_3\frac{\partial \varpi_1}{\partial \alpha_1}\right) \\
&\quad - \frac{f_{12}}{A_1A_2}\frac{\partial A_1}{\partial \alpha_2} + k_{11}g_{12} + k_{12}h_{12}, \\
\sqrt{\mathfrak{A}}\overset{*}{k}_{22} &= -\frac{1}{A_1}\left(\mathbb{S}_2\frac{\partial e_{22}}{\partial \alpha_1} + \mathbb{S}_1\frac{\partial e_{21}}{\partial \alpha_1} + \mathbb{S}_3\frac{\partial \varpi_2}{\partial \alpha_1}\right) \\
&\quad + \frac{f_{12}}{A_1A_2}\frac{\partial A_1}{\partial \alpha_2} - k_{11}h_{12} - k_{12}g_{12}.
\end{aligned} \tag{1.82}$$

Formulas (1.82) are obtained under the first Kirchhoff–Love hypothesis. The essence of the hypothesis is that normals to the undeformed middle surface S remain straight and normal to the deformed middle surface and undergo no extension, i.e. $\overline{m\overset{*}{r}_j} = \overline{m\overset{*}{\rho}_j} = g_{j3} = 0$ and $\varepsilon_{j3}^{z} = 0$. The hypotheses were first formulated by Kirchhoff for thin plates and later applied by Love for thin shells. They are known as the Kirchhoff–Love hypotheses and are fundamental in the theory of thin shells. Additional hypotheses will be introduced in the text as needed.

1.6 Equations of compatibility

For the surface to retain continuity during deformation, the parameters ε_{ik} and æ_{ik} $(i, k = 1, 2)$ must satisfy the three differential equations called the equations of continuity of deformations. They can be obtained by subtracting the Gauss–Codazzi equations formulated for the undeformed state from the corresponding equations for the deformed configuration. The Gauss formula for the deformed surface $\overset{*}{S}$ is given by (see equation (1.32))

$$\frac{\partial^2 \overset{*}{\chi}}{\partial\alpha_1\partial\alpha_2} + \frac{\partial}{\partial\alpha_1}\frac{\frac{\partial \overset{*}{A}_2}{\partial\alpha_1} - \cos\overset{*}{\chi}\frac{\partial \overset{*}{A}_1}{\partial\alpha_2}}{\overset{*}{A}_1 \sin\overset{*}{\chi}} + \frac{\partial}{\partial\alpha_2}\frac{\frac{\partial \overset{*}{A}_1}{\partial\alpha_2} - \cos\overset{*}{\chi}\frac{\partial \overset{*}{A}_2}{\partial\alpha_1}}{\overset{*}{A}_2 \sin\overset{*}{\chi}}$$
$$= \frac{\overset{*}{b}{}_{12}^2 - \overset{*}{b}_{11}\overset{*}{b}_{22}}{\overset{*}{A}_1\overset{*}{A}_2 \sin\overset{*}{\chi}}. \tag{1.83}$$

Substituting

$$\overset{*}{A}_1\overset{*}{A}_2 \sin\overset{*}{\chi} = A_1A_2\sqrt{\mathfrak{A}},$$
$$\cos\overset{*}{\chi} = 2\varepsilon_{12}/\sqrt{\mathbb{S}_{11}\mathbb{S}_{22}},$$
$$\sin\overset{*}{\chi} = \sqrt{\mathfrak{A}}/\sqrt{\mathbb{S}_{11}\mathbb{S}_{22}},$$
$$\frac{\partial\overset{*}{\chi}}{\partial\alpha_i} = -\frac{1}{\sin\overset{*}{\chi}}\frac{\partial\cos\overset{*}{\chi}}{\partial\alpha_i}$$
$$= \frac{1}{\sqrt{\mathfrak{A}}}\left[-2\frac{\partial\varepsilon_{12}}{\partial\alpha_i} + \varepsilon_{12}\frac{\partial}{\partial\alpha_i}\ln(\mathbb{S}_{11}\mathbb{S}_{22})\right]$$

into equation (1.83) we obtain

$$\frac{\partial}{\partial\alpha_1}\frac{1}{\sqrt{\mathfrak{A}}}\left[-\frac{\partial\varepsilon_{12}}{\partial\alpha_2} + \frac{\varepsilon_{12}}{2}\frac{\partial}{\partial\alpha_2}\ln(\mathbb{S}_{11}\mathbb{S}_{22}) + \frac{\overset{*}{A}_2}{A_1A_2}\left(\frac{\partial\overset{*}{A}_2}{\partial\alpha_1} - \cos\overset{*}{\chi}\frac{\partial\overset{*}{A}_1}{\partial\alpha_2}\right)\right]$$
$$+\frac{\partial}{\partial\alpha_2}\frac{1}{\sqrt{\mathfrak{A}}}\left[-\frac{\partial\varepsilon_{12}}{\partial\alpha_1} + \frac{\varepsilon_{12}}{2}\frac{\partial}{\partial\alpha_1}\ln(\mathbb{S}_{11}\mathbb{S}_{22}) + \frac{\overset{*}{A}_2}{A_1A_2}\left(\frac{\partial\overset{*}{A}_1}{\partial\alpha_2} - \cos\overset{*}{\chi}\frac{\partial\overset{*}{A}_2}{\partial\alpha_1}\right)\right] \tag{1.84}$$
$$= \frac{1}{\sqrt{\mathfrak{A}}}\frac{\overset{*}{b}{}_{12}^2 - \overset{*}{b}_{11}\overset{*}{b}_{22}}{A_1A_2}.$$

Further, using equations (1.65) and (1.66) in (1.84), the first Gauss formula is found to be

$$\frac{\partial}{\partial\alpha_1}\frac{1}{A_1\sqrt{\mathfrak{A}}}\left[\frac{A_1\varepsilon_{12}}{2}\frac{\partial}{\partial\alpha_1}\ln\frac{\mathbb{S}_{22}}{\mathbb{S}_{11}} + \frac{\partial A_2\varepsilon_{22}}{\partial\alpha_1} - \frac{\partial A_1\varepsilon_{12}}{\partial\alpha_2} - \varepsilon_{12}\frac{\partial A_1}{\partial\alpha_2}\right.$$
$$\left.+\,\varepsilon_{22}\frac{\partial A_2}{\partial\alpha_1} + \frac{\partial A_2}{\partial\alpha_1}\right] + \frac{\partial}{\partial\alpha_2}\frac{1}{A_2\sqrt{\mathfrak{A}}}\left[\frac{A_2\varepsilon_{21}}{2}\frac{\partial}{\partial\alpha_2}\ln\frac{\mathbb{S}_{11}}{\mathbb{S}_{22}} + \frac{\partial A_1\varepsilon_{11}}{\partial\alpha_2}\right.$$
$$\left.-\,\frac{\partial A_2\varepsilon_{21}}{\partial\alpha_1} - \varepsilon_{21}\frac{\partial A_2}{\partial\alpha_1} + \varepsilon_{11}\frac{\partial A_1}{\partial\alpha_2} + \frac{\partial A_1}{\partial\alpha_2}\right] = \frac{1}{\sqrt{\mathfrak{A}}}\frac{\overset{*}{b}{}_{12}^2 - \overset{*}{b}_{11}\overset{*}{b}_{22}}{A_1A_2}.$$

It can be written in more concise form as

$$\begin{aligned}&\frac{\partial}{\partial\alpha_1}\frac{1}{A_1\sqrt{\mathfrak{A}}}\left[\frac{A_1\varepsilon_{12}}{2}\frac{\partial}{\partial\alpha_2}\ln\frac{\mathbb{S}_{22}}{\mathbb{S}_{11}}+L_2'(\varepsilon_{ik})+(1+\varepsilon_{11}+\varepsilon_{22})\frac{\partial A_2}{\partial\alpha_1}\right]\\&+\frac{\partial}{\partial\alpha_2}\frac{1}{A_2\sqrt{\mathfrak{A}}}\left[\frac{A_2\varepsilon_{21}}{2}\frac{\partial}{\partial\alpha_2}\ln\frac{\mathbb{S}_{11}}{\mathbb{S}_{22}}+L_1'(\varepsilon_{ik})+(1+\varepsilon_{11}+\varepsilon_{22})\frac{\partial A_1}{\partial\alpha_2}\right]\\&=A_1A_2\frac{1}{\sqrt{\mathfrak{A}}}\left(\overset{*}{k}{}_{12}^2-\overset{*}{k}_{11}\overset{*}{k}_{22}\right),\end{aligned}\tag{1.85}$$

where the differential operators $L_j'(\varepsilon_{ik})$ are defined by

$$\begin{aligned}L_1'(\varepsilon_{ik})&=\frac{\partial A_1\varepsilon_{11}}{\partial\alpha_2}-\frac{\partial A_2\varepsilon_{12}}{\partial\alpha_1}-\varepsilon_{22}\frac{\partial A_1}{\partial\alpha_1}-\varepsilon_{12}\frac{\partial A_2}{\partial\alpha_1},\\L_2'(\varepsilon_{ik})&=\frac{\partial A_2\varepsilon_{22}}{\partial\alpha_1}-\frac{\partial A_1\varepsilon_{12}}{\partial\alpha_2}-\varepsilon_{11}\frac{\partial A_2}{\partial\alpha_1}-\varepsilon_{12}\frac{\partial A_1}{\partial\alpha_2}.\end{aligned}$$

Let $\overset{*}{K}$ be the Gaussian curvature of the deformed surface $\overset{*}{S}$

$$\overset{*}{K}=k_{12}^2-k_{11}k_{22}=\frac{1}{A_1A_2}\left[\frac{\partial}{\partial\alpha_1}\left(\frac{1}{A_1}\frac{\partial A_2}{\partial\alpha_1}\right)+\frac{\partial}{\partial\alpha_2}\left(\frac{1}{A_2}\frac{\partial A_1}{\partial\alpha_2}\right)\right].\tag{1.86}$$

With the help of equation (1.86), the first equation in (1.85) can be written as

$$\begin{aligned}&\frac{\partial}{\partial\alpha_1}\frac{1}{A_1\sqrt{\mathfrak{A}}}\left[\frac{A_1\varepsilon_{12}}{2}\frac{\partial}{\partial\alpha_2}\ln\frac{\mathbb{S}_{22}}{\mathbb{S}_{11}}+L_2'(\varepsilon_{ik})+(1+\varepsilon_{11}+\varepsilon_{22})\frac{\partial A_2}{\partial\alpha_1}\right]\\&+\frac{\partial}{\partial\alpha_2}\frac{1}{A_2\sqrt{\mathfrak{A}}}\left[\frac{A_2\varepsilon_{21}}{2}\frac{\partial}{\partial\alpha_2}\ln\frac{\mathbb{S}_{11}}{\mathbb{S}_{22}}+L_1'(\varepsilon_{ik})+(1+\varepsilon_{11}+\varepsilon_{22})\frac{\partial A_1}{\partial\alpha_2}\right]\\&=A_1A_2\frac{1}{\sqrt{\mathfrak{A}}}(K-K_0).\end{aligned}\tag{1.87}$$

The increment to the Gaussian curvature is defined by

$$K-\overset{*}{K}=æ_{12}^2-æ_{11}æ_{22}+2kæ_{12}-k_{11}æ_{11}-k_{22}æ_{11}.\tag{1.88}$$

To obtain the other two equations, recall the Codazzi formulas

$$\frac{\partial\overset{*}{b}_{11}}{\partial\alpha_2}-\frac{\partial\overset{*}{b}_{12}}{\partial\alpha_1}-\overset{*}{\Gamma}{}_{12}^1\overset{*}{b}_{11}-\left(\overset{*}{\Gamma}{}_{12}^2-\overset{*}{\Gamma}{}_{11}^1\right)\overset{*}{b}_{12}+\overset{*}{\Gamma}{}_{11}^2\overset{*}{b}_{22}=0.$$

Here $\overset{*}{\Gamma}{}^j_{ik}$ are the Christoffel symbols of $\overset{*}{S}$. Substituting $\overset{*}{b}_{ij} = -A_iA_j\overset{*}{k}_{ij} = A_iA_j(k_{ij} + \ae_{ij})$, we obtain

$$\begin{aligned}&\frac{\partial A_1A_2(k_{12} + \ae_{12})}{\partial\alpha_1} - \frac{\partial A_1^2(k_{11} + \ae_{11})}{\partial\alpha_2} + A_1^2\overset{*}{k}_{11}\overset{*}{\Gamma}{}^1_{12}\\ &+ A_1A_2\overset{*}{k}_{12}\left(\overset{*}{\Gamma}{}^2_{12} - \overset{*}{\Gamma}{}^1_{11}\right) - A_2^2\overset{*}{k}_{22}\overset{*}{\Gamma}{}^2_{11} = 0.\end{aligned} \tag{1.89}$$

Subtracting equation (1.37) and dividing the resultant equation by $-A_1$, the compatibility equations are found to be

$$\begin{aligned}&\frac{\partial A_1\ae_{11}}{\partial\alpha_2} - \frac{\partial A_2\ae_{12}}{\partial\alpha_1} - \ae_{12}\frac{\partial A_1}{\partial\alpha_2} + A_2\overset{*}{k}_{12}(A^1_{11} - A^2_{12})\\ &- A_1\overset{*}{k}_{11}A^1_{12} + \frac{A_2^2}{A_1}\overset{*}{k}_{22}A^2_{11} = 0,\\ &\frac{\partial A_2\ae_{22}}{\partial\alpha_1} - \frac{\partial A_1\ae_{12}}{\partial\alpha_2} - \ae_{12}\frac{\partial A_2}{\partial\alpha_1} + A_1\overset{*}{k}_{12}(A^2_{22} - A^1_{12})\\ &- A_2\overset{*}{k}_{22}A^2_{12} + \frac{A_1^2}{A_2}\overset{*}{k}_{11}A^1_{22} = 0.\end{aligned} \tag{1.90}$$

In the above we made use of the following formulas for derivatives

$$\begin{aligned}\frac{\partial A_1A_2(k_{12} + \ae_{12})}{\partial\alpha_1} &= A_1\frac{\partial A_2(k_{12} + \ae_{12})}{\partial\alpha_1} + A_2(k_{12} + \ae_{12})\frac{\partial A_1}{\partial\alpha_1},\\ \frac{\partial A_1^2(k_{11} + \ae_{11})}{\partial\alpha_2} &= A_1\frac{\partial A_1(k_{11} + \ae_{11})}{\partial\alpha_2} + A_1(k_{11} + \ae_{11})\frac{\partial A_1}{\partial\alpha_2}.\end{aligned}$$

Let A^j_{ik} be the components of the Christoffel deviator given by

$$A^j_{ik} = \overset{*}{\Gamma}{}^j_{ik} - \Gamma^j_{ik}. \tag{1.91}$$

Defining differential operators $L_j'(\ae_{ik})$ by

$$\begin{aligned}L_1'(\ae_{ik}) &= \frac{\partial A_1\ae_{11}}{\partial\alpha_2} - \frac{\partial A_2\ae_{12}}{\partial\alpha_1} - \ae_{12}\frac{\partial A_2}{\partial\alpha_1} - \ae_{22}\frac{\partial A_1}{\partial\alpha_2},\\ L_2'(\ae_{ik}) &= \frac{\partial A_2\ae_{22}}{\partial\alpha_1} - \frac{\partial A_1\ae_{12}}{\partial\alpha_2} - \ae_{12}\frac{\partial A_1}{\partial\alpha_2} - \ae_{11}\frac{\partial A_2}{\partial\alpha_1}.\end{aligned} \tag{1.92}$$

Equation (1.89) can be written in the form

$$\begin{aligned}&L_1'(\ae_{ik}) + A_2\overset{*}{k}_{12}(A^1_{11} - A^2_{12}) - A_1\overset{*}{k}_{11}A^1_{12} + \frac{A_2^2}{A_1}\overset{*}{k}_{22}A^2_{11} = 0,\\ &L_2'(\ae_{ik}) + A_1\overset{*}{k}_{12}(A^2_{22} - A^1_{12}) - A_2\overset{*}{k}_{22}A^2_{12} + \frac{A_1^2}{A_2}\overset{*}{k}_{22}A^1_{22} = 0.\end{aligned} \tag{1.93}$$

Substituting $\overset{*}{A}_i, \overset{*}{\chi}, \overset{*}{a}$ into equations (1.23), for $\overset{*}{\Gamma}{}^j_{ik}$ we obtain

$$\begin{aligned}
\overset{*}{a}\overset{*}{\Gamma}{}^1_{11} &= \overset{*}{A}_1\overset{*}{A}_2^{2}\frac{\partial \overset{*}{A}_1}{\partial \alpha_1} - \overset{*}{a}_{12}\left(\frac{\partial \overset{*}{a}_{12}}{\partial \alpha_1} - \overset{*}{A}_1\frac{\partial \overset{*}{A}_1}{\partial \alpha_2}\right),\\
\overset{*}{a}\overset{*}{\Gamma}{}^1_{12} &= \overset{*}{A}_1\overset{*}{A}_2^{2}\frac{\partial \overset{*}{A}_1}{\partial \alpha_2} - \overset{*}{A}_2\overset{*}{a}_{12}\frac{\partial \overset{*}{A}_1}{\partial \alpha_1},\\
\overset{*}{a}\overset{*}{\Gamma}{}^2_{11} &= \overset{*}{A}_1^{2}\frac{\partial \overset{*}{a}_{12}}{\partial \alpha_1} - \overset{*}{A}_1\overset{*}{a}_{12}\frac{\partial \overset{*}{A}_1}{\partial \alpha_1} - \overset{*}{A}_1^{3}\frac{\partial \overset{*}{A}_1}{\partial \alpha_2},\\
\overset{*}{a} &= a\mathfrak{A}, \quad \overset{*}{a}_{12} = \overset{*}{A}_1\overset{*}{A}_2\cos\overset{*}{\chi}.
\end{aligned} \tag{1.94}$$

Making use of equations (1.23) and (1.94) in (1.91), the final formulas for the Chrystoffel deviators become

$$\begin{aligned}
\mathfrak{A}A^1_{11} &= \frac{\varepsilon_{12}}{A_1A_2}\frac{\partial A_1^{2}\mathbb{S}_{11}}{\partial \alpha_2} - \frac{4\varepsilon_{12}}{A_2}\frac{\partial A_2\varepsilon_{12}}{\partial \alpha_1} + \mathbb{S}_{22}\frac{\partial \varepsilon_{11}}{\partial \alpha_1},\\
\mathfrak{A}A^2_{11} &= \frac{A_1 I}{A_2^2}\frac{\partial A_1}{\partial \alpha_2} + -\frac{\mathbb{S}_{11}}{A_2^2}\left(2A_1\frac{\partial A_2\varepsilon_{12}}{\partial \alpha_1} - \frac{1}{2}\frac{\partial A_1^{2}\mathbb{S}_{11}}{\partial \alpha_2}\right) - \frac{2A_2\varepsilon_{12}}{A_2}\frac{\partial \varepsilon_{11}}{\partial \alpha_1},\\
\mathfrak{A}A^2_{12} &= \mathbb{S}_{11}\frac{\partial \varepsilon_{22}}{\partial \alpha_1} - \frac{\varepsilon_{12}}{A_1A_2}\frac{\partial A_1^{2}\mathbb{S}_{11}}{\partial \alpha_2} + \frac{4\varepsilon_{12}^2}{A_2}\frac{\partial A_2}{\partial \alpha_1},\\
\mathfrak{A}A^2_{22} &= \frac{\varepsilon_{12}}{A_1\,A_2}\frac{\partial A_2^{1}\mathbb{S}_{22}}{\partial \alpha_1} - \frac{4\varepsilon_{12}}{A_1}\frac{\partial A_1\varepsilon_{12}}{\partial \alpha_2} + \mathbb{S}_{11}\frac{\partial \varepsilon_{22}}{\partial \alpha_2},\\
\mathfrak{A}A^1_{22} &= \frac{A_2 I}{A_1^1}\frac{\partial A_2}{\partial \alpha_1} - \frac{\mathbb{S}_{22}}{A_1^1}\left(2A_2\frac{\partial A_1\varepsilon_{12}}{\partial \alpha_2} - \frac{1}{2}\frac{\partial A_2^{1}\mathbb{S}_{22}}{\partial \alpha_1}\right) - \frac{2A_1\varepsilon_{12}}{A_1}\frac{\partial \varepsilon_{22}}{\partial \alpha_2},\\
\mathfrak{A}A^1_{12} &= \mathbb{S}_{22}\frac{\partial \varepsilon_{11}}{\partial \alpha_2} - \frac{\varepsilon_{12}}{A_1A_2}\frac{\partial A_2^{1}\mathbb{S}_{22}}{\partial \alpha_1} + \frac{4\varepsilon_{12}^2}{A_1}\frac{\partial A_1}{\partial \alpha_2}.
\end{aligned} \tag{1.95}$$

Further reading

Galimov K Z 1975 *Foundations of the Nonlinear Theory of Thin Shells* (Kazan: Kazan University Press)

Galimov K Z, Paimushin V N and Teregulov I G 1996 *Foundations of the Nonlinear Theory of Shells* (Kazan: ФЭН)

Norden A P 1950 *Proc. Kazan Branch Acad. Sci. USSR, Ser.: Phys-Maths and Tech. Sci.* **2** 12–37

IOP Publishing

Soft Biological Shells in Bioengineering

Roustem N Miftahof and Nariman R Akhmadeev

Chapter 2

Parameterization of shells of complex geometry

The method of fictitious deformation is introduced followed by examples of parameterization of the surface of complex geometry in preferred coordinates and on a plane.

2.1 Fictitious deformations

Most biological shells are of complex geometry. For example, the human stomach resembles a horn or a hook, the urine-filled bladder a prolate or oblate spheroid, whilst the pregnant uterus appears similar to a pear. Convenient parameterization of such shells is a difficult analytical task and may not even be feasible. On the other hand, all numerical methods are based on discretization of the computational domain and as such may appear secluded from the problem. However, computational algorithms are most efficient and accurate only when they operate in regular, canonical domains and they suffer a loss of accuracy in complex domains. Therefore, the question of parameterization of shells of complex geometry becomes of utmost importance.

Let an arbitrary point $M(\alpha_1, \alpha_2) \in S$ and its ε_M-domain be in one-to-one correspondence with a point $\overset{*}{M}(\overset{*}{\alpha}_1, \overset{*}{\alpha}_2)$ and its $\varepsilon_{\overset{*}{M}}$-domain on the deformed middle surface $\overset{*}{S}$ (figure 2.1). The transformation is defined analytically by

$$\overset{*}{\alpha}_i = \overset{*}{\alpha}_i(\alpha_1, \alpha_2), \tag{2.1}$$

where (α_1, α_2) and $(\overset{*}{\alpha}_1, \overset{*}{\alpha}_2)$ are the coordinates on S and $\overset{*}{S}$, respectively.

Assuming that equation (2.1) is continuously differentiable and $\det(\partial\overset{*}{\alpha}_i/\partial\alpha_k) \neq 0$ $(i, k = 1, 2)$, the inverse transformation is found to be

$$\alpha_i = \alpha_i(\overset{*}{\alpha}_1, \overset{*}{\alpha}_2). \tag{2.2}$$

doi:10.1088/2053-2563/ab1a9ech2

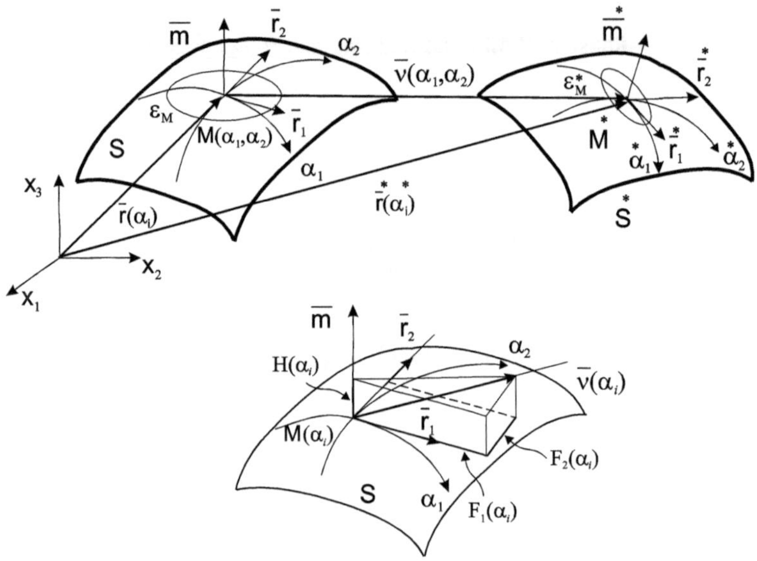

Figure 2.1. Continuous transformation of an ε_M-domain of the surface S. Decomposition of the displacement vector $\nu(\alpha_1, \alpha_2)$ in the undeformed base $\{\bar{r}_1, \bar{r}_2, \bar{m}\}$.

The coefficients of the direct and inverse transformations are given by

$$C_i^k = \frac{\partial \overset{*}{\alpha}_k}{\partial \alpha_i}, \qquad C = \det(C_i^k), \tag{2.3}$$

$$\overset{*}{C}{}_i^k = \frac{\partial \alpha_k}{\partial \overset{*}{\alpha}_i}, \qquad \overset{*}{C} = \det(\overset{*}{C}{}_i^k). \tag{2.4}$$

Assuming that $C \neq 0$, $C^* \neq 0$, we have

$$\sum_{i=1}^{2} C_i^k \overset{*}{C}{}_k^i = 1, \qquad \sum_{i=1}^{2} C_i^k \overset{*}{C}{}_j^k = 0 \quad (i \neq j),$$
$$C\overset{*}{C} = 1, \qquad \overset{*}{C}{}_i^k = [C_k^i]/C. \tag{2.5}$$

Here $[C_k^i]$ is the cofactor to the element C_k^i of the matrix (C_i^k).

It follows from the above considerations that the surface $\overset{*}{S}$ can also be referred to by the coordinates α_i. Then, the vector equations of S and $\overset{*}{S}$ are given by

$$
\begin{aligned}
\bar{r} &= \bar{r}(\alpha_1, \alpha_2), \\
\overset{*}{\bar{r}} &= \overset{*}{\bar{r}}(\overset{*}{\alpha}_1, \overset{*}{\alpha}_2) = \overset{*}{\bar{r}}[f_1(\alpha_1, \alpha_2), f_2(\alpha_1, \alpha_2)] \\
&= \bar{r}(\alpha_1, \alpha_2) + \bar{v}(\alpha_1, \alpha_2).
\end{aligned} \tag{2.6}
$$

Here use is made of equation (1.58) and $\bar{v}(\alpha_1, \alpha_2)$ is the displacement vector.

The lengths of a linear element ds, $\overset{*}{ds}$ before and after transformation are given by equations (1.11) and (1.63). Let the stretch ratio be defined by

$$
\lambda_i = \frac{\overset{*}{ds}}{ds} = \sqrt{\frac{\overset{*}{a}_{ik}}{a_{ik}}} \quad (i, k = 1, 2). \tag{2.7}
$$

If $\lambda_i > 1$ then the element experiences elongation during transformation and if $\lambda_i < 1$ it experiences contraction.

Similarly, the change of the area of a surface element is defined by

$$
\delta s_\Delta = \overset{*}{ds}_\Delta / ds_\Delta = \sqrt{\overset{*}{a}/a}\,, \tag{2.8}
$$

where areas ds_Δ, $\overset{*}{ds}_\Delta$ are calculated using equation (1.12). If $\delta s_\Delta > 1$ then the surface undergoes expansion and if $\delta s_\Delta < 1$, compression.

Expanding $\bar{v}(\alpha_1, \alpha_2)$ in the bases $\{\bar{r}_1, \bar{r}_2, \overline{m}\}$ and $\{\bar{r}^1, \bar{r}^2, \overline{m}\}$, we obtain (figure 2.1)

$$
\begin{aligned}
\bar{v}(\alpha_1, \alpha_2) &= \sum_{i=1}^{2} \mathrm{F}_i(\alpha_1, \alpha_2)\bar{r}^i + \mathrm{H}(\alpha_1, \alpha_2)\overline{m} \\
&= \sum_{i=1}^{2} \mathrm{F}^i(\alpha_1, \alpha_2)\bar{r}_i + \mathrm{H}(\alpha_1, \alpha_2)\overline{m}.
\end{aligned} \tag{2.9}
$$

Substituting equation (2.9) into (2.6) we obtain

$$
\begin{aligned}
\overset{*}{\bar{r}} &= \bar{r}(\alpha_1, \alpha_2) + \sum_{i=1}^{2} \mathrm{F}_i(\alpha_1, \alpha_2)\bar{r}^i + \mathrm{H}(\alpha_1, \alpha_2)\overline{m} \\
&= \bar{r}(\alpha_1, \alpha_2) + \sum_{i=1}^{2} \mathrm{F}^i(\alpha_1, \alpha_2)\bar{r}_i + \mathrm{H}(\alpha_1, \alpha_2)\overline{m}.
\end{aligned} \tag{2.10}
$$

Evidently, the transformation (2.10) can be achieved by deformation of the middle surface S. For the purpose of parameterization of the surface $\overset{*}{S}$ the transformation could be performed fictitiously. Therefore, such a transformation is called a fictitious deformation. The problem is to construct the three functions $\mathrm{F}_i(\alpha_i)$ and $\mathrm{H}(\alpha_i)$ $(i = 1, 2)$.

Differentiating equation (2.10) with respect to α_i and using equations (1.22) and (1.24), vectors $\overset{*}{\bar{r}}_i$ tangent to coordinate lines $\overset{*}{\alpha}_i$ on $\overset{*}{S}$ are found to be

$$\overset{*}{\bar{r}}_i = \sum_{k=1}^{2}(\delta_{ik} + \underline{e}_i^k)\bar{r}_k + \omega_i\bar{m} = \sum_{k=1}^{2}(a_{ik} + \underline{e}_{ik})\bar{r}^k + \underline{\omega}_i\bar{m}. \tag{2.11}$$

Here

$$\begin{aligned}\underline{e}_i^k &= \frac{\partial \mathrm{F}^k}{\partial \alpha_i} + \sum_{s=1}^{2}\Gamma_{is}^k \mathrm{F}^s(\alpha_i) - \mathrm{H}(\alpha_i)b_i^k := \nabla_i \mathrm{F}^k(\alpha_i) - \mathrm{H}(\alpha_i)b_i^k,\\ \underline{e}_{ki} &= \frac{\partial \mathrm{F}_k}{\partial \alpha_i} - \sum_{s=1}^{2}\Gamma_{ik}^s \mathrm{F}_s(\alpha_i) - \mathrm{H}(\alpha_i)b_{ik} := \nabla_i \mathrm{F}_k(\alpha_i) - \mathrm{H}(\alpha_i)b_{ik},\\ \underline{\omega}_i &= \frac{\partial \mathrm{H}(\alpha_i)}{\partial \alpha_i} + b_i^k \mathrm{F}_k(\alpha_i),\end{aligned} \tag{2.12}$$

and $\nabla_i(\ldots)$ is the covariant derivative in metric a_{jk}, δ_{ik} is the Kronecker delta, and b_{ik}, b_i^k are the components of the second fundamental form of S. Substituting equation (2.11) into (1.4) the components of the metric tensor $\overset{*}{\mathbf{A}}$ on $\overset{*}{S}$ are found to be

$$\overset{*}{a}_{ik} = a_{ik} + 2\underline{\varepsilon}_{ik}, \tag{2.13}$$

where $\underline{\varepsilon}_{ik}$ are the components of the tensor of tangent fictitious deformations given by

$$2\underline{\varepsilon}_{ik} = \overset{*}{\bar{r}}_i\overset{*}{\bar{r}}_k - \bar{r}_i\bar{r}_k = \underline{e}_{ik} + \underline{e}_{ki} + a_{js}\underline{e}_{ij}\underline{e}_{ks} + \underline{\varpi}_i\underline{\varpi}_k. \tag{2.14}$$

In just the same way as we introduced bending deformations $æ_{ik}$, we introduce bending fictitious deformations of the surface S,

$$\underline{æ}_{ik} = b_{ik} - \overset{*}{b}_{ik}. \tag{2.15}$$

The components $\underline{\varepsilon}_{ik}$ and $\underline{æ}_{ik}$ are interdependent and satisfy the conditions of continuity similar to those given by equations (1.85) and (1.90). Expressing $\underline{\varepsilon}_{ik}$ and $\underline{æ}_{ik}$ in terms of $\mathrm{F}_i(\alpha_i)$ and $\mathrm{H}(\alpha_i)$ we find that the continuity conditions require the existence of continuous derivatives of the functions up to order three at all regular points of the undeformed surface S.

2.2 Parameterization of the equidistant surface

Let a point $M(\alpha_1, \alpha_2) \in S$ be in one-to-one correspondence with point $M_z(\alpha_1, \alpha_2)$ on an equidistant surface S_z ($S_z \parallel S$). The position vector $\bar{\rho}$ of M_z is given by

$$\bar{\rho}(\alpha_1, \alpha_2) = \bar{r}(\alpha_1, \alpha_2) + \mathrm{H}^z\bar{m}, \tag{2.16}$$

where $\mathrm{H}^z = \text{const}$. Comparison of equations (2.16) and (2.10) shows that the surface S_z can be obtained from S by fictitious deformation, i.e. by continuous displacement of all points on S by H^z in the direction of the normal vector $\bar{m}$ ($\bar{m} \perp S$) (figure 1.5). Since $\mathrm{F}_i(\alpha_1, \alpha_2) = 0$ and $\partial \mathrm{H}^z/\partial \alpha_i = 0$ in equation (2.16), $\underline{e}_i^k$, $\underline{e}_{ki}$, $\underline{\omega}_i$ take the form

$$\underline{e}_i^{\,k} = -\mathrm{H}^z b_i^{\,k}, \quad \underline{e}_{ki} = -\mathrm{H}^z b_{ik}, \; \underline{\omega}_i = 0. \tag{2.17}$$

Basis vectors $\bar{\rho}_i$ on S_z are defined by

$$\bar{\rho}_i := \frac{\partial \bar{\rho}}{\partial \alpha_i} = \sum_{k=1}^{2} (\delta^k{}_i - \mathrm{H}^z b_i^{\,k}) \bar{r}_k = \sum_{k=1}^{2} \theta_i^{\,k} \bar{r}_k. \tag{2.18}$$

Hence, the components a_{ik}^z of the metric tensor on S_z are

$$a_{ik}^z = \bar{\rho}_i \bar{\rho}_k = \sum_{s=1}^{2} \sum_{n=1}^{2} \theta_i^{\,s} \theta_k^{\,n} a_{sn} = a_{ik} - 2\mathrm{H}^z b_{ik} + (\mathrm{H}^z)^2 \xi_{ik}, \tag{2.19}$$

where ξ_{ik} are the components of the third metric tensor of S given by

$$\xi_{ik} = \sum_{n=1}^{2} b^n{}_i b_{nk} = 2\Gamma b_{ik} - K a_{ik}. \tag{2.20}$$

Here Γ, K are the mean and the Gaussian curvature of S, respectively.

Since $\overline{m} = \overline{m}_z$ ($\overline{m}_z \perp S_z$),

$$\begin{aligned} b_{ik}^z &= -\bar{\rho}_i \overline{m}_z = -\bar{\rho}_i \overline{m} = -\bar{r}_n \overline{m}_k (\delta_i^{\,n} - \mathrm{H}^z b_i^{\,n}) \\ &= b_{nk}(\delta_i^{\,n} - \mathrm{H}^z b_i^{\,n}) = b_{ik} - \mathrm{H}^z \xi_{ik}. \end{aligned}$$

From the above with the help of equation (2.16), we find

$$b_{ik}^z = \sum_{n=1}^{2} b_{nk} \xi_i^{\,n} = b_{ik}(1 - 2\Gamma \mathrm{H}^z) + a_{ik} K \mathrm{H}^z. \tag{2.21}$$

Making use of equation (2.18) in the vector product $(\bar{\rho}_1 \times \bar{\rho}_2)$, we obtain

$$\begin{aligned} \bar{\rho}_1 \times \bar{\rho}_2 &= \sum_{k=1}^{2} \sum_{j=1}^{2} (\bar{r}_k \times \bar{r}_j) \theta^k{}_1 \theta^j{}_2 \\ &= (\bar{r}_1 \times \bar{r}_2)(\theta_1^{\,1} \theta_2^{\,2} - \theta_1^{\,2} \theta_2^{\,1}) \\ &= (\bar{r}_1 \times \bar{r}_2)(1 - 2\Gamma \mathrm{H}^z + K(\mathrm{H}^z)^2). \end{aligned} \tag{2.22}$$

Recalling that $(\bar{\rho}_1 \times \bar{\rho}_2)^2 = a^z$ and $(\bar{r}_1 \times \bar{r}_2)^2 = a$, we obtain, finally

$$a^z = a(1 - 2\Gamma \mathrm{H}^z + K(\mathrm{H}^z)^2)^2. \tag{2.23}$$

Thus, the change of a given surface element on S during transformation is found to be

$$\delta s_\Delta = \sqrt{a/a^z} = (1 - 2\Gamma \mathrm{H}^z + K(\mathrm{H}^z)^2) = (\theta_1^{\,1} \theta_2^{\,2} - \theta_1^{\,2} \theta_2^{\,1}). \tag{2.24}$$

The Gaussian curvature of S_z is determined by

$$a^z K^z := b_{11}^z b_{22}^z - b_{12}^z b_{21}^z = (\theta_1^{\,1} \theta_2^{\,2} - \theta_1^{\,2} \theta_2^{\,1})(b_1^{\,1} b_2^{\,2} - b_2^{\,1} b_1^{\,2}).$$

Using equation (2.24) in the above, for the Gaussian curvature of S_z we find

$$a^z K^z = a d_s^2 K. \tag{2.25}$$

The coefficients of the first and second fundamental forms of S_z satisfy the Gauss–Codazzi equations

$$a^z K^z = \frac{\partial \Gamma^z_{h,ij}}{\partial \alpha_k} - \frac{\partial \Gamma^z_{h,ik}}{\partial \alpha_j} + \sum_{s=1}^{2}\left(\Gamma^{(z)s}_{ik}\Gamma^z_{s,hj} - \Gamma^{(z)s}_{ij}\Gamma^z_{s,hk}\right), \tag{2.26}$$

$$\frac{\partial b^z_{ij}}{\partial \alpha_k} - \frac{\partial b^z_{ik}}{\partial \alpha_j} + \sum_{s=1}^{2}\left(\Gamma^{(z)s}{}_{ij} b^z_{sk} - \Gamma^{(z)s}{}_{ik} b^z_{sj}\right) = 0. \tag{2.27}$$

Here $\Gamma^z{}_{h,ij}$ and $\Gamma^{(z)s}{}_{ij}$ are the Christoffel symbols of the first and second kind, respectively, given by

$$\Gamma^z_{h,ij} = \frac{1}{2}\left(\frac{\partial a^z_{jh}}{\partial \alpha_i} + \frac{\partial a^z_{ih}}{\partial \alpha_j} - \frac{\partial a^z_{ij}}{\partial \alpha_h}\right),$$
$$\Gamma^{(z)s}_{ij} = a^{sh}\Gamma^z_{h,ij}. \tag{2.28}$$

2.3 A single function variant of the method of fictitious deformation

Complex biological shells may resemble classical canonical surfaces. For example, the large intestine where the goffered cylinder bears a resemblance to a circular cylinder, the urinary bladder where the prolate spheroid could be viewed as a sphere, and the antropyloric region of the stomach and the ureteropelvic junction of the kidney where the distorted funnel is similar to a cone, etc. Let S be a reference canonical surface for $\overset{*}{S}$. Assume that the vector $\bar{m}$ ($\bar{m} \perp S$) drawn at any point M on S intersects the surface $\overset{*}{S}$ only once (figure 2.2). Setting $F_i(\alpha_1, \alpha_2) = 0$ from equation (2.9) for the displacement vector we have

$$\bar{v}(\alpha_1, \alpha_2) = H(\alpha_1, \alpha_2)\bar{m}. \tag{2.29}$$

Here $H(\alpha_i)$ is the distance measured along $\bar{m}$ from the surface S to $\overset{*}{S}$. Evidently, the vector equation of $\overset{*}{S}$ can be written as

$$\overset{*}{\bar{r}} = \bar{r}(\alpha_1, \alpha_2) + H(\alpha_1, \alpha_2)\bar{m}. \tag{2.30}$$

Let

$$H(\alpha_1, \alpha_2) = H^z + \overset{*}{H}(\alpha_1, \alpha_2). \tag{2.31}$$

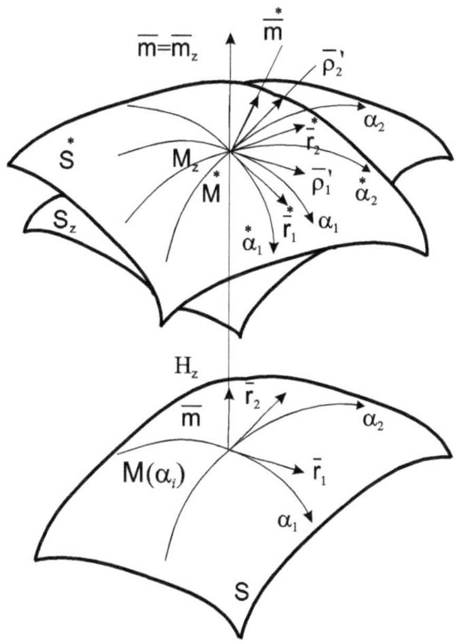

Figure 2.2. Fictitious deformation of the surface.

Then substituting equation (2.31) in (2.30) we obtain

$$\overset{*}{\bar{r}} = \bar{r}(\alpha_1, \alpha_2) + (\mathrm{H}^z + \overset{*}{\mathrm{H}}(\alpha_1, \alpha_2))\bar{m}. \tag{2.32}$$

Equation (2.32) describes the superimposition of two consecutive transformations: first, the transformation of the canonical surface S onto an equidistant surface S_z followed by the second transformation of S_z to $\overset{*}{S}$.

Differentiating equation (2.30) with respect to α_i and using $\bar{m}_i = -b_i^k \bar{r}_k$, basis vectors $\overset{*}{\bar{r}}_i$ onto $\overset{*}{S}$ are found to be

$$\overset{*}{\bar{r}}_i = \sum_{k=1}^{2} \bar{r}_k(\delta_i^k - \mathrm{H}(\alpha_i) b_i^k) + \frac{\partial \mathrm{H}(\alpha_i)}{\partial \alpha_i}\bar{m}. \tag{2.33}$$

Making use of equations (2.18), (2.31) in (2.33) we obtain

$$\overset{*}{\bar{r}}_i = \bar{\rho}_i' + \frac{\partial \overset{*}{\mathrm{H}}(\alpha_i)}{\partial \alpha_i}\bar{m}, \tag{2.34}$$

where

$$\bar{\rho}_i' = \bar{\rho}_i + \overset{*}{\mathrm{H}}(\alpha_i)\sum_{k=1}^{2} b_i^k \bar{r}_k.$$

Vectors $\bar{\rho}_i'$ lie in the tangent plane of the equidistant surface S_z and are collinear to vectors $\bar{r}_i \in S$. Therefore, at any point $\overset{*}{M}(\overset{*}{\alpha}_1, \overset{*}{\alpha}_2) \in \overset{*}{S}$ we can introduce two interrelated orthogonal bases, i.e. the main basis $\{\overset{*}{\bar{r}}_1, \overset{*}{\bar{r}}_2, \bar{m}\}$ with vectors $\overset{*}{\bar{r}}_i$ tangent to the coordinate lines $\overset{*}{\alpha}_i$ and the vector $\bar{m}$ normal to $\overset{*}{S}$, and an auxiliary basis $\{\bar{\rho}_1', \bar{\rho}_2', \bar{m}'\}$. The latter also serves as the main basis for the surface S_z that runs through $\overset{*}{M}$ parallel to S and $\bar{m}' = \bar{m}$.

Substituting equation (2.34) in (1.4) and using the fact that $\bar{\rho}_i'\bar{m} = 0$, for the components of the metric tensor $\overset{*}{\mathbf{A}}$ we find

$$\overset{*}{a}_{ik} = \overset{z}{a}_{ik} + \frac{\partial \overset{*}{\mathrm{H}}(\alpha_i)}{\partial \alpha_i}\frac{\partial \overset{*}{\mathrm{H}}(\alpha_i)}{\partial \alpha_k}. \tag{2.35}$$

Here

$$\begin{aligned} \overset{z}{a}_{ik} &= \sum_{s=1}^{2}\sum_{n=1}^{2}(\delta_i^s - \mathrm{H}(\alpha_i)b_i^s)(\delta_k^n - \mathrm{H}(\alpha_i)b_k^n)a_{sn} \\ &= a_{ik} - 2\mathrm{H}(\alpha_i)b_{ik} + \mathrm{H}(\alpha_i)^2\xi_{ik} \\ &= a_{ik}(1 + \overset{*}{\mathrm{H}}(\alpha_i)^2K) + 2(\Gamma\overset{*}{\mathrm{H}}(\alpha_i) - 1)\overset{*}{\mathrm{H}}(\alpha_i)b_k^i, \end{aligned} \tag{2.36}$$

where use is made of equations (2.19) and (2.20). Using equations (2.35) and (2.36) in (2.13) for the tensor of tangent fictitious deformations $2\underline{\varepsilon}_{ik}$, we obtain

$$\begin{aligned} 2\underline{\varepsilon}_{ik} &= 2\overset{z}{\underline{\varepsilon}}_{ik} + \frac{\partial \overset{*}{\mathrm{H}}(\alpha_i)}{\partial \alpha_i}\frac{\partial \overset{*}{\mathrm{H}}(\alpha_i)}{\partial \alpha_k}, \\ 2\overset{z}{\underline{\varepsilon}}_{ik} &= 2\mathrm{H}(\alpha_i)b_{ik} + \mathrm{H}(\alpha_i)^2\xi_{ik}. \end{aligned} \tag{2.37}$$

From equation (2.25) the determinant $\overset{*}{a}$ is found to be

$$\overset{*}{a} = a^z + \overset{z}{a}_{11}\left(\frac{\partial \overset{*}{\mathrm{H}}(\alpha_i)}{\partial \alpha_2}\right)^2 + \overset{z}{a}_{22}\left(\frac{\partial \overset{*}{\mathrm{H}}(\alpha_i)}{\partial \alpha_1}\right)^2 - 2\overset{z}{a}_{12}\frac{\partial \overset{*}{\mathrm{H}}(\alpha_i)}{\partial \alpha_1}\frac{\partial \overset{*}{\mathrm{H}}(\alpha_i)}{\partial \alpha_2}, \tag{2.38}$$

where the determinant a^z is given by equation (2.23).

Substituting equation (2.34) into formula $\overset{*}{\bar{m}} = (1/2)\overset{*ik}{c}(\overset{*}{\bar{r}}_i, \overset{*}{\bar{r}}_k)$ and using equations (1.8)–(1.10) for the normal vector $\overset{*}{\bar{m}}$ $(\overset{*}{\bar{m}} \perp \overset{*}{S})$ we have

$$\overset{*}{\overline{m}} = \frac{1}{2}\sqrt{\frac{a_z}{a}}c_z^{ik}\left[(\overline{\rho}_i', \overline{\rho}_k') + \frac{\partial \overset{*}{\mathrm{H}}(\alpha_i)}{\partial \alpha_k}(\overline{\rho}_i', \overline{m}) + \frac{\partial \overset{*}{\mathrm{H}}(\alpha_i)}{\partial \alpha_i}(\overline{m}, \overline{\rho}_k')\right]$$

$$= \frac{\mathrm{H}_0}{2}\sum_{i=1}^{2}\sum_{k=1}^{2}c_z^{ik}\left(\overline{m}c_{ik}^{z} + \sum_{j=1}^{2}\left(c_{ij}^{z}\overline{\rho}'^{j}\frac{\partial \overset{*}{\mathrm{H}}(\alpha_i)}{\partial \alpha_k} - c_{jk}^{z}\overline{\rho}'^{j}\frac{\partial \overset{*}{\mathrm{H}}(\alpha_i)}{\partial \alpha_i}\right)\right) \tag{2.39}$$

$$= \mathrm{H}_0\left(\overline{m} - \sum_{i=1}^{2}\overline{\rho}'^{i}\frac{\partial \overset{*}{\mathrm{H}}(\alpha_i)}{\partial \alpha_i}\right) = \mathrm{H}_0\left(\overline{m} - \sum_{k=1}^{2}\overline{\rho}_i' a_z^{ik}\frac{\partial \overset{*}{\mathrm{H}}(\alpha_i)}{\partial \alpha_k}\right),$$

where

$$a_z = a\mathrm{H}_0^2, \quad \mathrm{H}_0 = \left(1 + \sum_{i=1}^{2}\sum_{k=1}^{2}a_z^{ik}\frac{\partial \overset{*}{\mathrm{H}}(\alpha_i)}{\partial \alpha_i}\frac{\partial \overset{*}{\mathrm{H}}(\alpha_i)}{\partial \alpha_k}\right).$$

Further, substituting $\overline{\rho}_i' = \overline{\rho}_i + \overset{*}{\mathrm{H}}(\alpha_i)b_i^{k}\overline{r}_k$ into (2.39) for $\overset{*}{\overline{m}}$ in terms of basis vectors $\overline{r}_k \in S$ we obtain

$$\overset{*}{\overline{m}} = \mathrm{H}_0\left(\overline{m} - \overline{r}_k a_z^{ik}\frac{\partial \overset{*}{\mathrm{H}}(\alpha_i)}{\partial \alpha_k}(\delta_i^{k} - \mathrm{H}(\alpha_i)b_i^{k})\right). \tag{2.40}$$

Differentiating equation (2.39) with respect to α_i we obtain

$$\overset{*}{\overline{m}}_i = \mathrm{H}_0\left(\overline{m} - \sum_{k=1}^{2}\overline{\rho}'^{k}\frac{\partial \overset{*}{\mathrm{H}}(\alpha_i)}{\partial \alpha_k}\right)\frac{\partial \mathrm{H}_0}{\partial \alpha_i} + \mathrm{H}_0\frac{\partial}{\partial \alpha_i}\left(\overline{m} - \sum_{k=1}^{2}\overline{\rho}'^{k}\frac{\partial \overset{*}{\mathrm{H}}(\alpha_i)}{\partial \alpha_k}\right). \tag{2.41}$$

Using equation (2.39) the first term in the above can be written in the form

$$\left(\overline{m} - \overline{r}^{k}\frac{\partial \overset{*}{\mathrm{H}}(\alpha_i)}{\partial \alpha_k}\right) = \frac{\overset{*}{\overline{m}}_i}{\mathrm{H}_0}\frac{\partial \mathrm{H}_0}{\partial \alpha_i}. \tag{2.42}$$

In the second term we introduce the covariant derivative with respect to a_{ik}^{z} as (see equation (2.12))

$$\frac{\partial}{\partial \alpha_i}\left(\overline{m} - \sum_{k=1}^{2}\overline{\rho}'^k \frac{\partial \overset{*}{\mathrm{H}}(\alpha_i)}{\partial \alpha_k}\right) := \nabla_i^z\left(\overline{m} - \sum_{k=1}^{2}\overline{\rho}'^k \frac{\partial \overset{*}{\mathrm{H}}(\alpha_i)}{\partial \alpha_k}\right)$$
$$= \overline{m} - \sum_{k=1}^{2}\frac{\partial \overset{*}{\mathrm{H}}(\alpha_i)}{\partial \alpha_k}\nabla_i^z \overline{\rho}'^k - \sum_{k=1}^{2}\overline{\rho}'^k \nabla_i^z\left(\frac{\partial \overset{*}{\mathrm{H}}(\alpha_i)}{\partial \alpha_k}\right). \tag{2.43}$$

Derivatives of vectors $\overline{\rho}_i'$ and $\overline{m}$ can be found from equations (1.18) and (1.22) by substituting $\overline{\rho}_i'$ for $\overline{r}_i$. The components of the second fundamental form of S_z in terms of b_{ik} are given by

$$b_{ik}^z = \sum_{n=1}^{2} b_{nk}\theta_i^n = b_{ik}(1 - 2\Gamma\mathrm{H}(\alpha_i)) + a_{ik}K\mathrm{H}(\alpha_i),$$
$$b_i^{(z)k} = \sum_{s=1}^{2} a_z^{ks} b_{is}^z. \tag{2.44}$$

Thus, equation (2.43) can be written in the form

$$\frac{\partial}{\partial \alpha_i}\left(\overline{m} - \overline{\rho}'^k \frac{\partial \overset{*}{\mathrm{H}}(\alpha_i)}{\partial \alpha_k}\right) = \overline{m} - \sum_{k=1}^{2}\frac{\partial \overset{*}{\mathrm{H}}(\alpha_i)}{\partial \alpha_k} b_i^{(z)k}\overline{m}$$
$$- \sum_{k=1}^{2}\overline{\rho}'^k \nabla_i^z \frac{\partial \overset{*}{\mathrm{H}}(\alpha_i)}{\partial \alpha_k}. \tag{2.45}$$

Substituting equations (2.42) and (2.45) into (2.41) for $\overset{*}{\overline{m}}_i$ we obtain, finally,

$$\overset{*}{\overline{m}}_i = \frac{\overset{*}{\overline{m}}_i}{\mathrm{H}_0}\frac{\partial \mathrm{H}_0}{\partial \alpha_i} + \mathrm{H}_0\left(\overline{m} - \frac{\partial \overset{*}{\mathrm{H}}(\alpha_i)}{\partial \alpha_k} b_i^{(z)k}\overline{m} - \overline{\rho}'^k \nabla_i^z \frac{\partial \overset{*}{\mathrm{H}}(\alpha_i)}{\partial \alpha_k}\right). \tag{2.46}$$

The coefficients b_{ik} are found from equation (1.18) by substituting equations (2.34) and (2.46)

$$b_{ik} = \mathrm{H}_0 \sum_{j=1}^{2} \left(b_{ij}^{(z)} \left(\delta_k^j + a_z^{ji} \frac{\partial \overset{*}{\mathrm{H}}(\alpha_i)}{\partial \alpha_i} \frac{\partial \overset{*}{\mathrm{H}}(\alpha_i)}{\partial \alpha_k} \right) + \nabla_i^z \left(\frac{\partial \overset{*}{\mathrm{H}}(\alpha_i)}{\partial \alpha_k} \right) \right)$$

$$= \mathrm{H}_0 \sum_{j=1}^{2} \left(b_i^{(z)j} \left(a_{kj}^z - \frac{\partial \overset{*}{\mathrm{H}}(\alpha_i)}{\partial \alpha_k} \frac{\partial \overset{*}{\mathrm{H}}(\alpha_i)}{\partial \alpha_j} \right) + \nabla_i^z \left(\frac{\partial \overset{*}{\mathrm{H}}(\alpha_i)}{\partial \alpha_k} \right) \right) \tag{2.47}$$

$$= \mathrm{H}_0 \sum_{j=1}^{2} \left(b_i^{(z)j} a_{kj} + \nabla_i^z \left(\frac{\partial \overset{*}{\mathrm{H}}(\alpha_i)}{\partial \alpha_k} \right) \right).$$

The Christoffel symbols $\overset{*}{\Gamma}_{ij,k}$ of the first kind are calculated from $\overset{*}{\Gamma}_{ij,k} = \overset{*}{\bar{r}}_{ij} \overset{*}{\bar{r}}_k$. Thus differentiating equation (2.33) with respect to α_j and multiplying the resultant equation by $\overset{*}{\bar{r}}_k$, we find

$$\overset{*}{\Gamma}_{ij,k} = \Gamma_{ij,k}^{(z)} + \frac{\partial^2 \overset{*}{\mathrm{H}}(\alpha_i)}{\partial \alpha_i \partial \alpha_j} \frac{\partial \overset{*}{\mathrm{H}}(\alpha_i)}{\partial \alpha_k}, \tag{2.48}$$

where $\Gamma_{ij,k}^{(z)}$ are calculated using equation (2.28). The Christoffel symbols of the second kind $\overset{*}{\Gamma}{}_{ij}^{k}$ are found to be

$$\overset{*}{\Gamma}{}_{ij}^{k} = \overset{*}{a}{}^{\alpha k} \overset{*}{\Gamma}_{ij,\alpha} = \left(\Gamma_{ij,\alpha}^{(z)} + \frac{\partial^2 \overset{*}{\mathrm{H}}(\alpha_i)}{\partial \alpha_i \partial \alpha_j} \right) \times \left(a_z^{\alpha k} - \mathrm{H}_0^2 \sum_{m=1}^{2} \sum_{j=1}^{2} a_z^{\alpha m} a_z^{jk} \frac{\partial \overset{*}{\mathrm{H}}(\alpha_i)}{\partial \alpha_m} \frac{\partial \overset{*}{\mathrm{H}}(\alpha_i)}{\partial \alpha_j} \right), \tag{2.49}$$

where

$$\overset{*}{a}{}^{\alpha k} = a_z^{\alpha k} - \mathrm{H}_0^2 \sum_{j=1}^{2} \sum_{m=1}^{2} a_z^{\alpha m} a_z^{jk} \frac{\partial \overset{*}{\mathrm{H}}(\alpha_i)}{\partial \alpha_m} \frac{\partial \overset{*}{\mathrm{H}}(\alpha_i)}{\partial \alpha_j}.$$

2.4 Parameterization of a complex surface in preferred coordinates

The problem of parameterization of a complex surface simplifies significantly if the surface S is referred to by coordinate lines (α_1, α_2) that are the lines of curvature. Differentiating equation (2.30) with respect to α_i with the help of equation (1.30) the base vectors $\overset{*}{\bar{r}}_i \in \overset{*}{S}$ are found to be

$$\overset{*}{\bar{r}}_i = A_i^z (\bar{e}_i + y_i \overline{m}). \tag{2.50}$$

Here $A_i^z = A_i\theta_i = A_i[1 + \mathrm{H}(\alpha_i)/R_i]$, A_i are the Lamé parameters, R_i are the radii of the principal curvature, and $\bar{e}_i$ are the unit vectors on S. The coefficients y_i are given by

$$y_i = \frac{1}{A_i^z}\frac{\partial \mathrm{H}(\alpha_j)}{\partial \alpha_i} \equiv \frac{1}{A_i[1 + \mathrm{H}(\alpha_j)/R_i]}\frac{\partial \mathrm{H}(\alpha_j)}{\partial \alpha_i}. \tag{2.51}$$

The first term in equation (2.50) defines the basis vectors $\bar{\rho}_i'$ on the equidistant surface S_z. Hence, at any point $\overset{*}{M} \in \overset{*}{S}$ the unit vector $\bar{e}_i^z = \bar{\rho}_i/A_i^z$ ($\bar{e}_i^z \in S_z$) equals unit vector $\bar{e}_i$ defined on the canonical surface S: $\bar{e}_i^z = \bar{e}_i$.

By analogy to equation (2.40), for decomposition of the normal vector $\overset{*}{\bar{m}}$ we have

$$\overset{*}{\bar{m}} = \varsigma(\bar{m} - \varsigma_i\bar{e}_i). \tag{2.52}$$

Using equations (2.50) and (2.52) the scalar product of equation (2.52) by $\overset{*}{\bar{m}}$ and $\overset{*}{\bar{r}}_i$ yields

$$\varsigma_i = y_i, \qquad \varsigma = 1/\sqrt{1 + y_1^2 + y_2^2}.$$

Hence,

$$\overset{*}{\bar{m}} = \varsigma(\bar{m} - y_i\bar{e}_i) = \frac{1}{\sqrt{1 + y_1^2 + y_2^2}}(\bar{m} - y_1\bar{e}_1 - y_2\bar{e}_2). \tag{2.53}$$

Substituting equation (2.50) in $\overset{*}{a}_{ik} = \overset{*}{\bar{r}}_i \overset{*}{r} k_i$ we obtain

$$\overset{*}{a}_{ik} = A_i^z A_k^z(\delta_{ik} + y_i y_k). \tag{2.54}$$

The determinant of the metric tensor $\overset{*}{\mathbf{A}}$ on $\overset{*}{S}$ is found to be

$$\begin{aligned} \overset{*}{a} = \overset{*}{a}_{11}\overset{*}{a}_{22} - \overset{*}{a}{}_{12}^{2} &= a_{11}^z a_{22}^z(1 + y_1^2 + y_2^2 + y_1^2 y_2^2) \\ - a_{11}^z a_{22}^z y_1^2 y_2^2 &= a_{11}^z a_{22}^z(1 + y_1^2 + y_2^2) = \frac{a_{11}^z a_{22}^z}{\varsigma^2}. \end{aligned} \tag{2.55}$$

The contravariant components $\overset{*}{a}{}^{ik}$ of $\overset{*}{\mathbf{A}}$ are calculated as

$$\begin{aligned} \overset{*}{a}{}^{11} &= \frac{\overset{*}{a}_{22}}{\overset{*}{a}} = \frac{(1 + y_2^2)\varsigma^2}{a_{11}^z}, \\ \overset{*}{a}{}^{22} &= \frac{(1 + y_1^2)\varsigma^2}{a_{22}^z}, \\ \overset{*}{a}{}^{12} &= -\frac{a_{22}^z}{\overset{*}{a}} = -\frac{y_1 y_2 \varsigma^2}{A_1^z A_2^z}. \end{aligned} \tag{2.56}$$

Differentiating equation (2.53) with respect to α_i we obtain

$$\begin{aligned}\overset{*}{\bar{m}}_1 &= \frac{\partial \varsigma}{\partial \alpha_1}(\bar{m} - y_i \bar{e}_i) \\ &+ \varsigma\left[\frac{A_1}{R_1}\bar{e}_1 - \frac{\partial y_i}{\partial \alpha_1}\bar{e}_i + \frac{\partial \varsigma}{\partial \alpha_1}\left(\frac{A_1}{R_1}\bar{m} + \frac{\bar{e}_2}{A_2}\frac{\partial A_1}{\partial \alpha_2}\right) - \frac{\partial \varsigma}{\partial \alpha_2}\frac{\bar{e}_1}{A_2}\frac{\partial A_1}{\partial \alpha_2}\right], \\ \overset{*}{\bar{m}}_2 &= \frac{\partial \varsigma}{\partial \alpha_2}(\bar{m} - y_i \bar{e}_i) \\ &+ \varsigma\left[\frac{A_2}{R_2}\bar{e}_2 - \frac{\partial y_i}{\partial \alpha_2}\bar{e}_i + \frac{\partial \varsigma}{\partial \alpha_2}\left(\frac{A_2}{R_2}\bar{m} + \frac{\bar{e}_1}{A_1}\frac{\partial A_2}{\partial \alpha_1}\right) - \frac{\partial \varsigma}{\partial \alpha_1}\frac{\bar{e}_2}{A_1}\frac{\partial A_2}{\partial \alpha_1}\right],\end{aligned} \tag{2.57}$$

where use is made of equations (1.30). Substituting equations (2.49) and (2.57) into $\overset{*}{b}_{ik} = -\overset{*}{\bar{m}}_i \overset{*}{\bar{r}}_k$ we obtain

$$\begin{aligned}\overset{*}{b}_{11} &= -A_1^z\varsigma\left(\frac{A_1}{R_1}\sqrt{1 + y_1^2} - \frac{\partial y_1}{\partial \alpha_1} - \frac{y_2}{A_2}\frac{\partial A_1}{\partial \alpha_2}\right), \\ \overset{*}{b}_{22} &= -A_2^z\varsigma\left(\frac{A_2}{R_2}\sqrt{1 + y_2^2} - \frac{\partial y_2}{\partial \alpha_2} - \frac{y_1}{A_1}\frac{\partial A_2}{\partial \alpha_1}\right), \\ \overset{*}{b}_{12} &= -A_2^z\varsigma\left(y_1 y_2\frac{A_1}{R_1} - \frac{\partial y_2}{\partial \alpha_1} - \frac{y_1}{A_2}\frac{\partial A_1}{\partial \alpha_2}\right) = \overset{*}{b}_{21}.\end{aligned} \tag{2.58}$$

Formulas (2.48), (2.49), and (2.28) are used to calculate the Christoffel symbols $\overset{*}{\Gamma}{}_{ij}^{k}$ on $\overset{*}{S}$. $\Gamma_{ij}^{(z)k}$ are calculated from equations (1.27) by replacing A_i^z and their derivatives for A_i and $\partial A_i/\partial \alpha_{1,2}$, respectively.

For example, consider a shell of complex geometry $\overset{*}{S}$ as shown in figure 2.3. Let a cylinder of a constant radius R_0 be the reference surface for $\overset{*}{S}$. Its orientation with respect to $\overset{*}{S}$ is such that the function $\mathrm{H}(\alpha_i)$ and its derivatives satisfy the uniqueness of transformation (2.30).

Introduce polar coordinates α_1, α_2 on S, such that α_1 is the axial and α_2 is the polar angular coordinate. They are related to the global Cartesian coordinates by

$$\bar{r}(\alpha_i) = x\bar{i} + y\bar{j} + z\bar{k} = R_0(\bar{i}\sin\alpha_2 + \bar{k}\cos\alpha_2) + \alpha_1\bar{j}\,. \tag{2.59}$$

The Lamé parameters A_i and curvatures k_{ij} are given by

$$\begin{aligned}&A_1 = 1, \quad A_2 = R_0, \\ &k_{11} = 1/R_1 = 0, \\ &k_{12} = 0, \quad k_{22} = 1/R_2 = 1/R_0.\end{aligned} \tag{2.60}$$

For the coefficients $\theta_i = 1 + \mathrm{H}(\alpha_i)/R_i$ we have

$$\theta_1 = 1, \qquad \theta_2 = 1 + \mathrm{H}(\alpha_i)/R_0. \tag{2.61}$$

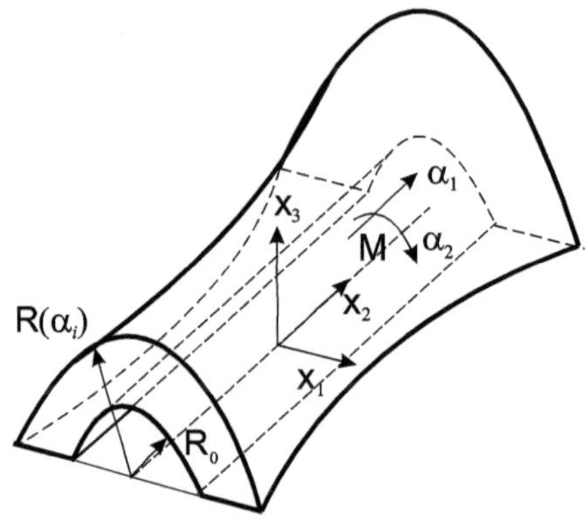

Figure 2.3. A shell of complex geometry in relation to the canonical cylindrical surface.

Hence, from equation (2.51) for y_i we obtain

$$y_1 = \frac{\partial \mathrm{H}(\alpha_i)}{\partial \alpha_1}, \quad y_2 = \frac{1}{R_0 + \mathrm{H}(\alpha_j)}. \tag{2.62}$$

Substituting equations (2.60)–(2.62) in (2.54) we find

$$\begin{aligned}
\overset{*}{a}_{11} &= 1 + y_1^2 = 1 + \left(\frac{\partial \mathrm{H}(\alpha_i)}{\partial \alpha_1}\right)^2, \\
\overset{*}{a}_{22} &= (R_0 + \mathrm{H}(\alpha_i))^2\left(1 + y_2^2\right) \\
&= (R_0 + \mathrm{H}(\alpha_i))^2 + \left(\frac{\partial \mathrm{H}(\alpha_i)}{\partial \alpha_2}\right)^2, \\
\overset{*}{a}_{12} &= \overset{*}{a}_{21} = (R_0 + \mathrm{H}(\alpha_i))^2 y_1 y_2 \\
&= \frac{\partial \mathrm{H}(\alpha_i)}{\partial \alpha_1}\frac{\partial \mathrm{H}(\alpha_i)}{\partial \alpha_2}.
\end{aligned} \tag{2.63}$$

The coefficients of the second fundamental form are found to be

$$\begin{aligned}
\overset{*}{b}_{11} &= \varsigma\frac{\partial y_1}{\partial \alpha_1} = \varsigma\frac{\partial^2 \mathrm{H}(\alpha_i)}{\partial \alpha_1^2}, \\
\overset{*}{b}_{12} &= \overset{*}{b}_{21} = \varsigma\left(\frac{\partial y_1}{\partial \alpha_2} - y_1 y_2\right) \\
&= \varsigma\left(\frac{\partial^2 \mathrm{H}(\alpha_i)}{\partial \alpha_1 \partial \alpha_2} - \frac{1}{R_0 + \mathrm{H}(\alpha_i)}\frac{\partial \mathrm{H}(\alpha_i)}{\partial \alpha_1}\frac{\partial \mathrm{H}(\alpha_i)}{\partial \alpha_2}\right), \\
\overset{*}{b}_{22} &= -\frac{1}{R_0 + \mathrm{H}(\alpha_i)} \\
&\quad \times \varsigma\left(1 - \frac{1}{R_0 + \mathrm{H}(\alpha_i)}\frac{\partial^2 \mathrm{H}(\alpha_i)}{\partial \alpha_1 \partial \alpha_2} + \left(\frac{\partial \mathrm{H}(\alpha_i)/\partial \alpha_2}{R_0 + \mathrm{H}(\alpha_i)}\right)^2\right).
\end{aligned} \tag{2.64}$$

Here

$$\varsigma = \sqrt{1 + \frac{\partial^2 \mathrm{H}(\alpha_i)}{\partial \alpha_1^2} + \left(\frac{\partial \mathrm{H}(\alpha_i)/\partial \alpha_2}{R_0 + \mathrm{H}(\alpha_i)}\right)^2}.$$

Substituting equation (2.63) into (2.47) after some algebra for $\overset{*}{\Gamma}{}^k_{ij}$ we have

$$\begin{aligned}
\overset{*}{a}\Gamma^1_{11} &= \frac{\partial \mathrm{H}(\alpha_i)}{\partial \alpha_1} \\
&\quad \times \left[(R_0 + \mathrm{H}(\alpha_i))^2 \frac{\partial^2 \mathrm{H}(\alpha_i)}{\partial \alpha_1^2} - 2\frac{\partial \mathrm{H}(\alpha_i)}{\partial \alpha_1}\frac{\partial \mathrm{H}(\alpha_i)}{\partial \alpha_2}\frac{\partial^2 \mathrm{H}(\alpha_i)}{\partial \alpha_1 \partial \alpha_2}\right], \\
\overset{*}{a}\Gamma^2_{11} &= \frac{\partial \mathrm{H}(\alpha_i)}{\partial \alpha_2}\frac{\partial^2 \mathrm{H}(\alpha_i)}{\partial \alpha_1^2}, \\
\overset{*}{a}\Gamma^1_{12} &= (R_0 + \mathrm{H}(\alpha_i))\frac{\partial \mathrm{H}(\alpha_i)}{\partial \alpha_1} \\
&\quad \times \left[(R_0 + \mathrm{H}(\alpha_i))\frac{\partial^2 \mathrm{H}(\alpha_i)}{\partial \alpha_1 \partial \alpha_2} - \frac{\partial \mathrm{H}(\alpha_i)}{\partial \alpha_1}\frac{\partial \mathrm{H}(\alpha_i)}{\partial \alpha_2}\right], \\
\overset{*}{a}\Gamma^1_{22} &= (R_0 + \mathrm{H}(\alpha_i))^3 \frac{\partial \mathrm{H}(\alpha_i)}{\partial \alpha_1} \\
&\quad \times \left[\frac{1}{(R_0 + \mathrm{H}(\alpha_i))}\frac{\partial^2 \mathrm{H}(\alpha_i)}{\partial \alpha_2^2} - 2\left(\frac{1}{(R_0 + \mathrm{H}(\alpha_i))}\frac{\partial \mathrm{H}(\alpha_i)}{\partial \alpha_2}\right)^2 - 1\right], \\
\overset{*}{a}\Gamma^2_{12} &= \frac{\partial^2 \mathrm{H}(\alpha_i)}{\partial \alpha_1 \partial \alpha_2}\frac{\partial \mathrm{H}(\alpha_i)}{\partial \alpha_2} + (R_0 + \mathrm{H}(\alpha_i))\frac{\partial \mathrm{H}(\alpha_i)}{\partial \alpha_1}\left(1 + \left(\frac{\partial \mathrm{H}(\alpha_i)}{\partial \alpha_1}\right)^2\right), \\
\overset{*}{a}\Gamma^2_{22} &= \frac{\partial \mathrm{H}(\alpha_i)}{\partial \alpha_2} \\
&\quad \times \left[R_0 + \mathrm{H}(\alpha_i) + \frac{\partial^2 \mathrm{H}(\alpha_i)}{\partial \alpha_2^2} - 2\frac{\partial \mathrm{H}(\alpha_i)}{\partial \alpha_1}\frac{\partial \mathrm{H}(\alpha_i)}{\partial \alpha_2}\frac{\partial^2 \mathrm{H}(\alpha_i)}{\partial \alpha_1 \partial \alpha_2}\right],
\end{aligned} \tag{2.65}$$

where $\overset{*}{a} = (R_0 + \mathrm{H}(\alpha_i))^2/\varsigma^2$, and use is made of equation (2.63).

To construct the unknown function $\mathrm{H}(\alpha_i)$ let the surface of revolution $\overset{*}{S}$ (figure 2.4) be defined by

$$\overset{*}{R} = \overset{*}{R}(x) = \overset{*}{R}(\alpha_i).$$

From geometric analysis of ΔOO_1B we have

$$\begin{aligned}
R_0 &= \mathrm{H}(\alpha_i) + \overline{O_1B}, \\
(\overline{OB})^2 &= (\overline{O_1B})^2 + (\overline{O_1O})^2 + 2\overline{O_1B} \cdot \overline{OB_1} \sin \alpha_2.
\end{aligned} \tag{2.66}$$

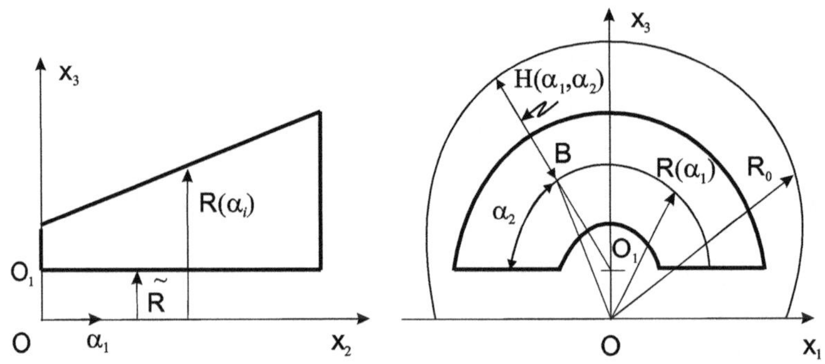

Figure 2.4. Parameterization of the shell of complex geometry and construction of $\mathrm{H}(\alpha_1, \alpha_2)$ function.

Since $\overline{OB} = \overset{*}{R}(\alpha_1)$, $\overline{OO_1} = \tilde{R}$ the last equation can be written as

$$(\overline{O_1B})^2 + 2\overline{O_1B} \cdot \tilde{R} \sin \alpha_2 + \tilde{R}^2 - \overset{*}{R}{}^2(\alpha_1) = 0.$$

Using equation (2.66) in the above, we obtain

$$\mathrm{H}(\alpha_1, \alpha_2) = R_0 + \tilde{R} \sin \alpha_2 \pm \sqrt{\overset{*}{R}{}^2(\alpha_1) - \tilde{R}^2 \cos^2 \alpha_2}\,. \tag{2.67a}$$

For $\tilde{R} = 0$ equation (2.67a) should satisfy the equality $\overline{O_1B} = \overset{*}{R}(\alpha_1)$. Therefore the final form for $\mathrm{H}(\alpha_i)$ is found to be

$$\mathrm{H}(\alpha_1, \alpha_2) = R_0 + \tilde{R} \sin \alpha_2 - \sqrt{\overset{*}{R}{}^2(\alpha_1) - \tilde{R}^2 \cos^2 \alpha_2}\,. \tag{2.67b}$$

Knowing $\mathrm{H}(\alpha_i)$ from equations (2.55)–(2.65) we find coefficients and parameters that characterize the geometry of the surface $\overset{*}{S}$. It is worth noting that equation (2.30) can also be used to parameterize composite shells of complex geometry with variable thicknesses of layers.

2.5 Parameterization of complex surfaces on a plane

Consider a complex planar surface $\overset{*}{S}$ that is referred to by coordinates $\overset{*}{\alpha}_1, \overset{*}{\alpha}_2$. Let S be the reference canonical surface to $\overset{*}{S}$ parameterized by orthogonal coordinates α_1, α_2 (figure 2.5). Assume that the coordinate lines are oriented along the contour C of S. Setting $\mathrm{H}(\alpha_1, \alpha_2) = 0$ in equation (2.10) and using equation (2.9) the position of a point $\overset{*}{M}(\alpha_1, \alpha_2) \in \overset{*}{S}$ is given by

$$\overset{*}{\bar{r}} = \bar{r}(\alpha_1, \alpha_2) + \bar{v}(\alpha_1, \alpha_2) = \bar{r}(\alpha_1, \alpha_2) + \sum_{i=1}^{2} \mathrm{F}_i(\alpha_1, \alpha_2)\bar{e}_i. \tag{2.68}$$

Here the meaning of parameters is as described by equations (1.4), (1.5), (2.9), and (2.10). Evidently, equation (2.68) describes the fictitious tangent deformation of the surface S onto $\overset{*}{S}$.

Differentiating equation (2.68) with respect to α_i, for tangent vectors $\overset{*}{\bar{r}_i}$ we obtain

$$\overset{*}{\bar{r}_i} = A_i \sum_{k=1}^{2} (\delta_{ik} + \underline{e}_{ik})\bar{e}_k, \tag{2.69}$$

where the rotation parameters are given by

$$\begin{aligned}
\underline{e}_{11} &= \frac{1}{A_1}\frac{\partial \mathrm{F}_1(\alpha_i)}{\partial \alpha_1} + \frac{\partial A_1}{\partial \alpha_2}\frac{\mathrm{F}_2(\alpha_i)}{A_1 A_2}, \\
\underline{e}_{22} &= \frac{1}{A_2}\frac{\partial \mathrm{F}_2(\alpha_i)}{\partial \alpha_2} + \frac{\partial A_2}{\partial \alpha_1}\frac{\mathrm{F}_1(\alpha_i)}{A_1 A_2}, \\
\underline{e}_{12} &= \frac{1}{A_1}\frac{\partial \mathrm{F}_2(\alpha_i)}{\partial \alpha_1} - \frac{\partial A_1}{\partial \alpha_1}\frac{\mathrm{F}_1(\alpha_i)}{A_1 A_2}, \\
\underline{e}_{21} &= \frac{1}{A_2}\frac{\partial \mathrm{F}_1(\alpha_i)}{\partial \alpha_2} - \frac{\partial A_2}{\partial \alpha_1}\frac{\mathrm{F}_2(\alpha_i)}{A_1 A_2}.
\end{aligned}$$

Using equation (2.69) the components of the tensor $\overset{*}{\mathbf{A}}$ at $\overset{*}{M}(\alpha_i) \in \overset{*}{S}$ are found to be

$$\overset{*}{a}_{ik} = A_i A_k(\delta_{ik} + 2\underline{\varepsilon}_{ik}), \tag{2.70}$$

where $\underline{\varepsilon}_{ik}$ are the physical components of the tensor of fictitious tangent deformation of S given by

$$2\underline{\varepsilon}_{ik} = \underline{e}_{ik} + \underline{e}_{ki} + \underline{e}_{is}\underline{e}_{ks}. \tag{2.71}$$

The determinant of $\overset{*}{\mathrm{A}}$ is calculated as

$$\overset{*}{a} = (A_1 A_2)^2[(1 + \underline{e}_{11})(1 + \underline{e}_{22}) - \underline{e}_{12}\underline{e}_{21}]. \tag{2.72}$$

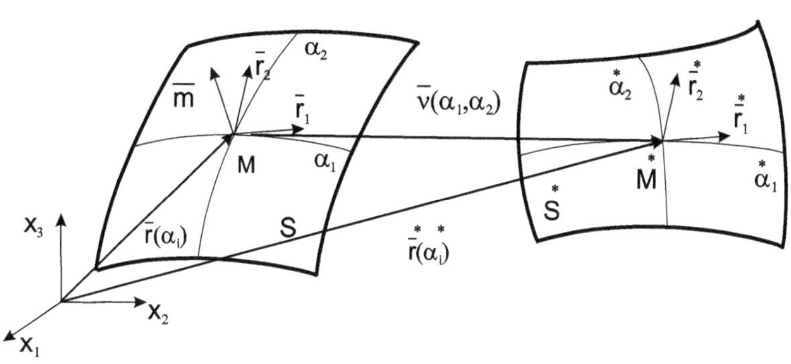

Figure 2.5. Parameterization of a planar surface of complex geometry.

Making use of equations (2.70) and (2.72) in the formulas $\overset{*}{a}{}^{ii} = \overset{*}{a}_{ii}/\overset{*}{a}$, $\overset{*}{a}{}^{12} = \overset{*}{a}{}^{21} = -\overset{*}{a}_{12}/\overset{*}{a}$, the contravariant components of $\overset{*}{\mathrm{A}}$ can be found. Using $\overset{*}{a}{}^{ik}$ and equations (2.69) and (2.70) for vectors of the reciprocal basis $\overset{*}{\bar{r}}{}^{i}$ we obtain

$$\overset{*}{\bar{r}}{}^{i} = \sum_{k=1}^{2} \overset{*}{a}{}^{ik} \overset{*}{\bar{r}}_k = \frac{1}{\overset{*}{a}} \sum_{s=1}^{2}\sum_{k=1}^{2} \operatorname{sgn} A_i A_k (\delta_{ik} + 2\underline{\varepsilon}_{ik})(\delta_{is} + \underline{e}_{is})\bar{e}_s. \tag{2.73}$$

Finally, with the help of equations (2.69) and (2.73) we calculate the Christoffel symbols of the first and second kind.

In the above derivations it is assumed that coordinates α_1, α_2 are linearly independent. To remain such after transformation the tangent vectors $\overset{*}{\bar{r}}_i$ should remain non-collinear $\forall\ \overset{*}{M}(\alpha_1, \alpha_2) \in \overset{*}{S}$. If at any point $\overset{*}{\bar{r}}_1 \times \overset{*}{\bar{r}}_2 = 0$ then transformation (2.68) at this point experiences singularity. Substituting equation (2.65) and using the fact that $\bar{e}_1 \times \bar{e}_2 = 0$, after some algebra, we obtain

$$A_i A_k[(1 + \underline{e}_{11})(1 + \underline{e}_{22}) - \underline{e}_{12}\underline{e}_{21}](e_1 \times e_2) = 0. \tag{2.74}$$

The condition of singularity then becomes

$$A_i A_k[(1 + \underline{e}_{11})(1 + \underline{e}_{22}) - \underline{e}_{12}\underline{e}_{21}] = \sqrt{\overset{*}{a}} = 0, \tag{2.75}$$

where use is made of equation (2.72).

As a final point of our discussion consider a problem of parameterization of a complex surface bounded by four smooth continuous lines (figure 2.6). Let the straight lines connecting corner points A, B and C, D intersect at point O.

Assume that the contour lines in polar coordinates (r, φ) $(r = \alpha_1, \varphi = \alpha_2)$ are given analytically by

$$\begin{gathered} C_1\colon \mathrm{F}_2^{(1)}(r), \quad C_2\colon R_c + \mathrm{F}_1^{(2)}(\varphi), \quad C_3\colon \mathrm{F}_2^{(3)}(\eta), \quad C_4\colon R_D + \mathrm{F}_1^{(4)}(\varphi), \\ (R_D \leqslant r \leqslant R_C,\ 0 \leqslant \varphi \leqslant \varphi_k,\ 0 \leqslant \eta \leqslant R_B - R_C), \end{gathered} \tag{2.76}$$

where $R_{A,B,C,D}$ are the radii and φ_k is the angle between the rays $\overline{OB}$ and $\overline{OC}$, and $\mathrm{F}_2^{(1)}(r)$, $\mathrm{F}_2^{(3)}(\eta)$ are the normal distances measured from $\overline{OC}$ and $\overline{OB}$ to the contour lines C_1, C_3, respectively.

The affine transformation of the line segment $\overline{AB}$ onto the line segment $\overline{A'B'}$ with coordinates $u = 0$, $u = R_B - R_A$, is given by

$$u = \xi_1 + \xi_2 r. \tag{2.77}$$

Making use of boundary conditions

$$r = R_D : u = 0; \quad r = R_C : \ u = R_B - R_A, \tag{2.78}$$

the coefficients ξ_1, ξ_2 are found to be

$$\xi_1 = -R_D\xi_2, \quad \xi_2 = (R_B - R_A)/(R_C - R_D).$$

Therefore, $u = \xi_2(r - R_D)$. This allows the equation for C_3 to be written in the form

$$F_2^{(3)}(u) = F_2^{(3)}[\xi_2(r - R_D)].$$

Expanding functions $F_i(r, \varphi)$ $(i = 1, 2)$ in the form

$$\begin{aligned} F_1(r, \varphi) &= \varsigma_1(\varphi) + r\varsigma_2(r), \\ F_2(r, \varphi) &= \varsigma_3(r) + \varphi\varsigma_4(r), \end{aligned} \tag{2.79}$$

and using boundary conditions given by equation (2.76), the coefficients of expansion ς_j are found to be

$$\begin{aligned} &r = R_D\colon\ F_1(R_D, \varphi) = F_1^{(4)}(\varphi), \\ &r = R_C\colon\ F_1(R_C, \varphi) = F_1^{(2)}(\varphi), \\ &\varphi = 0\colon\quad F_2(r, 0) = F_2^{(1)}(r), \\ &\varphi = \varphi_k\colon\ F_2(r, \varphi_k) = F_2^{(3)}[\xi_2(r - R_D)]. \end{aligned} \tag{2.80}$$

Here $\varphi_k = \angle COB$. From equations (2.79) and (2.80) we obtain

$$\begin{aligned} \varsigma_1(\varphi) &= F_1^{(4)}(\varphi) - \frac{R_D}{R_D - R_C}\left(F_1^{(4)}(\varphi) - F_1^{(2)}(\varphi)\right), \\ \varsigma_2(\varphi) &= \frac{1}{R_D - R_C}\left(F_1^{(4)}(\varphi) - F_1^{(2)}(\varphi)\right), \\ \varsigma_3(r) &= F_2^{(1)}(r) \\ \varsigma_4(r) &= \frac{1}{\varphi_k}\left(F_2^{(3)}[\xi_2(r - R_D)] - F_2^{(1)}(r)\right). \end{aligned}$$

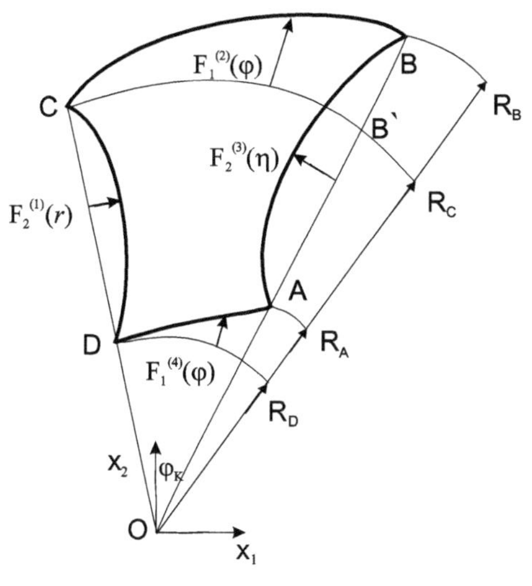

Figure 2.6. A complex surface bounded by four continuous lines and its parameterization.

Substituting the above into equation (2.79) we obtain

$$
\begin{aligned}
F_1(r,\varphi) &= F_1^{(4)}(\varphi) + \frac{r-R_D}{R_D-R_C}\left(F_1^{(4)}(\varphi) - F_1^{(2)}(\varphi)\right),\\
F_2(r,\varphi) &= F_2^{(1)}(r) + \frac{\varphi}{\varphi_k}\left(F_2^{(3)}[\xi_2(r-R_D)] - F_2^{(1)}(r)\right).
\end{aligned}
\tag{2.81}
$$

The unit base vectors $\bar{e}_{ik}$ are given by

$$
\begin{aligned}
\bar{e}_{11} &= \frac{R_D}{R_D-R_C}(F_1^{(4)}(\varphi) - F_1^{(2)}(\varphi)),\\
\bar{e}_{12} &= \frac{\varphi}{\varphi_k}\frac{d}{dr}(F_2^{(3)}[\xi_2(r-R_D)] - F_2^{(1)}(r)),\\
\bar{e}_{21} &= \frac{1}{r}\left(\frac{dF_1^{(4)}(\varphi)}{d\varphi} + \frac{r-R_D}{R_D-R_C}\frac{d}{d\varphi}(F_1^{(4)}(\varphi) - F_1^{(2)}(\varphi))\right.\\
&\quad \left. - F_2^{(1)}(r) - \frac{\varphi}{\varphi_k}(F_2^{(3)}[\xi_2(r-R_D)] - F_2^{(1)}(r))\right),\\
\bar{e}_{22} &= \frac{1}{r}\left(\frac{F_2^{(3)}[\xi_2(r-R_D)] - F_2^{(1)}(r)}{\varphi_k} + F_1^{(4)}(\varphi)\right.\\
&\quad \left. + \frac{r-R_D}{R_D-R_C}(F_1^{(4)}(\varphi) - F_1^{(2)}(\varphi))\right).
\end{aligned}
\tag{2.82}
$$

Making use of equation (2.82) in (2.71) we find the components of fictitious deformation $2\overset{*}{\underline{\varepsilon}}_{ik}$ and the Christoffel symbols $\overset{*}{\Gamma}{}^k_{ij}$ on $\overset{*}{S}$.

If the complex surface $\overset{*}{S}$ has three corner points such that $R_D \to 0$, $R_A \to 0$, $(F_1^{(4)}(\varphi) \equiv 0)$, then the corner points A and D would merge to a single point O. In this case the transformation would have had singularity at O, as discussed above.

Further reading

Galimov K Z and Paimushin V N 1985 *Theory of Shells of Complex Geometry: Geometrical Problems of the Theory of Shells* (Kazan: Kazan University Press)

Chapter 3

Nonlinear theory of thin shells

The fundamentals of the classic nonlinear theory of thin elastic shells based on the first Kirchhoff–Love hypothesis are presented. The analysis of the deformation, forces, and moments referred to the middle surface of the shell is provided. In conclusion, the equations of static and dynamic equilibrium are derived.

3.1 Deformation of a shell

All of the following discussion concerning the deformation of thin shells is based on the first Kirchhoff–Love hypothesis. Let the middle surface S of the undeformed thin shell be associated with the orthogonal curvilinear coordinates α_1, α_2. The position vector $\bar{\rho}$ of an arbitrary point M_z on the equidistant surface S_z ($S_z \| S$) is given by equation (1.39), where $z \in [-h/2, +h/2]$ and h is the thickness of the shell. The coordinate vectors and the Lamé coefficients satisfy equations (1.42) and (1.49).

The length of a line element on S_z is given by

$$(ds_z)^2 = H_1^2 d\alpha_1{}^2 + H_2^2 d\alpha_2^2 + dz^2, \tag{3.1}$$

where

$$(ds_z)_1 = H_1 d\alpha_1 \quad (ds_z)_2 = H_2 d\alpha_2, \tag{3.2}$$

are the lengths of line elements in the direction of α_1, α_2-coordinates.

In the deformed configuration the position vector $\overset{*}{\bar{\rho}}$ of point $\overset{*}{M}_z \in \overset{*}{S}_z$ is given by

$$\overset{*}{\bar{\rho}} = \bar{\rho}(\alpha_1, \alpha_2) + \bar{\nu}_z(\alpha_1, \alpha_2, z), \tag{3.3}$$

where $\bar{\nu}_z$ is the displacement vector. Since for thin shells $z \ll 1$ we assume $\overset{*}{z} \approx z$. The first fundamental form of $\overset{*}{S}_z$ is

doi:10.1088/2053-2563/ab1a9ech3

$$(d\overset{*}{s}_z)^2 = \overset{*}{g}_{11}d\alpha_1^2 + 2\overset{*}{g}_{12}d\alpha_1 d\alpha_2 + \overset{*}{g}_{22}d\alpha_2^2 + dz^2, \tag{3.4}$$

$$(d\overset{*}{s}_z)_1 = \sqrt{\overset{*}{g}_{11}}\,d\alpha_1, \quad (d\overset{*}{s}_z)_2 = \sqrt{\overset{*}{g}_{22}}\,d\alpha_2. \tag{3.5}$$

Here $\overset{*}{g}_{ik} = \overset{*}{\bar{\rho}}_i\overset{*}{\bar{\rho}}_k$ $(i, k = 1, 2)$ and vectors $\overset{*}{\bar{\rho}}_1$, $\overset{*}{\bar{\rho}}_2$ tangent to coordinate lines are obtained by differentiating equation (3.3) with respect to α_1, α_2,

$$\begin{aligned} \overset{*}{\bar{\rho}}_1 &= \overset{*}{\bar{r}}_1(1 - z\overset{*}{b}{}_1^1) - \overset{*}{\bar{r}}_2 z\overset{*}{b}{}_1^2 \\ \overset{*}{\bar{\rho}}_2 &= \overset{*}{\bar{r}}_2(1 - z\overset{*}{b}{}_2^2) - \overset{*}{\bar{r}}_1 z\overset{*}{b}{}_2^1 \\ \overset{*}{\bar{\rho}}_3 &= \overset{*}{\bar{m}}. \end{aligned} \tag{3.6}$$

Let ε_{11}^z, ε_{22}^z be deformations through point $M_z \in S_z$ in the direction of α_1, α_2 coordinates defined by

$$\varepsilon_{11}^z = \frac{(d\overset{*}{s}_z)_1 - (ds_z)_1}{(ds_z)_1}, \quad \varepsilon_{22}^z = \frac{(d\overset{*}{s}_z)_2 - (ds_z)_2}{(ds_z)_2}. \tag{3.7}$$

Substituting equations (3.1), (3.4) into (3.7), we obtain

$$\varepsilon_{11}^z = \left(\sqrt{\overset{*}{g}_{11}} - H_1\right)\Big/ H_1, \quad \varepsilon_{22}^z = \left(\sqrt{\overset{*}{g}_{22}} - H_2\right)\Big/ H_2. \tag{3.8}$$

Using equations (1.45), (1.53), the angle $\overset{*}{\chi}_z$ between the vectors $\overset{*}{\bar{\rho}}_1$ and $\overset{*}{\bar{\rho}}_2$ is found to be

$$\cos\overset{*}{\chi}_z = \frac{\overset{*}{\bar{\rho}}_1\overset{*}{\bar{\rho}}_2}{\left|\overset{*}{\bar{\rho}}_1\right|\left|\overset{*}{\bar{\rho}}_2\right|} = \frac{\overset{*}{g}_{12}}{\sqrt{\overset{*}{g}_{11}\overset{*}{g}_{22}}}, \tag{3.9}$$

where

$$\begin{aligned} \overset{*}{g}_{ii} &= \overset{*}{A}{}_i^2\left(1 + 2\overset{*}{k}_{ii}z\right) + \left(\overset{*}{\bar{m}}_i z\right)^2, \\ \overset{*}{g}_{12} &= \overset{*}{A}_1\overset{*}{A}_2\left(\cos\overset{*}{\chi} + 2\overset{*}{k}_{12}z\right) + \overset{*}{\bar{m}}_1\overset{*}{\bar{m}}_2 z^2. \end{aligned} \tag{3.10}$$

Let $\varepsilon^z{}_{12}$ be the shear deformation, i.e. the change in the angle between initially orthogonal coordinate lines $2\varepsilon_{12}^z = \pi/2 - \overset{*}{\chi}_z$. Evidently,

$$\cos \overset{*}{\chi}_z := \sin 2\varepsilon^z_{12} = \frac{\overset{*}{g}_{12}}{\sqrt{\overset{*}{g}_{22}\overset{*}{g}_{11}}}. \tag{3.11}$$

Making use of equation (3.6) and the fact $\overset{*}{\bar{r}}_1 \overset{*}{\bar{m}} = 0$, we find

$$\overset{*}{g}_{13} = \overset{*}{\bar{\rho}}_1 \overset{*}{\bar{m}} = 0, \quad \overset{*}{g}_{23} = \overset{*}{\bar{\rho}}_2 \overset{*}{\bar{m}} = 0, \quad \overset{*}{g}_{33} = \overset{*}{\bar{m}}\overset{*}{\bar{m}} = 1.$$

It follows from the above that the deformation over the thickness of the shell equals zero

$$2\varepsilon^z_{i3} = \frac{\overset{*}{g}_{i3}}{\sqrt{\overset{*}{g}_{ii}\overset{*}{g}_{33}}} = 0, \quad \varepsilon^z_{33} = \left(\sqrt{\overset{*}{g}_{33}} - H_3\right)\Big/ H_3 = 0, \quad (\overset{*}{g}_{i3} = 0,\ H_3 = 1).$$

In applications it is more convenient to use deformations ε^z_{ik} expressed in terms of the undeformed middle surface S. Thus, neglecting terms $O(z^2)$ in equation (2.10), we have

$$\overset{*}{g}_{ii} = \overset{*}{A}{}^2_i\left(1 + 2\overset{*}{k}_{ii}z\right), \quad \overset{*}{g}_{12} = \overset{*}{A}_1\overset{*}{A}_2\left(\cos\overset{*}{\chi} + 2\overset{*}{k}_{12}z\right). \tag{3.12}$$

Taking the square root of both sides

$$\sqrt{\overset{*}{g}_{ii}} \approx \overset{*}{A}_i\left(1 + \overset{*}{k}_{ii}z\right) + \cdots, \tag{3.13}$$

and substituting equations (3.13), (1.49) into (3.8), $\varepsilon^z{}_{ii}$ are found to be

$$\varepsilon^z_{ii} = \left[\overset{*}{A}_i - A_i + \left(\overset{*}{A}_i\overset{*}{k}_{ii} - A_i k_{ii}\right)z\right]\Big/ A_i(1 + k_{ii}z), \quad (i = 1, 2). \tag{3.13a}$$

Applying equations (1.65) and (1.69), the term in parenthesis can be written as

$$\begin{aligned}\overset{*}{A}_i\overset{*}{k}_{ii} - A_i k_{ii} &= A_i\sqrt{(1 + 2\varepsilon_{ii})}\overset{*}{k}_{ii} - A_i k_{ii} \\ &= A_i\left(\sqrt{(1 + 2\varepsilon_{ii})}\overset{*}{k}_{ii} - k_{ii}\right) = A_i\alpha_{ii}\sqrt{1 + 2\varepsilon_{ii}} + A_i k_{ii}\sqrt{1 + 2\varepsilon_{ii}}.\end{aligned}$$

Reverse substitution yields

$$\begin{aligned}\varepsilon^z_{ii} = {} & [A_i(\sqrt{1 + 2\varepsilon_{ii}} - 1) + A_i\alpha_{ii}z\sqrt{1 + 2\varepsilon_{ii}} \\ & + A_i k_{ii}z\sqrt{1 + 2\varepsilon_{ii}}]/A_i(1 + k_{ii}z).\end{aligned} \tag{3.13b}$$

Hence, deformation of the equidistant surface S_z of the shell is fully determined in terms of tangent deformations and curvatures of the middle surface S. Similarly, introducing $\overset{*}{g}_{12}$ and $\sqrt{\overset{*}{g}_{ii}}$ given by equations (3.12), (3.13) into (3.11), we obtain

$$\sin 2\varepsilon_{12}^{z} = \frac{\left(\cos \overset{*}{\chi} + 2\overset{*}{k}_{12}z\right)}{\left(1 + \overset{*}{k}_{11}z\right)\left(1 + \overset{*}{k}_{22}z\right)}.$$

Since $\overset{*}{k}_{12}z \approx \text{æ}_{12}z$, we have

$$\sin 2\varepsilon_{12}^{z} = \frac{\cos \overset{*}{\chi} + 2\text{æ}_{12}z}{\left(1 + \overset{*}{k}_{11}z\right)\left(1 + \overset{*}{k}_{22}z\right)}.$$

Since for thin shells $1 + k_{ii}z \approx 1$, $1 + \overset{*}{k}_{ii}z \approx 1$, the final formulas for tangent and shear deformations of S_z, take the form

$$\begin{aligned} \varepsilon_{ii}^{z} &= \sqrt{1 + 2\varepsilon_{ii}}\left(1 + z\overset{*}{k}_{ii}\right) - 1, \\ \sin 2\varepsilon_{12}^{z} &= \frac{1}{2}\left(\cos \overset{*}{\chi} + 2\text{æ}_{12}z\right). \end{aligned} \tag{3.14}$$

3.2 Forces and moments

Consider a differential element in the deformed shell bounded by the surfaces $\alpha_i =$ const, $\alpha_i + d\alpha_i =$ const, and $\overset{*}{z} \pm 0.5h$ (figure 3.1). Internal forces acting upon the element are given by $\bar{p}_1 \overset{*}{H}_2 d\alpha_2 dz$ and $\bar{p}_2 \overset{*}{H}_1 d\alpha_1 dz$. Here $\bar{p}_i$ are stress vectors, $\overset{*}{H}_2 d\alpha_2 dz$, $\overset{*}{H}_1 d\alpha_1 dz$ are the surface areas of differential boundary elements at $z =$ const. Integrating the internal forces over the thickness of the shell, we obtain the resultant of force vectors, $\bar{R}_1$, $\bar{R}_2$ in the form

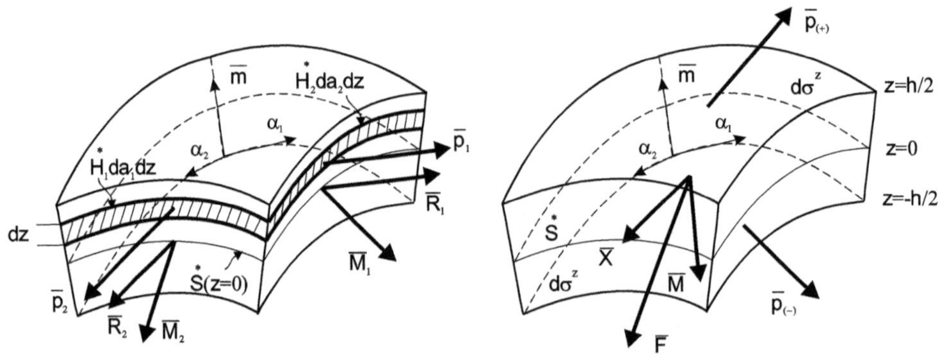

Figure 3.1. Forces and moments acting upon a three-dimensional solid.

$$\bar{R}_1 = \int_{z_1}^{z_2} \bar{p}_1 \overset{*}{H}_2 d\alpha_2 dz, \quad \bar{R}_2 = \int_{z_1}^{z_2} \bar{p}_2 \overset{*}{H}_1 d\alpha_1 dz, \quad (z_1 = -h/2,\ z_2 = +h/2).$$

Dividing $\bar{R}_i$ by the length of linear elements, $\overset{*}{A}_i d\alpha_i = A_i\sqrt{1 + 2\varepsilon_{ii}}\, d\alpha_i$ ($i = 1, 2$), we find

$$\bar{R}_1 = \frac{\int_{z_1}^{z_2} \bar{p}_1 \overset{*}{H}_2 dz}{A_2\sqrt{1 + 2\varepsilon_{22}}}, \quad \bar{R}_2 = \frac{\int_{z_1}^{z_2} \bar{p}_2 \overset{*}{H}_1 dz}{A_1\sqrt{1 + 2\varepsilon_{11}}}. \tag{3.15}$$

Similar reasoning leads to the definition of the resultant internal moment vectors. The moment of the force $\bar{p}_1$, acting on the face $\alpha_1 = \text{const}$, about the center of the middle surface $\overset{*}{S}$ is $\left(\overset{*}{\bar{m}z} \times \bar{p}_1 \overset{*}{H}_2 d\alpha_2 dz\right)$. Here $\overset{*}{\bar{m}z}$ is the radius vector of $\bar{p}_1$. Hence, the resultant moment vector of internal forces $\bar{M}_1$ is given by

$$\bar{M}_1 = \int_{z_1}^{z_2} \left(\overset{*}{\bar{m}z} \times \bar{p}_1 \overset{*}{H}_2 d\alpha_2 dz\right).$$

Dividing the above by the length of a line segment in the direction of the α_2-coordinate, $\overset{*}{A}_2 d\alpha_2 = A_2\sqrt{(1 + 2\varepsilon_{22})}\, d\alpha_2$, we obtain

$$\bar{M}_1 = \frac{1}{A_2\sqrt{(1 + 2\varepsilon_{22})}} \int_{z_1}^{z_2} \left(\overset{*}{\bar{m}z} \times \bar{p}_1\right) \overset{*}{H}_2 dz. \tag{3.16a}$$

Similarly, we define the resultant moment vector $\bar{M}_2$ as

$$\bar{M}_2 = \frac{1}{A_1\sqrt{1 + 2\varepsilon_{11}}} \int_{z_1}^{z_2} \left(\overset{*}{\bar{m}z} \times \bar{p}_2\right) \overset{*}{H}_1 dz. \tag{3.16b}$$

The above discussion implies that the internal forces acting on the differential element are statically equivalent to the resultant force and moment vectors, $\bar{R}_i$, $\bar{M}_i$.

Consider external forces acting on the free surfaces $z = \pm 0.5h$ of the shell. Let:

(i) $\bar{p}_{(+)}$ and $\bar{p}_{(-)}$ be the external forces applied on the surface of area $d\sigma^z$,

$$\begin{aligned} d\sigma^z &= \overset{*}{H}_1 \overset{*}{H}_2 d\alpha_1 d\alpha_2 \\ &\approx A_1 A_2 (1 + (k_{11} + \varkappa_{11})z)(1 + (k_{22} + \varkappa_{22})z)\sqrt{1 + 2\varepsilon_{11}}\sqrt{1 + 2\varepsilon_{22}}\, d\alpha_1 d\alpha_2, \end{aligned}$$

(ii) $\bar{F}$ be the vector of mass forces per unit volume $d\Omega$ of the deformed element

$$\begin{aligned} d\Omega &= \overset{*}{H}_1 \overset{*}{H}_2 d\alpha_1 d\alpha_2 d\overset{*}{z} \\ &\approx A_1 A_2 (1 + (k_{11} + \varkappa_{11})z)(1 + (k_{22} + \varkappa_{22})z)\sqrt{1 + 2\varepsilon_{11}}\sqrt{1 + 2\varepsilon_{22}}\, d\alpha_1 d\alpha_2 d\overset{*}{z}, \end{aligned}$$

where $H^{(+)}{}_1$, $H^{(-)}{}_2$ are the values of $\overset{*}{H}_i$ at $z = \pm 0.5h$, respectively.

Then, the resultant external force vectors are defined by

$$\bar{p}_{(+)} H^{(+)}{}_1 H^{(+)}{}_2 d\alpha_1 d\alpha_2 \quad \text{and} \quad \bar{p}_{(-)} H^{(-)}{}_1 H^{(-)}{}_2 d\alpha_1 d\alpha_2.$$

Their sum divided by the surface area of a deformed element, $\overset{*}{A}_1 \overset{*}{A}_2 d\alpha_1 d\alpha_2$, yields

$$\begin{aligned} &\frac{\bar{p}_{(+)} H^{(+)}{}_1 H^{(+)}{}_2 d\alpha_1 d\alpha_2 + \bar{p}_{(-)} H^{(-)}{}_1 H^{(-)}{}_2 d\alpha_1 d\alpha_2}{A_1 A_2 \sqrt{(1 + 2\varepsilon_{11})(1 + 2\varepsilon_{22})}\, d\alpha_1 d\alpha_2} \\ &= \frac{\bar{p}_z \overset{*}{H}_1 \overset{*}{H}_2}{A_1 A_2 \sqrt{(1 + 2\varepsilon_{11})(1 + 2\varepsilon_{22})}}. \end{aligned} \tag{3.17}$$

Here $(\bar{p}_z)_{z=0.5h} = \bar{p}_{(+)}$, $(\bar{p}_z)_{z=-0.5h} = -\bar{p}_{(-)}$, $\bar{p}_{-z} = -\bar{p}_z$.

Similarly, dividing the resultant of the mass force $\bar{F}$ given by

$$\int_{z_1}^{z_2} \bar{F} d\sigma^{z*} dz = \int_{z_1}^{z_2} \bar{F} \overset{*}{H}_1 \overset{*}{H}_2 d\alpha_1 d\alpha_2 dz,$$

by $\overset{*}{A}_1 \overset{*}{A}_2 d\alpha_1 d\alpha_2$ and taking the sum of the resultant with equation (3.17), we obtain

$$\bar{X} A_1 A_2 = \frac{\bar{p}_z \overset{*}{H}_1 \overset{*}{H}_2}{\sqrt{(1 + 2\varepsilon_{11})(1 + 2\varepsilon_{22})}} + \int_{z_1}^{z_2} \frac{\bar{F} \overset{*}{H}_1 \overset{*}{H}_2 dz}{\sqrt{(1 + 2\varepsilon_{11})(1 + 2\varepsilon_{22})}}. \tag{3.18}$$

$\bar{X}$ is the resultant external force vector referred to the deformed middle surface $\overset{*}{S}$ of the shell.

Moments of external forces about an arbitrary point on $\overset{*}{S}$ are given by

$$\left(\frac{\overset{*}{\bar{m}} h}{2} \times \bar{p}_{(+)} H^{(+)}{}_1 H^{(+)}{}_2 d\alpha_1 d\alpha_2\right) \quad \text{and} \quad \left(\frac{\overset{*}{\bar{m}} h}{2} \times \bar{p}_{(-)} H^{(-)}{}_1 H^{(-)}{}_2 d\alpha_1 d\alpha_2\right).$$

Their sum divided by the surface area $\overset{*}{A}_1 \overset{*}{A}_2 d\alpha_1 d\alpha_2$ yields

$$\left(\overset{*}{\bar{m}} z \times \bar{p}_{(z)} \frac{\overset{*}{H}_1 \overset{*}{H}_2}{A_1 A_2 \sqrt{(1 + 2\varepsilon_{11})(1 + 2\varepsilon_{22})}}\right)_{z_1}^{z_2}.$$

By analogy, the moment of $\bar{F}$ per unit area of the element $\overset{*}{S}$ is given by

$$\begin{aligned} &\int_{z_1}^{z_2} \left(\overset{*}{\bar{m}} z \times \bar{F}\right) \frac{\overset{*}{H}_1 \overset{*}{H}_2 d\alpha_1 d\alpha_2 dz}{A_1 A_2 \sqrt{(1 + 2\varepsilon_{11})(1 + 2\varepsilon_{22})}\, d\alpha_1 d\alpha_2} \\ &= \int_{z_1}^{z_2} \left(\overset{*}{\bar{m}} z \times \bar{F}\right) \frac{\overset{*}{H}_1 \overset{*}{H}_2 dz}{A_1 A_2 \sqrt{(1 + 2\varepsilon_{11})(1 + 2\varepsilon_{22})}}. \end{aligned}$$

Hence, the resultant external moment vector $\bar{M}$ of external forces is found to be

$$\bar{M}A_1A_2 = \left(\overset{*}{\overline{m}} z \times \bar{p}_{(z)} \frac{\overset{*}{H}_1 \overset{*}{H}_2}{\sqrt{(1 + 2\varepsilon_{11})(1 + 2\varepsilon_{22})}} \right)_{z_1}^{z_2} + \int_{z_1}^{z_2} \left(\overset{*}{\overline{m}} z \times \bar{F} \right) \frac{\overset{*}{H}_1 \overset{*}{H}_2 dz}{\sqrt{(1 + 2\varepsilon_{11})(1 + 2\varepsilon_{22})}}. \tag{3.19}$$

Again, the conclusion is that external forces acting upon the differential element are statically equivalent to the resultants of external force and moment vectors, $\bar{X}$ and $\bar{M}$.

Decomposing $\bar{p}_i$, $\bar{p}_z$, and $\bar{F}$ in the direction of unit vectors $\overset{*}{\bar{e}}{}_1^z = \overset{*}{\bar{\rho}}_1 / \overset{*}{H}_1$, $\overset{*}{\bar{e}}{}_2^z = \overset{*}{\bar{\rho}}_2 / \overset{*}{H}_2$, and $\overset{*}{\bar{e}}{}_3^z = \overset{*}{\overline{m}}$, we have

$$\begin{aligned} \bar{p}_1 &= \sigma_{11} \overset{*}{\bar{e}}{}_1^z + \sigma_{12} \overset{*}{\bar{e}}{}_2^z + \sigma_{13} \overset{*}{\overline{m}}, \\ \bar{p}_2 &= \sigma_{21} \overset{*}{\bar{e}}{}_1^z + \sigma_{22} \overset{*}{\bar{e}}{}_2^z + \sigma_{23} \overset{*}{\overline{m}}, \\ \bar{p}_z &= \sigma_{31} \overset{*}{\bar{e}}{}_1^z + \sigma_{32} \overset{*}{\bar{e}}{}_2^z + \sigma_{33} \overset{*}{\overline{m}}, \\ \bar{F} &= \overset{*}{F}_1 \overset{*}{\bar{e}}{}_1^z + \overset{*}{F}_2 \overset{*}{\bar{e}}{}_2^z + \overset{*}{F}_3 \overset{*}{\overline{m}}, \end{aligned} \tag{3.20}$$

where σ_{ij} $(i, j = 1, 2)$ are the internal stresses $(\sigma_{ij} = \sigma_{ji})$ and $\overset{*}{F}_j$ are the projections of $\bar{F}$ on the base $\left\{ \overset{*}{\bar{e}}{}_1^z, \overset{*}{\bar{e}}{}_2^z, \overset{*}{\overline{m}} \right\}$ (figure 3.2). Substituting equations (2.20) into (3.15) and (3.16), for $\bar{R}_i$ and $\bar{M}_i$, we find

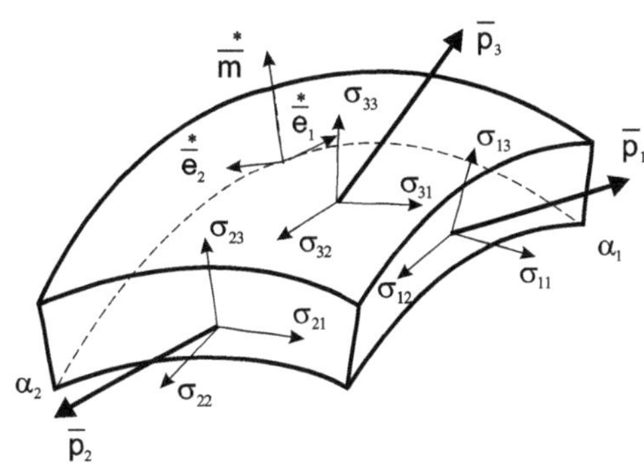

Figure 3.2. Internal stresses in the shell.

$$A_2\sqrt{(1+2\varepsilon_{22})}\,\bar{R}_1 = \int_{z_1}^{z_2}\left(\sigma_{11}\overset{*}{\bar{e}}{}_1^z + \sigma_{12}\overset{*}{\bar{e}}{}_2^z + \sigma_{13}\overset{*}{\bar{m}}\right)\overset{*}{H}_2 dz,$$

$$A_1\sqrt{(1+2\varepsilon_{11})}\,\bar{R}_2 = \int_{z_1}^{z_2}\left(\sigma_{21}\overset{*}{\bar{e}}{}_1^z + \sigma_{22}\overset{*}{\bar{e}}{}_2^z + \sigma_{23}\overset{*}{\bar{m}}\right)\overset{*}{H}_1 dz,$$

$$A_2\sqrt{(1+2\varepsilon_{22})}\,\bar{M}_1 = \int_{z_1}^{z_2}\left(\overset{*}{\bar{m}}z \times \left(\sigma_{11}\overset{*}{\bar{e}}{}_1^z + \sigma_{12}\overset{*}{\bar{e}}{}_2^z\right)\right)\overset{*}{H}_2 dz,$$

$$A_1\sqrt{(1+2\varepsilon_{11})}\,\bar{M}_2 = \int_{z_1}^{z_2}\left(\overset{*}{\bar{m}}z \times \left(\sigma_{21}\overset{*}{\bar{e}}{}_1^z + \sigma_{22}\overset{*}{\bar{e}}{}_2^z\right)\right)\overset{*}{H}_1 dz.$$

Since $\overset{*}{\bar{e}}{}_1^z = \overset{*}{\bar{e}}_1$, $\overset{*}{\bar{e}}{}_2^z = \overset{*}{\bar{e}}_2$, (equation (1.51)) we have

$$A_2\sqrt{(1+2\varepsilon_{22})}\,\bar{R}_1 = \int_{z_1}^{z_2}\left(\sigma_{11}\overset{*}{\bar{e}}_1 + \sigma_{12}\overset{*}{\bar{e}}_2 + \sigma_{13}\overset{*}{\bar{m}}\right)\overset{*}{H}_2 dz,$$

$$A_1\sqrt{(1+2\varepsilon_{11})}\,\bar{R}_2 = \int_{z_1}^{z_2}\left(\sigma_{21}\overset{*}{\bar{e}}_1 + \sigma_{22}\overset{*}{\bar{e}}_2 + \sigma_{23}\overset{*}{\bar{m}}\right)\overset{*}{H}_1 dz,$$

$$A_2\sqrt{(1+2\varepsilon_{22})}\,\bar{M}_1 = \int_{z_1}^{z_2}\left(\overset{*}{\bar{m}}z \times \left(\sigma_{11}\overset{*}{\bar{e}}_1 + \sigma_{12}\overset{*}{\bar{e}}_2\right)\right)\overset{*}{H}_2 dz$$

$$A_1\sqrt{(1+2\varepsilon_{11})}\,\bar{M}_2 = \int_{z_1}^{z_2}\left(\overset{*}{\bar{m}}z \times \left(\sigma_{21}\overset{*}{\bar{e}}_1 + \sigma_{22}\overset{*}{\bar{e}}_2\right)\right)\overset{*}{H}_1 dz,$$

where (see equations (1.61) and (1.72))

$$\begin{aligned}
\overset{*}{\bar{e}}_1 &= [\bar{e}_1(1+e_{11}) + \bar{e}_2 e_{22} + \bar{m}\varpi_1]/(1+2\varepsilon_{11}),\\
\overset{*}{\bar{e}}_2 &= [\bar{e}_1 e_{11} + \bar{e}_2(1+e_{22}) + \bar{m}\varpi_2]/(1+2\varepsilon_{22}),\\
\overset{*}{\bar{m}} &= (\bar{e}_1 E_1 + \bar{e}_2 E_2 + mE_3)/\sqrt{\mathfrak{A}}.
\end{aligned} \tag{3.21}$$

Using equations (1.57), $\bar{R}_i$ and $\bar{M}_i$ can be written in the form

$$\bar{R}_1 = \overset{*}{T}_{11}\overset{*}{\bar{e}}_1 + \overset{*}{T}_{12}\overset{*}{\bar{e}}_2 + \overset{*}{N}_1\overset{*}{\bar{m}}, \quad \bar{R}_2 = \overset{*}{T}_{21}\overset{*}{\bar{e}}_1 + \overset{*}{T}_{22}\overset{*}{\bar{e}}_2 + \overset{*}{N}_2\overset{*}{\bar{m}}, \tag{3.22}$$

$$\bar{M}_1 = \overset{*}{M}_{11}\overset{*}{\bar{e}}_2 - \overset{*}{M}_{12}\overset{*}{\bar{e}}_1, \quad \bar{M}_2 = \overset{*}{M}_{21}\overset{*}{\bar{e}}_2 - \overset{*}{M}_{22}\overset{*}{\bar{e}}_1, \tag{3.23}$$

where

$$
\begin{aligned}
A_2\sqrt{(1+2\varepsilon_{22})}\,\overset{*}{T}_{11} &= \int_{z_1}^{z_2} \overset{*}{\sigma}_{11}H_2dz, & A_2\sqrt{(1+2\varepsilon_{22})}\,\overset{*}{T}_{12} &= \int_{z_1}^{z_2} \overset{*}{\sigma}_{12}H_2dz,\\
A_2\sqrt{(1+2\varepsilon_{22})}\,\overset{*}{N}_1 &= \int_{z_1}^{z_2} \overset{*}{\sigma}_{13}H_2dz, & A_1\sqrt{(1+2\varepsilon_{11})}\,\overset{*}{T}_{21} &= \int_{z_1}^{z_2} \overset{*}{\sigma}_{21}H_1dz,\\
A_1\sqrt{(1+2\varepsilon_{11})}\,\overset{*}{T}_{22} &= \int_{z_1}^{z_2} \overset{*}{\sigma}_{22}H_1dz, & A_1\sqrt{(1+2\varepsilon_{11})}\,\overset{*}{N}_2 &= \int_{z_1}^{z_2} \overset{*}{\sigma}_{23}H_1dz,\\
A_2\sqrt{(1+2\varepsilon_{22})}\,\overset{*}{M}_{11} &= \int_{z_1}^{z_2} \overset{*}{\sigma}_{11}H_2zdz, & A_2\sqrt{(1+2\varepsilon_{22})}\,\overset{*}{M}_{12} &= \int_{z_1}^{z_2} \overset{*}{\sigma}_{12}H_2zdz,\\
A_1\sqrt{(1+2\varepsilon_{11})}\,\overset{*}{M}_{21} &= \int_{z_1}^{z_2} \overset{*}{\sigma}_{21}H_1zdz, & A_1\sqrt{(1+2\varepsilon_{11})}\,\overset{*}{M}_{22} &= \int_{z_1}^{z_2} \overset{*}{\sigma}_{22}H_1zdz.
\end{aligned}
\tag{3.24}
$$

Vectors $\overset{*}{T}_{i1}\overset{*}{\bar{e}}_1 + \overset{*}{T}_{i2}\overset{*}{\bar{e}}_2$ lie in the tangent plane of the deformed middle surface $\overset{*}{S}$. They are called the in-plane forces, namely: $\overset{*}{T}_{11}$, $\overset{*}{T}_{22}$ are normal forces, $\overset{*}{T}_{12}$, $\overset{*}{T}_{21}$ shear forces, and $\overset{*}{N}_i$ lateral (cut) forces. The moments $\overset{*}{M}_{11}$, $\overset{*}{M}_{22}$ are bending, and $\overset{*}{M}_{12}$, $\overset{*}{M}_{21}$ are twisting moments (figure 3.3). Since for thin shells, terms of order $O(h/R)$ can be neglected without loss of accuracy, from equation (3.24) we obtain

$$
\begin{aligned}
\sqrt{(1+2\varepsilon_{ik})}\,\overset{*}{T}_{ik} &= \int_{z_1}^{z_2} \sigma_{ik}dz,\\
\sqrt{(1+2\varepsilon_{ik})}\,\overset{*}{N}_i &= \int_{z_1}^{z_2} \sigma_{i3}dz,\\
\sqrt{(1+2\varepsilon_{ik})}\,\overset{*}{M}_{ik} &= \int_{z_1}^{z_2} \sigma_{ik}zdz.
\end{aligned}
\tag{3.25}
$$

Using equation (3.20) in (3.18) and (3.19) and neglecting terms $\overset{*}{k}_{ii}z \ll 1$, we find

$$
\begin{aligned}
\bar{X}A_1A_2 &= \overset{*}{X}_1\overset{*}{\bar{e}}_1 + \overset{*}{X}_2\overset{*}{\bar{e}}_2 + \overset{*}{X}_3\overset{*}{\bar{m}},\\
\overline{M} &= \overset{*}{M}_1\overset{*}{\bar{e}}_2 - \overset{*}{M}_2\overset{*}{\bar{e}}_1,
\end{aligned}
\tag{3.26}
$$

where

$$
\overset{*}{X}_i = \frac{\sigma_{i3}}{\sqrt{(1+2\varepsilon_{11})(1+2\varepsilon_{22})}} + \int_{z_1}^{z_2} \frac{\overset{*}{F}_i dz}{\sqrt{(1+2\varepsilon_{11})(1+2\varepsilon_{22})}},
$$

$$
\overset{*}{X}_3 = \frac{\sigma_{33}}{\sqrt{(1+2\varepsilon_{11})(1+2\varepsilon_{22})}} + \int_{z_1}^{z_2} \frac{\overset{*}{F}_3 dz}{\sqrt{(1+2\varepsilon_{11})(1+2\varepsilon_{22})}},
$$

$$
\overset{*}{M}_i = \frac{\sigma_{i3}z}{\sqrt{(1+2\varepsilon_{11})(1+2\varepsilon_{22})}} + \int_{z_1}^{z_2} \frac{\overset{*}{F}_i z dz}{\sqrt{(1+2\varepsilon_{11})(1+2\varepsilon_{22})}}.
$$

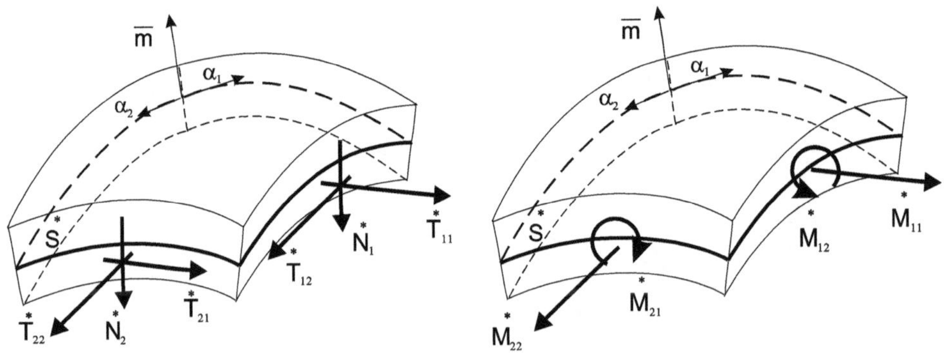

Figure 3.3. Forces and moments in a thin shell.

Here $\overset{*}{X}_i$ and $\overset{*}{M}_i$ are the projections of the external force and moment vectors on the base $\{\overset{*}{\bar{e}}_1, \overset{*}{\bar{e}}_2, \overset{*}{\bar{m}}\} \in \overset{*}{S}$.

3.3 Equations of equilibrium

From a modeling perspective, a thin shell can be treated as a three-dimensional solid. However, the complexity of the problem would be reduced significantly if its dimensionality could be reduced from three to two. To achieve this reduction, the second Kirchhoff–Love hypothesis is introduced. It states that 'the transverse normal stress is significantly smaller compared to other stresses in the shell, $\sigma_{33} \ll \sigma_{ik}$, $(i, k = 1, 2)$ and thus may be neglected'. In addition, recalling that the deformed state of the shell is completely defined in terms of deformations and curvatures of its middle surface, the shell can be regarded as a two-dimensional solid. Thus an analysis of the equilibrium conditions can be based on the study of the resultant forces and moments taken over the thickness of the shell.

Assume that the initial undeformed state of the shell is stress-free. The differential equations of equilibrium of a shell in terms of the deformed configuration can be derived as follows, proceeding from the vector equations of equilibrium for a three-dimensional solid given by

$$\frac{\partial \bar{p}_1 \overset{*}{H}_2}{\partial \alpha_1} + \frac{\partial \bar{p}_2 \overset{*}{H}_1}{\partial \alpha_2} + \frac{\partial \bar{p}_z \overset{*}{H}_1 \overset{*}{H}_2}{\partial z} + \bar{F} \overset{*}{H}_1 \overset{*}{H}_1 = 0, \tag{3.27}$$

$$\left(\overset{*}{\bar{p}}_1 \times \bar{p}_1\right) \overset{*}{H}_2 + \left(\overset{*}{\bar{p}}_2 \times \bar{p}_2\right) \overset{*}{H}_1 + \left(\overset{*}{\bar{m}} \times \bar{p}_z\right) \overset{*}{H}_1 \overset{*}{H}_2 = 0. \tag{3.28}$$

Multiplying equation (3.27) by dz and integrating it over the thickness of the shell, $z \in [z_1, z_2]$, we obtain

$$\frac{\partial A_2\bar{R}_1}{\partial\alpha_1}+\frac{\partial A_1\bar{R}_2}{\partial\alpha_2}+A_1A_2\bar{X}=0. \tag{3.29}$$

Here $\bar{R}_i$ and $\bar{X}$ satisfy equations (3.15) and (3.18).

Integrating the vector product of equation (3.27) and $\overset{*}{\bar{m}z}$ over z, we find

$$\int_{z_1}^{z_2}\left(\overset{*}{\bar{m}z}\times\left(\frac{\partial\bar{p}_1\overset{*}{H_2}}{\partial\alpha_1}+\frac{\partial\bar{p}_2\overset{*}{H_1}}{\partial\alpha_2}+\frac{\partial\bar{p}_z\overset{*}{H_1}\overset{*}{H_2}}{\partial z}+\bar{F}\overset{*}{H_1}\overset{*}{H_2}\right)\right)dz=0. \tag{3.30}$$

Since

$$\begin{aligned}
\int_{z_1}^{z_2}\left(\overset{*}{\bar{m}z}\times\frac{\partial\bar{p}_1\overset{*}{H_2}}{\partial\alpha_1}\right)dz &= \int_{z_1}^{z_2}\frac{\partial}{\partial\alpha_1}\left(\overset{*}{\bar{m}z}\times\bar{p}_1\overset{*}{H_2}\right)dz\\
&\quad-\int_{z_1}^{z_2}\frac{\partial}{\partial\alpha_1}\left(\overset{*}{\bar{m}_1z}\times\bar{p}_1H^{*}{}_2\right)dz\\
&=\frac{\partial A_2\bar{M}_1}{\partial\alpha_1}-\int_{z_1}^{z_2}\left(\left(\overset{*}{\bar{\rho}_1}-\overset{*}{\bar{r}_1}\right)\times\frac{\partial\bar{p}_1\overset{*}{H_2}}{\partial\alpha_1}\right)dz\\
&=\frac{\partial A_2\bar{M}_1}{\partial\alpha_1}+\left(\overset{*}{\bar{r}_1}\times\bar{R}_1\right)A_2-\int_{z_1}^{z_2}\left(\overset{*}{\bar{\rho}_1}\times\bar{p}_1\right)\overset{*}{H_2}dz,\\
\int_{z_1}^{z_2}\left(\overset{*}{\bar{m}z}\times\frac{\partial\bar{p}_2\overset{*}{H_1}}{\partial\alpha_2}\right)dz &= \frac{\partial A_1\bar{M}_2}{\partial\alpha_2}+\left(\overset{*}{\bar{r}_2}\times\bar{R}_2\right)A_1-\int_{z_1}^{z_2}\left(\overset{*}{\bar{\rho}_2}\times\bar{p}_2\right)\overset{*}{H_1}dz,\\
\overset{*}{\bar{m}_1z}=\overset{*}{\bar{\rho}_1}-\overset{*}{\bar{r}_1},&\quad \overset{*}{\bar{m}_2z}=\overset{*}{\bar{\rho}_2}-\overset{*}{\bar{r}_2},
\end{aligned} \tag{3.31}$$

substituting the left-hand sides of equation (3.31) into (3.30), with the help of equation (3.28), we obtain

$$\frac{\partial A_2\bar{M}_1}{\partial\alpha_1}+\frac{\partial A_1\bar{M}_2}{\partial\alpha_2}+A_1\left(\overset{*}{\bar{r}_1}\times\bar{R}_2\right)+A_2\left(\overset{*}{\bar{r}_2}\times\bar{R}_1\right)+A_1A_2\bar{M}=0. \tag{3.32}$$

Here $\bar{M}_i$ and $\bar{M}$ satisfy equations (3.16) and (3.19). Although equations (3.29) and (3.32) are derived under the assumption $h=\text{const}$, they are also valid for shells of variable thickness $h=h(\alpha_1,\alpha_2)$.

Substituting $\bar{R}_i$ and $\bar{X}$ given by equations (3.22), (3.27) into (3.29), for the equilibrium equations we have

$$
\begin{aligned}
&\frac{\partial A_2 \overset{*}{T}_{11}}{\partial \alpha_1} + \frac{\partial A_1 \overset{*}{T}_{21}}{\partial \alpha_2} + \overset{*}{T}_{12}\frac{A_2}{\overset{*}{A}_2}\frac{\partial \overset{*}{A}_1}{\partial \alpha_2} - \overset{*}{T}_{22}\frac{A_1}{\overset{*}{A}_1}\frac{\partial \overset{*}{A}_2}{\partial \alpha_1} \\
&\quad + \overset{*}{A}_1 A_2 \overset{*}{N}_1 \overset{*}{k}_{11} + A_1 \overset{*}{A}_2 \overset{*}{N}_2 \overset{*}{k}_{12} + A_1 A_2 \overset{*}{X}_1 = 0, \\
&\frac{\partial A_1 \overset{*}{T}_{22}}{\partial \alpha_2} + \frac{\partial A_2 \overset{*}{T}_{12}}{\partial \alpha_1} + \overset{*}{T}_{21}\frac{A_1}{\overset{*}{A}_1}\frac{\partial \overset{*}{A}_2}{\partial \alpha_1} - \overset{*}{T}_{11}\frac{A_2}{\overset{*}{A}_2}\frac{\partial \overset{*}{A}_1}{\partial \alpha_2} \\
&\quad + A_2 \overset{*}{A}_1 \overset{*}{N}_1 \overset{*}{k}_{21} + \overset{*}{A}_2 A_1 \overset{*}{N}_2 \overset{*}{k}_{22} + A_1 A_2 \overset{*}{X}_2 = 0,
\end{aligned}
\tag{3.33}
$$

$$
\begin{aligned}
&\frac{\partial A_2 \overset{*}{N}_1}{\partial \alpha_1} + \frac{\partial A_1 \overset{*}{N}_2}{\partial \alpha_2} - \overset{*}{A}_1 A_2 \overset{*}{T}_{11} \overset{*}{k}_{11} - A_1 \overset{*}{A}_2 \overset{*}{T}_{22} \overset{*}{k}_{22} \\
&\quad - A_1 \overset{*}{A}_2 \overset{*}{T}_{12} \overset{*}{k}_{12} - A_1 \overset{*}{A}_2 \overset{*}{T}_{21} \overset{*}{k}_{12} + A_1 A_2 \overset{*}{X}_3 = 0.
\end{aligned}
\tag{3.34}
$$

In deriving equations (3.33) and (3.34) use is made of the formulas for $\dfrac{\partial \overset{*}{\bar{e}}_i}{\partial \alpha_k}$ and $\overset{*}{\overline{m}}_i$,

$$
\begin{aligned}
&\frac{\partial \overset{*}{\bar{e}}_1}{\partial \alpha_1} = -\frac{\overset{*}{\bar{e}}_2}{\overset{*}{A}_2}\frac{\partial \overset{*}{A}_1}{\partial \alpha_2} - \overset{*}{A}_1 \overset{*}{k}_{11} \overset{*}{\overline{m}}, \quad \frac{\partial \overset{*}{\bar{e}}_1}{\partial \alpha_2} = \frac{\overset{*}{\bar{e}}_2}{\overset{*}{A}_1}\frac{\partial \overset{*}{A}_2}{\partial \alpha_1} - \overset{*}{A}_2 \overset{*}{k}_{12} \overset{*}{\overline{m}}, \\
&\frac{\partial \overset{*}{\bar{e}}_2}{\partial \alpha_1} = \frac{\overset{*}{\bar{e}}_1}{\overset{*}{A}_2}\frac{\partial \overset{*}{A}_1}{\partial \alpha_2} - \overset{*}{A}_1 \overset{*}{A}_{12} \overset{*}{\overline{m}}, \quad \frac{\partial \overset{*}{\bar{e}}_2}{\partial \alpha_2} = -\frac{\overset{*}{\bar{e}}_1}{\overset{*}{A}_1}\frac{\partial \overset{*}{A}_2}{\partial \alpha_1} - \overset{*}{A}_2 \overset{*}{k}_{22} \overset{*}{\overline{m}},
\end{aligned}
\tag{3.34a}
$$

$$
\overset{*}{\overline{m}}_i = \overset{*}{A}_i \left(\overset{*}{k}_{1i} \overset{*}{\bar{e}}_1 + \overset{*}{k}_{2i} \overset{*}{\bar{e}}_2 \right).
\tag{3.34b}
$$

By analogy, substituting $\bar{M}_i$, $\bar{M}$ given by equations (3.23) and (3.27) into (3.32) with the help of equations (3.22), (3.34a), and (3.34b), the equilibrium equations of moments take the form

$$
\begin{aligned}
&\frac{\partial A_2 \overset{*}{M}_{11}}{\partial \alpha_1} + \frac{\partial A_1 \overset{*}{M}_{21}}{\partial \alpha_2} + \overset{*}{M}_{12} \frac{A_2}{\overset{*}{A}_2} \frac{\partial \overset{*}{A}_1}{\partial \alpha_2} - \overset{*}{M}_{22} \frac{A_1}{\overset{*}{A}_1} \frac{\partial \overset{*}{A}_2}{\partial \alpha_1} \\
&\quad + \overset{*}{A}_1 \overset{*}{A}_2 \overset{*}{M}_1 - \overset{*}{A}_1 \overset{*}{A}_2 \overset{*}{N}_1 = 0, \\
&\frac{\partial A_2 \overset{*}{M}_{12}}{\partial \alpha_1} + \frac{\partial A_1 \overset{*}{M}_{22}}{\partial \alpha_2} + \overset{*}{M}_{21} \frac{A_1}{\overset{*}{A}_1} \frac{\partial \overset{*}{A}_2}{\partial \alpha_1} - \overset{*}{M}_{11} \frac{A_2}{\overset{*}{A}_2} \frac{\partial \overset{*}{A}_1}{\partial \alpha_2} \\
&\quad + \overset{*}{A}_2 \overset{*}{A}_1 \overset{*}{M}_2 - \overset{*}{A}_2 \overset{*}{A}_1 \overset{*}{N}_2 = 0,
\end{aligned}
\tag{3.35}
$$

$$
\begin{aligned}
&\overset{*}{A}_1 \overset{*}{A}_2 \overset{*}{T}_{12} - \overset{*}{A}_1 \overset{*}{A}_2 \overset{*}{T}_{21} + \overset{*}{A}_1 \overset{*}{A}_2 \overset{*}{M}_{12} k_{11} - \overset{*}{A}_1 \overset{*}{A}_2 \overset{*}{M}_{21} k_{22} \\
&\quad + \overset{*}{A}_1 \overset{*}{A}_2 \overset{*}{M}_{22} k_{12} - \overset{*}{A}_1 \overset{*}{A}_2 \overset{*}{M}_{11} k_{12} = 0.
\end{aligned}
\tag{3.36}
$$

The system of equations (3.33)–(3.36) contains six unknowns: $\overset{*}{T}_{ik}$, $\overset{*}{N}_i$, and $\overset{*}{M}_{ik}$ $(i, k = 1, 2)$. Introducing differential operators defined by

$$
\begin{aligned}
L_1\left(\overset{*}{T}_{ik}\right) &= \frac{\partial A_2 \overset{*}{T}_{11}}{\partial \alpha_1} + \frac{\partial A_1 \overset{*}{T}_{21}}{\partial \alpha_2} + \overset{*}{T}_{12} \frac{A_2}{\overset{*}{A}_2} \frac{\partial \overset{*}{A}_1}{\partial \alpha_2} - \overset{*}{T}_{22} \frac{A_1}{\overset{*}{A}_1} \frac{\partial \overset{*}{A}_2}{\partial \alpha_1}, \\
L_2\left(\overset{*}{T}_{ik}\right) &= \frac{\partial A_2 \overset{*}{T}_{12}}{\partial \alpha_1} + \frac{\partial A_1 \overset{*}{T}_{22}}{\partial \alpha_2} + \overset{*}{T}_{21} \frac{A_1}{\overset{*}{A}_1} \frac{\partial \overset{*}{A}_2}{\partial \alpha_1} - \overset{*}{T}_{11} \frac{A_2}{\overset{*}{A}_2} \frac{\partial \overset{*}{A}_1}{\partial \alpha_2},
\end{aligned}
\tag{3.37}
$$

$$
\begin{aligned}
L_1\left(\overset{*}{M}_{ik}\right) &= \frac{\partial A_2 \overset{*}{M}_{11}}{\partial \alpha_1} + \frac{\partial A_1 \overset{*}{M}_{21}}{\partial \alpha_2} + \overset{*}{M}_{12} \frac{A_2}{\overset{*}{A}_2} \frac{\partial \overset{*}{A}_1}{\partial \alpha_2} - \overset{*}{M}_{22} \frac{A_1}{\overset{*}{A}_1} \frac{\partial \overset{*}{A}_2}{\partial \alpha_1}, \\
L_2\left(\overset{*}{M}_{ik}\right) &= \frac{\partial A_2 \overset{*}{M}_{12}}{\partial \alpha_1} + \frac{\partial A_1 \overset{*}{M}_{22}}{\partial \alpha_2} + \overset{*}{M}_{21} \frac{A_1}{\overset{*}{A}_1} \frac{\partial \overset{*}{A}_2}{\partial \alpha_1} - \overset{*}{M}_{11} \frac{A_2}{\overset{*}{A}_2} \frac{\partial \overset{*}{A}_1}{\partial \alpha_2},
\end{aligned}
\tag{3.38}
$$

the first two equations in (3.33) and (3.35) can be written in the form

$$
\begin{aligned}
&L_1\left(\overset{*}{T}_{ik}\right) + \overset{*}{A}_1 \overset{*}{A}_2 \overset{*}{N}_1 k_{11} + \overset{*}{A}_1 \overset{*}{A}_2 \overset{*}{N}_2 k_{12} + A_1 \overset{*}{A}_2 X_1 = 0, \\
&L_2\left(\overset{*}{T}_{ik}\right) + \overset{*}{A}_2 \overset{*}{A}_1 \overset{*}{N}_2 k_{22} + \overset{*}{A}_2 \overset{*}{A}_1 \overset{*}{N}_1 k_{21} + A_1 \overset{*}{A}_2 X_2 = 0,
\end{aligned}
\tag{3.39}
$$

$$\frac{\partial A_2\overset{*}{N}_1}{\partial\alpha_1} + \frac{\partial A_1\overset{*}{N}_2}{\partial\alpha_2} - \overset{*}{A}_1 A_2 \overset{*}{T}_{11}\overset{*}{k}_{11} - A_1\overset{*}{A}_2\overset{*}{T}_{22}\overset{*}{k}_{22}$$
$$- A_1\overset{*}{A}_2\overset{*}{T}_{12}\overset{*}{k}_{12} - A_1\overset{*}{A}_2\overset{*}{T}_{21}\overset{*}{k}_{12} + A_1A_2\overset{*}{X}_3 = 0, \tag{3.40}$$

$$L_1\left(\overset{*}{M}_{ik}\right) + \overset{*}{A}_1A_2\overset{*}{M}_1 - A_1\overset{*}{A}_2\overset{*}{N}_1 = 0,$$
$$L_2\left(\overset{*}{M}_{ik}\right) + \overset{*}{A}_2A_1\overset{*}{M}_1 - A_2\overset{*}{A}_1\overset{*}{N}_1 = 0, \tag{3.41}$$

$$A_1\overset{*}{A}_2\overset{*}{T}_{12} - \overset{*}{A}_1A_2\overset{*}{T}_{21} + A_1\overset{*}{A}_2\overset{*}{M}_{12}\overset{*}{k}_{11} - \overset{*}{A}_1A_2\overset{*}{M}_{21}\overset{*}{k}_{22}$$
$$+ \overset{*}{A}_1A_2\overset{*}{M}_{22}\overset{*}{k}_{12} - A_1\overset{*}{A}_2\overset{*}{M}_{11}\overset{*}{k}_{12} = 0. \tag{3.42}$$

Equations (3.39)–(3.42) are nonlinear. The nonlinearity is introduced by the curvatures of the surface, $\overset{*}{k}_{ij} = k_{ij} + \text{æ}_{ij}$, projections of the forces and moments $\overset{*}{X}_i$, $\overset{*}{X}_3$, $\overset{*}{M}_i$, $\overset{*}{T}_{ik}$, $\overset{*}{N}_i$, $\overset{*}{M}_{ik}$ on the deformed axes, and, additionally, may be brought in by constitutive relations for the constructive material of a shell.

Proceeding from the second equation of equilibrium (3.29) and projecting it onto the orthogonal base $\{\bar{e}_1, \bar{e}_2, \bar{m}\}$, for the tangent T_{ik} and lateral forces N_i, we find

$$T_{11} = \bar{R}_1\bar{e}_1,\ T_{12} = \bar{R}_1\bar{e}_2,\ T_{21} = \bar{R}_2\bar{e}_1,\ T_{22} = \bar{R}_2\bar{e}_2,$$

$$N_i = \bar{R}_i\bar{m},\ X_i = \bar{X}\bar{e}_i,\ X_3 = \bar{X}\bar{m}.$$

Substituting expressions for $\bar{R}_i$, $\bar{X}$, and $\overset{*}{\bar{e}}_1$, $\overset{*}{\bar{e}}_2$, $\overset{*}{\bar{m}}$ given by equations (3.21), (3.23), and (3.27), we obtain

$$T_{11} = \left(\overset{*}{T}_{11}\overset{*}{\bar{e}}_1 + \overset{*}{T}_{12}\overset{*}{\bar{e}}_2 + \overset{*}{N}_1\overset{*}{\bar{m}}\right)\bar{e}_1 = \overset{*}{T}_{11}(1 + e_{11})/(1 + 2\varepsilon_{11})$$
$$+ \overset{*}{T}_{12}e_{12}/(1 + 2\varepsilon_{22}) + \overset{*}{N}_1\mathbb{S}_1/\sqrt{\mathfrak{A}},$$
$$T_{12} = \overset{*}{T}_{11}e_{12}/(1 + 2\varepsilon_{11}) + \overset{*}{T}_{12}(1 + e_{22})/(1 + 2\varepsilon_{22}) + \overset{*}{N}_1\mathbb{S}_2/\sqrt{\mathfrak{A}}, \tag{3.43}$$
$$T_{22} = \overset{*}{T}_{21}e_{12}/(1 + 2\varepsilon_{11}) + \overset{*}{T}_{22}(1 + e_{22})/(1 + 2\varepsilon_{22}) + \overset{*}{N}_2\mathbb{S}_2/\sqrt{\mathfrak{A}},$$
$$T_{21} = \overset{*}{T}_{21}(1 + e_{11})/(1 + 2\varepsilon_{11}) + \overset{*}{T}_{22}e_{21}/(1 + 2\varepsilon_{22}) + \overset{*}{N}_2\mathbb{S}_1/\sqrt{\mathfrak{A}},$$

$$
\begin{aligned}
N_1 &= \overset{*}{T}_{11}\varpi_1/(1+2\varepsilon_{11}) + \overset{*}{T}_{12}\varpi_2/(1+2\varepsilon_{22}) + \overset{*}{N}_1\mathbb{S}_3/\sqrt{\mathfrak{A}}, \\
N_2 &= \overset{*}{T}_{22}\varpi_2/(1+2\varepsilon_{22}) + \overset{*}{T}_{21}\varpi_1/(1+2\varepsilon_{11}) + \overset{*}{N}_2\mathbb{S}_3/\sqrt{\mathfrak{A}}, \\
X_1 &= \overset{*}{X}_1(1+e_{11})/(1+2\varepsilon_{11}) + \overset{*}{X}_2 e_{12}/(1+2\varepsilon_{22}) + \overset{*}{X}_3\varpi_1/\sqrt{\mathfrak{A}}, \\
X_2 &= \overset{*}{X}_1 e_{21}/(1+2\varepsilon_{11}) + \overset{*}{X}_2(1+e_{22})/(1+2\varepsilon_{22}) + \overset{*}{X}_3\varpi_2/\sqrt{\mathfrak{A}}, \\
X_3 &= \left(\overset{*}{X}_1\mathbb{S}_1 + \overset{*}{X}_2\mathbb{S}_2 + \overset{*}{X}_3\mathbb{S}_3\right)\Big/\sqrt{\mathfrak{A}}.
\end{aligned}
\tag{3.44}
$$

By analogy, substituting equations (1.19) and (1.23) into (3.29) we obtain the equilibrium equations for the thin shell in terms of the undeformed configuration,

$$
\begin{aligned}
&L_1(T_{ik}) + A_1A_2N_1k_{11} + A_1A_2N_2k_{12} + A_1A_2X_1 = 0, \\
&L_2(T_{ik}) + A_1A_2N_2k_{22} + A_1A_2N_1k_{21} + A_1A_2X_2 = 0,
\end{aligned}
\tag{3.45}
$$

$$
\begin{aligned}
&\frac{\partial A_2N_1}{\partial\alpha_1} + \frac{\partial A_1N_2}{\partial\alpha_2} - A_1A_2T_{11}k_{11} - A_1A_2T_{22}k_{22} \\
&\quad - A_1A_2T_{12}k_{12} - A_1A_2T_{21}k_{12} + A_1A_2X_2 = 0.
\end{aligned}
\tag{3.46}
$$

The resultant internal and external force vectors $\bar{R}_i$ and $\bar{X}$ are given by

$$
\begin{aligned}
\bar{R}_1 &= T_{11}\bar{e}_1 + T_{12}\bar{e}_2 + N_1\overline{m}, \\
\bar{R}_2 &= T_{21}\bar{e}_1 + T_{22}\bar{e}_2 + N_2\overline{m}, \\
\bar{X} &= X_1\bar{e}_1 + X_2\bar{e}_2 + X_3\overline{m}.
\end{aligned}
\tag{3.47}
$$

The equilibrium equations for moment equations (3.41) and (3.42) can be recast in similar way. The resultant equations are very bulky and are not given here.

Further reading

Amabili M 2018 *Nonlinear Mechanics of Shells and Plates in Composite, Soft and Biological Materials* (Cambridge: Cambridge University Press)

Galimov K Z, Paimushin V N and Teregulov I G 1996 *Foundations of the Nonlinear Theory of Shells* (Kazan: ФЭН)

Libai A and Simmonds J G 1998 *The Nonlinear Theory of Elastic Shells* 2nd edn (Cambridge: Cambridge University Press)

Taber L A 2004 *Nonlinear Theory of Elasticity: Applications in Biomechanics* (Singapore: World Scientific)

IOP Publishing

Soft Biological Shells in Bioengineering

Roustem N Miftahof and Nariman R Akhmadeev

Chapter 4

Boundary conditions

Boundary conditions, including clamped, simple, free, and freely supported edges with a single degree of freedom in the normal direction are considered. The Gauss–Codazzi equations for the undeformed boundary of the thin shell are obtained.

4.1 Geometry of the boundary

Consider the contour curve C on the boundary of the undeformed shell parameterized by arc length s

$$\bar{r} = \bar{r}(s) = \bar{r}(\alpha_1(s), \alpha_2(s)). \tag{4.1}$$

Let $\{\bar{n}, \bar{\tau}, \bar{m}\}$ be the orthogonal base of C (figure 4.1). Here $\bar{n}$, $\bar{\tau}$ are unit vectors normal and tangent to C, respectively, and $\bar{m}$ is the vector normal to the middle surface S. The three unit vectors are linearly independent

$$\bar{n} = \bar{\tau} \times \bar{m}, \quad \bar{\tau} = \bar{m} \times \bar{n}, \quad \bar{m} = \bar{n} \times \bar{\tau}. \tag{4.2}$$

Differentiating equation (4.1) with respect to s and using equation (1.13), the tangent vector $\bar{\tau}$ is found to be

$$\bar{\tau} = \frac{d\bar{r}}{ds} = \bar{r}_1\frac{d\alpha_1}{ds} + \bar{r}_2\frac{d\alpha_2}{ds} = \bar{e}_1\tau_1 + \bar{e}_2\tau_2. \tag{4.3}$$

Projections of $\bar{\tau}$ on unit vectors $\bar{e}_i \in S$ $(i = 1, 2)$ are given by

$$\tau_1 = A_1\frac{d\alpha_1}{ds}, \quad \tau_2 = A_2\frac{d\alpha_2}{ds}. \tag{4.4}$$

Decomposing the normal vector $\bar{n}$ in the direction of $\bar{e}_i$ yields

$$\bar{n} = (\bar{e}_1\tau_1 + \bar{e}_2\tau_2) \times \bar{m} = \bar{e}_1\tau_2 - \bar{e}_2\tau_1, \quad \bar{n} = \bar{e}_1 n_1 + \bar{e}_2 n_2. \tag{4.5}$$

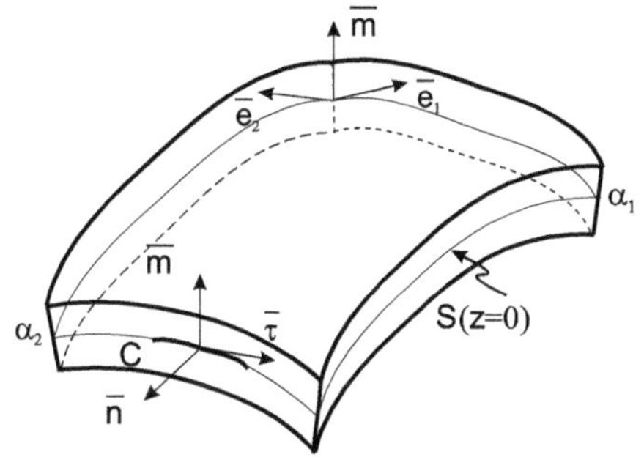

Figure 4.1. An orthonormal base $\{\bar{n}, \bar{\tau}, \bar{m}\}$ associated with the boundary.

From equations (4.4) and (4.5), projections of $\bar{n}$, are found to be

$$n_1 = \tau_2 = A_2\frac{d\alpha_2}{ds}, \quad n_2 = -\tau_1 = -A_1\frac{d\alpha_1}{ds}, \tag{4.6}$$

Since $\bar{n} \perp \bar{\tau}$, it follows that $\tau_1 n_1 + \tau_2 n_2 = 0$.

Let k_n, k_τ be normal curvatures in the direction of $\bar{n}$ and $\bar{\tau}$, and $k_{n\tau}$ be the twist of the contour line C

$$k_n = \sum_{i=1}^{2}\sum_{j=1}^{2} k_{ij}n_i n_j, \quad k_\tau = \sum_{i=1}^{2}\sum_{j=1}^{2} k_{ij}\tau_i\tau_j, \quad k_{n\tau} = \sum_{i=1}^{2}\sum_{j=1}^{2} k_{ij}\tau_i n_j, \tag{4.7}$$

where k_{ij} satisfy equations (1.21a) and (1.21b).

Let ds_z be the length of a line element on a contour curve C_z of the equidistant surface S_z ($S_z \| S$), and $\bar{\tau}^z$, $\bar{n}^z$ be unit tangent vectors to C_z. Then

$$\bar{\tau}^z = \bar{e}_1^z\tau_1^z + \bar{e}_2^z\tau_2^z, \quad \tau_1^z = H_1\frac{d\alpha_1}{ds_z}, \quad \tau_2^z = H_2\frac{d\alpha_2}{ds_z}, \tag{4.8}$$

$$n_1^z = H_2\frac{d\alpha_2}{ds_z}, \quad n_2^z = H_1\frac{d\alpha_1}{ds_z}, \tag{4.9}$$

where τ_i^z, n_i^z ($i = 1, 2$) are the projections of $\bar{\tau}^z$, $\bar{n}^z$ on vectors $\bar{e}_i^z \in S_z$. From equations (4.6) and (4.9) for projections of $\bar{n}$ on tangents to the coordinate lines on S_z, we have

$$n_1^z = \frac{H_2}{A_2}\frac{ds}{ds_z}n_1, \quad n_2^z = \frac{H_1}{A_1}\frac{ds}{ds_z}n_2. \tag{4.10}$$

Although equations (4.2)–(4.10) are obtained in terms of the undeformed shell, they are also valid for the deformed configuration. Thus,

$$\overset{*}{\tau}_i = \overset{*}{A}_i\frac{d\alpha_i}{d\overset{*}{s}}, \quad \overset{*}{n}_i = (-1)^{i+1}\overset{*}{A}_i\frac{d\alpha_i}{d\overset{*}{s}}, \quad (i = 1, 2), \tag{4.11}$$

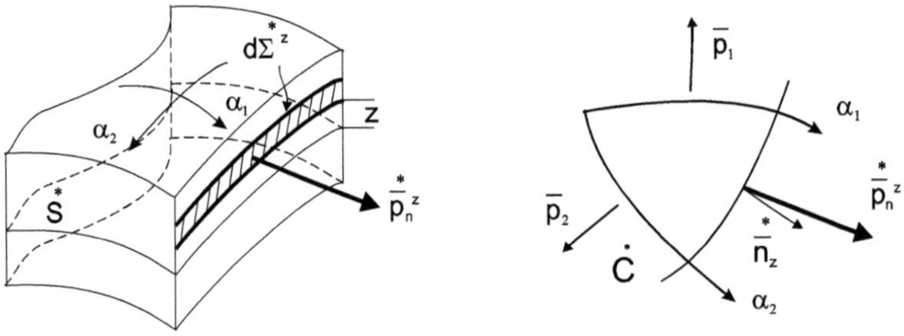

Figure 4.2. Stresses on the boundary of a shell.

where $\overset{*}{\tau}_i$, $\overset{*}{n}_i$, $\overset{*}{ds}$ are expressed in terms of the contour line $\overset{*}{C}$ and have the meaning as described above. Assuming that deformations on the boundary are small, $\overset{*}{A}_i \approx A_i$, $\overset{*}{ds} \approx ds$. Then from equation (4.1) we have

$$\overset{*}{\tau}_i \approx \tau_i, \quad \overset{*}{n}_i \approx n_i. \tag{4.12}$$

It implies that projections of $\overset{*}{\bar{\tau}}$ and $\overset{*}{\bar{n}}$ on the coordinate axes of the deformed middle surface $\overset{*}{S}$ equal projections of the same vectors on the undeformed middle surface S.

For curvatures k_n^*, k_τ^* in the direction of $\overset{*}{\bar{n}}$ and $\overset{*}{\bar{\tau}}$, and twist $k_{n\tau}^*$ of $\overset{*}{C}$ we have

$$\begin{aligned} k_n^* &= \sum_{i=1}^{2}\sum_{j=1}^{2} k_{ij}^* n_i^* n_j^* \approx \sum_{i=1}^{2}\sum_{j=1}^{2} k_{ij}^* n_i n_j, \\ k_\tau^* &= \sum_{i=1}^{2}\sum_{j=1}^{2} k_{ij}^* \tau_i^* \tau_j^* \approx \sum_{i=1}^{2}\sum_{j=1}^{2} k_{ij}^* \tau_i \tau_j, \\ k_{n\tau}^* &= \sum_{i=1}^{2}\sum_{j=1}^{2} k_{ij}^* \tau_i^* n_j^* \approx \sum_{i=1}^{2}\sum_{j=1}^{2} k_{ij}^* \tau_i n_j, \end{aligned} \tag{4.13}$$

where equations (4.7) and (4.12) are used. Formulas for the deformed contour are similar to those given by equation (4.10) and have the form

$$\overset{*}{n}{}_1^z = \frac{\overset{*}{H}_2}{\overset{*}{A}_2}\frac{\overset{*}{ds}}{\overset{*}{ds}_z}\overset{*}{n}_1, \quad \overset{*}{n}{}_2^z = \frac{\overset{*}{H}_1}{\overset{*}{A}_1}\frac{\overset{*}{ds}}{\overset{*}{ds}_z}\overset{*}{n}_2. \tag{4.14}$$

4.2 Stresses on the boundary

Let $\overset{*}{\bar{p}}{}_n^z$ be the normal stress vector acting upon a differential element of the boundary $\overset{*}{\Sigma}{}^z$ of the deformed shell located at a distance $\overset{*}{z} \approx z$ from the middle surface $\overset{*}{S}$ (figure 4.2),

$$\overset{*}{\bar{p}}{}_n^z = \bar{p}_1 \overset{*}{n}{}_1^z + \bar{p}_2 \overset{*}{n}{}_2^z + \bar{p}_3 \overset{*}{\bar{m}}. \tag{4.15}$$

Here $\overset{*}{n}{}_i^z$ are the projections of $\overset{*}{n}{}^z$ on $\overset{*}{\bar{e}}{}_i^z \in \overset{*}{S}$, and $\bar{p}_i$ are the stress vectors acting upon the faces $\alpha_1 = \text{const}$, $\alpha_2 = \text{const}$. Since $\overset{*}{n}{}^z \perp \overset{*}{\bar{m}}$, the third component in equation (4.15) vanishes, $\bar{p}_3 \overset{*}{\bar{m}} = 0$.

The surface area $d\overset{*}{\Sigma}_z$ of a differential element on the edge is given by

$$d\overset{*}{\Sigma}_z = d\overset{*}{s}_z \, d\overset{*}{z}. \tag{4.16}$$

The resultant force $\bar{R}_n^*$ and moment $\bar{M}_n^*$ vectors per unit length of $\overset{*}{C}$ acting upon $d\overset{*}{\Sigma}_z$ are given by

$$\bar{R}_n^* = \int_{z_1}^{z_2} \overset{*}{\bar{p}}{}_n^z \frac{d\overset{*}{\Sigma}_z}{d\overset{*}{s}}, \quad \bar{M}_n^* = \int_{z_1}^{z_2} \left(\overset{*}{\bar{m}} \overset{*}{z} \times \overset{*}{\bar{p}}{}_n^z \right) \frac{d\overset{*}{\Sigma}_z}{d\overset{*}{s}}. \tag{4.17}$$

Using equations (4.15) and (4.16) they can be written as

$$\bar{R}_n^* = \int_{z_1}^{z_2} \left(\bar{p}_1 \overset{*}{n}{}_1^z + \bar{p}_2 \overset{*}{n}{}_2^z \right) \frac{d\overset{*}{s}_z d\overset{*}{z}}{d\overset{*}{s}},$$

$$\bar{M}_n^* = \int_{z_1}^{z_2} \left(\overset{*}{\bar{m}} \overset{*}{z} \times \left(\bar{p}_1 \overset{*}{n}{}_1^z + \bar{p}_2 \overset{*}{n}{}_2^z \right) \right) \frac{d\overset{*}{s}_z d\overset{*}{z}}{d\overset{*}{s}}.$$

Substituting $\overset{*}{n}{}_i^z$ given by equation (4.14), and using approximations (4.12), $\bar{R}_n^*$, $\bar{M}_n^*$ on the skewed faces of the boundary are found to be

$$\begin{aligned} \bar{R}_n^* &= \bar{R}_1 \overset{*}{n}_1 + \bar{R}_2 \overset{*}{n}_2 \approx \bar{R}_1 n_1 + \bar{R}_2 n_2, \\ \bar{M}_n^* &= \bar{M}_1 \overset{*}{n}_1 + \bar{M}_2 \overset{*}{n}_2 \approx \bar{M}_1 n_1 + \bar{M}_2 n_2. \end{aligned} \tag{4.18}$$

Decomposing $\bar{R}_n^*$, $\bar{M}_n^*$ along the base $\{\overset{*}{\bar{n}}, \overset{*}{\bar{\tau}}, \overset{*}{\bar{m}}\}$ and substituting $\bar{R}_i$ and $\bar{M}_i$ given by equations (3.22) and (3.23), we obtain

$$\begin{aligned} \bar{R}_n^* &= \sum_{i=1}^{2} \sum_{k=1}^{2} \overset{*}{\bar{e}}_1 \overset{*}{T}_{ik} \overset{*}{n}_i + \overset{*}{\bar{m}} \left(\overset{*}{N}_1 \overset{*}{n}_1 + \overset{*}{N}_2 \overset{*}{n}_2 \right), \\ \bar{M}_n^* &= \overset{*}{\bar{e}}_2 \left(\overset{*}{M}_{11} \overset{*}{n}_1 + \overset{*}{M}_{21} \overset{*}{n}_2 \right) - \overset{*}{\bar{e}}_1 \left(\overset{*}{M}_{12} \overset{*}{n}_1 + \overset{*}{M}_{22} \overset{*}{n}_2 \right), \end{aligned} \tag{4.19}$$

where $\overset{*}{T}_{ik}$, $\overset{*}{N}_i$, and $\overset{*}{M}_{ik}$ are the in-plane forces and moments.

Let $T_{\overset{*}{n}}$, $T_{\overset{**}{n\tau}}$, and $\overset{*}{N}$ be the normal, tangent, and lateral forces acting on $\overset{*}{\Sigma}$

$$T_{\overset{*}{n}} = \bar{R}_{\overset{*}{n}}\overset{*}{\bar{n}}, \quad T_{\overset{**}{n\tau}} = \bar{R}_{\overset{*}{n}}\overset{*}{\bar{\tau}}, \quad \overset{*}{N} = \bar{R}_{\overset{*}{n}}\overset{*}{\bar{m}}.$$

Using $\bar{R}_{\overset{*}{n}}$ (4.19) and approximations (4.12), we find

$$\begin{aligned} T_{\overset{*}{n}} &= \sum_{i=1}^{2}\sum_{k=1}^{2} \overset{*}{T}_{ik}\overset{*}{n}_i\overset{*}{n}_k \approx \sum_{i=1}^{2}\sum_{k=1}^{2} \overset{*}{T}_{ik}n_i n_k \\ T_{\overset{**}{n\tau}} &= \sum_{i=1}^{2}\sum_{k=1}^{2} \overset{*}{T}_{ik}\overset{*}{n}_i\overset{*}{\tau}_k \approx \sum_{i=1}^{2}\sum_{k=1}^{2} \overset{*}{T}_{ik}n_i\tau_k \\ \overset{*}{N} &= \overset{*}{N}_1\overset{*}{n}_1 + \overset{*}{N}_2\overset{*}{n}_2 \approx \overset{*}{N}_1 n_1 + \overset{*}{N}_2 n_2. \end{aligned} \tag{4.20}$$

Projecting $\bar{M}_{\overset{*}{n}}$ on the tangent and normal planes to the boundary we obtain

$$\overset{*}{G} = \bar{M}_{\overset{*}{n}}\overset{*}{\bar{\tau}}, \overset{*}{H} = \bar{M}_{\overset{*}{n}}\overset{*}{\bar{n}},$$

where $\overset{*}{G}$, $\overset{*}{H}$ are the bending and twisting moments. Substituting $\bar{M}_{\overset{*}{n}}$ (equation (4.19)), we obtain

$$\overset{*}{G} = \overset{*}{\bar{\tau}}_2\left(\overset{*}{M}_{11}\overset{*}{n}_1 + \overset{*}{M}_{21}\overset{*}{n}_2\right) - \overset{*}{\bar{\tau}}_1\left(\overset{*}{M}_{21}\overset{*}{n}_1 + \overset{*}{M}_{22}\overset{*}{n}_2\right),$$

$$\overset{*}{H} = \overset{*}{\bar{n}}_2\left(\overset{*}{M}_{11}\overset{*}{n}_1 + \overset{*}{M}_{21}\overset{*}{n}_2\right) - \overset{*}{\bar{n}}_1\left(\overset{*}{M}_{21}\overset{*}{n}_1 + \overset{*}{M}_{22}\overset{*}{n}_2\right).$$

Making use of equation (4.6), after simple algebra, we find

$$\begin{aligned} \overset{*}{G} &= \sum_{i=1}^{2}\sum_{k=1}^{2} \overset{*}{M}_{ik}\overset{*}{n}_i\overset{*}{n}_k \approx \sum_{i=1}^{2}\sum_{k=1}^{2} \overset{*}{M}_{ik}n_i n_k \\ \overset{*}{H} &= -\sum_{i=1}^{2}\sum_{k=1}^{2} \overset{*}{M}_{ik}\overset{*}{n}_i\overset{*}{\tau}_k \approx -\sum_{i=1}^{2}\sum_{k=1}^{2} \overset{*}{M}_{ik}n_i\tau_k. \end{aligned} \tag{4.21}$$

Decomposing the resultant force and moment vectors in the directions of $\{\overset{*}{\bar{n}}, \overset{*}{\bar{\tau}}, \overset{*}{\bar{m}}\}$, we obtain

$$\bar{R}_{\overset{*}{n}} = T_{\overset{*}{n}}\overset{*}{\bar{n}} + T_{\overset{**}{n\tau}}\overset{*}{\bar{\tau}} + \overset{*}{N}\overset{*}{\bar{m}}, \quad \bar{M}_{\overset{*}{n}} = H_{\overset{*}{n}}\bar{n}^{*} + \overset{*}{G}\overset{*}{\bar{\tau}}. \tag{4.22}$$

The conclusion drawn from the considerations above is that the stressed state on the edge of the thin shell is determined in terms of five variables, namely, $T_{\overset{*}{n}}$, $T_{\overset{**}{n\tau}}$, $\overset{*}{N}$, $\overset{*}{G}$, and $\overset{*}{H}$. However, as will now be shown, the twisting moment $\overset{*}{H}$ can be replaced by a statically equivalent force $-\frac{\partial \overset{*}{H}\overset{*}{\bar{m}}}{\partial \overset{*}{s}}$ per unit arc length of c_0c_1 of the contour $\overset{*}{C}$. The substitution, according to the Saint-Venant principle, will have no effect on the stress state in the thin shell at distances sufficiently far from the boundary.

Let $\overset{*}{H}$ be the twisting moment vector acting at point $c_0 \in \overset{*}{C}$ (figure 4.3). Consider the vicinity of point c_0. Approximating the arc c_0c_1 by a straight line $\overline{c_0c_1}$ of a length $d\overset{*}{s}$ the resultant vector of twisting moment $\overset{*}{H}\overset{*}{\bar n}d\overset{*}{s}$ acting upon $\overline{c_0c_1}$ can be substituted by a statically equivalent couple given by $\left(-\overset{*}{H}\overset{*}{\bar m}, +\overset{*}{H}\overset{*}{\bar m}\right)$,

$$\overset{*}{H}\overset{*}{\bar n}d\overset{*}{s} \propto \left(-\overset{*}{H}\overset{*}{\bar m}, +\overset{*}{H}\overset{*}{\bar m}\right).$$

The vector $\overset{*}{\bar m}$ is orthogonal to $\overset{*}{S}$ and vector $\overset{*}{\bar n}$ is orthogonal to $\overset{*}{\bar m}$ at c_0 pointing towards the reader. The forces $\pm\overset{*}{H}\overset{*}{\bar m}$ are collinear with the vector $\overset{*}{\bar m}$ at c_{01}—the middle point of $\overline{c_0c_1}$. Then the moment of the couple about point c_{01} is indeed equal to

$$\overset{*}{\bar\tau}d\overset{*}{s} \times \overset{*}{H}\overset{*}{\bar m} = \left(\overset{*}{\bar\tau} \times \overset{*}{\bar m}\right)\overset{*}{H}d\overset{*}{s} = \overset{*}{H}\overset{*}{\bar n}d\overset{*}{s},$$

where $\overset{*}{\bar\tau}d\overset{*}{s} \approx \overline{c_0c_1}$.

In just the same way, it can be shown that the torque exerted on the segment $\overline{c_0c_2}$ is statically equivalent to the couple applied at points c_0 and c_2, respectively. These are oriented along $\overset{*}{\bar m}$ at c_{02} being the middle point of $\overline{c_0c_2}$, and equal

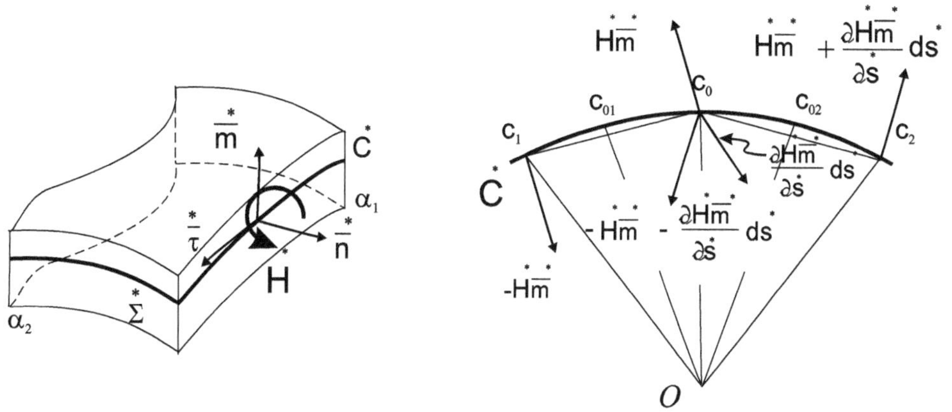

Figure 4.3. Substitution of the twist moment $\overset{*}{H}$ by a statically equivalent distributed force $\partial\overset{*}{H}\overset{*}{m}/\partial\overset{*}{s}$ acting on the boundary of a shell.

$$-\left(\overset{*}{H}\overset{*}{\overline{m}} + \frac{\partial \overset{*}{H}\overset{*}{\overline{m}}}{\partial \overset{*}{s}} d\overset{*}{s}\right), \quad \left(\overset{*}{H}\overset{*}{\overline{m}} + \frac{\partial \overset{*}{H}\overset{*}{\overline{m}}}{\partial \overset{*}{s}} d\overset{*}{s}\right).$$

The geometric sum of forces applied at point c_0 is $-\dfrac{\partial \overset{*}{H}\overset{*}{\overline{m}}}{\partial \overset{*}{s}} d\overset{*}{s}$. It follows that the twisting moment $\overset{*}{H}$ per unit length of the contour $\overset{*}{C}$ is indeed statically equivalent to the distributed force of density $-\dfrac{\partial \overset{*}{H}\overset{*}{\overline{m}}}{\partial \overset{*}{s}} d\overset{*}{s}$.

The resultant force and moment vectors $\bar{R}_{\overset{*}{n}}$ and $\bar{M}_{\overset{*}{n}}$ acting upon $\overset{*}{\Sigma}$ are statically equivalent to the generalized force vector

$$\bar{\Phi} = \bar{R}_{\overset{*}{n}} - \frac{\partial \overset{*}{H}\overset{*}{\overline{m}}}{\partial \overset{*}{s}} d\overset{*}{s}, \tag{4.23}$$

and the bending moment

$$\overset{*}{G} = \sum_{i=1}^{2}\sum_{k=1}^{2} \overset{*}{M}_{ik}\overset{*}{n}_i\overset{*}{n}_k \approx \sum_{i=1}^{2}\sum_{k=1}^{2} \overset{*}{M}_{ik} n_i n_k. \tag{4.24}$$

Here $\overset{*}{H}$ and $\bar{R}_{\overset{*}{n}}$ satisfy equations (4.21) and (4.22), respectively.

In the above derivations it is assumed that the boundary is non-singular and closed. If there are singularities, e.g. corner points along the edge of the boundary, then the force $-\partial \overset{*}{H}\overset{*}{\overline{m}}/\partial \overset{*}{s}$ should be supplemented by forces $\left(\pm \overset{*}{H}\overset{*}{\overline{m}}\right)$ acting at the corners.

4.3 Static boundary conditions

Since stresses on the boundary $\overset{*}{\Sigma}$ of the shell are statically equivalent to three forces $T_{\overset{*}{n}}$, $T_{\overset{*}{n}\overset{*}{\tau}}$, $\overset{*}{N}$ and two moments $\overset{*}{G}$, $\overset{*}{H}$, then five static conditions should be prescribed on the boundary. However, it was first shown by Kirchhoff in the case of thin shells, that the number of boundary conditions could be reduced to four. Kirchhoff based his proof on the assumption that stresses which produce the twisting moment $\overset{*}{H}$ are negligible and therefore can be substituted by the distributed force of density $-\partial \overset{*}{H}\overset{*}{\overline{m}}/\partial \overset{*}{s}$.

Let the deformed middle surface $\overset{*}{S}$ be parameterized by rectangular curvilinear coordinates. Assume that $\bar{\Phi}^s$, $\overset{*}{G^s}$ are applied external load and bending moment vectors per unit length of the deformed contour $\overset{*}{C}$. Now the static boundary conditions take the form

$$\bar{\Phi}^s = \bar{R}_{\overset{*}{n}} - \frac{\partial \overset{*}{H}\overset{*}{\overline{m}}}{\partial \overset{*}{s}}, \quad G^s = \sum_{i=1}^{2}\sum_{k=1}^{2} \overset{*}{M}_{ik}\overset{*}{n}_i\overset{*}{n}_k \approx \sum_{i=1}^{2}\sum_{k=1}^{2}\overset{*}{M}_{ik} n_i n_k, \tag{4.25}$$

where $\bar{R}_{\overset{*}{n}}$, $\overset{*}{H}$ satisfy equations (4.21) and (4.22), respectively. Projections of $\bar{\Phi}^s$ on $\{\overset{*}{\overline{n}}, \overset{*}{\overline{\tau}}, \overset{*}{\overline{m}}\}$ are given by

$$\overset{*}{\overline{n}}\Phi^s_{\overset{*}{n}} + \overset{*}{\overline{\tau}}\Phi^s_{\overset{*}{\tau}} + \overset{*}{\overline{m}}\Phi^s_{\overset{*}{m}} = \bar{R}_{\overset{*}{n}} - \frac{\partial \overset{*}{H}\overset{*}{\overline{m}}}{\partial \overset{*}{s}}.$$

The scalar product of the above by $\overset{*}{\overline{n}}$, $\overset{*}{\overline{\tau}}$, and $\overset{*}{\overline{m}}$ yields

$$\Phi^s_{\overset{*}{n}} = T_{\overset{*}{n}} - \overset{*}{\overline{n}}\overset{*}{H}\frac{\partial\overset{*}{\overline{m}}}{\partial\overset{*}{s}}, \qquad \Phi^s_{\overset{*}{\tau}} = T_{\overset{**}{n\tau}} - \overset{*}{\overline{\tau}}\overset{*}{H}\frac{\partial\overset{*}{\overline{m}}}{\partial\overset{*}{s}}, \qquad \Phi^s_{\overset{*}{m}} = N_{\overset{*}{n}} - \frac{\partial\overset{*}{H}}{\partial\overset{*}{s}}.$$

Here use is made of $\overset{*}{\overline{n}}\overset{*}{\overline{m}} = \overset{*}{\overline{\tau}}\overset{*}{\overline{m}} = \overset{*}{\overline{m}}\partial\overset{*}{\overline{m}}/\partial\overset{*}{s} = 0$. Since

$$\overline{m}^*_i = A^*_i(\bar{e}^*_1 k^*_{1i} + \bar{e}^*_2 k^*_{2i}), \qquad A^*_i \frac{\partial\alpha_i}{\partial s_*} = \tau^*_i, \tag{4.26}$$

for derivative $\partial\overset{*}{\overline{m}}/\partial\overset{*}{s}$ we have

$$\begin{aligned}\frac{\partial\overset{*}{\overline{m}}}{\partial\overset{*}{s}} &= \overset{*}{\overline{m}}_1\frac{\partial\alpha_1}{\partial\overset{*}{s}} + \overset{*}{\overline{m}}_2 \frac{\partial\alpha_2}{\partial\overset{*}{s}} \\ &= \sum_{i=1}^{2}\sum_{j=1}^{2} \overset{*}{A}_i\overset{*}{\bar{e}}_j\overset{*}{k}_{ij}\frac{\partial\alpha_i}{\partial s_*} = \sum_{i=1}^{2}\sum_{j=1}^{2} \overset{*}{\bar{e}}_j\overset{*}{k}_{ij}\overset{*}{\tau}_i.\end{aligned}$$

The scalar products of $\partial\overset{*}{\overline{m}}/\partial\overset{*}{s}$ by $\overset{*}{\overline{n}}$ and $\overset{*}{\overline{\tau}}$ are found to be

$$\begin{aligned}\overset{*}{\overline{n}}\frac{\partial\overset{*}{\overline{m}}}{\partial\overset{*}{s}} &= \sum_{i=1}^{2}\sum_{j=1}^{2}\left(\overset{*}{\overline{n}}\overset{*}{\bar{e}}_j\right)\overset{*}{k}_{ij}\overset{*}{\tau}_i = \overset{*}{k}_{n\tau} \\ \overset{*}{\overline{\tau}}\frac{\partial\overset{*}{\overline{m}}}{\partial\overset{*}{s}} &= \sum_{i=1}^{2}\sum_{j=1}^{2}\left(\overset{*}{\overline{\tau}}\overset{*}{\bar{e}}_j\right)\overset{*}{k}_{ij}\overset{*}{\tau}_i = \overset{*}{k}_{\tau},\end{aligned} \tag{4.27}$$

where use is made of approximations given by equation (4.12). Applying equation (4.27) in (4.23), boundary conditions are found to be

$$\Phi^s_{\overset{*}{n}} = T_{\overset{*}{n}} - \overset{*}{H}k^*_{n\tau}, \quad \Phi^s_{\overset{*}{\tau}} = T_{\overset{**}{n\tau}} - \overset{**}{H}k_\tau,$$
$$\Phi^s_{\overset{*}{m}} = N_{\overset{*}{n}} - \frac{\partial \overset{*}{H}}{\partial \overset{*}{s}} \approx N_{\overset{*}{n}} - \frac{\partial \overset{*}{H}}{\partial s}, \quad \overset{*}{G^s} \approx \sum_{i=1}^{2}\sum_{k=1}^{2} \overset{*}{M}_{ik}n_i n_k. \qquad (4.28)$$

In the above it is assumed that $d\overset{*}{s} \approx ds$. Equation (4.28) contain nonlinearities that are introduced by $\overset{*}{k}_{n\tau}$, $\overset{*}{k}_\tau$ and projections of the external load vector $\bar{\Phi}^s$. For example, if φ is the angle between the positive orientation of the α_1-axis and the vector $\bar{n}$, then the projections of $\bar{n}$ and $\bar{\tau}$ on the undeformed contour of the shell are given by

$$\tau_1 = -n_2 = -\sin\varphi, \quad \tau_2 = n_1 = \cos\varphi. \qquad (4.29)$$

Given below are some commonly used boundary conditions.

1. Clamped edge:

$$u_n = u_\tau = \omega = 0, \quad \frac{\partial\omega}{\partial n} = 0, \qquad (4.30)$$

   where u_n is the projection of the displacement vector $\bar{v}$ on the vector $\bar{n}$ perpendicular to the contour $C \in \Sigma$, $u\tau$ is the projection of $\bar{v}$ on the vector $\bar{\tau}$, and ω is the normal displacement (deflection),

$$u_n = \bar{v}\bar{n} = u_1 n_1 + u_2 n_2, \quad u_n = \bar{v}\bar{\tau} = u_1\tau_1 + u_2\tau_2.$$

   The last condition in equation (4.30) implies that the rotation about the vector $\bar{\tau}$ equals zero: $\bar{n}\overset{*}{\bar{m}} = 0$.

2. Simply supported edge:

$$u_n = u_\tau = \omega = 0, \quad \overset{*}{G^s} = \sum_{i=1}^{2}\sum_{k=1}^{2} \overset{*}{M}_{ik}\overset{*}{n}_i\overset{*}{n}_k \approx \sum_{i=1}^{2}\sum_{k=1}^{2} \overset{*}{M}_{ik}n_i n_k = 0, \qquad (4.31)$$

   where $\overset{*}{G^s}$ is the bending moment.

3. Freely supported edge with a single degree of freedom in the normal direction:

$$u_n = u_\tau = 0, \quad \overset{*}{G^s} = 0, \quad N_{\overset{*}{n}} - \frac{\partial \overset{*}{H}}{\partial \overset{*}{s}} \approx N_{\overset{*}{n}} - \frac{\partial \overset{*}{H}}{\partial s} = 0. \qquad (4.32)$$

4. Free edge:

$$\overset{*}{T}_{\overset{*}{n}} - \overset{*}{H}\overset{*}{k}_{n\tau} = 0, \quad \overset{*}{T}_{\overset{**}{n\tau}} - \overset{*}{H}\overset{*}{k}_{\tau} = 0,$$
$$N_{\overset{*}{n}} - \frac{\partial \overset{*}{H}}{\partial \overset{*}{s}} \approx N_{\overset{*}{n}} - \frac{\partial \overset{*}{H}}{\partial s} = 0, \tag{4.33}$$
$$\sum_{i=1}^{2}\sum_{k=1}^{2} \overset{*}{M}_{ik}\overset{*}{n}_i\overset{*}{n}_k \approx \sum_{i=1}^{2}\sum_{k=1}^{2} \overset{*}{M}_{ik}n_in_k = 0,$$

where the meaning of parameters is as above.

4.4 Deformations of the edge

Consider deformations of a line element on $d\Sigma$. Assume that it is orthogonal to the undeformed middle surface S of the shell. Tangents ε_n, ε_τ, bending $æ_n$, deformation $æ_\tau$, shear $\varepsilon_{n\tau}$, and twist $æ_{n\tau}$ of the edge of the shell are defined by

$$\varepsilon_n = \sum_{i=1}^{2}\sum_{k=1}^{2} \varepsilon_{ik}n_in_k, \quad \varepsilon_\tau = \sum_{i=1}^{2}\sum_{k=1}^{2} \varepsilon_{ik}\tau_i\tau_k, \quad \varepsilon_{n\tau} = \sum_{i=1}^{2}\sum_{k=1}^{2} \varepsilon_{ik}\tau_in_k, \tag{4.34}$$

$$æ_n = \sum_{i=1}^{2}\sum_{k=1}^{2} æ_{ik}n_in_k, \quad æ_\tau = \sum_{i=1}^{2}\sum_{k=1}^{2} æ_{ik}\tau_i\tau_k, \quad æ_{n\tau} = \sum_{i=1}^{2}\sum_{k=1}^{2} æ_{ik}\tau_in_k \tag{4.35}$$

where n_1, n_2 satisfy equation (4.29).

Applying equation (4.34) and expressions for the Lamé parameters

$$\overset{*}{A}_i^2 = A_i^2(1 + 2\varepsilon_{ii}), \quad \overset{*}{A}_1\overset{*}{A}_2 \cos\overset{*}{\chi} = 2\varepsilon_{12}A_1A_2, \quad \tau_i ds = A_i d\alpha_i,$$

the length of a line element $d\overset{*}{s}$ on $\overset{*}{C}$ is given by

$$(d\overset{*}{s})^2 = \overset{*}{A}_1^2 d\alpha_1{}^2 + 2\overset{*}{A}_1\overset{*}{A}_2 \cos\overset{*}{\chi}\, d\alpha_1 d\alpha_2 + \overset{*}{A}_2^2 d\alpha_2{}^2 = (1 + 2\varepsilon_\tau)ds^2. \tag{4.36}$$

Unit vectors $\overset{*}{\bar{\tau}}$ and $\bar{\tau}$ are given by

$$\overset{*}{\bar{\tau}} = \frac{d\overset{*}{\bar{r}}}{d\overset{*}{s}} = \frac{d\overset{*}{\bar{r}}}{ds}\frac{ds}{d\overset{*}{s}} = \left(\bar{\tau} + \frac{d\bar{v}}{ds}\right)\Big/\sqrt{1 + 2\varepsilon_\tau}, \quad \bar{\tau} = \frac{d\bar{r}}{ds}, \tag{4.37}$$

where use is made of equation (4.35).

The vector $\overset{*}{\overline{m}}$ normal to the surface $\overset{*}{S}$ is found from

$$\overset{*}{\overline{m}} = \left(\overset{*}{\overline{r}}_1 \times \overset{*}{\overline{r}}_2\right) \Big/ \sqrt{\overset{*}{a}}, \tag{4.38}$$

where $\overset{*}{a}$ is the invariant of the first fundamental form given by

$$\overset{*}{a} = (A_1 A_2)^2 \mathfrak{A}, \quad \mathfrak{A} = 1 + 2(\varepsilon_n + \varepsilon_\tau) + 4(\varepsilon_n \varepsilon_\tau - \varepsilon_{n\tau}^2). \tag{4.39}$$

Derivatives of the displacement vector in the direction of $\overline{n}$ and $\overline{\tau}$ are

$$\frac{d\overline{v}}{ds} = \frac{\overline{\tau}_1}{A_1}\frac{d\overline{v}}{d\alpha_1} + \frac{\overline{\tau}_2}{A_2}\frac{d\overline{v}}{d\alpha_2}, \quad \frac{d\overline{v}}{ds_n} = \frac{n_1}{A_1}\frac{d\overline{v}}{d\alpha_1} + \frac{n_2}{A_2}\frac{d\overline{v}}{d\alpha_2}. \tag{4.40}$$

Here s and s_n are the lengths of line elements on C and C_n, such that $C_n \perp C$, and $\overline{\tau} = \frac{d\overline{r}}{ds}$, $\overline{n} = \frac{d\overline{r}}{ds_n}$. Solving equation (4.40) for $d\overline{v}/d\alpha_i$ we find

$$\frac{1}{A_i}\frac{d\overline{v}}{d\alpha_i} = \tau_i \frac{d\overline{v}}{ds} + n_i \frac{d\overline{v}}{ds_n}. \tag{4.41}$$

Since $\overline{e}_i = \overline{\tau}\tau_i + \overline{n}n_i$, from equation (3.41) for vectors $\overset{*}{\overline{r}}_i$, we obtain

$$\overset{*}{\overline{r}}_i = \overset{*}{\overline{r}} + \frac{d\overline{v}}{d\alpha_i} = A_i\left(\overline{e}_i + \frac{1}{A_i}\frac{d\overline{v}}{ds}\right) = A_i(\underline{a}\tau_i + \underline{b}n_i). \tag{4.42}$$

Here we have introduced the following notations

$$\underline{a} = \frac{d\overset{*}{\overline{r}}}{ds} = \overline{\tau} + \frac{d\overline{v}}{ds}, \quad \underline{b} = \frac{d\overset{*}{\overline{r}}}{ds_n} = \overline{n} + \frac{d\overline{v}}{ds_n}. \tag{4.43}$$

Substituting equation (4.42) into (4.38), we obtain

$$\overset{*}{\overline{m}} = (b \times a)/\sqrt{\mathfrak{A}} = \left\{\overline{m} + \left(\overline{n} \times \frac{d\overline{v}}{ds}\right) + \left(\frac{d\overline{v}}{ds_n} \times \overline{\tau}\right) + \left(\frac{d\overline{v}}{ds_n} \times \frac{d\overline{v}}{ds}\right)\right\} \Big/ \sqrt{\mathfrak{A}}. \tag{4.44}$$

Using equation (4.42) and equality $\overline{r}_i = A_i(\overline{\tau}\tau_i + \overline{n}n_i)$, from $2A_i A_k \varepsilon_{ik} = \overset{*}{\overline{r}}_i \overset{*}{\overline{r}}_k - \overline{r}_i\overline{r}_k$ (see equations (1.67)) for deformation on the edge of the shell we have

$$2\varepsilon_{ik} = (\underline{a}\tau_i + \underline{b}n_i)(\underline{a}\tau_k + \underline{b}n_k) - (\overline{\tau}\tau_i + \overline{n}n_i)(\overline{\tau}\tau_k + \overline{n}n_k). \tag{4.45}$$

Further, with the help of equation (4.45) from equation (4.34), we obtain

$$\begin{aligned} \varepsilon_n &= \overline{n}\frac{d\overline{v}}{ds_n} + \frac{1}{2}\left(\frac{d\overline{v}}{ds_n}\right)^2, \quad \varepsilon_\tau = \overline{\tau}\frac{d\overline{v}}{ds_n} + \frac{1}{2}\left(\frac{d\overline{v}}{ds_n}\right)^2, \\ 2\varepsilon_{n\tau} &= \overline{n}\frac{d\overline{v}}{ds_n} + \overline{\tau}\frac{d\overline{v}}{ds_n} + \frac{d\overline{v}}{ds}\frac{d\overline{v}}{ds_n}, \end{aligned} \tag{4.46}$$

where use is made of the facts $\overline{n} \perp \overline{\tau}$, $n^2{}_1 + n^2{}_2 = \tau^2{}_1 + \tau^2{}_2 = 1$.

To express the vector $\overset{*}{\bar{n}}$ in terms of the displacements, we substitute $\overset{*}{\bar{\tau}}, \overset{*}{\bar{m}}$ given by equations (4.37) and (4.44) into equality $\overset{*}{\bar{n}} = \overset{*}{\bar{\tau}} \times \overset{*}{\bar{m}}$. After simple algebra we find

$$\overset{*}{\bar{n}}\sqrt{\mathfrak{A}(1 + 2\varepsilon_\tau)} = (1 + 2\varepsilon_\tau)\underline{b} - 2\varepsilon_{n\tau} \cdot \underline{a}. \tag{4.47}$$

To decompose the right-hand sides of equation (4.46) in the base $\{\bar{n}, \bar{\tau}, \bar{m}\}$ we proceed from the formulas for derivatives of $\bar{n}, \bar{\tau}, \bar{m}$ with respect to s and s_n, given by

$$\frac{d\bar{n}}{ds} = æ\bar{\tau} - \bar{m}k_{n\tau}, \quad \frac{d\bar{\tau}}{ds} = -\bar{m}k_\tau - æ\bar{n}, \quad \frac{d\bar{m}}{ds} = \bar{n}k_{n\tau} + \bar{\tau}k_\tau, \tag{4.48}$$

$$\frac{d\bar{n}}{ds_n} = -\bar{m}k_\tau - æ'\bar{\tau}, \quad \frac{d\bar{\tau}}{ds_n} = æ'\bar{n} - \bar{m}k_{n\tau}, \quad \frac{d\bar{m}}{ds_n} = \bar{\tau}k_{n\tau} + \bar{n}k_n. \tag{4.49}$$

Here $k_n, k_\tau, k_{n\tau}$ satisfy equation (4.7) and

$$\begin{aligned} k_n &= \bar{n}\frac{d\bar{\tau}}{ds_n} = -\bar{\tau}\frac{d\bar{n}}{ds_n}, \quad k_\tau = \bar{\tau}\frac{d\bar{m}}{ds_n} = -\bar{m}\frac{d\bar{\tau}}{ds_n}, \\ k_{n\tau} &= \bar{n}\frac{d\bar{m}}{ds_n} = -\bar{m}\frac{d\bar{n}}{ds_n}. \end{aligned} \tag{4.50}$$

$æ, æ'$ are the geodesic curvatures of the contour lines C, C_n ($C_n \perp C$) are described by

$$æ = \bar{\tau}\frac{d\bar{n}}{ds} = -\bar{n}\frac{d\bar{\tau}}{ds}, \quad æ' = \bar{\tau}\frac{d\bar{n}}{ds_n} = -\bar{n}\frac{d\bar{\tau}}{ds_n}, \tag{4.51}$$

or in the expanded form

$$\begin{aligned} æ &= \frac{d\varphi}{ds} + \frac{\cos\varphi}{A_1A_2}\frac{\partial A_2}{\partial\alpha_1} + \frac{\sin\varphi}{A_1A_2}\frac{\partial A_1}{\partial\alpha_2}, \\ æ' &= -\frac{d\varphi}{ds_n} - \frac{\sin\varphi}{A_1A_2}\frac{\partial A_2}{\partial\alpha_1} + \frac{\cos\varphi}{A_1A_2}\frac{\partial A_1}{\partial\alpha_2}. \end{aligned} \tag{4.52}$$

Expanding the displacement vector $\bar{v}$ along the base $\{\bar{n}, \bar{\tau}, \bar{m}\}$

$$\bar{v} = \bar{n}u_n + \bar{\tau}u_\tau + \bar{m}\omega, \tag{4.53}$$

and differentiating equation (4.53) with respect to s and s_n, we find

$$\frac{d\bar{v}}{ds} = \bar{n}e_{\tau n} + \bar{\tau}e_{\tau\tau} + \bar{m}\omega_\tau, \quad \frac{d\bar{v}}{ds_n} = \bar{n}e_{nn} + \bar{\tau}e_{n\tau} + \bar{m}\omega_n. \tag{4.54}$$

Here $e_{nn}, e_{n\tau}, e_{n\tau}, e_{\tau n}, \omega_n, \omega_\tau$ are the rotation angles given by

$$e_{\tau n} = \frac{du_n}{ds} - æu_\tau + \varpi k_{n\tau}, \quad e_{\tau\tau} = \frac{du_\tau}{ds} + æu_n + \varpi k_\tau, \tag{4.55}$$

$$e_{nn} = \frac{du_n}{ds_n} + \ae' u_\tau + \varpi k_n, \qquad e_{n\tau} = \frac{du_\tau}{ds_n} - \ae' u_n + \varpi k_{n\tau},$$
$$\omega_\tau = \frac{d\varpi}{ds} - k_{n\tau} u_n - k_\tau u_\tau, \qquad \omega_n = \frac{d\varpi}{ds_n} - k_n u_n - k_{n\tau} u_\tau. \tag{4.56}$$

In the above, use is made of equations (4.48) and (4.49). Substituting equation (4.54) into equation (4.44), we have

$$\overset{*}{\overline{m}}\sqrt{\mathfrak{A}} = \overline{n}\mathbb{S}_n + \overline{\tau}\mathbb{S}_\tau + \overline{m}\mathbb{S}_3, \tag{4.57}$$

where

$$\begin{aligned} \mathbb{S}_n &= \omega_\tau e_{n\tau} - \omega_n (1 + e_{\tau\tau}), \\ \mathbb{S}_\tau &= \omega_n e_{\tau n} - \omega_\tau (1 + e_{nn}), \\ \mathbb{S}_3 &= (1 + e_{\tau\tau})(1 + e_{nn}) - e_{\tau n} e_{n\tau}. \end{aligned} \tag{4.58}$$

Let $\overset{*}{k}_n$, $\overset{*}{k}_\tau$, $\overset{*}{k}_{n\tau}$ be the curvature and twist of the contour $\overset{*}{C}$ (see equation (4.13))

$$\begin{aligned} \overset{*}{k}_n &= \sum_{i=1}^{2}\sum_{j=1}^{2} \overset{*}{k}_{ij} n_i n_j = \underline{b}\frac{d\overset{*}{\overline{m}}}{ds_n} = -\overset{*}{\overline{m}}\frac{d\underline{b}}{ds_n}, \\ \overset{*}{k}_\tau &= \sum_{i=1}^{2}\sum_{j=1}^{2} \overset{*}{k}_{ij} \tau_i \tau_j = \underline{a}\frac{d\overset{*}{\overline{m}}}{ds} = -\overset{*}{\overline{m}}\frac{d\underline{a}}{ds}, \\ \overset{*}{k}_{n\tau} &= \sum_{i=1}^{2}\sum_{j=1}^{2} \overset{*}{k}_{ij} \tau_i n_j = \underline{b}\frac{d\overset{*}{\overline{m}}}{ds} = -\overset{*}{\overline{m}}_i\frac{d\underline{b}}{ds}. \end{aligned} \tag{4.59}$$

Using equation (4.59), the bending deformation of the shell boundary is found to be

$$\ae_n = \overset{*}{k}_n - k_n = \overline{m}\frac{d\overline{n}}{ds_n} - \overset{*}{\overline{m}}\frac{d\underline{b}}{ds_n}, \qquad \ae_\tau = \overline{m}\frac{d\overline{\tau}}{ds} - \overset{*}{\overline{m}}\frac{d\underline{a}}{ds},$$
$$\ae_{n\tau} = \overline{m}\frac{d\overline{n}}{ds} - \overset{*}{\overline{m}}\frac{d\underline{b}}{ds}. \tag{4.60}$$

Curvatures of $\overset{*}{C}$ are calculated as

$$\begin{aligned} \overset{*}{k}{}_\tau^{*} &= -\overset{*}{\overline{m}}\frac{d\overset{*}{\overline{\tau}}}{d\overset{*}{s}} = -\frac{\overset{*}{\overline{m}}}{\sqrt{(1 + 2\varepsilon_\tau)}}\frac{d\overset{*}{\overline{\tau}}}{d\overset{*}{s}}, \\ \overset{*}{k}{}_{n\tau}^{**} &= -\overset{*}{\overline{m}}\frac{d\overset{*}{\overline{n}}}{d\overset{*}{s}} = -\frac{\overset{*}{\overline{m}}}{\sqrt{(1 + 2\varepsilon_\tau)}}\frac{d\overset{*}{\overline{n}}}{d\overset{*}{s}}. \end{aligned} \tag{4.61}$$

Substituting $\overset{*}{\overline{\tau}}$ and $\overset{*}{\overline{n}}$ given by equations (4.37) and (4.47) into (4.61) and recalling the fact that $\overset{*}{\overline{m}}\underline{a} = \overset{*}{\overline{m}}\underline{b} = 0$, we obtain

$$\overset{*}{k}{}_{\tau}^{*} = -\frac{\overset{*}{k}_{\tau}}{\sqrt{(1 + 2\varepsilon_{\tau})}}, \quad \overset{*}{k}{}_{n\tau}^{**} = -\frac{(\overset{*}{k}_{n\tau} + 2\overset{*}{k}_{n\tau}\varepsilon_{\tau} - 2\overset{*}{k}_{\tau}\varepsilon_{n\tau})}{\sqrt{\mathfrak{A}(1 + 2\varepsilon_{\tau})}}. \tag{4.62}$$

Here $\overset{*}{k}_{\tau} = k_{\tau} + æ_{\tau}$, $\overset{*}{k}_{n\tau} = k_{n\tau} + æ_{n\tau}$ and satisfy equation (4.59).

4.5 Equations of Gauss–Codazzi for the boundary

As a final point of this discussion, the Gauss–Codazzi equations for the undeformed boundary of the thin shell are derived. For the integral of a vector (scalar) function $f(\alpha_1, \alpha_2)$ to exist, the following should hold:

$$\frac{\partial}{\partial s_n}\left(\frac{\partial f}{\partial s}\right) - \frac{\partial}{\partial s}\left(\frac{\partial}{\partial s_n}\right) = æ'\frac{\partial f}{\partial s_n} - æ\frac{\partial f}{\partial s}. \tag{4.63}$$

Substituting vector $\bar{m}$ ($\bar{m} \perp S$) for f and using equations (4.48) and (4.49), we obtain

$$\frac{\partial}{\partial s_n}(\bar{n}k_{n\tau} + \bar{\tau}k_{\tau}) - \frac{\partial}{\partial s}(\bar{\tau}k_{n\tau} + \bar{n}k_n) = æ'(\bar{\tau}k_{n\tau} + \bar{n}k_n) - æ(\bar{n}k_{n\tau} + \bar{\tau}k_{\tau}). \tag{4.64}$$

Carrying differentiation (4.64) and equating the coefficients of $\bar{n}$, $\bar{\tau}$, and $\bar{m}$ to zero, the Codazzi formulas are found to be

$$\begin{aligned} \frac{\partial k_{n\tau}}{\partial s_n} - \frac{\partial k_n}{\partial s} + æ'(k_{\tau} - k_n) + 2æk_{n\tau} = 0, \\ \frac{\partial k_{\tau}}{\partial s_n} - \frac{\partial k_{n\tau}}{\partial s} + æ(k_{\tau} - k_n) - 2æ'k_{n\tau} = 0. \end{aligned} \tag{4.65}$$

Similarly, substituting $\bar{\tau}$ for f, we find

$$-\frac{\partial}{\partial s_n}(\bar{m}k_{\tau} + æ\bar{n}) - \frac{\partial}{\partial s}(æ'\bar{n} - \bar{m}k_{n\tau}) = æ'(\bar{n}æ' - \bar{m}k_{n\tau}) + æ(\bar{m}k_{\tau} + \bar{n}æ),$$

from where after differentiation and setting to zero the coefficients of $\bar{n}$, we obtain the Gauss formula

$$\frac{\partial æ}{\partial s_n} - \frac{\partial æ'}{\partial s} + æ'^2 + æ^2 = k_{n\tau}^2 + k_n k_{\tau}. \tag{4.66}$$

If the coefficients of $\bar{m}$ to zero are equated, the Codazzi formulas are obtained once again. Formulas (4.63)–(4.66) can also be expressed in terms of the deformed boundary of the shell.

Further reading

Galimov K Z 1975 *Foundations of the Nonlinear Theory of Thin Shells* (Kazan: Kazan University Press)

IOP Publishing

Soft Biological Shells in Bioengineering

Roustem N Miftahof and Nariman R Akhmadeev

Chapter 5

Soft shells

This chapter presents the basics of the theory of the dynamics of soft shells. A special class of soft shells, structurally related to nets, is considered and the governing system of equations in the general curvilinear and special coordinates are derived.

5.1 Deformation of a soft shell

A class of thin shells, $h/L \sim 10^{-5}$–10^{-2}, in which h is thickness and L is the characteristic dimension of a shell:

(i) possesses low resistance to stretching and zero-order flexural rigidity;
(ii) undergoes finite deformations;
(iii) can withstand only stretch but not compression forces;
(iv) have an actual configuration defined by internal/external loads per unit surface area only;
(v) have stress–strain states fully described by in-plane membrane forces per unit length.

Such shells are known as soft shells. Soft shells acquire multiple forms in the absence of loads. Therefore it is instructive to consider the cut configuration $\overset{0}{S}$ of the shell, in addition to the undeformed S and deformed $\overset{*}{S}$ configurations (figure 5.1). This defines the configuration of bending in the absence of loads with more accuracy.

Assume that the middle surface S of an undeformed soft shell coincides with its cut surface $\overset{0}{S}$ ($\overset{0}{S} \equiv S$). Let S be parameterized by curvilinear coordinates α_1, α_2. A point $M(\alpha_1, \alpha_2) \in S$ is described by the position vector $\bar{r}(\alpha_1, \alpha_2)$. In response to the action of external and/or internal loads the shell will deform to attain a new configuration $\overset{*}{S}$. It is assumed that the deformation is such that $\forall\ M(\alpha_1, \alpha_2) \to \overset{*}{M}(\overset{*}{\alpha}_1, \overset{*}{\alpha}_2)$ and is a homeomorphism. Thus, the inverse transformation exists.

doi:10.1088/2053-2563/ab1a9ech5

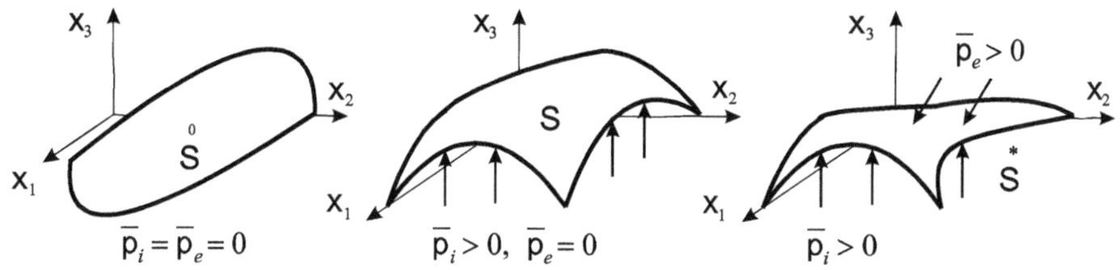

Figure 5.1. Definition of the cut (ironed out), initial (undeformed), and actual (deformed) configurations of the soft shell.

Deformation of linear elements along the α_1, α_2-coordinate lines is described by stretch ratios λ_i ($i = 1, 2$) and elongations $e_{\alpha i}$ given by equations (1.68) and (2.3), respectively,

$$e_{\alpha i} = \frac{d\overset{*}{s}_i - ds_i}{ds_i} = \lambda_i - 1 = \frac{\sqrt{\overset{*}{a}_{ii}}}{\sqrt{a_{ii}}} - 1. \tag{5.1}$$

Changes in the angle between coordinate lines and the surface area are described by equations (1.69) and (2.4) or in equivalent form

$$\gamma = \overset{(0)}{\chi} - \overset{*}{\chi} = \overset{(0)}{\chi} - \cos^{-1}\frac{a_{12}}{\sqrt{a_{11}a_{22}}} \tag{5.2}$$

$$\delta s_\Delta = \frac{d\overset{*}{s}_\Delta}{ds_\Delta} = \frac{\sqrt{\overset{*}{a}}}{\sqrt{a}} = \frac{\sqrt{\overset{*}{a}_{11}\overset{*}{a}_{22}}\,\sin\overset{*}{\chi}}{\sqrt{a_{11}a_{22}}\,\sin\overset{(0)}{\chi}} = \lambda_1\lambda_2\frac{\sin\overset{*}{\chi}}{\sin\overset{(0)}{\chi}}. \tag{5.3}$$

In the above use is made of equations (1.4), (1.12), and (2.3).

Vectors $\bar{r}_i$ and $\overset{*}{\bar{r}}_i$ tangent to coordinate lines on S and $\overset{*}{S}$ are defined by equations (1.3) and (1.4). Making use of equations (2.3) and (2.4), we have

$$\bar{r}_i = \sum_{k=1}^{2} C_i^k \overset{*}{\bar{r}}_k, \quad \overset{*}{\bar{r}}_i = \sum_{k=1}^{2} \overset{*}{C}{}_i^k \bar{r}_k. \tag{5.4}$$

Hence, the unit vectors $\bar{e}_i \in S$, $\overset{*}{\bar{e}}_i \in \overset{*}{S}$ are found to be

$$\begin{aligned} \bar{e}_i &= \frac{\bar{r}_i}{|\bar{r}_i|} = \frac{\bar{r}_i}{\sqrt{a_{ii}}} = \sum_{k=1}^{2} C_i^k\left(\overset{*}{\bar{r}}_k\sqrt{\frac{a_{ii}}{\overset{*}{a}_{kk}}}\right) = \sum_{k=1}^{2} \hat{C}_i^k \overset{*}{\bar{e}}_k, \\ \overset{*}{\bar{e}}_i &= \sum_{k=1}^{2} \hat{C}_i^k \bar{e}_k, \end{aligned} \tag{5.5}$$

where the following notations are introduced

$$\hat{C}_i^{\,k} = C_i^k \sqrt{\frac{\overset{*}{a}_{kk}}{a_{ii}}}, \quad \overset{*}{\hat{C}}{}_i^{\,k} = \overset{*}{C}{}_i^k \sqrt{\frac{a_{kk}}{\overset{*}{a}_{ii}}}. \tag{5.6}$$

With the help of equation (5.6), the scalar and vector products of unit vectors $\overset{*}{\bar{e}}_i$ and $\overset{*}{\bar{e}}_k$ are found to be

$$\begin{aligned} \overset{*}{\bar{e}}_i \cdot \overset{*}{\bar{e}}_k &:= \cos \overset{*}{\chi}_{ik} = \sum_{j=1}^{2}\sum_{n=1}^{2} \bar{e}_j \cdot \bar{e}_n \overset{*}{\hat{C}}{}_i^{\,j} \overset{*}{\hat{C}}{}_k^{\,n} \\ &= \sum_{j=1}^{2}\sum_{n=1}^{2} \overset{*}{\hat{C}}{}_i^{\,j} \overset{*}{\hat{C}}{}_k^{\,n} \cos \overset{(0)}{\chi}_{jn}, \\ \overset{*}{\bar{e}}_i \times \overset{*}{\bar{e}}_k &:= \overset{*}{\bar{m}} \sin \overset{*}{\chi}_{ik} = \sum_{j=1}^{2}\sum_{n=1}^{2} \bar{e}_j \times \bar{e}_n \overset{*}{\hat{C}}{}_i^{\,j} \overset{*}{\hat{C}}{}_k^{\,n} \\ &= \sum_{j=1}^{2}\sum_{n=1}^{2} \overset{*}{\hat{C}}{}_i^{\,j} \overset{*}{\hat{C}}{}_k^{\,n} \overset{*}{\bar{m}} \sin \overset{(0)}{\chi}_{jn}. \end{aligned} \tag{5.7}$$

In just the same way, proceeding from the scalar and vector multiplication of $\bar{e}_i$ by $\bar{e}_k$, it can be shown that

$$\begin{aligned} \cos \overset{(0)}{\chi}_{ik} &= \sum_{j=1}^{2}\sum_{n=1}^{2} \hat{C}_i^{\,j} \hat{C}_k^{\,n} \cos \overset{*}{\chi}_{jn}, \\ \sin \overset{(0)}{\chi}_{ik} &= \sum_{j=1}^{2}\sum_{n=1}^{2} \hat{C}_i^{\,j} \hat{C}_k^{\,n} \sin \overset{*}{\chi}_{jn}. \end{aligned} \tag{5.8}$$

To calculate the coefficients C_i^k, $\overset{*}{\hat{C}}{}_i^{\,k}$, we proceed from geometric considerations. Let vectors $\bar{e}_i$, $\overset{*}{\bar{e}}_i$ at point $\overset{*}{M}(\overset{*}{\alpha}_1, \overset{*}{\alpha}_2) \in \overset{*}{S}$ be oriented as shown (figure 5.2). Decomposing $\overset{*}{\bar{e}}_i$ in the directions of $\bar{e}_k$, we have

$$\overset{*}{\hat{C}}{}_1^{\,1} = \overline{MC}, \quad \overset{*}{\hat{C}}{}_1^{\,2} = \overline{CD}, \quad \overset{*}{\hat{C}}{}_2^{\,1} = -\overline{AB}, \quad \overset{*}{\hat{C}}{}_2^{\,2} = \overline{MB}. \tag{5.9}$$

Solving ΔMCD and ΔMBA, we find

$$\begin{aligned} &\overset{*}{\hat{C}}{}_1^{\,1} = \sin\left(\overset{*}{\chi} - \overset{*}{\chi}_2\right) \Big/ \sin \overset{*}{\chi}, \qquad \overset{*}{\hat{C}}{}_1^{\,2} = \sin \overset{*}{\chi}_2 \Big/ \sin \overset{*}{\chi}, \\ &\overset{*}{\hat{C}}{}_2^{\,1} = -\sin\left(\overset{*}{\chi}_1 + \overset{*}{\chi}_2 - \overset{*}{\chi}\right) \Big/ \sin \overset{*}{\chi}, \; \overset{*}{\hat{C}}{}_2^{\,2} = \sin\left(\overset{*}{\chi}_1 + \overset{*}{\chi}_2\right) \Big/ \sin \overset{*}{\chi}, \\ &\overset{*}{\hat{C}} = \det \overset{*}{\hat{C}}{}_i^{\,k} = \sin \overset{*}{\chi}_2 \Big/ \sin \overset{*}{\chi}. \end{aligned} \tag{5.10}$$

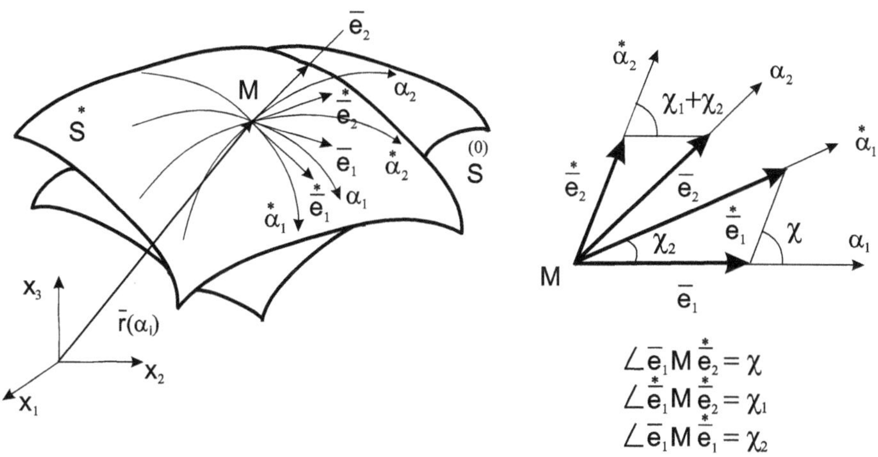

Figure 5.2. Deformation of an element of the soft shell.

Similarly, expanding unit vectors $\bar{e}_i$ along $\overset{*}{\bar{e}}_k$, we obtain

$$\begin{aligned} &\hat{C}_1^1 = \sin\left(\overset{0}{\chi}_1 + \overset{0}{\chi}_2\right)\Big/\sin\overset{0}{\chi}_1, \qquad \hat{C}_1^2 = -\sin\overset{0}{\chi}_2\Big/\sin\overset{0}{\chi}_1, \\ &\hat{C}_2^1 = \sin\left(\overset{0}{\chi}_1 + \overset{0}{\chi}_2 - \overset{0}{\chi}\right)\Big/\sin\overset{0}{\chi}_1, \hat{C}_2^2 = \sin\left(\overset{0}{\chi} - \overset{0}{\chi}_2\right)\Big/\sin\overset{0}{\chi}_1, \\ &\hat{C} = \det\hat{C}_i^k = \sin\overset{0}{\chi}\Big/\sin\overset{0}{\chi}_1. \end{aligned} \tag{5.11}$$

Note, that the coefficients C_i^k, $\overset{*}{\hat{C}}_i^k$ are the functions of $\overset{0}{\chi}_i$ and $\overset{*}{\chi}_i$, while $\hat{C}_i^k$, $\overset{*}{\hat{C}}_i^k$ depend on $\bar{r}_i$ and $\overset{*}{\bar{r}}_i$ and the actual configuration of a shell.

Let the cut configuration of a soft shell $\overset{0}{S}$ be different from the undeformed configuration S. We introduce the coefficients of transformation $\bar{r}_i \in \overset{0}{S} \to \overset{*}{S}$ by

$$\hat{\hat{C}}_i^k = C_i^k\sqrt{\frac{\overset{*}{a}_{kk}}{\overset{0}{a}_{ii}}}, \qquad \overset{*}{\hat{\hat{C}}}_i^k = \overset{*}{C}_i^k\sqrt{\frac{\overset{0}{a}_{kk}}{\overset{*}{a}_{ii}}}, \tag{5.12}$$

where $\overset{0}{a}_{ii}$, $\overset{*}{a}_{ii}$ are the components of the metric tensor **A** on $\overset{0}{S}$ and $\overset{*}{S}$, respectively. Eliminating C_i^k, $\overset{*}{C}_i^k$ from equation (5.6), for the coefficients of the cut and deformed surfaces we obtain

$$\hat{C}_i^k = \hat{\hat{C}}_i^k\frac{\overset{*}{\lambda}_k}{\lambda_i}, \qquad \overset{*}{\hat{C}}_i^k = \overset{*}{\hat{\hat{C}}}_i^k\frac{\lambda_k}{\overset{*}{\lambda}_i}. \tag{5.13}$$

By analogy to equations (5.12), we introduce the coefficients

$$\overset{*}{\hat{C}}{}_i^k = \left[\hat{C}_k^i\right] \Big/ \hat{C}, \quad \overset{*}{\hat{\hat{C}}}{}_i^k = \left[\hat{\hat{C}}{}_k^i\right] \Big/ \hat{\hat{C}}, \tag{5.14}$$

where

$$\hat{C} = C\sqrt{\frac{\overset{*}{a}_{11}\overset{*}{a}_{22}}{\overset{0}{a}_{11}\overset{0}{a}_{22}}}, \quad \hat{\hat{C}} = C\sqrt{\frac{\overset{*}{a}_{11}\overset{*}{a}_{22}}{\overset{0}{a}_{11}\overset{0}{a}_{22}}}. \tag{5.15}$$

Finally, from equations (5.12)–(5.15), we obtain

$$\hat{C} = \hat{\hat{C}}\frac{\overset{*}{\lambda}_1\overset{*}{\lambda}_2}{\lambda_1\lambda_2}. \tag{5.16}$$

Let $\mathbf{E}$ be the tensor of deformation of $S(S = \overset{0}{S})$ given by

$$\mathbf{E} = \sum_{i=1}^{2}\sum_{k=1}^{2} \varepsilon_{ik}\bar{r}^i\bar{r}^k, \tag{5.17}$$

where

$$\varepsilon_{ik} = \frac{\overset{*}{a}_{ik} - a_{ik}}{2}. \tag{5.18}$$

Substituting equations (1.4), (2.3) into (5.18) for ε_{ik}, we find

$$\varepsilon_{ik} = \frac{\left(\lambda_i\lambda_k \cos\overset{*}{\chi} - \cos\chi\right)\sqrt{a_{ii}a_{kk}}}{2}. \tag{5.19}$$

It is easy to show that the following relations hold

$$\begin{aligned} \varepsilon_{ik} &= \sum_{j=1}^{2}\sum_{n=1}^{2} \overset{*}{\varepsilon}_{jn} C_i^j C_k^n, \quad & \varepsilon^{ik} &= \sum_{j=1}^{2}\sum_{n=1}^{2} \overset{*}{\varepsilon}{}^{jn} C_j^i C_n^k, \\ \overset{*}{\varepsilon}_{ik} &= \sum_{j=1}^{2}\sum_{n=1}^{2} \varepsilon_{jn} \overset{*}{C}{}_i^j \overset{*}{C}{}_k^n, \quad & \overset{*}{\varepsilon}{}^{ik} &= \sum_{j=1}^{2}\sum_{n=1}^{2} \varepsilon^{jn} C_j^i C_n^k. \end{aligned} \tag{5.20}$$

In the theory of soft thin shells, stretch ratios and membrane forces per unit length of a differential element are preferred to traditional deformations and stresses per unit cross-sectional area of the shell. Thus, dividing equation (5.19) by the surface area $\sqrt{a_{ii}a_{kk}}$ of an element, we obtain

$$\tilde{\varepsilon}_{ik} := \frac{\varepsilon_{ik}}{\sqrt{a_{ii}a_{kk}}} = \frac{\left(\lambda_i\lambda_k \cos\overset{*}{\chi} - \cos\chi\right)}{2}, \tag{5.21}$$

where $\tilde{\varepsilon}_{ik}$ are called the physical components of **E**. Using equation (5.20), for $\overset{*}{\tilde{\varepsilon}}_{ik}$ in terms of the deformed configuration, we obtain

$$\overset{*}{\tilde{\varepsilon}}_{ik} = \sum_{j=1}^{2}\sum_{n=1}^{2} \tilde{\varepsilon}_{jn} \overset{*}{C}_i^j \overset{*}{C}_k^n \frac{\sqrt{a_{jj}a_{nn}}}{\sqrt{\overset{*}{a}_{jj}\overset{*}{a}_{nn}}}, \tag{5.22}$$

where the coefficients $\overset{*}{C}_i^j$ satisfy equations (2.3) and (2.4).

Making use of equation (5.21) in (2.3) and (5.2) for λ_i and γ, we find

$$\begin{aligned} &\lambda_i = 1 + \varepsilon_i = \sqrt{1 + 2\tilde{\varepsilon}_{ii}}, \\ &\gamma = \overset{(0)}{\chi} - \cos^{-1}\frac{2\tilde{\varepsilon}_{12} + \cos\overset{(0)}{\chi}}{\sqrt{(1 + 2\tilde{\varepsilon}_{11})}\sqrt{(1 + 2\tilde{\varepsilon}_{22})}}. \end{aligned} \tag{5.23}$$

Substituting $\hat{C}_i^k$, $\overset{*}{\hat{C}}_i^k$ given by equations (5.12) in (5.22), we have

$$\overset{*}{\tilde{\varepsilon}}_{ik} = \sum_{j=1}^{2}\sum_{n=1}^{2} \tilde{\varepsilon}_{jn} \overset{*}{\hat{C}}_i^j \overset{*}{\hat{C}}_k^n \quad \tilde{\varepsilon}_{ik} = \sum_{j=1}^{2}\sum_{n=1}^{2} \tilde{\varepsilon}_{jn}^m \hat{C}_i^j \hat{C}_k^n. \tag{5.24}$$

Finally, formulas for $\overset{*}{\tilde{\varepsilon}}_{ik}$ in terms of the $\overset{0}{S}$-configuration of the soft shell take the form

$$\begin{aligned} \overset{*}{\tilde{\varepsilon}}_{11} = &\Big[\tilde{\varepsilon}_{11}\sin^2\Big(\overset{0}{\chi} - \overset{0}{\chi}_2\Big) + \tilde{\varepsilon}_{22}\sin^2\overset{0}{\chi}_2 \\ &+ 2\tilde{\varepsilon}_{12}\sin\Big(\overset{0}{\chi} - \overset{0}{\chi}_2\Big)\sin\overset{0}{\chi}_2\Big]\Big/\sin^2\overset{0}{\chi}, \\ \overset{*}{\tilde{\varepsilon}}_{12} = &\Big[-\tilde{\varepsilon}_{11}\sin\Big(\overset{0}{\chi} - \overset{0}{\chi}_2\Big)\sin\Big(\overset{0}{\chi}_1 + \overset{0}{\chi}_2 - \overset{0}{\chi}\Big) + \tilde{\varepsilon}_{22}\sin\overset{0}{\chi}_2\sin\Big(\overset{0}{\chi}_1 + \overset{0}{\chi}_2\Big) \\ &- \tilde{\varepsilon}_{12}\Big(\cos\Big(\overset{0}{\chi}_1 + 2\overset{0}{\chi}_2 - \overset{0}{\chi}\Big) - \cos\overset{0}{\chi}\cos\overset{0}{\chi}_1\Big)\Big]\Big/\sin^2\overset{0}{\chi}, \\ \overset{*}{\tilde{\varepsilon}}_{22} = &\Big[\tilde{\varepsilon}_{11}\sin^2\Big(\overset{0}{\chi}_1 + \overset{0}{\chi}_2 - \overset{0}{\chi}\Big) + \tilde{\varepsilon}_{22}\sin^2\Big(\overset{0}{\chi}_1 + \overset{0}{\chi}_2\Big) \\ &- 2\tilde{\varepsilon}_{12}\sin\Big(\overset{0}{\chi}_1 + \overset{0}{\chi}_2 - \overset{0}{\chi}\Big)\sin\Big(\overset{0}{\chi}_1 + \overset{0}{\chi}_2\Big)\Big]\Big/\sin^2\overset{0}{\chi}. \end{aligned} \tag{5.25}$$

With the help of equation (5.21) in (5.24) the physical components can also be expressed in terms of stretch ratios and shear angles as

$$\overset{*}{\lambda}_i\overset{*}{\lambda}_k\cos\overset{*}{\chi}_{ik} - \cos\overset{0}{\chi}_{ik} = \sum_{j=1}^{2}\sum_{n=1}^{2}\Big(\lambda_j\lambda_n\cos\chi_{jn} - \cos\overset{0}{\chi}_{jn}\Big)\overset{*}{\hat{C}}_i^j\overset{*}{\hat{C}}_k^n. \tag{5.26}$$

Further, using equations (5.7) and (5.10), equation (5.26) in terms of $\overset{0}{S}$-configuration takes the form

$$\overset{*}{\lambda}_i\overset{*}{\lambda}_k \cos\overset{*}{\chi}_{ik} = \sum_{j=1}^{2}\sum_{n=1}^{2}\lambda_j\lambda_n \overset{*}{\hat{C}}{}_i^{\,j}\,\overset{*}{\hat{C}}{}_k^{\,n}\cos\overset{0}{\chi}_{jn}, \tag{5.27}$$

or in expanded form

$$\begin{aligned}
\overset{*}{\lambda}_1 &= \Big[\lambda_1^2\sin^2\big(\overset{0}{\chi} - \overset{0}{\chi}_2\big) + \lambda_2^2\sin^2\overset{0}{\chi}_2 \\
&\quad + 2\lambda_1\lambda_2\sin\big(\overset{0}{\chi} - \gamma\big)\sin\big(\overset{0}{\chi} - \overset{0}{\chi}_2\big)\sin\overset{0}{\chi}_2\Big]^{1/2}\Big/\sin^2\overset{0}{\chi}, \\
\overset{*}{\gamma} &= \overset{0}{\chi}_1 - \cos^{-1}\Big[\Big(-\lambda_1^2\sin\big(\overset{0}{\chi} - \overset{0}{\chi}_2\big)\sin\big(\overset{0}{\chi}_1 + \overset{0}{\chi}_2 - \overset{0}{\chi}\big) \\
&\quad + \lambda_2^2\sin\overset{0}{\chi}_2\sin\big(\overset{0}{\chi}_1 + \overset{0}{\chi}_2\big) + \lambda_1\lambda_2\Big(\cos\big(\overset{\wedge}{\delta} + 2\overset{0}{\chi}_2 - \overset{0}{\chi}\big) \\
&\quad - \cos\overset{0}{\chi}\cos\overset{0}{\chi}_1\Big)\cos\big(\overset{0}{\chi} - \gamma\big)\Big)\Big(\overset{*}{\lambda}_1\overset{*}{\lambda}_2\sin^2\overset{0}{\chi}\Big)^{-1}\Big] \\
\overset{*}{\lambda}_2 &= \Big[\lambda_1^2\sin^2\big(\overset{0}{\chi}_1 + \overset{0}{\chi}_2 - \overset{0}{\chi}\big) + \lambda_2^2\sin^2\big(\overset{0}{\chi}_1 + \overset{0}{\chi}_2\big) \\
&\quad - 2\lambda_1\lambda_2\cos\big(\overset{0}{\chi} - \Delta\overset{*}{\chi}\big)\sin\big(\overset{0}{\chi}_1 + \overset{0}{\chi}_2 - \overset{0}{\chi}\big)\sin\big(\overset{0}{\chi}_1 + \overset{0}{\chi}_2\big)\Big]^{1/2}\Big/\sin^2\overset{0}{\chi}.
\end{aligned} \tag{5.28}$$

Formulas (5.27) and (5.28) are preferred in practical applications particularly when dealing with finite deformations of shells.

5.2 Principal deformations

At any point $\overset{*}{M} \in \overset{*}{S}$, there exist two mutually orthogonal directions that remain orthogonal during deformation and along which the components of $\mathbf{E}$, attain the maximum and minimum value. They are called the principal directions.

To find the orientation of the principal axes, we proceed as follows. Let $\overset{(0)}{\varphi}$, $\overset{*}{\varphi}$ be the angles of the direction away from the base vectors $\bar{e}_1 \in \overset{(0)}{S}$, $\overset{*}{\bar{e}}_1 \in \overset{*}{S}$, respectively. We assume that the cut and undeformed configurations are indistinguishable, $\overset{0}{S} = S$. Then, setting $\overset{0}{\chi}_2 = \overset{0}{\varphi}$ in the first equation of (5.31), we have

$$\overset{*}{\tilde{\varepsilon}}_{11}\sin^2\overset{0}{\chi} = \tilde{\varepsilon}_{11}\sin^2\big(\overset{0}{\chi} - \overset{0}{\varphi}\big) + 2\tilde{\varepsilon}_{12}\sin\big(\overset{0}{\chi} - \overset{0}{\varphi}\big)\sin\overset{0}{\varphi} + \tilde{\varepsilon}_{22}\sin^2\overset{0}{\varphi}. \tag{5.29}$$

After simple rearrangements it can be written in the form

$$\varepsilon = a_0 + b_0\cos 2\overset{0}{\varphi} + c_0\sin 2\overset{0}{\varphi}, \tag{5.30}$$

where

$$a_0 = \left[\frac{1}{2}(\tilde{\varepsilon}_{11} + \tilde{\varepsilon}_{22}) - \tilde{\varepsilon}_{12}\cos\overset{0}{\chi}\right]\Big/\sin^2\overset{0}{\chi},$$
$$b_0 = \left[\frac{1}{2}(\tilde{\varepsilon}_{11} - \tilde{\varepsilon}_{22}) + \left(\tilde{\varepsilon}_{12} - \tilde{\varepsilon}_{11}\cos\overset{0}{\chi}\right)\Big/\cos\overset{0}{\chi}\right]\Big/\sin^2\overset{0}{\chi}, \tag{5.31}$$
$$c_0 = \left(\tilde{\varepsilon}_{12} - \tilde{\varepsilon}_{11}\cos\overset{0}{\chi}\right)\Big/\sin\overset{0}{\chi}.$$

Differentiating equation (5.30) with respect to $\overset{0}{\varphi}$ and equating the resultant equation to zero, for the principal axes on the surface $\overset{(0)}{S}$, we find ($b_0 \neq 0$)

$$\tan 2\overset{0}{\varphi} = \frac{c_0}{b_0} = \frac{2\left(\tilde{\varepsilon}_{11}\cos\overset{0}{\chi} - \tilde{\varepsilon}_{12}\right)\sin\overset{0}{\chi}}{\tilde{\varepsilon}_{11}\cos 2\overset{0}{\chi} - 2\tilde{\varepsilon}_{12}\cos\overset{0}{\chi} + \tilde{\varepsilon}_{22}}. \tag{5.32}$$

Substituting equation (5.32) into (5.30), we obtain the principal physical components ε_1, ε_2 of $\mathbf{E}$

$$\varepsilon_{1,2} = a_0^2 \pm \sqrt{b_0^2 + c_0^2} = \frac{(\tilde{\varepsilon}_{11} + \tilde{\varepsilon}_{22}) - 2\tilde{\varepsilon}_{12}\cos\overset{0}{\chi}}{2\sin^2\overset{0}{\chi}}$$
$$\pm \frac{1}{\sin^2\overset{0}{\chi}}\sqrt{\frac{(\tilde{\varepsilon}_{11} - \tilde{\varepsilon}_{22})^2}{4} + \tilde{\varepsilon}_{12}^2 + \tilde{\varepsilon}_{11}\tilde{\varepsilon}_{22}\cos^2\overset{0}{\chi} - \tilde{\varepsilon}_{12}(\tilde{\varepsilon}_{11} + \tilde{\varepsilon}_{22})\cos\overset{0}{\chi}}. \tag{5.33}$$

Henceforth, we assume that $\max\varepsilon_1$ is achieved in the direction of the principal axis defined by the angle $\overset{0}{\varphi}_1 = \overset{0}{\varphi}$, and $\min\varepsilon_2$—along the axis, defined by the angle $\overset{0}{\varphi}_2 = \overset{0}{\varphi} + \pi/2$. Since for the principal directions $\overset{0}{\chi}_1 \equiv \pi/2$, from the second equation (5.25), we find

$$\overset{*}{\tilde{\varepsilon}}_{12} = -b_0\sin 2\overset{0}{\varphi} + c_0\cos 2\overset{0}{\varphi}. \tag{5.34}$$

Dividing both sides of equation (5.34) by $c_0\cos 2\overset{0}{\varphi}$ and using equation (5.32), we find $\overset{*}{\tilde{\varepsilon}}_{12} = 0$. Thus, there exist indeed two mutually orthogonal directions at $\forall\, M(\alpha_i) \in \overset{(0)}{S}$ that remain orthogonal throughout deformation. A similar result, i.e. $\overset{*}{\gamma} = 0$, can be obtained from equation (5.9) by setting $\overset{0}{\chi} = \pi/2$.

Substituting equation (5.21) in (5.32) and (5.33) for the orientation of the principal axes on $\overset{0}{S}$ and the principal stretch ratios, we obtain

$$\tan 2\overset{0}{\varphi}_1 = \frac{2\left[\lambda_1\lambda_2\cos\left(\overset{0}{\chi} - \overset{*}{\gamma}\right) - \lambda_1^2\cos\overset{0}{\chi}\right]\sin\overset{0}{\chi}}{\lambda_1^2 - \lambda_2^2 + 2\left[\lambda_1\lambda_2\cos\left(\overset{0}{\chi} - \overset{*}{\gamma}\right) - \lambda_1^2\cos\overset{0}{\chi}\right]\cos\overset{0}{\chi}}, \tag{5.35}$$

$$\overset{0}{\varphi}_2 = \overset{0}{\varphi}_1 + \pi/2,$$

$$\begin{aligned}\boldsymbol{\Lambda}_{1,2}^2 = \Bigg[&\left(\lambda_1^2 + \lambda_2^2\right)/2 - \lambda_1\lambda_2\cos\left(\overset{0}{\chi} - \overset{*}{\gamma}\right)\cos\overset{0}{\chi} \\ &\pm\Bigg(\left(\lambda_1^2 + \lambda_2^2\right)^2/4 + \lambda^2{}_1\lambda^2{}_2\cos\left(2\overset{0}{\chi} - \overset{*}{\gamma}\right)\cos\overset{*}{\gamma} \\ &- \lambda_1\lambda_2\left(\lambda_1^2 + \lambda_2^2\right)\cos\left(\overset{0}{\chi} - \overset{*}{\gamma}\right)\cos\overset{0}{\chi}\Bigg)^{1/2}\Bigg]^{1/2} \Bigg/ \sin\overset{0}{\chi}.\end{aligned} \tag{5.36}$$

To find the orientation of the principal axes on the deformed surface $\overset{*}{S}$, consider a triangular element on S bounded by the two principal axes and the α_1-coordinate line (figure 5.3).

Geometric analysis leads to the following obvious equalities

$$\cos\overset{*}{\varphi}_1 = \frac{d\overset{*}{s}_1}{ds_1} = \frac{\boldsymbol{\Lambda}_1}{\lambda_1}\cos\overset{(0)}{\varphi}_1, \quad \sin\overset{*}{\varphi}_1 = \frac{d\overset{*}{s}_2}{ds_1} = \frac{\boldsymbol{\Lambda}_2}{\lambda_1}\sin\overset{(0)}{\varphi}_1.$$
$$\tan\overset{*}{\varphi}_1 = \frac{d\overset{*}{s}_2}{d\overset{*}{s}_1} = \frac{\boldsymbol{\Lambda}_2}{\boldsymbol{\Lambda}_1}\tan\overset{(0)}{\varphi}_1. \tag{5.37}$$

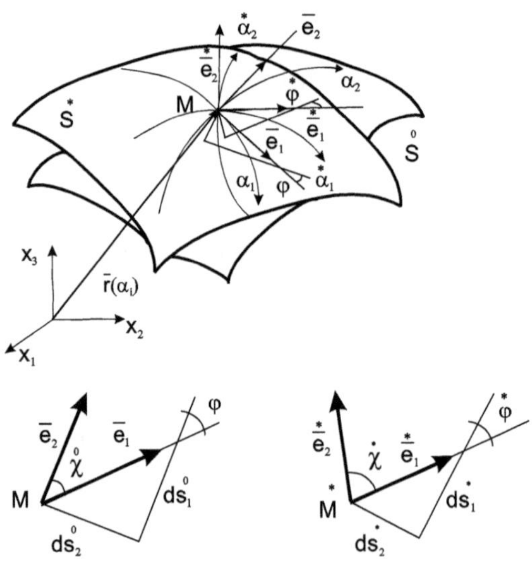

Figure 5.3. Principal deformations.

Using equations (5.35) and (5.36) from the above, we find the angles for the principal axes $\overset{*}{\varphi}_1$ and $\overset{*}{\varphi}_2 = \overset{*}{\varphi}_1 + \pi/2$.

Finally, substituting equations (5.3) and (5.21) into expressions for the first and second invariants of the tensor of deformation **E** defined by

$$
\begin{aligned}
I^{(\mathrm{E})}{}_1 &= \overset{*}{\varepsilon}_1 + \overset{*}{\varepsilon}_2 = \tilde{\varepsilon}_{11} + \tilde{\varepsilon}_{22} = \left[\tilde{\varepsilon}_{11} - 2\tilde{\varepsilon}_{12}\cos\overset{0}{\chi} + \tilde{\varepsilon}_{22}\right] \Big/ \sin^2\overset{0}{\chi}, \\
I^{(\mathrm{E})}{}_2 &= \overset{*}{\varepsilon}_1\overset{*}{\varepsilon}_2 = \overset{*}{\tilde{\varepsilon}}_{11}\tilde{\varepsilon}_{22} - (\tilde{\varepsilon}_{12})^2 = [\tilde{\varepsilon}_{11}\tilde{\varepsilon}_{22} - (\tilde{\varepsilon}_{12})^2]/\sin^2\overset{0}{\chi}.
\end{aligned}
\tag{5.38}
$$

For the principal stretch ratios and the shear angle, we obtain

$$
\begin{aligned}
\Lambda^2{}_1 + \Lambda^2{}_2 &= \left(\overset{*}{\lambda}_1\right)^2 + \left(\overset{*}{\lambda}_2\right)^2 \\
&= \left(\lambda_1^2 + \lambda_2^2 - 2\lambda_1\lambda_2\cos\left(\overset{0}{\chi} - \gamma\right)\cos\overset{0}{\chi}\right) \Big/ \sin^2\overset{0}{\chi}, \\
\Lambda_1\Lambda_2 &= \sqrt{1 + 2I^{(\mathrm{E})}{}_1 + 4I^{(\mathrm{E})}{}_2} = \overset{*}{\lambda}_1\overset{*}{\lambda}_2\cos\gamma \\
&= \lambda_1\lambda_2\sin\left(\overset{0}{\chi} - \gamma\right) \Big/ \sin\overset{0}{\chi}.
\end{aligned}
\tag{5.39}
$$

The last equation is also used to calculate the change of the surface area of S.

5.3 Membrane forces

The stress state of a differential element of the soft shell is described entirely by in-plane tangent $T_{ii}(T^{ii})$ and shear $T_{ik}(T^{ik})$ $(i \neq k)$ forces per unit length of the element. To study the equilibrium of the shell, we proceed from consideration of triangular elements ΔMAB and ΔMCD on $\overset{*}{S}$ (figure 5.4). Analysis of force distribution in the elements yields

$$
\begin{aligned}
-\overline{MA}\sum_{k=1}^{2} T^{1k}\overset{*}{\bar{e}}_k + \overline{MB}\sum_{i=1}^{2} T^{1i}\bar{e}_i + \overline{AB}\sum_{i=1}^{2} T^{2i}\bar{e}_i &= 0, \\
\overline{MD}\sum_{k=1}^{2} T^{2k}\overset{*}{\bar{e}}_k + \overline{CD}\sum_{i=1}^{2} T^{1i}\bar{e}_i - \overline{MC}\sum_{i=1}^{2} T^{2i}\bar{e}_i &= 0,
\end{aligned}
\tag{5.40}
$$

where $\overset{*}{\hat{C}}{}_1^1 = \overline{MC}$, $\overset{*}{\hat{C}}{}_1^2 = \overline{CD}$, $\overset{*}{\hat{C}}{}_2^1 = -\overline{AB}$, $\overset{*}{\hat{C}}{}_2^2 = \overline{MB}$ (equation (5.9)). The scalar product of equation (5.40) and $\overset{*}{\bar{e}}{}^k$ yields

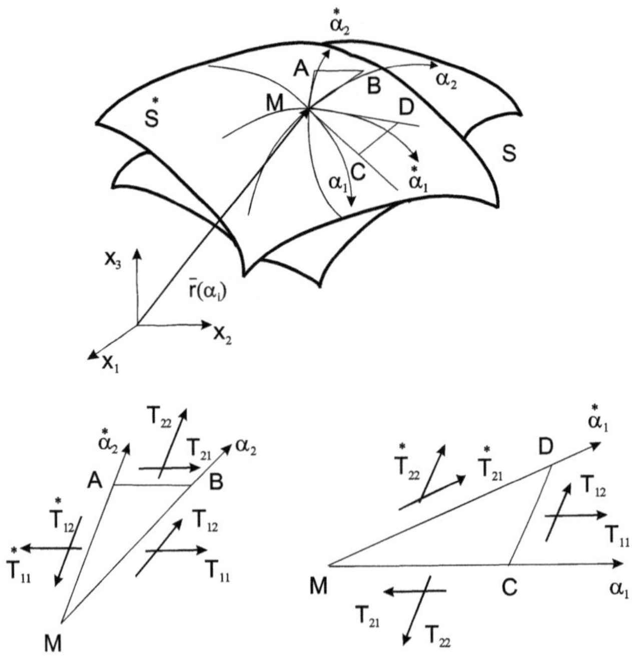

Figure 5.4. Membrane forces in the soft shell.

$$\overset{*}{T}{}^{1k} = \sum_{i=1}^{2}\left(T^{1i}\hat{C}_i^{\,k}\overset{*}{\hat{C}}{}_2^{2} - T^{2i}\hat{C}_i^{\,k}\overset{*}{\hat{C}}{}_2^{1} \right),$$

$$\overset{*}{T}{}^{2k} = \sum_{i=1}^{2}\left(-T^{1i}\hat{C}_i^{\,k}\overset{*}{\hat{C}}{}_1^{2} + T^{2i}\hat{C}_i^{\,k}\overset{*}{\hat{C}}{}_1^{1} \right),$$

where use is made of equation (5.5). Substituting $\overset{*}{\hat{C}}{}_i^{k}$ given by equation (5.14) for $\hat{C}_i^{\,k}$, we find

$$\overset{*}{T}{}^{ik} = \frac{1}{C}\sum_{j=1}^{2}\sum_{n=1}^{2} T^{jn}\hat{C}_j^{\,i}\hat{C}_n^{\,k}. \tag{5.41}$$

Using equation (5.11), the components of the membrane forces are found to be

$$
\begin{aligned}
\overset{*}{T}{}^{11} &= \Big\{T^{11}\sin^2\big(\overset{0}{\chi}_1 + \overset{0}{\chi}_2\big) + T^{22}\sin^2\big(\overset{0}{\chi}_1 + \overset{0}{\chi}_2 - \overset{0}{\chi}\big) \\
&\quad + 2T^{12}\sin\big(\overset{0}{\chi}_1 + \overset{0}{\chi}_2 - \overset{0}{\chi}\big)\sin\big(\overset{0}{\chi}_1 + \overset{0}{\chi}_2\big)\Big\} \Big/ \sin\overset{0}{\chi}\sin\overset{0}{\chi}_1 \\
\overset{*}{T}{}^{12} &= \Big\{-T^{11}\sin\overset{0}{\chi}_2\sin\big(\overset{0}{\chi}_1 + \overset{0}{\chi}_2\big) + T^{22}\sin\big(\overset{0}{\chi}_1 + \overset{0}{\chi}_2 - \overset{0}{\chi}\big)\sin\big(\overset{0}{\chi} - \overset{0}{\chi}_2\big) \\
&\quad + T^{12}\Big[\cos\big(\overset{0}{\chi}_1 + 2\overset{0}{\chi}_2 - \overset{0}{\chi}\big) - \cos\overset{0}{\chi}\cos\overset{0}{\chi}_1\Big]\Big\} \Big/ \sin\overset{0}{\chi}\sin\overset{0}{\chi}_1, \\
\overset{*}{T}{}^{22} &= \Big\{T^{11}\sin^2\overset{0}{\chi}_2 - 2T^{12}\sin\big(\overset{0}{\chi} - \overset{0}{\chi}_2\big)\sin\overset{0}{\chi}_2 \\
&\quad + T^{22}\sin^2\big(\overset{0}{\chi} - \overset{0}{\chi}_2\big)\Big\} \Big/ \sin\overset{0}{\chi}\sin\overset{0}{\chi}_1.
\end{aligned}
\tag{5.42}
$$

Introducing the tensor of membrane forces **T**

$$
\mathbf{T} = \sum_{j=1}^{2}\sum_{n=1}^{2} T^{ik}\bar{r}_i\bar{r}_k = \frac{1}{\sin\overset{*}{\chi}}\sum_{j=1}^{2}\sum_{n=1}^{2}\tilde{T}^{ik}\bar{e}_i\bar{e}_k, \tag{5.43}
$$

where $\tilde{T}^{ik}$ are the physical components of **T**, and using equation (5.5), $\tilde{T}^{ik}$ can be expressed in terms of $\overset{*}{\tilde{T}}{}^{ik}$ as

$$
\mathbf{T} = \frac{1}{\sin\overset{*}{\chi}}\sum_{j=1}^{2}\sum_{n=1}^{2}\tilde{T}^{ik}\bar{e}_i\bar{e}_k = \frac{1}{\sin\overset{*}{\chi}_1}\sum_{j=1}^{2}\sum_{n=1}^{2}\overset{*}{\tilde{T}}{}^{jn}\overset{*}{\bar{e}}_i\overset{*}{\bar{e}}_k = \frac{1}{\sin\overset{*}{\chi}_1}\sum_{j=1}^{2}\sum_{n=1}^{2}\overset{*}{\tilde{T}}{}^{jn}\bar{e}_i\bar{e}_k\overset{*}{\hat{C}}{}^{i}_{j}\overset{*}{\hat{C}}{}^{k}_{n}.
$$

Furthermore, making use of equation (5.11), we obtain

$$
T = \frac{1}{\overset{*}{C}}\sum_{j=1}^{2}\sum\nolimits_{n=1}^{2}\overset{*}{\tilde{T}}{}^{jn}\overset{*}{\hat{C}}{}^{i}_{j}\overset{*}{\hat{C}}{}^{k}_{n}. \tag{5.44}
$$

Substituting $\overset{*}{\hat{C}}{}^{i}_{j}$ given by equations (5.10), we obtain

$$
\begin{aligned}
\tilde{T}^{11} &= \Big\{ \overset{*}{\tilde{T}}{}^{11} \sin^2\big(\overset{*}{\chi} - \overset{*}{\chi}_2\big) + \overset{*}{\tilde{T}}{}^{22} \sin^2\big(\overset{*}{\chi}_1 + \overset{*}{\chi}_2 - \overset{*}{\chi}\big) \\
&\quad - 2\overset{*}{\tilde{T}}{}^{12} \sin\big(\overset{*}{\chi}_1 + \overset{*}{\chi}_2 - \overset{*}{\chi}\big) \sin\big(\overset{*}{\chi} - \overset{*}{\chi}_2\big) \Big\} \Big/ \sin \overset{*}{\chi} \sin \overset{*}{\chi}_1, \\
\tilde{T}^{12} &= \Big\{ \overset{*}{\tilde{T}}{}^{11} \sin \overset{*}{\chi}_2 \sin\big(\overset{*}{\chi} - \overset{*}{\chi}_2\big) + \overset{*}{\tilde{T}}{}^{22} \sin\big(\overset{*}{\chi}_1 + \overset{*}{\chi}_2 - \overset{*}{\chi}\big) \sin\big(\overset{*}{\chi}_1 + \overset{*}{\chi}_2\big) \\
&\quad + \overset{*}{\tilde{T}}{}^{12} \Big[\cos\big(\overset{*}{\chi}_1 + 2\overset{*}{\chi}_2 - \overset{*}{\chi}\big) - \cos \overset{*}{\chi} \cos \overset{*}{\chi}_1 \Big] \Big\} \Big/ \sin \overset{*}{\chi} \sin \overset{*}{\chi}_1, \\
\tilde{T}^{22} &= \Big\{ \overset{*}{\tilde{T}}{}^{11} \sin \overset{*}{\chi}_2 - 2\overset{*}{\tilde{T}}{}^{12} \sin\big(\overset{*}{\chi}_1 + \overset{*}{\chi}_2\big) \sin \overset{*}{\chi}_2 \\
&\quad + \tilde{T}^{*22} \sin^2\big(\overset{*}{\chi}_1 + \overset{*}{\chi}_2\big) \Big\} \Big/ \sin \overset{*}{\chi} \sin \overset{*}{\chi}_1.
\end{aligned}
\tag{5.45}
$$

Using equations (5.13) after simple rearrangements, equation (5.44) takes the form

$$
\frac{\lambda_1 \lambda_2}{\lambda_i \lambda_k} \tilde{T}^{ik} = \frac{1}{\hat{\overset{*}{C}}} \sum_{j=1}^{2} \sum_{n=1}^{2} \frac{\overset{*}{\lambda}_1 \overset{*}{\lambda}_2}{\overset{*}{\lambda}_j \overset{*}{\lambda}_n} \overset{*}{\tilde{T}}{}^{jn} \hat{C}_j^{*j} \hat{C}_n^{*k}. \tag{5.46}
$$

The formula (5.46) is preferred to (5.44) in applications. First, the coefficients $\hat{C}_n^{*k}$ are used in calculations of both deformations and membrane forces. Second, $\hat{C}_n^{*k}$ depend only on parameterization of the initial configuration of the shell. Therefore, once calculated they can be used throughout.

5.4 Principal membrane forces

As in the case of principal deformations at any point $\overset{*}{M} \in \overset{*}{S}$, there exist two mutually orthogonal directions that remain orthogonal throughout deformation and along which **T** attains extreme values. They are called the principal directions and the principal membrane forces, respectively.

Assuming that the coordinates $\overset{*}{\alpha}_i \in \overset{*}{S}$ and $\alpha_i \in S$ are related by the angle $\overset{*}{\psi}$, then, setting $\overset{*}{\chi}_1 = \pi/2$ and $\overset{*}{\chi}_2 = \psi$ in equation (5.42), we find

$$\overset{*}{T}{}^{11} = \left\{ T^{11}\cos^2\overset{*}{\psi} + T^{22}\cos^2\left(\overset{*}{\chi} - \overset{*}{\psi}\right) + 2T^{12}\cos\overset{*}{\psi}\cos\left(\overset{*}{\chi} - \overset{*}{\psi}\right) \right\} \Big/ \sin\overset{*}{\chi}$$

$$\begin{aligned} \overset{*}{T}{}^{12} = \Big\{ &-T^{11}\cos\overset{*}{\psi}\sin\overset{*}{\psi} + T^{12}\sin\left(\overset{*}{\chi} - 2\overset{*}{\psi}\right) \\ &+ T^{22}\cos\left(\overset{*}{\chi} - \overset{*}{\psi}\right)\sin\left(\overset{*}{\chi} - \overset{*}{\psi}\right) \Big\} \Big/ \sin\overset{*}{\chi}, \end{aligned} \tag{5.47}$$

$$\overset{*}{T}{}^{22} = \left\{ T^{11}\sin^2\overset{*}{\psi} - 2T^{12}\sin\left(\overset{*}{\chi} - \overset{*}{\psi}\right)\sin\overset{*}{\psi} + T^{22}\sin^2\left(\overset{*}{\chi} - \overset{*}{\psi}\right) \right\} \Big/ \sin\overset{*}{\chi}.$$

Equations (5.47) can be written in the form

$$\begin{aligned} \overset{*11}{T} &= a_1 + b_1\cos 2\overset{*}{\psi} + c_1\sin 2\overset{*}{\psi}, \\ \overset{*12}{T} &= -b_1\sin 2\overset{*}{\psi} + c_1\cos 2\overset{*}{\psi}, \\ \overset{*22}{T} &= a_1 - b_1\cos 2\overset{*}{\psi} - c_1\sin 2\overset{*}{\psi}, \end{aligned} \tag{5.48}$$

where the following notations are introduced

$$\begin{aligned} a_1 &= \left[\frac{1}{2}(T^{11} + T^{22}) - T^{12}\cos\overset{*}{\chi}\right] \Big/ \sin\overset{*}{\chi}, \\ b_1 &= \left[\frac{1}{2}(T^{11} + T^{22}) + \left(T^{12} + T^{22}\cos\overset{*}{\chi}\right)\cos\overset{*}{\chi}\right] \Big/ \sin\overset{*}{\chi}, \\ c_1 &= T^{12} + T^{22}\cos\overset{*}{\chi}. \end{aligned}$$

Differentiating $\overset{*}{T}{}^{ii}$ with respect to $\overset{*}{\psi}$ and equating the result to zero, we obtain

$$\tan 2\overset{*}{\psi} = \frac{c_1}{b_1} = \frac{2\left(T^{12} + T^{22}\cos\overset{*}{\chi}\right)\sin\overset{*}{\chi}}{T^{11} + 2T^{12}\cos\overset{*}{\chi} + T^{22}\cos 2\overset{*}{\chi}}. \tag{5.49}$$

Solving the above for $\overset{*}{\psi}$ for the directional angles of the principal axes, we obtain

$$\begin{aligned} \tan 2\overset{*}{\psi}_1 &= \frac{2\left(T^{12} + T^{22}\cos\overset{*}{\chi}\right)\sin\overset{*}{\chi}}{T^{11} + 2T^{12}\cos\overset{*}{\chi} + T^{22}\cos 2\overset{*}{\chi}}, \\ \overset{*}{\psi}_2 &= \overset{*}{\psi}_1 + \pi/2. \end{aligned} \tag{5.50}$$

Substituting equation (5.49) into (5.48), we have

$$\overset{*}{T}{}^{11} = a_1 + \sqrt{b_1^2 + c_1^2}, \quad \overset{*}{T}{}^{12} = 0, \quad \overset{*}{T}{}^{22} = a_1 - \sqrt{b_1^2 + c_1^2}.$$

From equation (5.54) the principal membrane forces T_1, T_2 are found to be

$$T_{1,2} = a_1^2 \pm \sqrt{b_1^2 + c_1^2} = \frac{1}{\sin\overset{*}{\chi}}\left\{\frac{(T^{11} + T^{22})}{2} + T^{12}\cos\overset{*}{\chi}\right.$$
$$\left. \pm\sqrt{1/4(T^{11} - T^{22})^2 + (T^{12})^2 + T^{12}(T^{11} + T^{22})\cos\overset{*}{\chi} + T^{11}T^{22}\cos^2\overset{*}{\chi}}\right\}. \tag{5.51}$$

Thus, at each point of the surface of the soft shell there are two mutually orthogonal directions that remain orthogonal throughout deformation. Henceforth, we assume that $T_1 \geqslant T_2$, i.e. the maximum stress is in the direction of the principal axis defined by the angle $\overset{*}{\psi}_1$, and the minimum by the angle $\overset{*}{\psi}_2$.

By analogy to the invariants of the tensor of deformation described by equations (5.38), we introduce the first and second invariants of **T**,

$$I^{(T)}{}_1 = T_1 + T_2 = \overset{*}{T}{}^{11} + \overset{*}{T}{}^{22} = \left(T^{11} + T^{22} + 2T^{12}\cos\overset{*}{\chi}\right)\Big/\sin\overset{*}{\chi},$$
$$I^{(T)}{}_2 = T_1T_2 = \overset{*}{T}{}^{11}\overset{*}{T}{}^{22} - \left(\overset{*}{T}{}^{12}\right)^2 = T^{11}T^{22} - (T^{12})^2. \tag{5.52}$$

5.5 Corollaries of the fundamental assumptions

The fundamental assumptions stated at the beginning of the chapter have several corollaries specific to thin soft shells.

1. The zero-flexural rigidity state is natural and unique to thin soft shells in contrast to thin elastic shells with finite bending rigidity.
2. Soft shells do not resist compression forces and thus $T_1 \geqslant 0$, $T_2 \geqslant 0$ and $I^{(T)}{}_1 \geqslant 0$, $I^{(T)}{}_2 \geqslant 0$.
3. Shear membrane forces are significantly smaller compared to stretch forces, $T_{12} \approx 10^{-3} \max T_{ii}$.
4. Areas of the soft shell, where $\mathbf{\Lambda}_1 \leqslant 1$ and $\mathbf{\Lambda}_2 \leqslant 1$, attain multiple configurations and are treated as the zero-stressed areas.
5. Stress states of the soft shell are classified as: (i) biaxial, if $T_1 > 0$, $T_2 > 0$, ($I^{(T)}{}_1 > 0$, $I^{(T)}{}_2 > 0$); (ii) uniaxial, if either $T_1 = 0$, $T_2 > 0$ or $T_1 > 0$, $T_2 = 0$, ($I^{(T)}{}_1 > 0$, $I^{(T)}{}_2 = 0$); and (iii) unstressed, if $T_1 = 0$ and $T_2 = 0$, ($I^{(T)}{}_1 = I^{(T)}{}_2 = 0$).
6. Constitutive relations for the uniaxial stress–strain state (figure 5.5) are functions of either $\mathbf{\Lambda}_1$ or $\mathbf{\Lambda}_2$ and empirical mechanical constants c_m given by

$$T_1 = f_1(\mathbf{\Lambda}_1, c_1, \ldots c_m, Z_{ij}) \quad \text{for} \quad \mathbf{\Lambda}_1 \geqslant 1,\ \mathbf{\Lambda}_2 < 1,$$
$$T_2 = f_2(\mathbf{\Lambda}_2, c_1, \ldots c_m, Z_{ij}) \quad \text{for} \quad \mathbf{\Lambda}_1 < 1,\ \mathbf{\Lambda}_2 \geqslant 1. \tag{5.53}$$

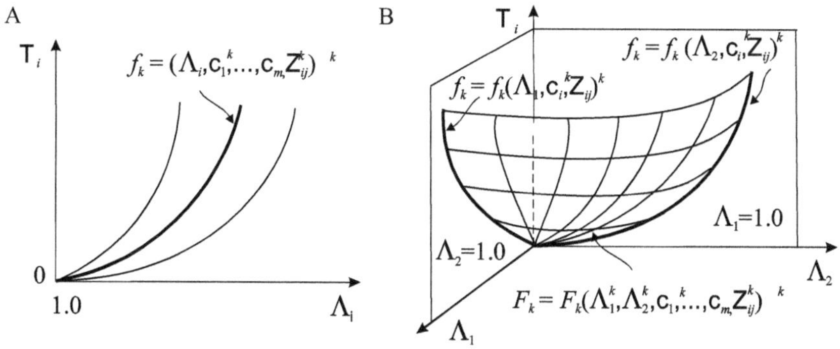

Figure 5.5. Uniaxial (A) and biaxial (B) constitutive relations for soft biological tissues.

7. Constitutive relations for the in-plane biaxial state (figure 5.5), $\Lambda_1 > 1$, $\Lambda_2 > 1$ ($T_1 > 0$, $T_2 > 0$) have the form

$$\begin{aligned} T_1 &= F_1(\Lambda_1, \Lambda_2, \varphi, c_1, \ldots c_m, Z_{ij}), \\ T_2 &= F_2(\Lambda_1, \Lambda_2, \varphi, c_1, \ldots c_m, Z_{ij}), \\ \psi &= \psi(\Lambda_1, \Lambda_2, \varphi, c_1, \ldots c_m, Z_{ij}). \end{aligned} \tag{5.54}$$

In general $f_n(\ldots) \neq F_n(\ldots)$, however, $f_n(\ldots)$ can be defined uniquely if $F_n(\ldots)$ is known.

Constitutive relations for biological tissues are derived either analytically or obtained experimentally. Continuum models typically allow greater computational efficiency and are easily integrated into multicomponent mathematical models. However, the identification of homogenized parameters and constants of the models can be a formidable challenge. Therefore, it is common practice to use approximations of experimental results from uniaxial, biaxial, and shear tests conducted on isolated tissue samples. Constitutive relations for soft biological tissues, e.g. the skin, the stomach, and the gallbladder, are usually obtained along structurally preferred directions defined by the orientation of reinforced smooth muscle, collagen, and elastin fibers, thus making them easy to use in calculations.

If constitutive relations are obtained in directions different from the actual parameterization of the shell, then the task is to learn to calculate membrane forces in the principal directions. Consider two typical situations:

Case 1. Constitutive relations are given by equation (5.54). Then,

(i) from equations (5.35) and (5.37), we calculate the principal deformations Λ_1, Λ_2 and the angle φ^*_1;

(ii) using equations (5.61), we compute the principal membrane forces T_1 and T_2 and the angle ψ;

(iii) finally, setting $\overset{*}{\chi}_1 = \pi/2$, $\overset{*}{\chi}_2 = \psi$, $\overset{*11}{T} = T_1$, $\overset{*22}{T} = T_2$, $\overset{*12}{T} = 0$ in equation (5.45), we find

$$\begin{aligned}\tilde{T}^{11} &= \{T_1 \sin^2(\chi - \psi) + T_2 \cos^2(\chi - \psi)\}/\sin\chi,\\ \tilde{T}^{12} &= \{T_1 \sin\psi \sin(\chi - \psi) - T_2 \cos\psi \cos(\chi - \psi)\}/\sin\chi,\\ \tilde{T}^{22} &= \{T_1 \sin^2\psi + T_2 \cos^2\psi\}/\sin\chi.\end{aligned} \tag{5.55}$$

Case 2. Constitutive relations are formulated for the orientation of reinforced fibers, superscript r,

$$\begin{aligned}T^r{}_1 &= F^r{}_1(\lambda^r{}_1, \lambda^r{}_2, \gamma^r, c_1, \ldots c_m, Z_{ij}),\\ T^r{}_2 &= F^r{}_2(\lambda^r{}_1, \lambda^r{}_2, \gamma^r, c_1, \ldots c_m, Z_{ij}),\\ S^r &= S^r(\lambda^r{}_1, \lambda^r{}_2, \gamma^r, c_1, \ldots c_m, Z_{ij}).\end{aligned} \tag{5.56}$$

Let $\overset{*}{\alpha}_i \in \overset{*}{S}$ be an auxiliary orthogonal coordinate system oriented with respect to a set of reinforced fibers by $\overset{*}{\psi}$. Then,

(i) setting $\chi_1 = \pi/2$, $\chi_2 = \psi$, $\overset{*}{\chi}_1 = \pi/2 - \gamma^r$ in equation (5.28), where $\lambda_1^r := \overset{*}{\lambda}_1$, $\lambda_2^r := \overset{*}{\lambda}_2$, for the stretch ratios and the shear angle γ^r, we have

$$\begin{aligned}\lambda_1^r &= \left(\lambda_1^2 \sin^2\left(\overset{0}{\chi} - \overset{0}{\psi}\right) + \lambda_2^2 \sin^2\overset{0}{\psi}\right.\\ &\quad \left. + 2\lambda_1\lambda_2 \cos\overset{0}{\chi} \sin\left(\overset{0}{\chi} - \overset{0}{\psi}\right) \sin\overset{0}{\psi}\right)^{1/2} \Big/ \sin\overset{0}{\chi},\\ \gamma^r &= \sin^{-1}\left(\frac{1}{\lambda_1\lambda_2 \sin^2\overset{0}{\chi}}\left(-\frac{1}{2}\lambda^2{}_1 \sin 2\left(\overset{0}{\chi} - \overset{0}{\psi}\right)\right.\right.\\ &\quad \left.\left. + \frac{1}{2}\lambda_2^2 \sin 2\overset{0}{\psi} + \lambda_1\lambda_2 \cos\overset{0}{\chi} \sin\left(\overset{0}{\chi} - \overset{0}{\psi}\right)\right)\right)\\ \lambda_2^r &= \left(\lambda_1^2 \cos^2\left(\overset{0}{\chi} - \overset{0}{\psi}\right) + \lambda_2^2 \cos^2\overset{0}{\psi}\right.\\ &\quad \left. - 2\lambda_1\lambda_2 \cos\left(\overset{0}{\chi} - \overset{0}{\psi}\right) \cos\overset{0}{\chi} \cos\overset{0}{\psi}\right)^{1/2} \Big/ \sin\overset{0}{\chi};\end{aligned} \tag{5.57}$$

(ii) using equations (5.63) we find $T^r{}_1$, $T^r{}_2$, and S^r;

(iii) the angle $\overset{*}{\psi}$ is found from equation (5.28) by putting $\overset{*}{\chi}_1 = \overset{*}{\psi}$,

$$\begin{aligned}&\overset{*}{\lambda}_1 = \lambda_1,\ \overset{*}{\lambda}_2 = \lambda_1^r,\\ &\overset{*}{\psi} = \cos^{-1}\left(\frac{1}{\lambda_1^r \sin\overset{0}{\chi}}\left(\lambda_1 \sin\left(\overset{0}{\chi} - \overset{0}{\psi}\right) + \lambda_2 \cos\overset{0}{\chi} \sin\overset{0}{\psi}\right)\right);\end{aligned} \tag{5.58}$$

(iv) finally, setting $\overset{*}{\chi}_1 = \pi/2 - \gamma^r$, $\overset{*}{\chi}_2 = \overset{*}{\psi}$, $T_1^r := \overset{*}{\tilde{T}}{}^{11}$, $T_2^r := \overset{*}{\tilde{T}}{}^{22}$, $S^r := \overset{*}{\tilde{T}}{}^{12}$ in equations (5.45), we obtain

$$\begin{aligned}
\tilde{T}^{11} &= \Big\{ T^r{}_1 \sin^2\!\big(\overset{*}{\chi} - \overset{*}{\psi}\big) + T^r{}_2 \cos^2\!\big(\overset{*}{\chi} - \overset{*}{\psi} + \gamma^r\big) \\
&\quad - 2S^r \cos\!\big(\overset{*}{\chi} - \overset{*}{\psi} + \gamma^r\big) \sin\!\big(\overset{*}{\chi} - \overset{*}{\psi}\big)\Big\} \Big/ \sin\overset{*}{\chi} \cos\gamma^r, \\
\tilde{T}^{12} &= \Big\{ T^r{}_1 \sin\mu \sin\!\big(\overset{*}{\chi} - \overset{*}{\psi}\big) - T^r{}_2 \cos\!\big(\overset{*}{\psi} + \gamma^r\big) \cos\!\big(\overset{*}{\chi} - \overset{*}{\psi} + \gamma^r\big) \\
&\quad + S^r\Big[\sin\!\big(\overset{*}{\chi} - 2\overset{*}{\psi} + \gamma^r\big) - \cos\overset{*}{\chi} \sin\gamma^r\Big]\Big\} \Big/ \sin\overset{*}{\chi} \cos\gamma^r, \\
\tilde{T}^{22} &= \Big\{ T^r{}_1 \sin^2\overset{*}{\psi} - 2S^r \sin\!\big(\overset{*}{\psi} - \gamma^r\big) \sin\overset{*}{\psi} + T^r{}_2 \cos^2\!\big(\overset{*}{\psi} - \gamma^r\big)\Big\} \Big/ \sin\overset{*}{\chi} \cos\gamma^r.
\end{aligned} \tag{5.59}$$

Formulas (5.59) can be written in more concise form if we introduce generalized forces defined by $N^{ik} = T^{ik}\frac{\lambda_k}{\lambda_i}$,

$$\overset{*}{N}{}^{11} = T_1^r \frac{\lambda_2^r}{\lambda_1^r}, \quad \overset{*}{N}{}^{22} = T_2^r \frac{\lambda_1^r}{\lambda_2^r}, \quad \overset{*}{N}{}^{12} = S^r.$$

Then, equation (5.46) takes the form

$$N^{ik} = \frac{1}{\hat{\hat{C}}{}^*} \sum_{j=1}^{2}\sum_{n=1}^{2} \overset{*}{N}{}^{jn} \hat{\hat{C}}{}_j^{*i} \hat{\hat{C}}{}_n^{*k}. \tag{5.60}$$

Substituting $\hat{\hat{C}}{}_j^{*i}$ given by equations (5.12) and (5.14), we find

$$\begin{aligned}
N^{11} &= \Big\{ \overset{*}{N}{}^{11} \sin^2\!\big(\overset{0}{\chi} - \overset{0}{\chi}_2\big) + \overset{*}{N}{}^{22} \sin^2\!\big(\overset{0}{\chi}_1 + \overset{0}{\chi}_2 - \overset{0}{\chi}\big) \\
&\quad - 2\overset{*}{N}{}^{12} \sin\!\big(\overset{0}{\chi}_1 + \overset{0}{\chi}_2 - \overset{0}{\chi}\big) \sin\!\big(\overset{0}{\chi} - \overset{0}{\chi}_2\big)\Big\} \Big/ \sin\overset{0}{\chi} \sin\overset{0}{\chi}_1 \\
N^{12} &= \Big\{ \overset{*}{N}{}^{11} \sin\overset{0}{\chi}_2 \sin\!\big(\overset{0}{\chi} - \overset{0}{\chi}_2\big) + \overset{*}{N}{}^{22} \sin\!\big(\overset{0}{\chi}_1 + \overset{0}{\chi}_2 - \overset{0}{\chi}\big) \sin\!\big(\overset{0}{\chi}_1 + \overset{0}{\chi}_2\big) \\
&\quad + \overset{*}{N}{}^{12}\Big[\cos\!\big(\overset{0}{\chi}_1 + 2\overset{0}{\chi}_2 - \overset{0}{\chi}\big) - \cos\overset{0}{\chi} \cos\overset{0}{\chi}_1\Big]\Big\} \Big/ \sin\overset{0}{\chi} \sin\overset{0}{\chi}_1, \\
N^{22} &= \Big\{ \overset{*}{N}{}^{11} \sin^2\overset{0}{\chi}_2 - 2\overset{*}{N}{}^{12} \sin\!\big(\overset{0}{\chi}_1 + \overset{0}{\chi}_2\big) \sin\overset{0}{\chi}_2 \\
&\quad + \overset{*}{N}{}^{22} \sin^2\!\big(\overset{0}{\chi}_1 + \overset{0}{\chi}_2\big)\Big\} \Big/ \sin\overset{0}{\chi} \sin\overset{0}{\chi}_1.
\end{aligned} \tag{5.61}$$

Putting $\overset{0}{\chi}_1 = \pi/2$, $\overset{0}{\chi}_2 = \overset{0}{\psi}$ in equations (5.61), for the membrane forces in terms of the undeformed surface S ($\overset{0}{S} = S$), we have

$$\tilde{T}^{11} = \frac{\lambda_1}{\lambda_2}\left(T_1^r\frac{\lambda_2^r}{\lambda_1^r}\sin^2\left(\overset{0}{\chi} - \overset{0}{\psi}\right) + T_2^r\frac{\lambda_1^r}{\lambda_2^r}\cos^2\left(\overset{0}{\chi} - \overset{0}{\psi}\right)\right.$$
$$\left.- 2S^r \sin 2\left(\overset{0}{\chi} - \overset{0}{\psi}\right)\right)\Big/\sin\overset{0}{\chi},$$
$$\tilde{T}^{12} = \left(T_1^r\frac{\lambda_2^r}{\lambda_1^r}\sin^2\left(\overset{0}{\chi} - \overset{0}{\psi}\right)\sin\overset{0}{\psi} - T_2^r\frac{\lambda_1^r}{\lambda_2^r}\cos^2\left(\overset{0}{\chi} - \overset{0}{\psi}\right)\cos\overset{0}{\psi}\right. \tag{5.62}$$
$$\left.+ S^r \sin\left(\overset{0}{\chi} - 2\overset{0}{\psi}\right)\right)\Big/\sin\overset{0}{\chi},$$
$$\tilde{T}^{22} = \frac{\lambda_2}{\lambda_1}\left(T_1^r\frac{\lambda_2^r}{\lambda_1^r}\sin^2\overset{0}{\psi} + T_2^r\frac{\lambda_1^r}{\lambda_2^r}\cos^2\overset{0}{\psi} + S^r\sin 2\overset{0}{\psi}\right)\Big/\sin\overset{0}{\chi}.$$

Formulas (5.62) depend only on parameterization of S and the axes of anisotropy and are therefore less computationally demanding compared to equations (5.58) and (5.59).

5.6 Nets

A special class of soft shell in which discrete reinforced fibers are the main structural and weight bearing elements is called nets. Depending on their engineering design and practical needs, the fibers may remain discrete or embedded in the connective matrix. Although nets have a distinct discrete structure, they are modeled as a solid continuum. Since nets have very low resistance to shear forces, $T_{12} = 0$ ($S^r \equiv 0$) and the resultant formulas obtained in the previous paragraphs are valid in modeling nets.

Consider a net with the cell structure of a parallelogram. Let the sides of the cell be formed by two distinct families of reinforced fibers (figure 5.6). Their mechanical properties are described by

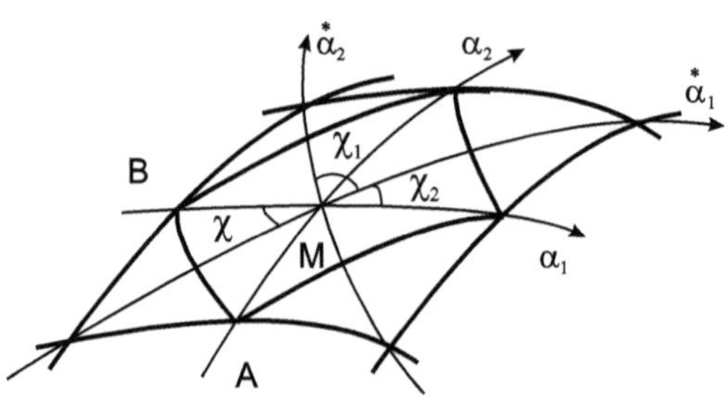

Figure 5.6. A structural element of the net formed by two distinct types of reinforced fibers.

$$T_1^r = F_1^r(\lambda_1^r, \lambda_2^r, \gamma^r, c_1, \ldots c_m, Z_{ij}),$$
$$T_2^r = F_2^r(\lambda_1^r, \lambda_2^r, \gamma^r, c_1, \ldots c_m, Z_{ij}), \tag{5.63}$$

where the meaning of parameters and constants are as discussed above.

Let the undeformed ($S \equiv \overset{0}{S}$) configuration of the net be parameterized by $\overset{*}{\alpha}_1$, $\overset{*}{\alpha}_2$ coordinates oriented along the reinforced fibers. For force distribution in the net we have to:

(i) find the stretch ratios $\lambda_1^r = \overset{*}{\lambda}_1$, $\lambda_2^r = \overset{*}{\lambda}_2$, using equations (5.28);

(ii) substitute $\lambda_1^r = \overset{*}{\lambda}_1$, $\lambda_2^r = \overset{*}{\lambda}_2$ in equation (5.70) to calculate T_1^r, T_2^r;

(iii) make use of equations (5.59) or (5.62) to find the membrane forces in terms of the S-configuration

$$\tilde{T}^{11} = \frac{\lambda_1}{\lambda_2}\left(T_1^r\frac{\lambda_2^r}{\lambda_1^r}\sin^2\left(\overset{0}{\chi} - \overset{0}{\psi}\right) + T_2^r\frac{\lambda_1^r}{\lambda_2^r}\cos^2\left(\overset{0}{\chi} - \overset{0}{\psi}\right)\right)\Big/\sin\overset{0}{\chi},$$
$$\tilde{T}^{12} = \left(T_1^r\frac{\lambda_2^r}{\lambda_1^r}\sin^2\left(\overset{0}{\chi} - \overset{0}{\psi}\right)\sin\overset{0}{\psi} - T_2^r\frac{\lambda_1^r}{\lambda_2^r}\cos^2\left(\overset{0}{\chi} - \overset{0}{\psi}\right)\cos\overset{0}{\psi}\right)\Big/\sin\overset{0}{\chi}, \tag{5.64}$$
$$\tilde{T}^{22} = \frac{\lambda_2}{\lambda_1}\left(T_1^r\frac{\lambda_2^r}{\lambda_1^r}\sin^2\overset{0}{\psi} + T_2^r\frac{\lambda_1^r}{\lambda_2^r}\cos^2\overset{0}{\psi}\right)\Big/\sin\overset{0}{\chi}.$$

The principal membrane forces and their directions are found from equations (5.50) and (5.51) by putting $T^{12} = S^r = 0$, $T^{11} = T_1^r$, $T^{22} = T_2^r$:

$$T_{1,2} = \frac{(T_1^r + T_2^r) \pm \sqrt{(T_1^r - T_2^r)^2 + 4T_1^rT_2^r\cos^2\overset{*}{\chi}}}{2\sin\overset{*}{\chi}},$$
$$\tan 2\overset{*}{\psi}_1 = \frac{T_2^r\sin 2\overset{*}{\chi}}{T_1^r + T_2^r\cos 2\overset{*}{\chi}}, \tag{5.65}$$
$$\overset{*}{\psi}_2 = \overset{*}{\psi}_1 + \pi/2.$$

In particular,

(i) if $\overset{*}{\chi} = \pi/2$ then $\overset{*}{\psi}_1 = 0$, $T_1 = T_1^r$, $T_2 = T_2^r$;

(ii) if $T_1^r = 0$ then $\overset{*}{\psi}_1 = 0$, $T_1 = T_1^r/\sin\overset{*}{\chi}$, $T_2 = 0$;

(iii) if $T_2^r = 0$ then $\overset{*}{\psi}_1 = \overset{*}{\chi}$, $T_1 = T_2^r/\sin\overset{*}{\chi}$, $T_2 = 0$.

Corollary 5 of the fundamental assumptions for the nets is given by

$$I^{(\mathrm{T})}{}_1 = T_1 + T_2 = \frac{1}{\sin \overset{*}{\chi}}(T_1^r + T_2^r) \geqslant 0,$$
$$I^{(\mathrm{T})}{}_2 = T_1 T_2 = T_1^r T_2^r \geqslant 0. \tag{5.66}$$

5.7 Equations of motion in general curvilinear coordinates

Let $\Delta\overset{(*)}{\sigma}$ and $\Delta\overset{(*)}{m}$ be the surface area and mass of a differential element of the soft shell in undeformed and deformed configurations. The position of a point $\overset{*}{M} \in \overset{*}{S}$ at any moment of time t is given by vector $\bar{r}(\alpha_1, \alpha_2, t)$. Densities of the material in undeformed, ρ, and deformed, $\overset{*}{\rho}$, states are defined by

$$\rho = \lim_{\Delta\sigma \to 0} \frac{\Delta m}{\Delta \sigma} = \frac{dm}{d\sigma} \quad \text{and} \quad \overset{*}{\rho} = \lim_{\Delta\overset{*}{\sigma} \to 0} \frac{\Delta \overset{*}{m}}{\Delta \overset{*}{\sigma}} = \frac{d\overset{*}{m}}{d\overset{*}{\sigma}}, \tag{5.67}$$

where

$$d\sigma = \sqrt{a}\, d\alpha_1 d\alpha_2, \quad d\overset{*}{\sigma} = \sqrt{\overset{*}{a}}\, d\alpha_1 d\alpha_2.$$

Applying the law of conservation of the mass to equation (5.74) we find

$$dm = d\overset{*}{m} = \overset{*}{\rho}\, d\overset{*}{\sigma} = \overset{*}{\rho}\sqrt{\overset{*}{a}}\, d\alpha_1 d\alpha_2 = \rho\sqrt{\overset{*}{a}}\, d\alpha_1 d\alpha_2.$$

It follows that

$$\overset{*}{\rho} = \rho\sqrt{a/\overset{*}{a}}. \tag{5.68}$$

Let $\bar{p}_s(\alpha_1, \alpha_2, t)$ be the resultant of the external, $\bar{p}_{(+)}(\alpha_1, \alpha_2, t)$, and internal, $\bar{p}_{(-)}(\alpha_1, \alpha_2, t)$, forces distributed over the outer and inner surfaces of the shell

$$\bar{p}_s(\alpha_1, \alpha_2, t) = \bar{p}_{(+)}(\alpha_1, \alpha_2, t) + \bar{p}_{(-)}(\alpha_1, \alpha_2, t).$$

The density of the resultant force per unit area of a deformed element $\bar{p}_s$ is defined by

$$\bar{p}(\alpha_1, \alpha_2, t) = \lim_{\Delta\sigma^* \to 0} \frac{\bar{p}_s}{\Delta\overset{*}{\sigma}}. \tag{5.69}$$

Similarly, we introduce the density of the mass force $\bar{F}(\alpha_1, \alpha_2, t)$ by

$$\bar{f}(\alpha_1, \alpha_2, t) = \lim_{\Delta m \to 0} \frac{\bar{F}}{\Delta m} = \frac{d\bar{F}}{dm} = \frac{1}{\rho}\frac{d\bar{F}}{d\sigma}. \tag{5.70}$$

The resultant stress vectors $\bar{R}_i$ acting upon the differential element are found to be

$$\begin{aligned}
\overline{R}_1 &= -\,(T^{11}\bar{e}_1 + T^{12}\bar{e}_2)\sqrt{\overset{*}{a}_{22}}\,d\alpha_2,\\
\overline{R}_2 &= -\,(T^{21}\bar{e}_1 + T^{22}\bar{e}_2)\sqrt{\overset{*}{a}_{11}}\,d\alpha_1,\\
-\left(\overline{R}_1 + \frac{\partial \overline{R}_1}{\partial \alpha_1}d\alpha_1\right) &= -\,(T^{11}\bar{e}_1 + T^{12}\bar{e}_2)\sqrt{\overset{*}{a}_{22}}\,d\alpha_2\\
&\quad - \frac{\partial}{\partial \alpha_1}(T^{11}\bar{e}_1 + T^{12}\bar{e}_2)\sqrt{\overset{*}{a}_{22}}\,d\alpha_1 d\alpha_2,\\
-\left(\overline{R}_2 + \frac{\partial \overline{R}_2}{\partial \alpha_2}d\alpha_2\right) &= -\,(T^{21}\bar{e}_1 + T^{22}\bar{e}_2)\sqrt{\overset{*}{a}_{11}}\,d\alpha_1\\
&\quad - \frac{\partial}{\partial \alpha_2}(T^{21}\bar{e}_1 + T^{22}\bar{e}_2)\sqrt{\overset{*}{a}_{11}}\,d\alpha_1 d\alpha_2.
\end{aligned} \tag{5.71}$$

Applying the law of conservation of momentum to equations (5.69)–(5.71), for the equation of motion of the soft shell we obtain

$$\overset{*}{\rho}\frac{d^2\bar{r}(\alpha_1, \alpha_2, t)}{dt^2} = -\frac{\partial \overline{R}_1}{\partial \alpha_1}d\alpha_1 - \frac{\partial \overline{R}_2}{\partial \alpha_2}d\alpha_2 + \bar{p} + \bar{f}\,\overset{*}{\rho}, \tag{5.72}$$

where $\frac{d^2\bar{r}}{dt^2}$ is acceleration. Substituting $\bar{R}_i$ and $\overset{*}{\rho}$ given by equations (5.75) and (5.78) into (5.72), we obtain

$$\begin{aligned}
\rho\sqrt{a}\frac{d^2\bar{r}}{dt^2} &= \frac{\partial}{\partial \alpha_1}\left[(T^{11}\bar{e}_1 + T^{12}\bar{e}_2)\sqrt{\overset{*}{a}_{22}}\right]\\
&\quad + \frac{\partial}{\partial \alpha_2}\left[(T^{21}\bar{e}_1 + T^{22}\bar{e}_2)\sqrt{\overset{*}{a}_{11}}\right] + \bar{p}\sqrt{\overset{*}{a}} + \bar{f}\,\rho\sqrt{a}.
\end{aligned} \tag{5.73}$$

Let $\bar{G}_i$, $\bar{M}_p$, and $\bar{M}_f$ be the resultant moment vectors acting on the element of the shell defined by

$$\begin{aligned}
&\overline{G}_1 = \bar{r} \times \overline{R}_1, \quad \overline{G}_2 = \bar{r} \times \overline{R}_2\\
&\quad -\left(\overline{G}_1 + \frac{\partial \overline{G}_1}{\partial \alpha_1}d\alpha_1\right), \quad -\left(\overline{G}_2 + \frac{\partial \overline{G}_2}{\partial \alpha_2}d\alpha_2\right) \quad (\alpha_i + d\alpha_i = \text{const})\\
&\overline{M}_p = (\bar{r} \times \bar{p})\sqrt{\overset{*}{a}}\,d\alpha_1 d\alpha_2, \quad \overline{M}_f = (\bar{r} \times \bar{f}\,)\rho\sqrt{\overset{*}{a}}\,d\alpha_1 d\alpha_2.
\end{aligned} \tag{5.74}$$

Assuming the shell is in equilibrium, the sum of the moments vanishes. Hence

$$-\frac{\partial \overline{G}_1}{\partial \alpha_1}d\alpha_1 - \frac{\partial \overline{G}_2}{\partial \alpha_2}d\alpha_2 + \overline{M}_p + \overline{M}_q = 0. \tag{5.75}$$

Substituting $\bar{G}_i$, $\bar{M}_p$, and $\bar{M}_f$ in equation (5.75), we obtain

$$\left[-\left(\bar{r}\times\frac{\partial\bar{R}_1}{\partial\alpha_1}d\alpha_1\right)-\left(\bar{r}\times\frac{\partial\bar{R}_2}{\partial\alpha_2}d\alpha_2\right)+(\bar{r}\times\bar{p})+(\bar{r}\times\bar{f})\right]$$
$$-(\bar{r}\times\bar{R}_1)d\alpha_1-(\bar{r}\times\bar{R}_2)d\alpha_2=0.$$

Further, using equation (5.78), we find

$$[\bar{e}_1\times(T^{11}\bar{e}_1+T^{12}\bar{e}_2)+\bar{e}_2\times(T^{21}\bar{e}_1+T^{22}\bar{e}_2)]\sqrt{\overset{*}{a}_{11}}\sqrt{\overset{*}{a}_{22}}\,d\alpha_1 d\alpha_2$$
$$-\bar{r}\times\left[\underline{-\frac{\partial\bar{R}_1}{\partial\alpha_1}d\alpha_1-\frac{\partial\bar{R}_2}{\partial\alpha_2}d\alpha_2+\bar{p}+\bar{f}}\right]=0. \tag{5.76}$$

Since the underlined term equals zero, we have

$$(\bar{e}_1\times\bar{e}_2)T^{12}+(\bar{e}_2\times\bar{e}_1)T^{21}=0. \tag{5.77}$$

It follows immediately from the above the $T^{12}=T^{21}$.

Remarks

1. If a soft shell is parameterized along the principal axes then $T^{11}=T_1$, $T^{22}=T_2$, $T^{12}=0$, $\overset{*}{a}_{12}=a_{12}=0$ and the equation of motion (5.73) takes the simplest form

$$\rho\sqrt{a}\frac{d^2\bar{r}}{dt^2}=\frac{\partial}{\partial\alpha_1}\left[T_1\sqrt{\overset{*}{a}_{22}}\,\bar{e}_1\right]+\frac{\partial}{\partial\alpha_2}\left[T_2\sqrt{\overset{*}{a}_{11}}\,\bar{e}_2\right]$$
$$+\bar{p}\sqrt{\overset{*}{a}}+\bar{f}\rho\sqrt{a}. \tag{5.78}$$

2. During the dynamic process of deformation different parts of the soft shell may undergo different stress–strain states. The biaxial stress state occurs when $I^{(T)}{}_1=T_1+T_2>0$, $I^{(T)}{}_2=T_1T_2>0$, the uniaxial state develops in areas where $I^{(T)}{}_1>0$, $I^{(T)}{}_2=0$, and the zero stress state takes place anywhere in the shell where $I^{(T)}{}_1=I^{(T)}{}_2=0$. The uniaxially stressed area ($T_2=0$) will develop wrinkles oriented along the action of the positive principal membrane force T_1. The equation of motion for the wrinkled area becomes

$$\rho\sqrt{a}\frac{d^2\bar{r}}{dt^2}=\frac{\partial}{\partial\alpha_1}\left[T_1\sqrt{\overset{*}{a}_{22}}\,\bar{e}_1\right]+\bar{p}\sqrt{\overset{*}{a}}+\bar{f}\rho\sqrt{a}. \tag{5.79}$$

To preserve smoothness and continuity of the surface $\overset{*}{S}$, the uniaxially stressed area is substituted by an ironed surface made out of an array of closely packed reinforced fibers. Such an approach permits the use of the equations of motion (5.72) throughout the deformed surface $\overset{*}{S}$.

The governing system of equations of dynamics of the soft shell includes the equations of motion (5.80) and (5.85), constitutive relations (5.53), (5.54) or (5.63), initial and boundary conditions, and the conditions given by corollary 5.

5.8 Governing equations in orthogonal Cartesian coordinates

Let a soft shell be associated with an orthogonal Cartesian coordinate system x_1, x_2, x_3:

$$\begin{aligned} x_1 &= x_1(\alpha_1, \alpha_2, t), \\ x_2 &= x_2(\alpha_1, \alpha_2, t), \\ x_3 &= x_3(\alpha_1, \alpha_2, t). \end{aligned} \tag{5.80}$$

The position vector of point $M(\alpha_1, \alpha_2) \in S$ and its derivatives are given by

$$\bar{r} = \bar{i}_1 x_1 + \bar{i}_2 x_2 + \bar{i}_3 x_3 = \sum_{k=1}^{3} x_k \bar{i}_k, \tag{5.81}$$

$$\bar{r}_i = \frac{\partial \bar{r}}{\partial \alpha_i} = \sum_{k=1}^{3} \frac{\partial x_k}{\partial \alpha_i} \bar{i}_k = \sum_{k=1}^{3} \bar{r}_{ik} \bar{i}_k, \quad (i = 1, 2), \tag{5.82}$$

where $\bar{r}_{ik} = \frac{\partial x_k}{\partial \alpha_i}$ is the projection of the ith basis vector on the x_1, x_2, x_3 axes. Decomposing the unit vectors $\bar{e}_i = \bar{r}_i / |\bar{r}_i|$ along the base $\{\bar{i}_1, \bar{i}_2, \bar{i}_3\}$, we obtain

$$\bar{e}_i = \sum_{k=1}^{3} l_{ik} \bar{i}_k = \frac{\bar{r}_i}{\sqrt{\overset{*}{a}_{ii}}} = \frac{\bar{r}_{ik}}{\sqrt{\overset{*}{a}_{ii}}} \bar{i}_k = l_{ik} \bar{i}_k, \tag{5.83}$$

where l_{ik} are the direction cosines defined by

$$l_{ik} := \cos(\bar{e}_i, \bar{i}_k) = \bar{r}_{ik} / \sqrt{\overset{*}{a}_{ii}}. \tag{5.84}$$

The vector $\bar{m}$ normal to $\bar{e}_i$ ($\bar{m} \perp \bar{e}_i$) is given by

$$\bar{m} = (\bar{e}_1 \times \bar{e}_2) \frac{\sqrt{\overset{*}{a}_{11} \overset{*}{a}_{22}}}{\sqrt{\overset{*}{a}}}. \tag{5.85}$$

With the help of equations (5.90) and (5.92), the direction cosines $l_{3k} = \cos(\bar{m}, \bar{i}_k)$ are found to be

$$\begin{aligned} l_{31} &= (l_{12} l_{23} - l_{13} l_{22}) \sqrt{\overset{*}{a}_{11} \overset{*}{a}_{22}} \Big/ \sqrt{\overset{*}{a}}, \\ l_{32} &= (l_{13} l_{21} - l_{11} l_{23}) \sqrt{\overset{*}{a}_{11} \overset{*}{a}_{22}} \Big/ \sqrt{\overset{*}{a}}, \\ l_{33} &= (l_{11} l_{22} - l_{12} l_{21}) \sqrt{\overset{*}{a}_{11} \overset{*}{a}_{22}} \Big/ \sqrt{\overset{*}{a}}. \end{aligned} \tag{5.86}$$

Scalar products $\bar{e}_i\bar{e}_k$ yield

$$\begin{aligned}
\bar{e}_1\bar{e}_2 &= l_{11}l_{21} + l_{12}l_{22} + l_{13}l_{23} = \cos\overset{*}{\chi} = \overset{*}{a}_{12}\Big/\sqrt{\overset{*}{a}_{11}\overset{*}{a}_{22}} \\
\bar{e}_i\bar{e}_2 &= l_{i1}l_{31} + l_{i2}l_{32} + l_{i3}l_{33} = 0, \\
\bar{e}_k\bar{e}_k &= l_{k1}^2 + l_{k2}^2 + l_{k3}^2 = 1.
\end{aligned} \tag{5.87}$$

Expanding $\bar{p}, \bar{f}$ in the direction of $\bar{e}_i$ and $\bar{i}_i$, respectively, we obtain

$$\bar{p} = \bar{e}_1p_1 + \bar{e}_2p_2 + \bar{m}p_3, \tag{5.88}$$

$$\bar{f} = \bar{i}_1f_1 + \bar{i}_2f_2 + \bar{i}_3f_3. \tag{5.89}$$

Substituting equations (5.84), (5.86), (5.88), and (5.89) in (5.77), the equation of motion of the soft shell takes the form

$$\begin{aligned}
\rho\sqrt{a}\frac{d^2x_1}{dt^2} &= \frac{\partial}{\partial\alpha_1}\left[(T^{11}l_{11} + T^{12}l_{21})\sqrt{\overset{*}{a}_{22}}\right] + \frac{\partial}{\partial\alpha_2}\left[(T^{12}l_{11} + T^{22}l_{21})\sqrt{\overset{*}{a}_{11}}\right] \\
&\quad + (p_1l_{11} + p_2l_{21})\sqrt{\overset{*}{a}} + p_3(l_{21}l_{23} - l_{13}l_{22})\sqrt{\overset{*}{a}_{11}\overset{*}{a}_{22}} + \rho f_1\sqrt{a}, \\
\rho\sqrt{a}\frac{d^2x_2}{dt^2} &= \frac{\partial}{\partial\alpha_1}\left[(T^{11}l_{12} + T^{12}l_{22})\sqrt{\overset{*}{a}_{22}}\right] + \frac{\partial}{\partial\alpha_2}\left[(T^{12}l_{12} + T^{22}l_{22})\sqrt{\overset{*}{a}_{11}}\right] \\
&\quad + (p_1l_{12} + p_2l_{22})\sqrt{\overset{*}{a}} + p_3(l_{13}l_{21} - l_{11}l_{23})\sqrt{\overset{*}{a}_{11}\overset{*}{a}_{22}} + \rho f_2\sqrt{a}, \\
\rho\sqrt{a}\frac{d^2x_3}{dt^2} &= \frac{\partial}{\partial\alpha_1}\left[(T^{11}l_{13} + T^{12}l_{23})\sqrt{\overset{*}{a}_{22}}\right] + \frac{\partial}{\partial\alpha_2}\left[(T^{12}l_{13} + T^{22}l_{23})\sqrt{\overset{*}{a}_{11}}\right] \\
&\quad + (p_1l_{13} + p_2l_{23})\sqrt{\overset{*}{a}} + p_3(l_{11}l_{22} - l_{12}l_{21})\sqrt{\overset{*}{a}_{11}\overset{*}{a}_{22}} + \rho f_3\sqrt{a}.
\end{aligned} \tag{5.90}$$

Here d^2x_i/dt^2 ($i = 1, 2, 3$) are the components of the vector of acceleration. Equation (5.90) should be complemented by constitutive relations (5.53), (5.54) or (5.63), initial and boundary conditions, and the conditions given by corollary 5.

5.9 Governing equations in cylindrical coordinates

Let a soft shell be associated with a cylindrical coordinate system $\{r, \varphi, z\}$

$$\begin{aligned}
r &= r(\alpha_1, \alpha_2, t), \\
\varphi &= \varphi(\alpha_1, \alpha_2, t), \\
z &= z(\alpha_1, \alpha_2, t).
\end{aligned} \tag{5.91}$$

It is related to the orthogonal Cartesian coordinates $\{x_1, x_2, x_3\}$ as

$$x_1 = r\cos\varphi, \quad x_2 = r\sin\varphi, \quad x_3 = z.$$

The position vector $\bar{r}$ of point $M(r, \varphi, z) \in S$ is given by

$$\bar{r} = r\bar{k}_1 + z\bar{k}_3, \tag{5.92}$$

where

$$\bar{k}_1 = \bar{i}_1 \cos\varphi + \bar{i}_2 \sin\varphi, \quad \bar{k}_2 = -\bar{i}_1 \sin\varphi + \bar{i}_2 \cos\varphi. \tag{5.93}$$

Differentiating equation (5.92) with respect to α_i with the help of equation (5.93), we find

$$\begin{aligned} \bar{r}_i = \frac{\partial \bar{r}}{\partial \alpha_i} &= \frac{\partial r}{\partial \alpha_i}\bar{k}_1 + r\frac{\partial \bar{k}_1}{\partial \alpha_i} + \frac{\partial z}{\partial \alpha_i}\bar{k}_3 \\ &= \frac{\partial r}{\partial \alpha_i}\bar{k}_1 + r\frac{\partial \varphi}{\partial \alpha_i}\bar{k}_2 + \frac{\partial z}{\partial \alpha_i}\bar{k}_3, \end{aligned} \tag{5.94}$$

where

$$\begin{aligned} \frac{\partial \bar{k}_1}{\partial \alpha_i} &= \frac{\partial}{\partial \alpha_i}(\bar{i}_1 \cos\varphi + \bar{i}_2 \sin\varphi) \\ &= \frac{\partial \varphi}{\partial \alpha_i}(-\bar{i}_1 \sin\varphi + \bar{i}_2 \cos\varphi) = \frac{\partial \varphi}{\partial \alpha_i}\bar{k}_2. \end{aligned} \tag{5.95}$$

Projections of $\bar{r}_i$ in the direction of the r, φ, and z axes are given by

$$\bar{r}_{ir} = \frac{\partial r}{\partial \alpha_i}, \quad \bar{r}_{i\varphi} = \frac{\partial \varphi}{\partial \alpha_i}, \quad \bar{r}_{iz} = \frac{\partial z}{\partial \alpha_i}.$$

Hence,

$$\bar{r}_i = \bar{r}_{ik}\bar{k}_1 + \bar{r}_{i\varphi}\bar{k}_2 + \bar{r}_{iz}\bar{k}_3. \tag{5.96}$$

Decomposing $\bar{e}_i$ along the base $\{\bar{k}_1, \bar{k}_2, \bar{k}_3\}$, we find

$$\bar{e}_i = l_{ir}\bar{k}_1 + l_{i\varphi}\bar{k}_2 + l_{iz}\bar{k}_3, \tag{5.97}$$

here the direction cosines l_{ij} $(i = 1, 2, 3; j = r, \varphi, z)$ are given by

$$\begin{aligned} &\bar{e}_1\bar{e}_2 = l_{1r}l_{2r} + l_{1\varphi}l_{2\varphi} + l_{1z}l_{2z} = \cos\overset{*}{\chi} = \overset{*}{a}_{12}\Big/\sqrt{\overset{*}{a}_{11}\overset{*}{a}_{22}}, \\ &\bar{e}_i\bar{e}_3 = l_{ir}l_{3r} + l_{i\varphi}l_{3\varphi} + l_{iz}l_{3z} = 0, \\ &\bar{e}_n\bar{e}_n = l_{n1}^2 + l_{n2}^2 + l_{n3}^2 = 1, \quad (n = 1, 2, 3). \end{aligned} \tag{5.98}$$

Expanding the resultant of external, $\bar{p}$, and mass, $\bar{f}$, forces in the direction of unit vectors $\bar{e}_i$, we obtain

$$\bar{p} = \bar{e}_1 p_1 + \bar{e}_2 p_2 + \bar{e}_3 p_3, \tag{5.99}$$

$$\bar{f} = \bar{k}_1 f_r + \bar{k}_2 f_\varphi + \bar{k}_3 f_z. \tag{5.100}$$

The vector of acceleration $\bar{a}(a_r, a_\varphi, a_z)$ in cylindrical coordinates is given by

$$a_r = -\frac{d^2 r}{dt^2} - r\left(\frac{d\varphi}{dt}\right)^2, \quad a_\varphi = -r\frac{d^2\varphi}{dt^2} + 2r\frac{dr}{dt}\frac{d\varphi}{dt}, \quad a_z = -\frac{d^2 z}{dt^2}. \tag{5.101}$$

Substituting equations (5.97), (5.99)–(5.101) in (5.77), the equations of motion of the soft shell in cylindrical coordinates take the form

$$\begin{aligned}
\rho\sqrt{a}\left(\frac{d^2 r}{dt^2} - r\left(\frac{d\varphi}{dt}\right)^2\right) &= \frac{\partial}{\partial\alpha_1}\left[(T^{1r}l_{1r} + T^{2r}l_{2r})\sqrt{\overset{*}{a}_{22}}\right] \\
&\quad + \frac{\partial}{\partial\alpha_2}\left[(T^{1r}l_{1r} + T^{2r}l_{2r})\sqrt{\overset{*}{a}_{11}}\right] + (p_1 l_{1r} + p_2 l_{2r})\sqrt{\overset{*}{a}} \\
&\quad + p_3(l_{2\varphi}l_{2z} - l_{1z}l_{2\varphi})\sqrt{\overset{*}{a}_{11}\overset{*}{a}_{22}} + \rho f_r\sqrt{a}, \\
\rho\sqrt{a}\left(r\frac{d^2\varphi}{dt^2} + 2r\frac{dr}{dt}\frac{d\varphi}{dt}\right) &= \frac{\partial}{\partial\alpha_1}\left[(T^{1\varphi}l_{1\varphi} + T^{1\varphi}l_{2\varphi})\sqrt{\overset{*}{a}_{22}}\right] \\
&\quad + \frac{\partial}{\partial\alpha_2}\left[(T^{1\varphi}l_{1\varphi} + T^{2\varphi}l_{2\varphi})\sqrt{\overset{*}{a}_{11}}\right] + (p_1 l_{1\varphi} + p_2 l_{2\varphi})\sqrt{\overset{*}{a}} \\
&\quad + p_3(l_{1z}l_{2r} - l_{1r}l_{2z})\sqrt{\overset{*}{a}_{11}\overset{*}{a}_{22}} + \rho f_\varphi\sqrt{a}, \\
\rho\sqrt{a}\frac{d^2 z}{dt^2} &= \frac{\partial}{\partial\alpha_1}\left[(T^{1z}l_{1z} + T^{2z}l_{2z})\sqrt{\overset{*}{a}_{22}}\right] + \frac{\partial}{\partial\alpha_2}\left[(T^{1z}l_{1z} + T^{2z}l_{2z})\sqrt{\overset{*}{a}_{11}}\right] \\
&\quad + (p_1 l_{1z} + p_2 l_{2z})\sqrt{\overset{*}{a}} + p_3(l_{1r}l_{2\varphi} - l_{1\varphi}l_{2r})\sqrt{\overset{*}{a}_{11}\overset{*}{a}_{22}} + \rho f_z\sqrt{a}.
\end{aligned} \tag{5.102}$$

Finally, to close the mathematical problem, equations (5.102) should be complemented by constitutive relations (5.53), (5.54), or (5.63), initial and boundary conditions, and the conditions given by corollary 5.

Further reading

Ridel V V and Gulin B V 1990 *Dynamics of Soft Shells* (Moscow: Nauka)

IOP Publishing

Roustem N Miftahof and Nariman R Akhmadeev

Chapter 6

A continuum model of biological tissue

Exercising the principles of thermodynamics, a model of a three-phase biomaterial is developed as a mechanochemically and electrogenically active continuum. All constitutive relations are formulated for the averaged parameters.

6.1 Histomorphology of tissue

The effectiveness and diversity of the physiological responses of various organs to internal and external stimuli depend on the inherent activity of histomorphological elements: the smooth muscle cells (SMCs), connective tissue matrix, neurons, and interstitial cells, along with their topographical organization in tissue. The innermost lining consists of sheets of epithelial cells that primarily have secretory, absorptive, and protective functions. Their role in the biodynamics of the organ, i.e. force–stretch development, propulsion, etc, is negligible.

The fibrillary connective tissue is formed from insoluble high-molecular-weight polymers of the proteins collagen and elastin, surrounded by a large amount of extracellular matrix. The extracellular matrix (ECM) is comprised of three major types of macromolecules, i.e. fibers (elastin and collagen), proteoglycans, and glycolproteins. It provides the biochemically stable micro-environment for the tissue through soluble and insoluble mediators guaranteeing its strength and elasticity through structural and mechanical constraints. Elastin is composed of flexible cross-linked polypeptides and has a linear stress–strain relation of up to 200%. Collagen, on the other hand, has a more organized structure with both crystalline and amorphous phases. Its fibers have a diameter in the range of 25–50 nm giving fiber bundles a diameter of several hundred micrometers. The fibers are undulated in the undeformed state becoming stiff when straightened under the action of externally applied loads. Collagen exhibits a highly nonlinear stress–strain curve. The overall strength of soft tissues is strongly correlated with the elastin–collagen content and the morphological characteristics of fibril length, diameter, distribution, and orientation. The collagen and elastin fibers are loosely woven and densely packed in an ordered

doi:10.1088/2053-2563/ab1a9ech6

way to form a three-dimensional supportive network for smooth muscle bundles and other multiple cellular elements. Such structural organization provides the required stability of the tissue, allowing organs to undergo reversible changes in length, while also offering remarkable properties of stiffness and elasticity.

The smooth muscle cell (myocyte) has a characteristic spindle-like shape measuring ~100–250 μm in length and ~5–6 μm in diameter. Its cytoplasm contains a centrally located nucleus, intracellular thin α- and β-actin (~6 nm), intermediate (mainly desmin; ~10 nm) and thick (~20–25 nm) filaments, mitochondria, and fairly sparse elements of the sarcoplasmic reticulum. The thin α- and β-actin filaments are arranged into a lattice attached to the cell membrane at the sites of dense bands (plaques). They guarantee the integrity, strength, and high degree of deformability of the wall and provide binding sites for myosin thick filaments.

Regularly spaced dense bands are comprised of multifunctional proteins: integrins, desmin, vincullin, tensin, calponin, nonmuscle β- and γ-actins, and filamin. They establish direct structural and functional contacts between the intracellular cytoskeleton and the ECM. The anchoring plaques play an essential role in transmitting forces of contraction–relaxation in the tissue, and act as mechanosensors in gene expression, signaling pathways, cell migration, growth, and adaptation.

Myocytes are arranged into SM fasciculi, $\simeq$300 ± 100 μm, and further assembled into bundles that are $\simeq$1–2 mm in length. These are embedded into a network of collagenous and elastin fibers and are coupled, via gap junctions, into syncytia.

The contractile apparatus of myocytes consists of thin-actin and thick-myosin filaments, a family of special proteins and kinases including: light chain myosin, tropomyosin, calmodulin, h-caldesmon, calponin, myosin light chain kinase, and myosin phosphatase. Actin filaments are single helical coils of actin associated with tropomyosin and caldesmon. Myosin filaments are made out of two coil rod-like structures of heavy chains with a globular head domain.

Nervous tissue provides communication among organs and systems predominantly by electrical signals. Neurons are responsible for the production and propagation of the waves of depolarization in the myelinated and unmyelinated nerve fibers, smooth muscle syncytia, and other cell aggregates. Each neuron has a soma, a number of branching dendrites, and the unmyelinated axon. They are arranged in planar neuronal networks via neuronal junctions called synapses. Neuroglial cells are a diverse group of morphoelements that play a supportive, mainly, trophic role.

6.2 A biocomposite as a mechanochemical continuum

The connection between the geometrical and statistical quantities studied in the previous chapters must be complemented by equations establishing relationships among the stresses and deformations and the rates, temperature, and structural changes of constructive materials, e.g. the tissue that forms the wall of a biological shell. The complete theoretical formulation is best achieved by applying the principles of thermodynamics supported by extensive experimentation, including in-plane and complex loading testing. The advantage of such an approach is that it employs generalized quantities, such as entropy, free energy, and Gibb's potential, as fundamental descriptors. Specific problems are encountered because of the discrete morphological structure of the biological tissue and the continuum scale, which is typically ~1 μm. For example, owing to existing anisotropy, multidimensional strain data from the uniaxial experiments are not enough to extrapolate to the fully three-dimensional constitutive equations. Furthermore, small specimen sizes, tethering effects, heterogeneity of deformation, and the difficulty in maintaining constant force distribution along specimen edges make experiments on soft tissues very difficult. Additionally since these are heterogeneous, anisotropic, non-linear, viscoelastic, incompressible composites (biocomposites), they defy simple material models. Accounting for these particulars in both constitutive models and experimental evaluations presents a huge challenge.

In this book the phenomenological approach towards modeling a soft biocomposite has been adopted. Derivations are based on the following histological assumptions:

(i) The biomaterial is a three-phase, multicomponent, mechanochemically active, anisotropic medium—phase 1 comprises the connective tissue net, phase 2 the mechanochemically active smooth muscle fibers, and phase 3 the inert myofibrils (figure 6.1).
(ii) The phase interfaces are semipermeable to certain substrates.
(iii) Smooth muscle, collagen, and elastin fibers are the main weight bearing and active force generating elements.
(iv) The biocomposite endows properties of general curvilinear anisotropy and viscoelasticity, the viscous properties are due to smooth muscle fiber mechanics while the elastic properties depend mainly on the collagen and elastin fibers.
(v) Active forces of contraction–relaxation produced by smooth muscle are the result of multicascade intracellular mechanochemical reactions—the reactions run in a large number of small loci that are evenly distributed throughout the whole volume of the tissue; the sources of chemical reagents are uniformly dispersed within the volume of the composite and are ample.
(vi) There are no temperature and/or deformation gradients within the tissue.
(vii) The biocomposite is incompressible and statistically homogeneous.

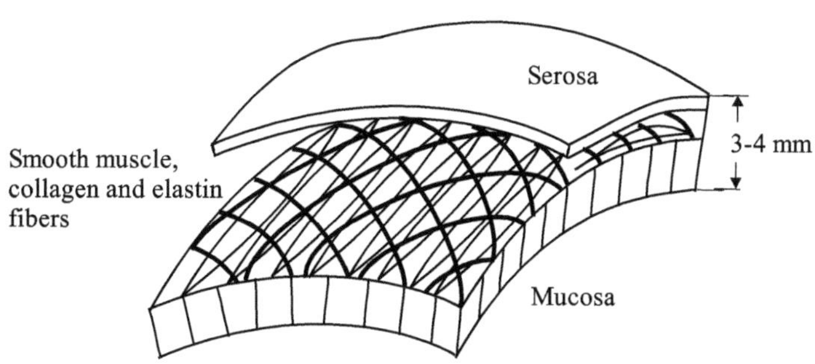

Figure 6.1. The tissue as a biological composite. Reprinted from Miftahof R N 2017 *Biomechanics of the Human Stomach* (Berlin: Springer) by permission of Springer Nature. Copyright 2017.

All the equations that follow are written for the averaged parameters. The quantities obtained by averaging the volume of a particular phase are contained in the angle brackets, and those free of brackets are attained by averaging the entire volume.

Let ρ be the mean density of the tissue. The partial density of the ζth substrate ($\zeta = \overline{1, n}$) in the β phase ($\beta = 1, 2, 3$) is defined as

$$\rho_\zeta^\beta = m_\zeta^\beta / \upsilon,$$

where m_ζ^β is the mass of the ζth substrate, υ is the total elementary volume of the tissue $\upsilon = \sum_{\beta=1}^{3} \upsilon^\beta$. The mass and the effective concentrations of substrates are

$$c_\zeta^\beta = \rho_\zeta^\beta / \rho, \quad \langle c^\beta \rangle = m_\zeta^\beta / \upsilon^\beta \rho^\beta. \tag{6.1}$$

Assuming $\rho = \langle \rho^\beta \rangle = \text{const}$, we have

$$\langle \rho^\beta \rangle = \sum_{\zeta=1}^{n} \frac{m_\zeta^\beta}{\upsilon^\beta}. \tag{6.2}$$

Setting $\beta = 1$ we find

$$\langle \rho^1 \rangle = \sum_{\zeta=1}^{n} \frac{m_\zeta^1}{\upsilon^1} = \sum_{\zeta=1}^{n} \frac{\rho_\zeta^1 \upsilon}{\upsilon^1} = \sum_{\zeta=1}^{n} \frac{c_\zeta^1 \rho \upsilon}{\upsilon^1} = \rho \sum_{\zeta=1}^{n} \frac{c_\zeta^1}{\eta},$$

where η is the porosity of phase β ($\eta = \upsilon / \upsilon^\beta$). It is easy to show that

$$\eta = \sum_{\zeta=1}^{n} c_\zeta^1 \equiv c^1. \tag{6.3}$$

Hence the mass c_ζ^β and the effective $\left\langle c_\zeta^\beta \right\rangle$ concentrations are interrelated by $c_\zeta^\beta = \eta \left\langle c_\zeta^\beta \right\rangle$. The sum of all concentrations c_ζ^β in the medium equals $\sum_{\zeta=1}^{n} c_\zeta^\beta = 1$.

The change in the concentration of constituents in different phases is due to the exchange of the matter among phases, external fluxes, chemical reactions, and diffusion. Since chemical reactions run only in phase 2 and the substrates move at the same velocity, there is no diffusion within phases. Hence, the equations of the conservation of mass of the ζth substrate in the medium is given by

$$\rho \frac{dc_\zeta^1}{dt} = Q_\zeta^1, \quad \rho \frac{dc_\zeta^2}{dt} = Q_\zeta^2 + \sum_{j=1}^{r} \nu_{\zeta j} J_j, \quad \rho \frac{dc_\zeta^3}{dt} = Q_\zeta^3. \tag{6.4}$$

Here Q_ς^β is the velocity of influx of the ζth substrate into the phase α, and $\nu_{\zeta j} J_j$ is the rate of ζth formation in the jth chemical reaction ($j = \overline{1, r}$). The quantity $\nu_{\zeta j}$ is related to the molecular mass M_ζ of the substrate ζ and is analogous to the stoichiometric coefficient in the jth reaction. $\nu_{\zeta j}$ takes positive values if the substrate is formed but becomes negative if the substrate disassociates. Since the mass of reacting components is conserved in each chemical reaction, we have

$$\sum_{\zeta=1}^{n} \nu_{\zeta j} = 0.$$

Assume that there is a flux Q_ζ^β of the matter into: (i) phase 1 from external sources and phase 3; (ii) phase 2 from phases 1 and 3 only; and (iii) phase 3 from phase 2. Hence, we have

$$Q_\zeta^1 = -Q_\zeta + Q_\zeta^e, \quad Q_\zeta^2 = Q_\zeta + Q_\zeta^m, \quad Q_\zeta^3 = -Q_\zeta^m, \tag{6.5}$$

where Q_ζ^e is the flux of externally distributed sources, Q_ζ is the exchange flux between phases, and Q_ζ^m is the flux of the matter from phase 3 into phase 2 (figure 6.2). Applying the incompressibility condition to (6.5), we have

$$\sum_{\zeta=1}^{n} Q_\zeta^e = 0.$$

Let also $\sum_{\zeta=1}^{n} Q_\zeta = 0$. Assuming that the effective concentration of substrates in phase 3 remains constant throughout, $\langle c_\zeta^3 \rangle = \text{const}$ and using equation (6.5) in (6.4), we obtain

$$\rho \frac{dc_\zeta^1}{dt} = -Q_\zeta + Q_\zeta^e, \quad \rho \frac{\partial c_\zeta^2}{\partial t} = Q_\zeta - Q_\zeta^3 + \sum_{j=1}^{r} \nu_{\zeta j} J_j, \quad \rho \frac{\partial c_\zeta^3}{\partial t} = -Q_\zeta. \tag{6.6}$$

In the above, we have neglected the convective transport of the matter within phases.

The equations of continuity and the conservation of momentum for the tissue treated as a three-dimensional solid in a fixed Cartesian coordinate system (x_1, x_2, x_3) is given by

$$\frac{\partial u}{\partial x_1} + \frac{\partial v}{\partial x_2} + \frac{\partial w}{\partial x_3} = 0, \tag{6.7}$$

$$\rho \frac{\partial^2 u_i}{\partial t^2} = \frac{\partial \sigma_{ij}}{\partial x_j} + \rho f_i\,. \tag{6.8}$$

Here u, v, w are the components of the displacement vector, f_i is the mass force, and σ_{ij} $(i, j = x_1, x_2, x_3)$ are stresses.

Let $U^{(\beta)}$, $s^{(\beta)}$, σ_{ij}^α be the free energy, entropy, and stresses of each phase. Hence the Gibbs relations for each phase are defined by

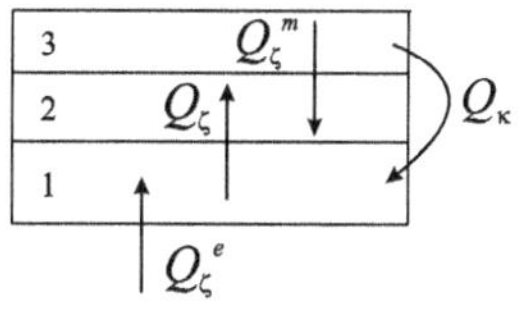

Figure 6.2. Flux exchanges in a three-phase biocomposite. Reprinted from Miftahof R N 2017 *Biomechanics of the Human Stomach* (Berlin: Springer) by permission of Springer Nature. Copyright 2017.

$$c^1\langle U^1\rangle = U^1{}_0\left(c_\zeta^1, T\right) + \frac{1}{2\rho}E_{ijlm}\varepsilon_{ij}\varepsilon_{lm} \tag{6.9}$$

$$c^\beta\langle U^\beta\rangle = U_0^\beta\left(c_\zeta^\beta, T\right) + \frac{1}{2\rho}Y_{ijlm}\varsigma_{ij}^\beta\varsigma_{lm}^\beta \tag{6.10}$$

$$d(c^1\langle U^1\rangle) = dU^1 = \frac{1}{\rho}c^1\langle\sigma^1\rangle_{ij}d\varepsilon_{ij}^1 - c^1\langle s^1\rangle dT + \sum_{\varsigma=1}^{n}\left\langle\mu_\zeta^1\right\rangle d\left\langle c_\zeta^1\right\rangle \tag{6.11}$$

$$\begin{gathered} d(c^\beta\langle U^\beta\rangle) = dU^\beta = \frac{1}{\rho}c^\beta\langle\sigma^\beta\rangle_{ij}d\varsigma_{ij}^\beta - c^\beta\langle s^\beta\rangle dT + \sum_{\varsigma=1}^{n}\left\langle\mu_\zeta^\beta\right\rangle d\left\langle c_\zeta^\beta\right\rangle \\ \left\langle\mu_\zeta^\beta\right\rangle = \partial\langle U^\beta\rangle/\partial\left\langle c_\zeta^\beta\right\rangle, \quad \langle s^\beta\rangle = \partial\langle U^\beta\rangle/\partial T, \quad (\beta = 2, 3), \end{gathered} \tag{6.12}$$

where T is temperature, μ_ζ^β is the chemical potential of the ζth substrate in the β phase, $\mu_\zeta^\beta = \partial c^\beta\langle U^\beta\rangle/\partial c_\zeta^\beta$, and ς_{ij} is the elastic and Δ_{ij} is the viscous part of deformation $\left(\varepsilon_{ij}^\beta = \varsigma_{ij}^\beta + \Delta_{ij}^\beta, \beta = 2, 3\right)$. Making use of equality

$$\partial(c^\beta\langle U^\beta\rangle)/\partial c_\zeta^\beta = \left\langle\mu_\zeta^\beta\right\rangle + \langle U^\beta\rangle - \sum_{\varsigma=1}^{n}\left\langle\mu_\zeta^\beta\right\rangle\left\langle c_\zeta^\beta\right\rangle.$$

Equations (6.11) and (6.12) can be written as

$$\begin{gathered} d(c^1\langle U^1\rangle) = \frac{1}{\rho}c^1\langle\sigma^1\rangle_{ij}d\varepsilon_{ij}^1 - c^1\langle s^1\rangle dT + \sum_{\varsigma=1}^{n}\mu_\zeta^1 dc_\zeta^1 \\ d(c^\beta\langle U^\beta\rangle) = \frac{1}{\rho}c^\beta\langle\sigma^\beta\rangle_{ij}d\varsigma_{ij}^\beta - c^\beta\langle s^\beta\rangle dT + \sum_{\varsigma=1}^{n}\mu_\zeta^\beta dc_\zeta^\beta \ (\beta = 2, 3). \end{gathered} \tag{6.13}$$

Assuming that the mass sources are present only in phases 1 and 2, the general heat flux and the second law of thermodynamics for the tissue are described by

$$dU = \frac{1}{\rho}\sigma_{ij}d\varepsilon_{ij} - sdT - dq' + \frac{1}{\rho}\sum_{\varsigma=1}^{n}\frac{\partial F}{\partial c^1{}_\varsigma}Q_\zeta^e dt, \tag{6.14}$$

$$Tds = dq^e + dq' + \sum_{\varsigma=1}^{n} TS^1{}_{\varsigma} \frac{Q_\zeta^e}{\rho} dt,$$
$$S_\zeta^1 = \left(\frac{\partial s}{\partial c_\zeta^1} \right)_{T, c^i{}_\vartheta(\vartheta \neq \zeta), \varsigma_{ij}, \varepsilon_{ij}} = \frac{\partial^2 F}{\partial T \partial c_\zeta^1}. \tag{6.15}$$

Here $U = \sum_{\beta=1}^{3} c^\beta \langle U^\beta \rangle$, $s = \sum_{\beta=1}^{3} c^\beta \langle s^\beta \rangle$, $\sigma_{ij} = \sum_{\alpha=1}^{3} c^\beta \langle \sigma^\beta \rangle_{ij}$, and S_ζ^1 is the partial entropy of the biocomposite.

To complete the formulation of the model we need to specify thermodynamic fluxes Q_ζ^e, Q_ζ, J_j and stresses $\sigma_{ij}^{(\beta)}$.

Let the heart flux $\bar{q}$ be given by

$$\rho dq^{(e)} = -\left(\frac{\partial q_x}{\partial x} + \frac{\partial q_y}{\partial y} + \frac{\partial q_z}{\partial z} \right) dt \equiv -\mathrm{div}\, \bar{q} dt.$$

Using equation (6.13) in (6.14), (6.15), the equation of the balance of entropy of the composite takes the form

$$\rho \frac{ds}{dt} - \sum_{\zeta=1}^{n} \frac{\partial s}{\partial c_\zeta^1} Q_\zeta^e = -\mathrm{div}\, \frac{\bar{q}}{T} + \frac{\boldsymbol{R}}{T}, \tag{6.16}$$

$$\boldsymbol{R} = -\frac{\bar{q}}{T} \left(\frac{\partial T}{\partial x} + \frac{\partial T}{\partial y} + \frac{\partial T}{\partial z} \right) + \sigma_{ij}^2 \frac{d\Delta_{ij}^2}{dt} + \sigma^3{}_{ij} \frac{d\Delta_{ij}^3}{dt}$$
$$+ \sum_{\varsigma=1}^{n} \left(\mu_\zeta^1 - \mu_\zeta^2 \right) Q_\zeta^e + \sum_{\varsigma=1}^{n} \left(\mu_\zeta^3 - \mu_\zeta^2 \right) Q_\zeta^e - \sum_{j=1}^{r} J_j \Lambda_j, \tag{6.17}$$

$$\Lambda_j = \sum_{\zeta=1}^{n} v_{\varsigma j} \mu_\zeta^2. \tag{6.18}$$

Here $\boldsymbol{R}$ is the dissipative function, Λ_j is the affinity constant of the jth chemical reaction.

Let thermodynamic forces acting in the system be

$$-\frac{1}{T^2} \left(\frac{\partial T}{\partial x} + \frac{\partial T}{\partial y} + \frac{\partial T}{\partial z} \right), \quad \frac{1}{T} \frac{d\Delta_{ij}^2}{dt}, \quad \frac{1}{T} \frac{d\Delta_{ij}^3}{dt},$$
$$\frac{\left(\mu_\varsigma^1 - \mu_\varsigma^2 \right)}{T}, \quad \frac{\left(\mu_\varsigma^3 - \mu_\varsigma^2 \right)}{T}, \quad -\frac{\Lambda_j}{T}. \tag{6.19}$$

Assuming linear relationship among thermodynamics fluxes $\bar{q}$, $\sigma_{ij}^{(\alpha)}$, Q_{ζ}^{e}, Q_{ζ}, J_j and thermodynamic forces, we have

$$q_i = -W_{ij}\frac{\partial T}{\partial x_j}, \tag{6.20}$$

$$\sigma_{kl}^{1} = E_{ijkl}\varepsilon_{ij}, \tag{6.21}$$

$$\begin{aligned}\sigma_{kl}^{2} = {} & B_{ijkl}\frac{d\Delta_{ij}^{2}}{dt} + B_{klij}^{*}\frac{d\Delta_{ij}^{3}}{dt} + \sum_{\beta=1}^{r} D_{\beta kl}^{*}\Lambda_{\beta} \\ & - \sum_{\alpha=1}^{n} O_{\alpha kl}^{*}\left(\mu_{\alpha}^{1} - \mu_{\alpha}^{2}\right) - \sum_{\alpha=1}^{n} Y_{\alpha kl}^{*}\left(\mu_{\alpha}^{3} - \mu_{\alpha}^{2}\right),\end{aligned} \tag{6.22}$$

$$\begin{aligned}\sigma_{ij}^{3} = {} & B_{ijkl}^{*}\frac{d\Delta_{ij}^{2}}{dt} + B_{ijkl}\frac{d\Delta_{ij}^{3}}{dt} + \sum_{\beta=1}^{r} D_{\beta ij}^{*}\Lambda_{\beta} \\ & - \sum_{\alpha=1}^{n} O_{\alpha kl}^{*}\left(\mu_{\alpha}^{1} - \mu_{\alpha}^{2}\right) - \sum_{\alpha=1}^{n} V_{\alpha kl}^{*}\left(\mu_{\alpha}^{3} - \mu_{\alpha}^{2}\right),\end{aligned} \tag{6.23}$$

$$\begin{aligned}J_{\beta} = {} & D_{\beta ij}\frac{d\Delta_{ij}^{2}}{dt} + D_{\beta kl}^{*}\frac{d\Delta_{ij}^{2}}{dt} - \sum_{\gamma=1}^{r} {}^{1}l_{\beta\gamma}\Lambda_{\beta} \\ & + \sum_{\alpha=1}^{n} {}^{2}l_{\alpha\beta}\left(\mu_{\alpha}^{1} - \mu_{\alpha}^{2}\right) + \sum_{\alpha=1}^{n} {}^{3}l_{\alpha\beta}\left(\mu_{\alpha}^{3} - \mu_{\alpha}^{2}\right),\end{aligned} \tag{6.24}$$

$$\begin{aligned}Q_{\alpha} = {} & O_{\alpha ij}\frac{d\Delta_{ij}^{2}}{dt} + O_{\alpha kl}^{*}\frac{d\Delta_{ij}^{3}}{dt} - \sum_{\beta=1}^{r} {}^{2}l_{\alpha\beta}\Lambda_{\beta} \\ & + \sum_{\beta=1}^{n} {}^{4}l_{\alpha\beta}\left(\mu_{\beta}^{1} - \mu_{\beta}^{2}\right) + \sum_{\gamma=1}^{n} {}^{5}l_{\beta\gamma}\left(\mu_{\gamma}^{3} - \mu_{\gamma}^{2}\right),\end{aligned} \tag{6.25}$$

$$\begin{aligned}Q_{n}^{e} = {} & Y_{nij}\frac{d\Delta_{ij}^{2}}{dt} + Y_{nkl}^{*}\frac{d\Delta_{ij}^{3}}{dt} - \sum_{\beta=1}^{r} {}^{3}l_{n\beta}\Lambda_{\beta} \\ & + \sum_{\alpha=1}^{n} {}^{5}l_{n\alpha}\left(\mu_{\alpha}^{1} - \mu_{\alpha}^{2}\right) - \sum_{\alpha=1}^{n} {}^{6}l_{n\alpha}\left(\mu_{\alpha}^{3} - \mu_{\alpha}^{2}\right).\end{aligned} \tag{6.26}$$

Here ${}^{m}l_{n\alpha,n\beta,\alpha\beta,\beta\gamma}$ ($m = \overline{1, 6}$) are scalars and $B^{(*)}_{ijkl}$, E_{ijkl}, $D^{(*)}_{nij}$, $Y^{(*)}_{\alpha ij}$, $O^{(*)}_{\alpha ij}$, W_{ij} are the parameters of tensorial nature. They satisfy the Onsager reciprocal relations

$$B^{(*)}_{ijkl} = B^{(*)}_{klij}, \quad D^{*}_{nij} = -D_{nij}, \quad W_{ji} = W_{ij}$$
$$V^{*}_{\alpha ij} = -V_{\alpha ij}, \quad O^{*}_{\alpha ij} = -O_{\alpha ij}, \quad {}^{m}l_{n\alpha,n\beta,\alpha\beta,\beta\gamma} = {}^{m}l_{\alpha n,\beta n,\beta\alpha,\gamma\beta}.$$

For example, assuming that the tissue is transversely anisotropic, then B_{ijkl}, D_{nij} are defined by

$$\begin{aligned} B_{ikjl} &= \lambda_1(\delta_{ik}\delta_{jl} + \delta_{il}\delta_{jk} - 2/3\delta_{ij}\delta_{kl}) \\ &\quad + \lambda_2(\delta_{ij}b_{kl} + \delta_{kl}b_{ij} - 1/3\delta_{ij}\delta_{kl} - 3b_{ij}b_{kl}) \\ &\quad + \lambda_3(\delta_{ik}b_{jl} + \delta_{jk}b_{il} + \delta_{il}b_{jk} + \delta_{jl}b_{ik} - 4b_{ij}b_{kl}) \\ D_{nij} &= D_n(\delta_{ij} - 3b_{ij}) \ (n = 1, 2, \ldots, r). \end{aligned}$$

Multiple experimental data on uniaxial and biaxial loading show that collagen and elastin fibers possess nonlinear elastic and muscle tissue, i.e. viscoelastic characteristics. Hence, for stresses we have

$$\sigma_{ij} = \sum_{\alpha=1}^{3} \sigma^{\alpha}_{ij} = c^1 E_{ijkl}\varepsilon_{kl} + c^2 E^{ve}_{ijkl}(\varepsilon_{kl} - \Delta^2_{kl}) + c^3 E^{ve}_{ijkl}(\varepsilon_{kl} - \Delta^3_{kl}), \tag{6.27}$$

where E^{ve}_{ijkl} is the tensor of viscous characteristics $\left(E^{ve}_{ijkl} = E^{ve}_{klij}\right)$. Differentiating the above with respect to time, the constitutive relations of the mechanochemically active biological tissue are found to be

$$\begin{aligned} & B^{*}_{klij}\underline{E}^{ve}_{ijmn}\frac{d\sigma_{kl}}{dt} + \left(\mathbf{I} - \frac{1}{c^3}B^{*}_{klij}\underline{E}^{ve}_{ijmn}\frac{dc^3}{dt}\right)\sigma_{kl} \\ &= c^1 E_{ijmn}\varepsilon_{ij} - \left(\frac{c^1}{c^3}B^{*}_{klij}\underline{E}^{ve}_{ijmn}E_{mnkl}\frac{dc^3}{dt} + B^{*}_{klij}\underline{E}^{ve}_{ijmn}E_{mnkl}\frac{dc^1}{dt}\right)\varepsilon_{mn} \\ &\quad - \frac{c^2}{c^3}B^{*}_{klij}\frac{dc^3}{dt}\varepsilon_{mn} + B^{*}_{ijmn}\left(c^1\underline{E}^{ve}_{ijkl}E_{klmn} + c^2 + c^3\right)\frac{d\varepsilon_{ij}}{dt} \\ &\quad - B^{*}_{ijmn}\left(\frac{dc^2}{dt} - \frac{c^2}{c^3}\frac{dc^3}{dt}\right)\frac{d\Delta^2_{ij}}{dt} + c^2 Z_{mn} + c^3 Z^{*}_{mn}, \end{aligned}$$

$$\begin{aligned} & B^{*}_{ijmn}\underline{E}^{ve}_{ijkl}\frac{d\Delta^2{}_{kl}}{dt} - \varsigma^2_{mn} + \underline{E}^{ve}_{ijmn}Z_{ij} = 0, \\ & B^{*}_{ijmn}\underline{E}^{ve}_{ijkl}\frac{d\Delta^3_{kl}}{dt} - \varsigma^3_{mn} + \underline{E}^{ve}_{ijmn}Z^{*}_{ij} = 0, \end{aligned}$$

$$
\begin{aligned}
c^2\frac{dZ_{mn}}{dt} &= B^T_{mnij}\frac{d\Delta^3_{ij}}{dt} + \sum_{\beta=1}^{r} D^*_{\beta mn}\Lambda_\beta - \sum_{\alpha=1}^{n} O^*_{\alpha mn}\left(\mu^1_\alpha - \mu^2_\alpha\right) \\
&\quad - \sum_{\alpha=1}^{n} Y^*_{\alpha mn}\left(\mu^3_\alpha - \mu^2_\alpha\right), \\
c^3\frac{dZ^*_{mn}}{dt} &= B_{mnij}\frac{d\Delta^2_{ij}}{dt} + \sum_{\beta=1}^{r} D_{\beta mn}\Lambda_\beta - \sum_{\alpha=1}^{n} O_{\alpha mn}\left(\mu^1_\alpha - \mu^2_\alpha\right) \\
&\quad - \sum_{\alpha=1}^{n} Y_{\alpha mn}\left(\mu^3_\alpha - \mu^2_\alpha\right), \\
&\quad (\mathbf{B}^{\mathrm{T}} = \mathbf{B}).
\end{aligned}
\tag{6.28}
$$

Here $\underline{\mathbf{E}}$ is the tensor inverse to $\mathbf{E}$ ($\underline{\mathbf{E}}\mathbf{E} = \mathbf{I}$), $\mathbf{I}$ is the identity tensor and Z^*_{ij} is the 'biofactor' which accounts for various biological phenomena, including electromechanical, chemical, remodeling, aging, etc, in the tissue.

Although the system of equation (6.28) describes the mechanics of biocomposites, it does not provide the required relationships between in-plane forces, moments, and deformations in the thin shell. To establish the missing link, we need to consider the distribution of ε^z_{ik} and stresses σ_{ik} $(i, k = 1, 2, 3)$ in the shell. Recalling the first Kirchhoff–Love geometric hypothesis, $\varepsilon^z_{13} = \varepsilon^z_{23} = 0$, it would be appealing to exclude the shear stresses and lateral forces from the equilibrium equations by neglecting the terms $\sigma_{13} = \sigma_{23} = 0$, $\overset{*}{N}_1 = \overset{*}{N}_2 = 0$. However, it would strongly violate the equilibrium conditions. Accepting the second Kirchhoff–Love hypothesis, which states that the normal stress σ_{33} is significantly smaller when compared to σ_{ij} $(i, k = 1, 2)$, we can eliminate only the terms containing σ_{33}. Then, equation (6.28) takes the form

$$
\begin{aligned}
&B^*_{klij}\underline{E}^{ve}_{ijmn}\frac{d\sigma_{kl}}{dt} + \left(\mathbf{I} - \frac{1}{c^3}B^*_{klij}\underline{E}^{ve}_{ijmn}\frac{dc^3}{dt}\right)\sigma_{kl} \\
&= c^1\underline{E}^{ve}_{ijmn}\varepsilon^z_{ij} - B^*_{klij}\underline{E}^{ve}_{ijmn}E_{mnkl}\left(\frac{c^1}{c^3}\frac{dc^3}{dt} + \frac{dc^1}{dt}\right)\varepsilon^z_{mn} \\
&\quad - \frac{c^2}{c^3}B^*_{klij}\frac{dc^3}{dt}\varepsilon^z_{mn} + B^*_{ijmn}\left(c^1\underline{E}^{ve}_{ijkl}E_{klmn} + c^2 + c^3\right)\frac{d\varepsilon^z_{ij}}{dt} \\
&\quad - B^*_{ijmn}\left(\frac{dc^2}{dt} - \frac{c^2}{c^3}\frac{dc^3}{dt}\right)\frac{d\Delta^{z2}_{ij}}{dt} + c^2 Z_{mn} + c^3 Z^*_{mn},
\end{aligned}
$$

$$
\begin{aligned}
&B^*_{ijmn}\underline{E}^{ve}_{ijkl}\frac{d\Delta^{z2}_{kl}}{dt} - \varsigma^{z2}_{mn} + \underline{E}^{ve}_{ijmn}Z_{ij} = 0, \\
&B^*_{ijmn}\underline{E}^{ve}_{ijkl}\frac{d\Delta^{z3}_{kl}}{dt} - \varsigma^{z3}_{mn} + \underline{E}^{ve}_{ijmn}Z^*_{ij} = 0,
\end{aligned}
\tag{6.29}
$$

$$c^2\frac{dZ_{mn}}{dt} = B^T_{ijmn}\frac{d\Delta^{z3}_{ij}}{dt} + \sum_{\beta=1}^{r} D^*_{\beta mn}\Lambda_\beta - \sum_{\alpha=1}^{n} O^*_{\alpha mn}\left(\mu^1_\alpha - \mu^2_\alpha\right)$$
$$- \sum_{\alpha=1}^{n} Y^*_{\alpha mn}\left(\mu^3_\alpha - \mu^2_\alpha\right),$$
$$c^3\frac{dZ^*_{mn}}{dt} = B_{mnij}\frac{d\Delta^{z2}_{ij}}{dt} + \sum_{\beta=1}^{r} D_{\beta mn}\Lambda_\beta - \sum_{\alpha=1}^{n} O_{\alpha mn}\left(\mu^1_\alpha - \mu^2_\alpha\right)$$
$$- \sum_{\alpha=1}^{n} Y_{\alpha mn}\left(\mu^3_\alpha - \mu^2_\alpha\right).$$

Finally, substituting $\varepsilon^{\bar{z}}_{ik}$ given by equation (6.14) and solving the resultant equations for σ_{11}, σ_{22}, and σ_{12}, we obtain constitutive relations for the mechanochemically active biocomposite in terms of deformations, curvature, and twist in the middle surface of the shell. Applying σ_{ik} in equations (3.25) and integrating it over the thickness of the shell, we find explicit relations for the in-plane forces $\overset{*}{T}_{ij}$ and moments $\overset{*}{M}_{ij}$.

6.3 Biofactor Z_{ij}

The essential mechanical functions of the abdominal viscera such as peristalsis, propulsion, grinding, and expulsion are closely related to electromechanical wave processes and the coordinated propagation of the waves of contraction–relaxation within electrically excitable smooth muscle syncytia. From Ohm's law we have

$$\bar{J}_i = -\left(\hat{g}_{i1}\frac{\partial \Psi_i}{\partial x_1}\bar{e}_1 + \hat{g}_{i2}\frac{\partial \Psi_i}{\partial x_2}\bar{e}_2\right), \tag{6.30}$$

$$\bar{J}_o = -\left(\hat{g}_{o1}\frac{\partial \Psi_o}{\partial x_1}\bar{e}_1 + \hat{g}_{o2}\frac{\partial \Psi_o}{\partial x_2}\bar{e}_2\right), \tag{6.31}$$

where $\bar{J}_i$, $\bar{J}_o$ are the intra- (i) and extracellular (o) currents, Ψ_i, Ψ_o are the scalar electrical potentials, $\hat{g}_{ij}$, $\hat{g}_{oj}$ (j = 1, 2) are the conductivities, and $\bar{e}_1$, $\bar{e}_2$ are the unit vectors in the directions of the α_1, α_2 coordinate lines. Both cellular spaces are coupled through the transmembrane current I_{m1} and potential V_m as

$$I_{m1} = -\text{div}\,\bar{J}_i = \text{div}\,\bar{J}_o, \tag{6.32}$$

$$V_m = \Psi_i - \Psi_o. \tag{6.33}$$

Substituting equations (6.30) and (6.31) into (6.32), we obtain

$$I_{m1} = \hat{g}_{i1}\frac{\partial^2 \Psi_i}{\partial \alpha_1^2}\bar{e}_1 + \hat{g}_{i2}\frac{\partial^2 \Psi_i}{\partial \alpha_2^2}\bar{e}_2, \tag{6.34}$$

$$I_{m1} = -\hat{g}_{o1}\frac{\partial^2 \Psi_o}{\partial \alpha_1^2}\bar{e}_1 + \hat{g}_{o2}\frac{\partial^2 \Psi_o}{\partial \alpha_2^2}\bar{e}_2. \tag{6.35}$$

Equating equations (6.34) and (6.35), we find

$$(\hat{g}_{i1} + \hat{g}_{o1})\frac{\partial^2 \Psi_i}{\partial \alpha_1^2} + (\hat{g}_{i2} + \hat{g}_{o2})\frac{\partial^2 \Psi_i}{\partial \alpha_2^2} = \hat{g}_{o1}\frac{\partial^2 V_m}{\partial \alpha_1^2} + \hat{g}_{o2}\frac{\partial^2 V_m}{\partial \alpha_2^2}. \tag{6.36}$$

Solving equation (6.36) for Ψ_i, we obtain

$$\Psi_i = \frac{1}{4\pi}\iint\left(\frac{\hat{g}_{o1}}{\hat{g}_{i1} + \hat{g}_{o1}}\frac{\partial^2 V_m}{\partial X'^2} + \frac{\hat{g}_{o2}}{\hat{g}_{i2} + \hat{g}_{o2}}\frac{\partial^2 V_m}{\partial Y'^2}\right) + [\log((X - X')^2 + (Y - Y')^2)]dX'dY',$$

where the following substitutions are used: $X = \alpha_1/\sqrt{g_{i1} + g_{o1}}$, $Y = \alpha_2/\sqrt{\hat{g}_{i2} + \hat{g}_{o2}}$. Here the integration variables are primed, and the unprimed variables indicate the space point (α_1', α_2') at which Ψ_i is evaluated. The reverse substitution of X and Y gives

$$\Psi_i = \frac{1}{4\pi}\iint\left(\hat{g}_{o1}\frac{\partial^2 V_m}{\partial X'^2} + \hat{g}_{o2}\frac{\partial^2 V_m}{\partial Y'^2}\right) + \left[\log\left(\frac{(\alpha_1 - \alpha_1')^2}{\hat{g}_{i1} + \hat{g}_{o1}} + \frac{(\alpha_2 - \alpha_2')^2}{\hat{g}_{i2} + \hat{g}_{o2}}\right)\right]\frac{d\alpha_1' d\alpha_2'}{\sqrt{(\hat{g}_{i1} + \hat{g}_{o1})(\hat{g}_{i2} + \hat{g}_{o2})}}. \tag{6.37}$$

Introducing equation (6.37) into (6.34), after some algebra we obtain

$$I_{m1} = \frac{\tilde{\mu}_1 - \tilde{\mu}_2}{2\pi G(1 + \tilde{\mu}_1)(1 + \tilde{\mu}_2)}\iint\left(\hat{g}_{o1}\frac{\partial^2 V_m}{\partial X'^2} + \hat{g}_{o2}\frac{\partial^2 V_m}{\partial Y'^2}\right) \times\left[\left(\frac{(\alpha_1 - \alpha_1')^2}{G_1} - \frac{(\alpha_2 - \alpha_2')^2}{G_2}\right)\Big/\left(\frac{(\alpha_1 - \alpha_1')^2}{G_1} + \frac{(\alpha_2 - \alpha_2')^2}{G_2}\right)^2\right] \times d\alpha_1' d\alpha_2', \tag{6.38}$$

where

$$G_1 = \hat{g}_{i1} + \hat{g}_{o1}, \quad G_2 = \hat{g}_{i2} + \hat{g}_{o2},$$
$$G = \sqrt{G_1 G_2}, \quad \tilde{\mu}_1 = \hat{g}_{o1}/\hat{g}_{i1}, \quad \tilde{\mu}_2 = \hat{g}_{o2}/\hat{g}_{i2}.$$

Substituting equation (6.37) into (6.34), we find the contribution of an ε-neighborhood of $(\alpha_1' = 0, \alpha_2' = 0)$ to I_{m1}. Using the transformations given by $X = \alpha_1/\sqrt{\hat{g}_{i1}}$, $Y = \alpha_2/\sqrt{\hat{g}_{i2}}$, we find

$$I_{m2} = \frac{\sqrt{\hat{g}_{i1}\hat{g}_{i2}}}{4\pi G}\left(\hat{g}_{o1}\frac{\partial^2 V_m}{\partial X'^2} + \hat{g}_{o2}\frac{\partial^2 V_m}{\partial Y'^2}\right)_{\alpha_1'=\alpha_2'=0} \times \int \mathrm{divgrad}\left[\log\left(\frac{X'^2}{G_1/\hat{g}_{i1}} + \frac{Y'^2}{G_2/\hat{g}_{i2}}\right)\right]d\alpha_1' d\alpha_2'. \tag{6.39}$$

Applying the divergence theorem and performing the gradient operation, the integral in equation (6.39) is converted to a line integral

$$\int \frac{(2X'\hat{g}_{i1}/G_1)\bar{e}_1 + (2Y'\hat{g}_{i2}/G_2)\bar{e}_2}{(X'^2\hat{g}_{i1}/G_1) + (Y'^2\hat{g}_{i2}/G_2)} \cdot \bar{n}dC', \tag{6.40}$$

where dC' is an element of the ε-contour. The result of integration yields

$$I_{m2} = \left(\hat{g}_{o1}\frac{\partial^2 V_m}{\partial \alpha_1'^2} + \hat{g}_{o2}\frac{\partial^2 V_m}{\partial \alpha_2'^2}\right)\left(\frac{\hat{g}_{i2}}{G_2} + \frac{2(\tilde{\mu}_1 - \tilde{\mu}_2)}{\pi(1+\tilde{\mu}_1)(1+\tilde{\mu}_2)}\tan^{-1}\sqrt{\frac{G_1}{G_2}}\right). \tag{6.41}$$

To simulate the excitation and propagation pattern in the anisotropic smooth muscle syncytium we employ the Hodgkin–Huxley formalism described by

$$C_m\frac{\partial V_m}{\partial t} = -(I_{m1} + I_{m2} + I_{\text{ion}}),$$

where C_m is the membrane capacitance and I_{ion} is the total ion current through the membrane. Substituting expressions for I_{m1} and I_{m2} given by (6.38) and (6.41), we obtain

$$\begin{aligned} C_m\frac{\partial V_m}{\partial t} = &-\frac{\tilde{\mu}_1 - \tilde{\mu}_2}{2\pi G(1+\tilde{\mu}_1)(1+\tilde{\mu}_2)}\iint\left(\hat{g}_{o1}\frac{\partial^2 V_m}{\partial X'^2} + \hat{g}_{o2}\frac{\partial^2 V_m}{\partial Y'^2}\right) \\ &\times\left[\left(\frac{(\alpha_1 - \alpha_1')^2}{G_1} - \frac{(\alpha_2 - \alpha_2')^2}{G_2}\right)\right. \\ &\left.\Big/\left(\frac{(\alpha_1 - \alpha_1')^2}{G_1} + \frac{(\alpha_2 - \alpha_2')^2}{G_2}\right)^2\right]d\alpha_1' d\alpha_2' \\ &-\left(\hat{g}_{o1}\frac{\partial^2 V_m}{\partial \alpha_1'^2} + \hat{g}_{o2}\frac{\partial^2 V_m}{\partial \alpha_2'^2}\right)\left(\frac{\hat{g}_{i2}}{G_2} + \frac{2(\tilde{\mu}_1 - \tilde{\mu}_2)}{\pi(1+\tilde{\mu}_1)(1+\tilde{\mu}_2)}\right. \\ &\left.\times\tan^{-1}\sqrt{\frac{G_1}{G_2}}\right) - I_{\text{ion}}, \end{aligned} \tag{6.42}$$

where I_{ion} is the function depending on the type and ion channel properties of the tissue.

In the case of electrical isotropy, $\tilde{\mu}_1 = \tilde{\mu}_2 = \tilde{\mu}$, the integral in equation (6.42) vanishes and we obtain

$$C_m\frac{\partial V_m}{\partial t} = -\frac{1}{(1+\tilde{\mu})}\left(\hat{g}_{o1}\frac{\partial^2 V_m}{\partial \alpha_1^2} + \hat{g}_{o2}\frac{\partial^2 V_m}{\partial \alpha_2^2}\right) - I_{\text{ion}}. \tag{6.43}$$

Finally, the constitutive relations of mechanochemically active electrogenic biological medium include equations (6.6)–(6.8), (6.29), (6.42), and/or (6.43). The system is closed by providing the free energy, ion currents, initial and boundary conditions, and the function $Z_{ij} = Z_{ij}(V_m, \mu_i, \hat{g}_{ij}, \hat{g}_{oj})$. It is worth noting that the closed system of equations describes the development of stresses in the absence of active strains and vice versa. This is a condition unique to all biological materials.

Further reading

Nikitin N L 1980 *Mech. Comp. Mater.* **1** 113–20

Plonsey R L and Barr R G 1984 *Biophys. J.* **43** 557–71

Tester J W and Modell M 1996 *Thermodynamics and its Applications* 3rd edn (Englewood Cliffs, NJ: Prentice Hall)

Usik P I 1973 *J. Appl. Math. Mech. (Trans. Prikladnaya Matematika i Mechanika)* **37** 428–39

IOP Publishing

Soft Biological Shells in Bioengineering

Roustem N Miftahof and Nariman R Akhmadeev

Chapter 7

Neurons and neuronal assemblies

This chapter focuses on the mathematical modeling of both neurons and the interstitial cells of Cajal along with their assemblies in excitable neuronal circuits and networks.

7.1 The intrinsic regulatory system in the gut

The enteric nervous system (ENS) is comprised of a large number of neurons, 46 260 ± 3.829 neurons/cm^2. The neurons possess two major morphological forms, i.e. uniaxonal and multiaxonal, respectively, although bipolar, ovoid, polygonal, and stellar shapes have also been described. Morphofunctional and projectile classification reflects on intrinsic primary afferent, ascending (orally)/descending (aborally) inter-, motor, intestinofugal, secretomotor, and vasomotor neurons. In contrast, electrophysiological taxonomy is based mainly on firing pattern characteristics. Thus S-type neurons exhibit brief action potentials and lack a prolonged slow post-after-hyperpolarization phase, whilst AH-type neurons show prominent long lasting (up to 20 s) hyperpolarization dynamics.

The primary afferent (sensory) neurons have not been definitely identified and there is still considerable controversy concerning their location and projections. They have smooth cell bodies, and could be adendritic, pseudo-uniaxonal, or multiaxonal (with two or more long processes). There is a tendency towards primary and secondary branching of the neurites close to the soma with few or even no synaptic inputs. The receptive fields, mechanoreceptors, are free nerve endings located in the mucosa and the submucous layer.

Motor neuron cells are uniaxonal and multidendritic. Dendrites are of intermediate length, with relatively little branching and project to SIP. The distinguishing characteristic of their electrical behavior is that they discharge long trains of spikes. These patterns resemble all-or-nothing events and are independent of the initial stimulus.

doi:10.1088/2053-2563/ab1a9ech7

The neurons group together to form morphofunctional units known as ganglia. Ganglia are diverse in terms of their number, morphology, size, and the number of neurons they contain. The density of ganglia distribution is not constant, e.g. it is relatively sparse in the fundus of the stomach but denser in the antrum and pylorus, whilst it is evenly distributed in the small intestine. Quantitative analysis reveals that an average ganglion is formed of 3.4–5.4 neurons that are spread over a surface area of $(1.8 \pm 0.3) \times 10^2$ mm^2. The actual size of matured neurons ranges within $(29.6 \pm 2.25) \times 10$ μm^2.

The ENS is organized in a strict hierarchical manner. Their ganglia are assembled in three anatomically distinct spatially dispersed plexi (the myenteric (Auerbach's), the submucous (Meissner's), and the mucous nervous plexus). These are unevenly represented throughout the organs of the gastrointestinal tract. Whereas Auerbach's and Meissner's plexi are equally prominent in the small intestine, the former is dominant in the human stomach whilst the latter appears very sparse in this organ. Confocal microscopy studies show that the plexi structure resembles a rectangular network with an average spacing between ganglia of ~200–500 μm. Numerous overlapping polysynaptic pathways ensure the effective and efficient transmission of information coded in the form of electrochemical signals within each plexus.

Immunoreactivity studies have demonstrated that matured neuronal cells in the ENS can co-localize multiple neurotransmitters and/or modulators. Thus a quantitative analysis of co-localization shows that 8.3% ± 3.1% of all neurons are positive both for ACh and SP, 4.9% ± 12.6% for ACh/VIP, 3.1% ± 1.8% for ACh/NO, 3.1% ± 1.8% for ACh/NO/VIP, and 1.1% ± 0.7% for ACh/NO/VIP/SP. Such coexistence suggests that cells may simultaneously release more than one substrate and that co-transmission may take place. Indeed, the co-release of neurotransmitters (ACh, 5-HT, NO, SP, galanin, enkephaline, glutamate, γ-amino butyric acid, and dopamine) and peptides (vasoactive intestinal peptide (VIP), calcitonin gene-related peptide, adenosine triphosphate (ATP)) have been recorded in the gastrointestinal tract. The process is highly regulated in response to various physiological, chemical, and pathological signals. However, the exact mechanisms and how these occur remains an open question.

The histoarchitecture of the ENS, as described above, allows the ad hoc formation of intrinsic neuronal circuits within, and guarantees the stability and high degree reliability of its function. Despite the fact that the human stomach is under the control of the central nervous system via the *vagus* nerve, the possibility of generating intrinsic reflexes independently from the CNS places Auerbach's plexus in a unique position to operate autonomously.

7.2 Interstitial cells of Cajal

A class of interstitial cells of Cajal (ICC) and platelet-derived growth factor receptor α cells (PDGFRα^+), that are distinct in their origin, phenotype, morphology, and ultrastructure, are present within smooth muscle syncytia of the human stomach, the small intestine, and the colon. Deriving embryologically from the mesencymal lineage, they possess typical features attributed either to primitive smooth muscle or the 'fibroblast-like' interstitial cells. The recent advance in antibody labeling has shown that only cells expressing the gene product of *c-Kit*, a proto-oncogene that encrypts a tyrosine kinase receptor (Kit), differentiate and mature into ICC. No specific markers for PDGFRα^+ precursor cells have been identified and their role in the development of a Kit-positive precursor into a functional ICC or a SMC, remains to be discovered.

Immunochemical studies on matured ICC have confirmed: (i) the presence of soluble guanylate cyclase, the physiological receptor for NO; (ii) the translocation of PKC isozymes from the cytoplasm to the membrane in response to cholinergic stimulation and activation of μ_2 and μ_3, receptors, and anoctamin-1 (ANO1), Ca^{2+}-activated Cl^- channels; (iii) the internalization of neurokinin type 1 and 3 (NK_1, NK_3) receptors after the application of exogenous SP; (iv) the presence of VIP receptors as well as non-selective cation channels TRP4 and TRP6. Currently there is no strong functional evidence to support the hypothesis of the involvement of P2X, P2Y, and $VPAC_{1/2}$ receptors in signal transduction on ICC. Additionally, L-, and possibly T-type, Ca^{2+} as well as tetrodotoxin-insensitive Na^+ transmembrane ion channels have been implemented in the mechanosensitivity of ICC in response to applied axial/shear stretches and positive/negative pressures. PDGFRα^+ cells have both P2Y1 receptors and SK3 channels, suggesting that these cells are purinergic mediators of ATP, ADP, and β-nicotinamide adenine dinucleotide.

A set of ICC/PDGFRα^+ cells that is present intramuscularly, mainly in the circular smooth muscle layer of the gastrointestinal tract, is referred to as ICC/PDGFRα^+–IM. ICC, possessing both bipolar and multipolar morphology, are connected through multiple electrical synapses to form an extensive network of their own. Owing to its location and close proximity to Auerbach's plexus, the network is termed ICC-MY. It is worth noting that the ICC-MY anastomosing network enfolds myenteric ganglia but is not intrinsic to them.

7.3 Electrical activity in neurons

Electrical activity in neurons is ubiquitous. It is manifested both through a variety of patterns of discharges and the specificity of transduction mechanisms that enable the system to integrate and to coordinate the overall behaviors in space and time. For the purpose of the mathematical modeling of neuronal activity two types of complexity must be dealt with: the interplay of ion channel dynamics that underlie the excitability, and the neuronal morphology that allows neurons to communicate signals amongst them. Despite significant advancements in simulation that have put forward a large number of proposed mathematical models of excitable media, the only biologically plausible and accurate model remains the Hodgkin–Huxley (H–H) model (1952). It contains a current balance equation that satisfies Kirchoff's law

$$C_m^f \frac{dV}{dt} = -\sum_{i=1}^{n} g_i x_i^p y_i^p (V - V_i) + I_{\text{appl}}(t), \tag{7.1}$$

and relaxation equations for ionic conductances

$$\frac{dx_i}{dt} = \frac{x_{i\infty}(V) - x_i}{\tau_{x_i}(V)}, \qquad i = \overline{1, n},$$
$$\frac{dy_i}{dt} = \frac{y_{i\infty}(V) - y_i}{\tau_{y_i}(V)}, \qquad i = \overline{1, n}. \tag{7.2}$$

Here C_m^f is the membrane capacitance, V is the membrane potential, V_i is the Nernst potential for the ith ion, g_i is the maximal conductance of the channel for the different ion-selective channels, $x_i^p(x_{i\infty})$, $y_i^p(y_{i\infty})$ are the actual (steady) state activation and inactivation variables, respectively, τ_{x_i} and τ_{y_i} are the relaxation time constants, and $I_{\mathrm{appl}}(t)$ is the applied current. The nonlinear system (7.1), (7.2) accurately reproduces the rich dynamic behavior in various excitable tissues ranging both from tonic bursting to chaos, and from stationary to traveling wave phenomena. Such versatility and reliability are the result of a mathematical formulation that incorporates both explicitly and implicitly the intrinsic properties of the cell membrane. Dynamic systems analysis has provided insights into how cell activity is shaped by individual parameters. Thus, it has been demonstrated that a qualitative change from large amplitude and stable periodic behavior to small amplitude and unstable periodic oscillations—a subcritical Hopf bifurcation—can be achieved by an increase in $[Ca_0^{2+}]$, a reduction in membrane maximal K^+ conductance, or by a shift of the Nernst potential for K^+ in the depolarizing direction.

Much recent research has been directed at understanding the impact of anatomical architecture on signal integration within a neuron and neuronal ensembles. Initially, a single, electrically equivalent cable model was used to simulate the generation and propagation of voltage waves and current changes in the axon and dendrites

$$C_m^f \frac{dV}{dt} = \frac{d_{\mathrm{f}}}{2R_a^f} \frac{\partial^2 V}{\partial \alpha^2} - \sum_{i=1}^{n} g_i x_i^p y_i^p (V - V_i) + I_{\mathrm{appl}}(t), \tag{7.3}$$

where R_a^f is the membrane resistance, d_{f} is the cross-sectional diameter of the nerve fiber, and α is the Lagrange coordinate $(0 \leqslant \alpha \leqslant L^s)$ of the axon. The meaning of other parameters and constants is as described above. However, it does not answer questions related to the synaptic transmission. As an extension, compartmental models have been developed to explore the role of evolving dendritic morphology and to embrace biological mechanisms at molecular and cellular levels that support the temporal and spatial stability of signaling in diverse neuronal topologies.

7.4 Neuronal circuits

A framework for investigating the informational and computational capabilities of neuronal networks is based on the general scheme with one-layer feedback or multi-layer feed-forward performance and 'artificial' neurons linked by 'artificial' synapses. Being a drastic simplification with respect to a biological prototype the models have predicted many clinical effects with some rate of success. However, such approaches do not encompass the existing complexity of nonlinear dynamic interactions among intertwined signaling polysynaptic pathways. Awareness of the nonlinear correlation of these interactions becomes of paramount importance with a burgeoning understanding of cellular mechanisms of multiple neurotransmission.

A brief outline of existing and proposed neuronal elements and circuits that include synaptic connections along with mathematical descriptions of their dynamics are given below.

7.4.1 A neuronal network—ICC circuit

Consider a neuronal arrangement as shown in figure 7.1.

Mechanoreceptors convert mechanical stimuli (stretch deformation) to the receptor potential via activation of Na^+ selective ion channels. The dynamics of the dendritic receptor potential is given by

$$\begin{aligned} C_m^e \frac{dV^e}{dt} &= -(\tilde{I}_{Na} + \tilde{I}_K + \tilde{I}_{Cl}) - (V^d - V^e)/R_m \\ \gamma \frac{dV^d}{dt} &= -V^d + k(V^d - V^e)/R_m, \end{aligned} \tag{7.4}$$

where V^d, V^e are the nerve ending and dendritic receptor potentials, respectively, C_m^e is the dendritic membrane capacitance, R_m is the membrane resistance, and γ, k are the membrane time and numerical constants. $\tilde{I}_{Na}$, $\tilde{I}_K$, $\tilde{I}_{Cl}$ are the sodium, potassium, and chloride currents

$$\begin{aligned} \tilde{I}_{Na} &= \tilde{g}_{Na}\tilde{m}^3\tilde{h}(\tilde{V}^e - \tilde{V}_{Na}), \\ \tilde{I}_K &= \tilde{g}_K\tilde{n}^4(\tilde{V}^e - \tilde{V}_K), \\ \tilde{I}_{Cl} &= \tilde{g}_{Cl}(\tilde{V}^e - \tilde{V}_{Cl}). \end{aligned} \tag{7.5}$$

Here $\tilde{g}_{Na}$, $\tilde{g}_K$, $\tilde{g}_{Cl}$ are the maximal conductances for the Na^+, K^+, Cl^- channels, $\tilde{m}$, $\tilde{h}$, $\tilde{n}$ are probabilities of opening these channels, and $\tilde{V}_{Na}$, $\tilde{V}_K$, $\tilde{V}_{Cl}$ are the reversal

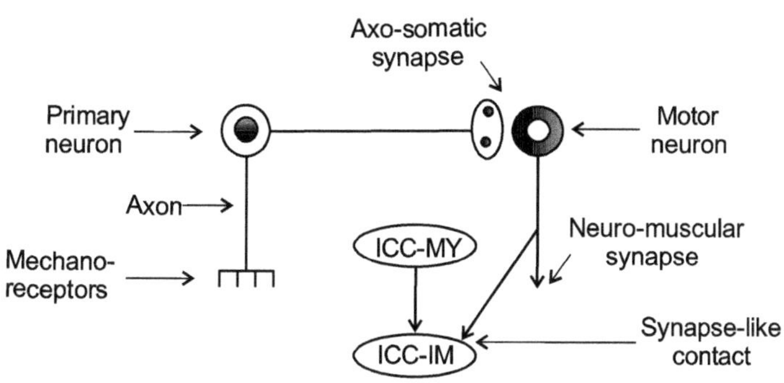

Figure 7.1. A neuronal network—ICC circuit.

potentials of the Na^+, K^+, Cl^- currents. The activation and deactivation of ion channels is described by

$$\frac{dy^*}{dt} = \psi(\tilde{\alpha}_y(1 - y^*) - \tilde{\beta}_y y^*) \qquad (y^* = \tilde{m}, \tilde{h}, \tilde{n}), \tag{7.6}$$

where ψ is the temperature scale factor, $\tilde{\alpha}_y$ is the rate of switching channels from a closed to an open state, and $\tilde{\beta}_y$ is the rate of reverse. They are obtained from the approximation of experimental data

$$\begin{aligned} \tilde{\alpha}_m &= 0.221 \exp(\varepsilon(t) + 0.01 V^e), \quad \tilde{\beta}_{m\infty} = 4.5 \exp(-V^e/18) \\ \tilde{\alpha}_h &= 0.048 \exp(-V^e/36), \quad \tilde{\beta}_h = 0.12/(1 + \exp(3.4 - 0.2 V^e)) \\ \tilde{\alpha}_n &= 0.33 \exp(1.1 - 0.1 V^e), \quad \tilde{\beta}_n = 0.185 \exp(-V^e/80). \end{aligned} \tag{7.7}$$

Here $\varepsilon(t)$ is the applied deformation.

The dynamics of action potentials at the soma of neuronal and interstitial cells of Cajal is given by

$$C_n^s \frac{dV_n^s}{dt} = -\sum_j I_j + I_{\text{ext}}, \tag{7.8}$$

where C_n^s is the membrane capacitance of the soma of a cell, I_j ($j = Ca^{2+}$, Ca^{2+}–K^+, Na^+, K^+, Cl^-) are ion currents carried through specified ion channels (their choice and inclusion in the model depends on the biological characteristics of the cell), $I_{\text{ext}} = V/R_{\text{ICC}}$ is the external membrane current, and R_{ICC} is the input cellular resistance. Thus the ion currents are defined as

$$\begin{aligned} I_{\text{Ca}} &= g_{\text{Ca}(i)} z_{\text{Ca}} \left(V_n^s - V_{\text{Ca}(i)}\right) / \left(1 + \vartheta_{\text{Ca}}[\text{Ca}_i^{2+}]\right), \\ I_{\text{Ca-K}} &= g_{\text{Ca-K}(i)} \rho_\infty \left(V_n^s - V_{\text{Ca-K}(i)}\right) / \left(0.5 + [\text{Ca}_i^{2+}]\right), \\ I_{\text{Na}} &= g_{\text{Na}(i)} m_{\text{Na}}^3 h_{\text{Na}} \left(V_n^s - V_{\text{Na}(i)}\right), \\ I_{\text{K}} &= g_{\text{K}(i)} n_{\text{K}}^4 \left(V_n^s - V_{\text{K}(i)}\right), \\ I_{\text{Cl}} &= g_{\text{Cl}(i)} \left(V_n^s - V_{\text{Cl}(i)}\right), \end{aligned} \tag{7.9}$$

where $V_{\text{Ca}(i)}$, $V_{\text{Ca-K}(i)}$, $V_{\text{Na}(i)}$, $V_{\text{K}(i)}$, $V_{\text{Cl}(i)}$ are the reversal potentials and $g_{\text{Ca}(i)}$, $g_{\text{Ca-K}(i)}$, $g_{\text{Na}(i)}$, $g_{\text{K}(i)}$, $g_{\text{Cl}(i)}$ are the maximal conductances of channels, ϑ_{Ca} is the parameter of calcium inhibition of the Ca^{2+} channels, and $[\text{Ca}_i^{2+}]$ is the intracellular concentration of free calcium. Here subscript i refers to a respective neuron/ICC.

Dynamic variables z_{Ca}, ρ_∞, m_{Na}, h_{Na} and n_{K} are

$$\begin{aligned} & dz_{\text{Ca}}/dt = (z_\infty - z_{\text{Ca}})/\tau_z, \quad dh_{\text{Na}}/dt = \lambda_h(h_\infty - h_{\text{Na}})/\tau_h, \\ & dn_{\text{K}}/dt = \lambda_n(n_\infty - n_{\text{K}})/\tau_n, \quad \rho_\infty = [1 + \exp 0.15(V_i + 47)]^{-1}, \\ & m_{\text{Na}} = m_\infty(V_i). \end{aligned} \tag{7.10}$$

In the above m_∞, h_∞, n_∞, z_∞ are calculated as

$$y_{y\infty} = \alpha_{y\infty}/(\alpha_{y\infty} + \beta_{y\infty}), \quad (y = m, h, n)$$
$$\tau_y = 1/(\alpha_y + \beta_y) \tag{7.11}$$
$$z_\infty = [1 + \exp(-0.15(V_i + 42))]^{-1},$$

where

$$\alpha_{m\infty} = \frac{0.12(V_i + 27)}{1 - \exp(-(V_i + 27)/8)}, \quad \beta_{m\infty} = 4\exp(-(V_i + 47)/15)$$
$$\alpha_{h\infty} = 0.07\exp(-(V_i + 47)/17), \quad \beta_{h\infty} = [1 + \exp(-(V_i + 22)/8)]^{-1} \tag{7.12}$$
$$\alpha_{n\infty} = \frac{0.012(V_i + 12)}{1 - \exp(-(V_i + 12)/8)}, \quad \beta_{n\infty} = 0.125\exp(-(V_i + 20)/67).$$

These relationships refer mainly to neurons of the ENS. In the case of ICC they are different.

Initial conditions assume the physiological status of a cell at rest. It is assumed that ICC discharge electrical signals of given amplitude $\overset{0}{V_i}$ and duration t_i^d, and receive input signals, excitatory (EPSP) or inhibitory (IPSP) postsynaptic potentials, from the myenteric neurons

$$\text{at } t = 0: \quad V_i = \begin{cases} \text{EPSP or IPSP}, & 0 < t < t_i^d \\ \overset{0}{V_i}, & t \geqslant t_i^d \end{cases}, \tag{7.13}$$
$$[\mathrm{Ca}_i^{2+}] = [\overset{0}{\mathrm{Ca}_i^{2+}}], \quad z = z_\infty, \quad h_{\mathrm{Na}} = h_{\mathrm{Na}\infty}, \quad n_{\mathrm{Na}} = n_{\mathrm{Na}\infty}.$$

Finally, a single, electrically equivalent cable model to simulate the generation and propagation of waves of depolarization in the axon and dendrites must be taken into consideration along with the synaptic neurotransmission.

7.4.2 An inhibitory neuronal circuit

The relative temporal and spatial integration of excitatory and inhibitory signals at any individual neuron depends on the synapse and properties of the neuron *per se*. The adrenergic and nonadrenergic inhibitory nerves reduce the excitability and firing frequency and suppress the intrinsic reflex pathways. The following nomenclature of synapses is adopted depending on their location on the neuron: axo-axonic, axo-somatic, axo-dendritic, and dendro-denritic. The particular combination of neurotransmitters and receptors involved in the dynamics of transduction correlates with the specific functional classes of the nerves.

Consider a two neuronal circuit composed of an excitatory and inhibitory neuron which interact at the axo-axonal synapse as shown in figure 7.2. Assume that the action potential propagating along the axon and the IPSP sum up linearly

$$V_{\mathrm{sum}} = V|_{s=s^*} + V_{\mathrm{syn}}^{(-)}, \tag{7.14}$$

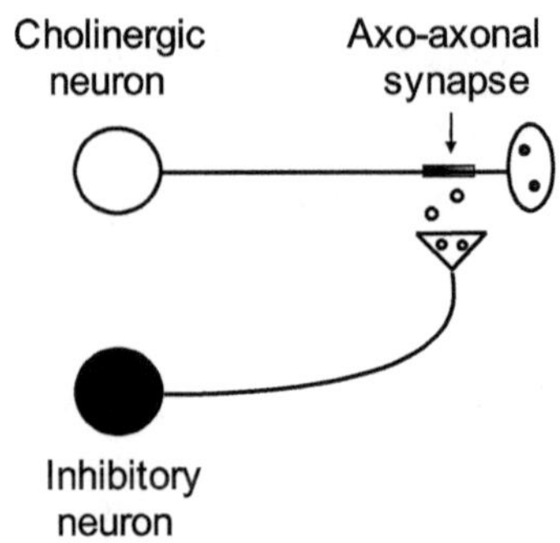

Figure 7.2. A two neuronal assembly with an axo-axonal inhibitory synapse.

where $s = s^*$ is the Lagrange coordinate of the synapse. The mathematical formulation of the problem includes the system of equations for: the action potential propagation along the axons (8.1)–(8.4); electrochemical signal transduction mechanisms at the synapse (8.5), (8.6), (8.8), (8.10); the inhibitory postsynaptic potential development; and synaptic interaction at the axo-axonal synapse (7.14) with specified initial and boundary conditions (8.7), (8.8), (8.12).

7.4.3 A neuronal network of excitable cells

Currently little is known about the histomorphological topology of interganglionic connectivity within Auerbach's and Meissner's plexi. Although it is impossible to provide accurate morphofunctional correlations in the plexi, it is reasonable to assume the following neuronal interrelationships (figure 7.3):

(i) *direct*—connects n and the adjacent, oral or aboral, $(n + 1)$ neurons;
(ii) *transitory*—passes signals from n to $(n + 2)$ neurons;
(iii) *divergent*—communicates signals from n to $(n + i)$ $(i = 1, 2, \ldots)$ interneurons;
(iv) *convergent*—transmits signals from $(n + i)$ interneurons to n neuron;
(v) *local inhibitory*—provides self-inhibition within a ganglion.

Such a discrete network architecture enables a dynamic framework for universal (stability, phase-locked oscillatory activity) and intrinsic (action potentials, electrochemical coupling) patterns of physiological behavior. The spatio-temporal symmetry of connectivity guarantees the occurrence of rhythmic activities including slow waves of different frequencies and amplitude along with traveling waves. The spontaneous desynchronization of firing activity of cells and consequent breaking of symmetry may enhance a network's ability to generate a variety of irregular myoelectrical rhythms, e.g. reverberating waves. However, the nonlinear delayed feedback control mechanisms counteract abnormal interactions and thereby restore the natural frequencies of oscillation in the system.

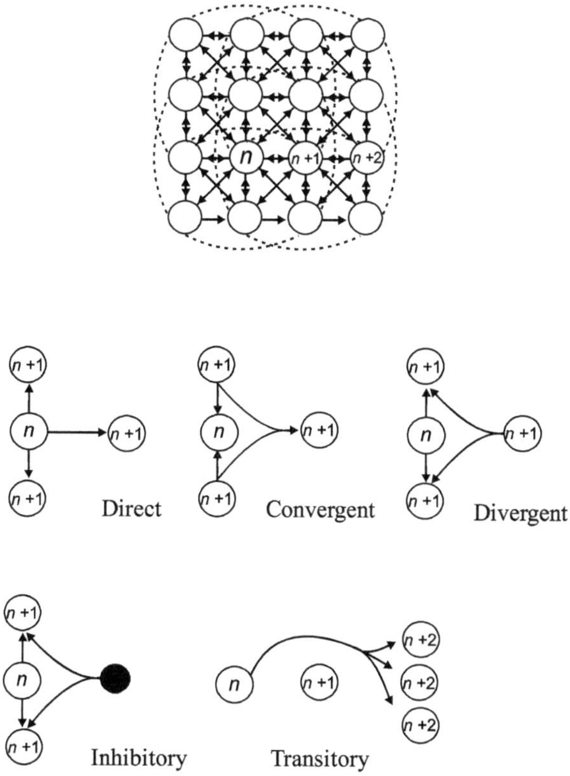

Figure 7.3. The structure of a functional element of the neuronal network and exercised interneuronal arrangements.

Further reading

Dayan P and Abbott L F 2001 *Theoretical Neuroscience: Computational and Mathematical Modeling of Neural Systems* (MA: MIT Press)

Fausett L V 1993 *Fundamentals of Neural Networks: Architectures, Algorithms And Applications* (London: Pearson)

Gerstner W and Kistler W I 2002 *Spiking Neuron Models. Single Neurons, Populations, Plasticity* (Cambridge: Cambridge University Press)

Hodgkin A L and Huxley A F 1952 *J. Physiol.* **117** 500–44

Hoppenstedt F C and Izhikevich E M 1997 *Weakly Connected Neural Networks* (New York: Springer)

IOP Publishing

Soft Biological Shells in Bioengineering

Roustem N Miftahof and Nariman R Akhmadeev

Chapter 8

Chemical synapse

A three compartmental mathematical model of the chemical synapse, essential in the exchange of information within biological systems, is constructed. The kinetics of a single and multiple neurotransmission and the involvement of transmembrane and G-protein coupled receptors are analyzed in detail.

8.1 A mathematical model

Neurohormonal modulation and electromechanical coupling in biological tissues involve a cascade of chemical processes including synthesis, storage, stimulation, release, diffusion, and the binding of various substrates to specific receptors with the activation of intracellular second messenger systems and the generation of a variety of physiological responses. Qualitative analysis and quantitative evaluation of each and every step experimentally is very difficult, and sometimes practically impossible.

Let a synapse (neuronal or neuromuscular) be an open three compartmental system. Compartment 1 comprises presynaptic elements where synthesis and storage of a neurotransmitter occurs. For example, in the case of cholinergic or adrenergic synapses it corresponds morphologically with a nerve terminal of the unmyelinated axon; for SP, it is comprised of the endoplasmic reticulum, the Golgi apparatus and the membrane transport system for exocytotic release and large dense core vesicles for storage, and for serotonin (enterochromaffin cells).

Ligands, i.e. ACh, AD, 5-HT, SP, etc, are released upon neural stimulation by exocytosis to the synaptic cleft and bloodstream. The common sequence of events involved in the dynamics of their transduction includes:

(i) depolarization of the nerve terminal or cell membrane;
(ii) influx of extracellular calcium through voltage-gated Ca^{2+} channels;
(iii) binding of free cytosolic Ca_i^{2+} to transmitter-containing vesicles;
(iv) release of vesicular/granular stored ligand, L_v, into the synaptic cleft.

doi:10.1088/2053-2563/ab1a9ech8

Propagation of the wave of depolarization, V^f, in the nerve terminal is accurately described by the modified Hodgkin–Huxley system of equations

$$C_m^f \frac{\partial V^f}{\partial t} = \frac{1}{2R_a^f} \frac{\partial}{\partial \alpha}\left(d_f^2(\alpha)\frac{\partial V^f}{\partial \alpha}\right) - (I_{Na}^f + I_K^f + I_{Cl}^f),$$
$$d_f(\alpha) = \begin{cases} d_f, & L^s < \alpha \leqslant L^s - L^s{}_0 \\ 2d_f & \alpha > L^s - L^s{}_0,\ t > 0,\ \ \alpha \in (0, L^s). \end{cases} \tag{8.1}$$

Here L^s, $L^s{}_0$ are the lengths of the axon and the terminal, respectively, while the meaning of the other parameters and constants is as described above. The above ion currents are defined by

$$\begin{aligned} I_{\mathrm{Na}}^f &= g_{\mathrm{Na}}^f m_f^3 h_f (V^f - V_{\mathrm{Na}}^f) \\ I_{\mathrm{K}}^f &= g_{\mathrm{K}}^f n_f^4 h_f (V^f - V_{\mathrm{K}}^f) \\ I_{\mathrm{Cl}}^f &= g_{\mathrm{Cl}}^f (V^f - V_{\mathrm{Cl}}^f), \end{aligned} \tag{8.2}$$

where g_{Na}^f, g_{K}^f, g_{Cl}^f are the maximal conductances for the Na^+, K^+, and Cl^- currents, respectively, V_{Na}^f, V_{K}^f, V_{Cl}^f are the equilibrium potentials for the respective ion currents and m_f, n_f, h_f are the state variables that are calculated from

$$dy/dt = \alpha_y(1 - y) - \beta_y y \quad y = (m_f, n_f, h_f). \tag{8.3}$$

The activation, α_y, and deactivation, β_y, parameters satisfy the following empirical relations:

$$\begin{aligned} \alpha_{m,f} &= \frac{0.1T(2.5 - V^f)}{\exp(2.5 - 0.1V^f)}, & \beta_{m,f} &= 4T\exp(-V^f/18) \\ \alpha_{h,f} &= 0.07T\exp(-0.05V^f), & \beta_{h,f} &= T/(1 + \exp(3 - 0.1V^f)), \\ \alpha_{n,f} &= \frac{0.1T(10 - V^f)}{\exp(1 - 0.1V^f) - 1}, & \beta_{n,f} &= 0.125T\exp(-0.125V^f). \end{aligned} \tag{8.4}$$

Here T is temperature.

The cytosolic calcium turnover is given by

$$\frac{d[\mathrm{Ca}_i^{2+}]}{dt} = g_{\mathrm{syn}}^{\mathrm{Ca}} V^f(t)[\mathrm{Ca}_0^{2+}] - k_b[\mathrm{Ca}_i^{2+}], \tag{8.5}$$

where $g_{\mathrm{syn}}^{\mathrm{Ca}}$ is the conductivity of the voltage-gated Ca^{2+}-channel at the synaptic end and k_b is the intracellular buffer system constant.

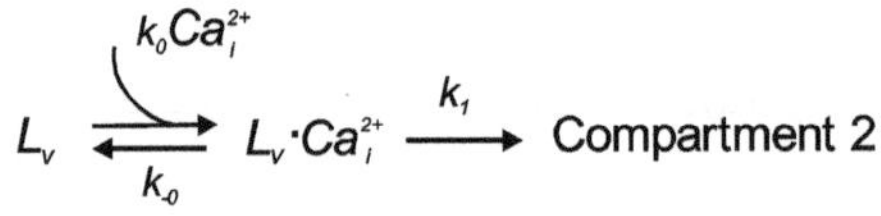

Figure 8.1. The diagram of transmitter release from the presynaptic nerve terminal. Reprinted from Miftahof R N 2017 *Biomechanics of the Human Stomach* (Berlin: Springer) by permission of Springer Nature. Copyright 2017.

The release of a stored fraction of the ligand, L_v, is described by the state diagram (figure 8.1) given by

$$\frac{d[X_2]}{dt} = -k_0[X_1][X_2]. \tag{8.6}$$

Here $X_1 := [Ca_i^{2+}]$, $X_2 := [L_v]$ are concentrations of the cytosolic Ca^{2+} and vesicular stored ligand, respectively, k_0 is the rate constant of the association of Ca_i^{2+} with calcium-dependent centers on the vesicles, and k_1 is the diffusion constant.

At $t = 0$ the nerve axon and the synapse are assumed to be at a state of rest and the concentrations of reacting components are known

$$m_f(0) = m_{f,0},\ h_f(0) = h_{f,0},\ n_f(0) = n_{f,0},\ V^f(0, \alpha) = 0,\ L_v(0) = L_{v,0}. \tag{8.7}$$

The synapse is excited at the free end ($\alpha = 0$) by an electrical impulse of an amplitude $\overset{0}{V^f}$ and duration t^d, while the presynaptic terminal end ($\alpha = L$) remains unexcited throughout:

$$V^f(0, t) = \begin{cases} \overset{0}{V^f}, & 0 < t < t^d \\ 0, & t \geqslant t^d \end{cases}, \quad V^f(L, t) = 0. \tag{8.8}$$

The dynamics of the release of various neuromediators is highly specific and depends entirely on the particular intrinsic cellular processes involved. For example, the dynamics of exocytosis of SP and the specific transporter mediated release of prostaglandins $F_{2\alpha}$ and E_2, as a first approximation, could be described by

$$\frac{d[X_i]}{dt} = \frac{B_{tr}([X_i] - [X_o])}{K_{tr} + [X_i]}, \quad X_i(0) = X_{i0} \tag{8.9}$$

where B_{tr}, K_{tr} are the parameters that refer to the process of exocytosis/transporter, and $[X]_{i,o}$ are the concentrations of SP and prostaglandins $F_{2\alpha}$ and E_2, respectively, both inside (subscript i) and outside (o) the cell. In contrast, progesterone is constantly produced and secreted into the bloodstream as an active hormone and its concentration is tightly regulated and maintained at a constant level. This means it is reasonable to assume that [PR] = constant throughout.

Upon their release, neurotransmitters and hormones passively diffuse through the synaptic cleft (compartment 2) towards the postsynaptic membrane. The synaptic cleft has a width of ≈12–20 nm across many synaptic types. It contains N-cadherin, adhesion molecules, and microtubules organized in periodic transsynaptic complexes and roughly regular patches.

Compartment 3—the postsynaptic membrane—contains a complex network of surface membrane proteins which modulate the transmission. Additionally, this involves the following processes:

(v) binding of a free ligand in the cleft, L_c, to the G-protein coupled receptor, R, and its conformational change, $L_c \cdot R$;
(vi) active configuration of the receptor, R^*, (the $L_c \cdot R^*$ reactive complex is able to produce a biological effect, i.e. the postsynaptic potential, V_{syn});
(vii) binding of $L_c \cdot R^*$ to G protein, the formation of the $L_c \cdot R^* \cdot G$-complex and the initiation of guanosine diphosphate/guanosine triphosphate (GDP/GTP) exchange;
(viii) the dissociation of G protein α and $\beta\gamma$ subunits with the subsequent release of G_{act} protein that interacts with downstream effector pathways;
(ix) enzymatic, E, clearance of the excess of L_c in the synaptic cleft through the formation of intermediate complexes, $L_c \cdot E$ and ES, and the final metabolite, S.

They are described by the following state diagram (figure 8.2).

Assuming that:

(i) the distribution of reactive substrates is uniform throughout and no chemical gradients exist;
(ii) the total enzyme concentration does not change over time, E_0 = constant;
(iii) the total ligand concentration is much larger than the total enzyme concentration;
(iv) no product is present at the beginning of the reaction; and
(v) the maximum rate of chemical reaction occurs when the enzyme is saturated, i.e. all enzyme molecules are tied up with a substrate,

then all reactions are of the first order and satisfy the Michaelis–Menten kinetics. Hence the system of equations for the ligand conversion is given by

$$d\mathbf{X}/dt = \mathbf{AX}(t), \tag{8.10}$$

where the vector $\mathbf{X}(t) = (X_j)^T (j = \overline{1, 20})$ has the components

$$\begin{array}{llll}
X_1 = [\text{Ca}_i^{2+}], & X_2 = [L_v], & X_3 = [L_v \cdot \text{Ca}_i^{2+}], & X_4 = [L_c], \\
X_5 = [R], & X_6 = [R^*], & X_7 = [L_c \cdot R^*], & X_8 = [L_c \cdot R], \\
X_9 = [L_c \cdot R^* \cdot G], & X_{10} = [R^* \cdot G], & X_{11} = [A_c \cdot E], & X_{12} = [G], \\
X_{13} = [C_1], & X_{14} = [C_2], & X_{15} = [C_3], & X_{16} = [C_4], \\
X_{17} = [G'], & X_{18} = [G_{\text{act}}], & X_{19} = [ES], & X_{20} = [S].
\end{array}$$

The matrix $\mathbf{A}(a_{ij})$ $(i, j = \overline{1, 20})$ has the non-zero elements

$$a_{11} = g_{\text{syn}}^{\text{Ca}} V^f(t)[\text{Ca}_0^{2+}], \qquad a_{12} = -k_0[X_1],$$
$$a_{13} = k_{-0}, \qquad a_{22} = -k_0[X_1],$$
$$a_{23} = k_{-0}, \qquad a_{32} = k_0[X_1],$$
$$a_{33} = -(k_{-0} + k_1), \qquad a_{43} = k_1,$$
$$a_{44} = k_2([E_0] - [X_8]) + k_6[X_5] + k_{-8}[X_6] + k_{-11}[X_{10}],$$
$$a_{47} = k_8, \qquad a_{48} = k_{-6},$$
$$a_{49} = k_{11}, \qquad a_{4,11} = k_{-2},$$
$$a_{55} = -(k_{-5} + k_6)[X_4], \qquad a_{56} = k_5[X_{12}],$$
$$a_{58} = k_{-6}, \qquad a_{65} = k_{-5},$$
$$a_{66} = -k_{-8}[X_4] - (k_5 + k_{-10}k_{19}[X_{18}])[X_{12}],$$
$$a_{67} = k_8[X_{12}], \qquad a_{6,10} = k_{10},$$
$$a_{6,16} = k_{17}, \qquad a_{76} = k_{-8}[X_4],$$
$$a_{77} = -(k_{-7} + k_8 + k_9)k_{19}[X_{12}][X_{18}],$$
$$a_{78} = k_7, \qquad a_{79} = k_{-9}k_{12}[X_{40}],$$
$$a_{7,14} = k_{16}, \qquad a_{85} = k_6[X_4],$$
$$a_{87} = k_{-7}[X_{12}], \qquad a_{88} = -k_{-6} - k_7,$$
$$a_{97} = k_9k_{19}[X_{12}][X_{18}], \qquad a_{99} = -k_{-9} - k_{11} - k_{12}[X_{40}],$$
$$a_{9,10} = k_{-11}[X_4], \qquad a_{10,6} = k_{-10}[X_{12}],$$
$$a_{10,9} = k_{11}, \qquad a_{10,10} = -(k_{10} + k_{-11})[X_4] - k_{13}[X_{40}],$$
$$a_{11,4} = k_2([X_{41}] - [X_8]), \qquad a_{11,11} = -(k_{-2} + k_3),$$
$$a_{11,19} = k_3, \qquad a_{12,6} = k_{-5} + k_{-8}[X_4],$$
$$a_{12,8} = k_7, \qquad a_{12,9} = k_{-9},$$
$$a_{12,12} = -(k_5 + k_{-10}k_{19}[X_{18}])[X_6] - (k_{-7} + k_8 + k_9k_{19}[X_{18}])[X_7],$$
$$a_{12,10} = k_{10}, \qquad a_{13,9} = k_{12}[X_{40}],$$
$$a_{13,13} = -k_{14}[X_{39}], \qquad a_{13,14} = k_{-14},$$
$$a_{14,13} = k_{14}[X_{39}], \qquad a_{14,14} = -(k_{-14} + k_{16}),$$
$$a_{15,10} = k_{13}[X_{40}], \qquad a_{15,15} = -k_{15}[X_{39}],$$
$$a_{15,16} = k_{-15}, \qquad a_{16,15} = k_{15}[X_{39}],$$
$$a_{16,16} = -(k_{17} + k_{-15}), \qquad a_{17,14} = k_{16},$$
$$a_{17,16} = k_{17}, \qquad a_{17,17} = -k_{18},$$
$$a_{18,17} = k_{18}, \qquad a_{18,18} = -k_{19},$$
$$a_{19,11} = k_3, \qquad a_{19,19} = -(k_{-3} + k_4),$$
$$a_{19,20} = k_{-4}([X_{41}] - [X_8]), \qquad a_{20,19} = k_4,$$
$$a_{20,20} = -k_{-4}([X_{41}] - [X_8]).$$

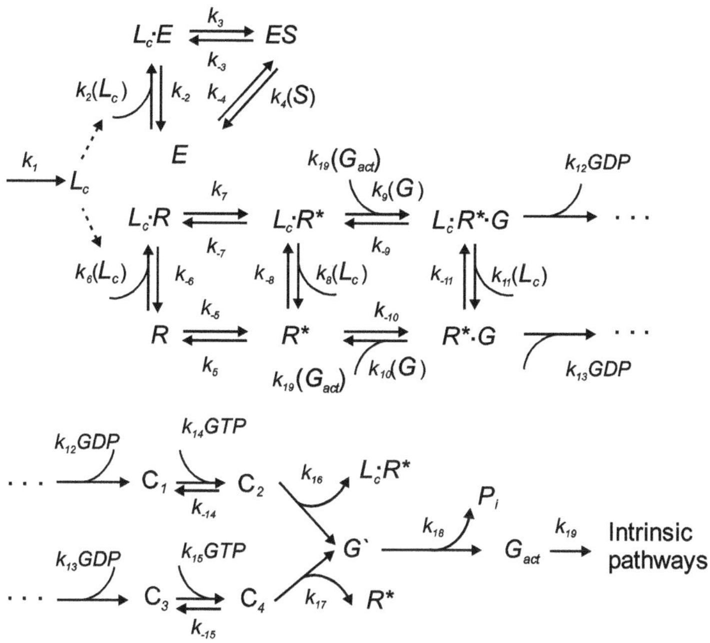

Figure 8.2. A diagram of neurotransmitter conversion at the postsynaptic membrane.

Here $k_{\pm i}$ are the forward $(+i)$ and backward $(-i)$ rate constants of chemical reactions, C_j $(j = \overline{1, 4})$ are the intermediate complexes, and $[X_{39}]$, $[X_{40}]$, $[X_{41}]$ are the given concentrations of the *GTP*, *GDP*, and *E* enzymes, respectively. Note that in the case of $PGF_{2\alpha}$ and PGE_2 their release is described by equation (8.6).

Finally, the generation of the excitatory/inhibitory postsynaptic potential, $V_{\text{syn}}^{(+,-)}$ is given by

$$C_p \frac{dV_{\text{syn}}^{(+,-)}}{dt} + V_{\text{syn}}(\mp\Omega[X_9] + R_v^{-1}) = \frac{V_{\text{syn},0}}{R_v}, \tag{8.11}$$

where C_p is the capacitance of the postsynaptic membrane, R_v is the resistance of the synaptic structures, Ω is the empirical constant, and $V_{syn,0}$ is the resting postsynaptic potential.

Given the concentrations of reacting components and the state of the synapse

$$\mathbf{X}(0) = \mathbf{X}_0, \quad V_{\text{syn}} = 0. \tag{8.12}$$

Equations (8.1)–(8.12) provide the mathematical formulation for the dynamics of the common pathway of neurotransmission at the synaptic site.

The quantitative assessment of the velocities of reactions shows that the rates, k_{12}, k_{13}, of exchange of *G* protein for GDP at $L_c{\cdot}R^*\cdot G$ and $R^*\cdot G$ sites, respectively, are significantly smaller compared to the rates of other reactions. Hence, the system (figures 8.1 and 8.2) can be viewed as a combination of rapid equilibrium segments interconnected through slow, rate-limiting steps. The characteristic feature of such a system is that it attains the steady state when the rapid segment has already reached quasi-equilibrium. This fact allows us to simplify the system as follows.

Let $\tilde{f}_1$ and $\tilde{f}_2$ be the fractional concentration factors of the rapid segment 'product'-substrates

$$\tilde{f}_1 = [X_9]/[Y], \quad \tilde{f}_2 = [X_{10}]/[Y], \tag{8.13}$$

where Y is

$$[Y] = [X_9] + [X_{10}] + [X_{12}].$$

Define the association constant as

$$\begin{aligned} K_1 &= [X_6][X_{12}]/[X_{10}], \qquad & K_2 &= [X_4][X_{10}]/[X_9], \\ K_3 &= [X_7][X_{10}]/[X_9], \qquad & K_4 &= [X_4][X_6]/[X_9], \end{aligned}$$

and after simple algebra, for $\tilde{f}_1$, we have

$$\begin{aligned} \tilde{f}_1 &= \frac{[X_4][X_6]/K_1K_2}{1 + [X_4][X_6]/K_1K_2 + [X_6]K_1} = \frac{[X_4][X_6]}{K_1K_2 + [X_6]([X_4] + K_2)}, \\ \tilde{f}_2 &= \frac{[X_6]/K_1}{1 + [X_4][X_6]/K_1K_2 + [X_6]/K_1} = \frac{K_2[X_6]}{K_{10}K_{11} + [X_6]([X_4] + K_2)}. \end{aligned} \tag{8.14}$$

Now the concentration distribution equations for the main reactants can be obtained in the form

$$\begin{aligned} (D)\frac{[Y]}{[Y']} &= k_{14}k_{15}k_{16}k_{17}k_{18}k_{19}[X_{39}]^2 \\ (D)\frac{[X_{13}]}{[Y']} &= k_{12}k_{15}k_{17}k_{18}k_{19}\tilde{f}_1[X_{39}](k_{-14} + k_{16}) \\ (D)\frac{[X_{14}]}{[Y']} &= k_{12}k_{14}k_{15}k_{17}k_{18}k_{19}\tilde{f}_1[X_{39}]^2 \\ (D)\frac{[X_{15}]}{[Y']} &= k_{11}k_{14}k_{16}k_{18}k_{19}\tilde{f}_2[X_{39}](k_{-15} + k_{17}) \\ (D)\frac{[X_{16}]}{[Y]} &= k_{11}k_{14}k_{15}k_{16}k_{18}k_{19}\tilde{f}_2[X_{39}]^2 \\ (D)\frac{[X_{17}]}{[Y']} &= k_{14}k_{15}k_{16}k_{17}\tilde{f}_2[X_{39}]^2(k_{12}\tilde{f}_1 + k_{11}\tilde{f}_2), \end{aligned} \tag{8.15}$$

where

$$[Y'] = [Y] + [X_{13}] + [X_{14}] + [X_{15}] + [X_{16}] + [X_{17}],$$

and D is the sum of all the values on the right side of equation (8.14). Note that these are algebraic equations. The initial velocity equation for Y complex formation is given by

$$d[Y]/dt = k_{18}k_{19}[X_{17}]. \tag{8.16}$$

Finally, substituting X_{17} from equation (8.15) and making use of equation (8.14) we arrive at

$$\frac{1}{[Y']}\frac{d[Y]}{dt} = \frac{k_{14}k_{15}k_{16}k_{17}k_{18}k_{19}[X_{39}]^2\left[\frac{k_{12}[X_4][X_6]/K_1K_2 + k_{11}[X_6]/K_1}{1 + [X_4][X_6]/K_1K_2 + [X_6]/K_1}\right]}{[\ldots]},$$

where

$$\begin{aligned}
[\ldots] = {} & k_{14}k_{15}k_{16}k_{17}k_{18}k_{19}[X_{39}]^2 \\
& + \left[\frac{[X_4][X_6]/K_1K_2}{1 + [X_4][X_6]/K_1K_2 + [X_6]/K_1}\right] \\
& \times (k_{12}k_{15}k_{17}k_{18}k_{19}[X_{39}](k_{-14} + k_{16}) \\
& + k_{12}k_{14}k_{15}k_{17}k_{18}k_{19}[X_{39}]^2) \\
& + \left[\frac{k_{12}[X_4][X_6]/K_1K_2 + k_{11}[X_6]/K_1}{1 + [X_4][X_6]/K_1K_2 + [X_6]/K_1}\right] \\
& \times (k_{14}k_{15}k_{16}k_{17}[X_{39}]^2) \\
& + \left[\frac{[X_6]/K_1}{1 + [X_4][X_6]/K_1K_2 + [X_6]/K_1}\right] \\
& \times (k_{11}k_{14}k_{15}k_{16}k_{18}k_{19}[X_{39}]^2 \\
& + k_{11}k_{14}k_{16}k_{18}k_{19}[X_{39}](k_{-15} + k_{17}))
\end{aligned}$$

or, after some algebraic rearrangements, in the form

$$\begin{aligned}
& \frac{1}{[Y']}\frac{d[Y]}{dt} \\
& = \frac{k_{14}k_{15}k_{16}k_{17}k_{18}k_{19}[X_{39}][k_{12}[X_4] + k_{11}K_2]}{\left\{\begin{aligned} & [X_4][X_{39}]k_{14}k_{15}k_{17}[k_{16}k_{18}k_{19} + k_{12}k_{18}k_{19} + k_{12}k_{16}] \\ & + [X_{39}]k_{14}k_{15}k_{16}K_2\left[k_{17}k_{18}k_{19}\left(1 + \frac{K_1}{[X_6]}\right) + k_{11}k_{17} + k_{11}k_{18}k_{19}\right] \\ & + [X_4][k_{12}k_{15}k_{17}k_{18}k_{19}(k_{-14} + k_{16})] + k_{11}k_{14}k_{16}k_{18}k_{19}K_2(k_{-15} + k_{17}) \end{aligned}\right\}}.
\end{aligned} \tag{8.17}$$

Both of these mathematical formulations, i.e. the system of differential equation (8.10) or a simplified model given by (8.17), when supplemented by initial and boundary conditions, provide a detailed description of electrochemical coupling at a synapse. In practice, the preference for either of them depends on the intended application and is entirely the researcher's choice.

8.2 cAMP-dependent pathway

Stimulation of cholinergic μ_2 and adrenergic β-receptors leads to the production of cAMP. cAMP influences a wide range of physiological effects including: (i) the increase in Ca^{2+} channel conductance; (ii) the activation of protein kinase C (PKC) and protein kinase A (PKA) enzymes; and (iii) the regulation of GDP-GTP exchange factor (Rho-GEF), RhoA and RhoK kinases.

The production of cAMP is controlled by a number of adenylate cyclase (AC) enzymes. These are dually regulated by a family of G proteins, forskolin, and other class-specific substrates. The diversity and expression of AC isoforms provides a mechanism for integrating, positively or negatively, the responses to various transmitters. The isoforms V and VI of ACs have a high affinity to $G\beta\gamma$ subunits of inhibitory proteins. Their functionality is affected by phosphorylation with PKC whilst types V and VI are inhibited directly by low levels of Ca^{2+}. Adenylyl cyclase isoforms I, III, and VIII are shown to be up-regulated by a calmodulin dependent protein kinase in response to the elevation in Ca_i^{2+}. By contrast, the isoforms II, IV, and IX are stimulated by in the presence of $G\alpha_s$ subunits. Although the exact presence and distribution of the specific types of AC isoforms in the human body are not known, it is obvious that the same stimulus may trigger different physiological responses depending not only on the type of receptors involved but also on the type of adenylyl cyclase to which they are coupled.

The proposed structure of AC consists of a short amino terminal region and two cytoplasmic domains. The latter are separated by two extremely hydrophobic domains which take the form of six transmembrane helices. The catalytic core of the enzyme consists of a pseudosymmetric heterodimer composed of two highly conserved portions of the cytoplasmic domains. It binds one molecule of $G\alpha_{i-q}$ which, in turn, catalyzes the conversion of ATP into cyclic adenosine monophosphate.

In addition to AC, the level of cAMP is controlled by the activity of phosphodiesterases (PDEs) that degrade it to 5′-AMP. At least 11 families of PDE isoenzymes are identified. Their hydrolytic activity is determined by the catalytic domain and conserved areas of amino acids specific to each family. For example, PDE3 and PDE4 hydrolyze cAMP whilst PDE5 demonstrates dual specificity to cAMP and cGMP. Another mechanism that reduces the production of cAMP is the activation of $G\alpha_{i-q/11}$ proteins which directly inhibit adenylyl cyclase through the MAPK signaling cascade.

Protein kinase C enzymes comprise a family of eleven isoenzymes that are divided into three subfamilies, conventional, novel, and atypical. This classification is based on their second messenger requirements for activation. For example, conventional PKCs (α, β_1, β_2, γ) require free Ca^{2+} and 1,2-diacylglycerol (DAG) for activation; novel PKCs (δ, ε, η, θ, μ) need only DAG whilst atypical PKCs ($\zeta\imath$, λ) require none of these for activation.

PKCs consist of a variable regulatory and a highly conserved catalytic domain, tethered together by a hinge region. The regulatory domain contains two subregions, namely C1 and C2. The C1 subregion has a binding site for DAG and phorbol esters. C2 acts as a Ca^{2+} sensor and is functional only in PKCs α, β_1, β_2, and γ. On activation, kinases are translocated to the plasma membrane by RACK proteins where they remain active for a long period of time. The effect is attributed to the property of diacyglycerol *per se*. The binding of cAMP to the regulatory subunit causes the release of catalytic subunits and the transfer of ATP terminal phosphates to PKC-potentiated inhibitory protein (CPI-17) at T38. This in turn inhibits the catalytic subunit of myosin light chain phosphatase (MLCP). The result is an increase in the affinity of MLCK for the calcium–calmodulin complex and SM contraction.

Protein kinase A is a holoenzyme that consisting of two regulatory and two catalytic subunits. Its activity is controlled entirely by high concentrations of cAMP. On binding to the two binding sites on the regulatory subunits of the holoenzyme, cAMP causes the transfer of ATP terminal phosphates to myosin light chain kinase. The result is a decrease in the affinity of MLCK for the calcium–calmodulin complex and SM relaxation. Additionally, PKA may promote relaxation by inhibiting phospholipase C, intracellular Ca^{2+} entry, and by activating BK_{Ca} channels and calcium pumps. Under low levels of cAMP, PKA enzyme remains intact and catalytically inactive.

The state diagram of the cAMP-dependent pathway as described above is shown in figure 8.3.

The system of equations for the cAMP-pathway activation is given by

$$d\mathbf{X}/dt = \mathbf{B}\mathbf{X}(t), \tag{8.18}$$

where $\mathbf{X}(t) = (X_j)^{\mathrm{T}}$ $(j = \overline{21, 26})$ has the components

$$X_{21} = [\mathrm{AC}],\ X_{22} = [\mathrm{ATP}],\ X_{23} = [\mathrm{cAMP}],$$
$$X_{24} = [\mathrm{PKC}],\ X_{25} = [\mathrm{PKC}^*],\ X_{26} = [5'-\mathrm{AMP}],$$

and the square matrix $\mathbf{B}(b_{ij})$ $(i, j = \overline{6, 6})$ has the non-zero elements

$$b_{11} = -k_{19}k_{20}[X_{18}],\quad b_{22} = -k_{21}[X_{27}],\quad b_{32} = k_{21}[X_{27}],$$
$$b_{33} = -k_{23}[X_{28}]_0,\quad b_{44} = -k_{22}[X_{23}],\quad b_{54} = k_{22}[X_{23}],$$
$$b_{55} = -k_{24},\quad b_{63} = k_{23}[X_{28}]_0,\quad b_{66} = -k_{25}.$$

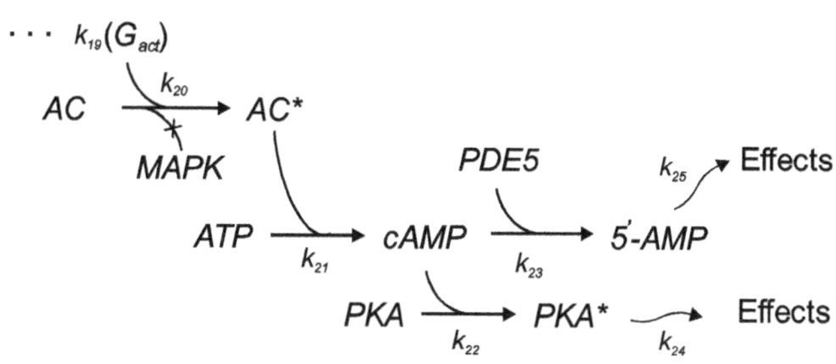

Figure 8.3. The state diagram of activation of the cAMP-dependent intrinsic pathway.

The active form of adenylyl cyclase, $X_{27} := \text{AC}^*$, is obtained from

$$[X_{27}](t) = [X_{21}]_0 - [X_{21}](t), \tag{8.19}$$

where $[X_{21}]_0 = \text{const}$ is the initial concentration of the enzyme. It is also assumed that the level of phosphodiesterase enzyme, $[X_{28}]_0 := \text{PDE}$, remains constant.

The initial conditions provide concentrations of the reacting components, thus

$$\mathbf{X}(0) = \mathbf{X}_0. \tag{8.20}$$

8.3 PLC-dependent pathway

Activation of cholinergic μ_3, oxytocin, and/or prostaglandin receptors, results in downstream stimulation of the intracellular phospholipase C (PLC) pathway. Four β, two γ, four δ, and ε isoforms of PLC enzymes have been isolated from within the human body. PLCβ members are triggered by Ca^{2+}, but are differently regulated by G proteins. PLCβ1 and PLCβ4 are sensitive to $G\alpha_{q/11}$, whereas PLCβ2 and PLCβ3 can be activated by $G\alpha_{q/11}$ and $G\beta\gamma$ subunits. Without exception, their activation leads to the breakdown of inositide-4,5-biphosphate (PIP_2) and the generation of second messenger molecules—IP_3 and DAG. IP_3 is a highly soluble structure and it quickly diffuses through the cytosol towards the sarcoplasmic reticulum. Here it binds to R_{IP3} surface receptors and triggers the mobilization of stored Ca^{2+}.

The simplified state diagram of the PLC pathway is outlined in figure 8.4.

The corresponding system of equations is given by

$$d\mathbf{X}/dt = \mathbf{C}\mathbf{X}(t) + \mathbf{C}_0, \tag{8.21}$$

where $\mathbf{X}(t) = (X_j)^T$ $(j = \overline{29, 34})$ has the components

$$X_{29} = [\text{PIP}_2],\ X_{30} = [\text{IP}_3],\ X_{31} = [\text{DAG}],$$
$$X_{32} = [\text{DAGT}],\ X_{33} = [\text{PKC}],\ X_{34} = [\text{R}_{\text{IP3}}].$$

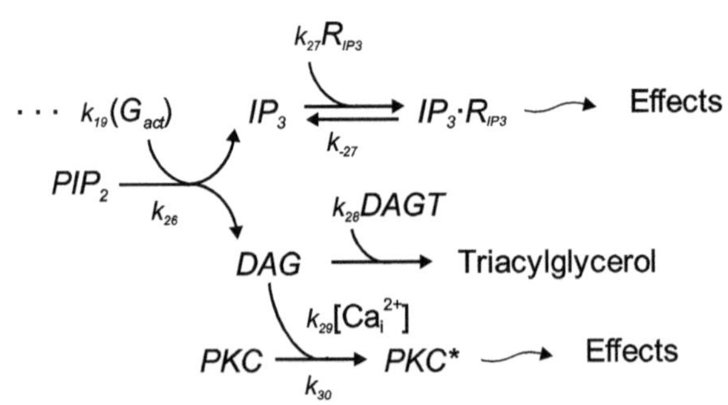

Figure 8.4. The state diagram of activation of the PLC pathway.

The matrix $\mathbf{C}(c_{ij})$ $(i, j = \overline{6, 6})$ has the non-zero elements

$$\begin{aligned}
&c_{11} = -k_{19}k_{26}[X_{18}], \quad c_{22} = -k_{27},\\
&c_{21} = -c_{11}, \quad c_{33} = -k_{28}[X_{32}] - k_{29}k_{30}[X_1][X_{33}],\\
&c_{31} = c_{21}, \quad c_{55} = -k_{29}k_{30}[X_1][X_{31}],\\
&c_{66} = -k_{27}[X_{30}] - k_{-27}, \quad c_{44} = -k_{28}[X_{31}],
\end{aligned}$$

and the vector-column is $\mathbf{C_0} = (0, k_{-27}[X_{37}], 0, 0, 0, k_{-27}[X_{37}])^{\mathrm{T}}$.

Concentrations of the active form of protein kinase C, $X_{35} := \mathrm{PKC}^*$, and the activated $\mathrm{IP_3}$–$\mathrm{R_{IP3}}$ complex, $X_{36} := \mathrm{IP_3} \cdot \mathrm{R_{IP3}}$, can be obtained from the algebraic relations

$$\begin{aligned}
&[X_{35}](t) = [X_{38}]_0 - [X_{33}](t)\\
&[X_{36}](t) = [X_{37}]_0 - [X_{34}](t).
\end{aligned} \tag{8.22}$$

Here $[X_{37}]_0$, $[X_{38}]_0$ are the initial concentrations of the $\mathrm{IP_3}$-receptor on the endoplasmic reticulum and PKC enzyme, respectively.

The dynamics of intracellular calcium release from the stores is described by

$$\frac{d[X_1]}{dt} = \tilde{k}_0\left(\tilde{k}_1 - \tilde{k}_2[X_{36}]^3[X_1] - [\mathrm{Ca}^{2+}_{\mathrm{SR}}]\right) - \frac{\tilde{k}_3[X_1]}{[X_1]^2 - \tilde{k}_4}, \tag{8.23}$$

where $\tilde{k}_i$ $(i = 0{,}4)$ are the kinetic parameters related to the release of sarcoplasmic $\mathrm{Ca}^{2+}_{\mathrm{SR}}$.

Provided that initial concentrations of reactive substrates are known, the system of equations (8.21)–(8.23) models the PLC pathway dynamics.

8.4 Co-localization and co-transmission

The phenomenon of co-localization by multiple neurotransmitters is ubiquitous in biology and is therefore considered the rule rather than the exception. Functional co-transmission implies that various postsynaptic receptors exist in the vicinity of the presynaptic terminal or an adjacent cell. In the context of such a configuration, one transmitter/modulator could affect the action of another. For example, it may shunt and modify the time course of excitation/inhibition signals. It may also provide presynaptic neuromodulation and/or synapse-specific adaptation, control the differential modulation of the neuro-effector circuit, and activate synergistically multiple receptors of the same or different postjunctional cells. In addition, it adds a safety factor to the communication process and thus compensates for activity and/or pathology-dependent alterations in postsynaptic receptor subunits. These mechanisms appear to be extremely useful since cell-to-cell signaling is not fully constrained by synaptic wiring and synapse independence.

The quantitative features of integrative physiological phenomena in the human body are defined by contributions from the myriad of interconnecting cross-talk intracellular signaling pathways. The combined state diagram of ligand–receptor binding, activation of second messenger systems, and the exertion of electromechanical effects in the case of multiple neurotransmission is given in figure 8.5.

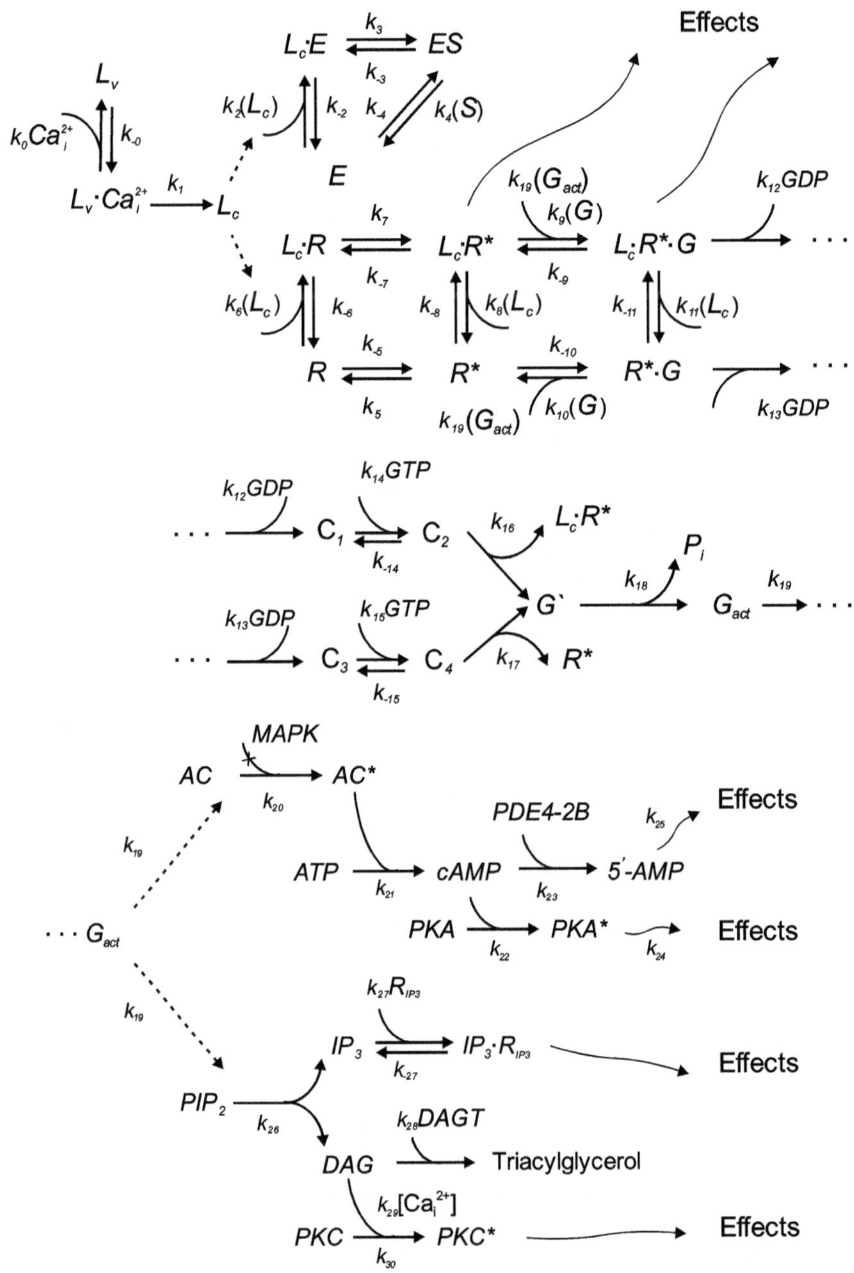

Figure 8.5. A scheme of multiple pathway neurotransmission.

From the diagram, it is apparent that elements of one pathway cross-regulate and share components with another pathway in the transduction process. The corresponding governing system of equations is given by

$$d\mathbf{X}/dt = \mathbf{DX}(t) + \mathbf{C_0}, \tag{8.24}$$

where

$$\mathbf{D}(m \times n) = \begin{pmatrix} \begin{matrix} a_{ij} \\ (i, j = 1, 20) \end{matrix} & 0 & 0 \\ 0 & \begin{matrix} b_{kl} \\ (k, l = 1, 6) \end{matrix} & 0 \\ 0 & 0 & c_{kl} \end{pmatrix}, \quad \mathbf{X} = \begin{pmatrix} X_1 \\ \vdots \\ X_{26} \\ X_{29} \\ \vdots \\ X_{34} \end{pmatrix}, \quad \mathbf{C}_0 = \begin{pmatrix} 0 \\ \vdots \\ 0 \\ C_{30} \\ \vdots \\ C_{34} \end{pmatrix}.$$

The elements of **D**, **X**, and $\mathbf{C_0}$ are defined by equations (8.10), (8.18), and (8.21). Algebraic relationships (8.19), (8.22) are used to calculate current concentrations of the reactants X_{27}, X_{35}, and X_{36}, while the values of $X_{28,37-41}$ refer to initial concentrations of substrates and are defined *a priori*.

Assuming the level of separate or conjoint activation of final components, i.e. $L_c \cdot R^*$, $5'$ – AMP, PKA^*, PKC^* and $IP_3 \cdot R_{IP3}$, is taken as a measure of pathway output, responses of the myometrium to stimulatory signals may be:

(i) depolarization of the cell membrane, which is described by equation (8.8);

(ii) increase in permeability of ion channels

$$g_p(t) = g_p[X_q]/[X_q]_{\max}, \tag{8.25}$$

where the channel selectivity (p) depends on the transmitter and the receptor type (q) involved, e.g. $(p, q) \propto$ (BK_{Ca}, NO/PKA^*), (Ca_i^{2+}, SP), (T-Ca_i^{2+}, OTR^*), (L-Ca_i^{2+}, $PrF_{2\alpha}$/5-HT), (L-Ca_i^{2+}, PrE_2);

(iii) augmentation of contraction/relaxation, which in a one-dimensional case, T^a, and in the case of in-plane forces, $T^p_{l(c)}$.

Further reading

Cha S 1998 *J. Biol. Chem.* **25** 820–5

Kandel E, Jessell T and Schwartz J H 2013 *Principles of Neural Science* 5th edn (Norwalk: Appleton and Lange)

Kenakin T 2004 *Trends Pharmacol. Sci.* **25** 186–92

King E L and Altman C 1956 *J. Phys. Chem.* **60** 1375–8

Nusbaum M P, Blitz D M, Swensen A M, Wood D and Marder E 2001 *Trends Neurosci.* **24** 146–54

Teschemacher A G and Christopher D J 2008 Cotransmission in the autonomic nervous system *Exp. Physiol.* **94** 18–9

Trudeau L-E and Gutiérrez R 2007 On cotransmission and neurotransmitter phenotype plasticity *Mol. Int.* **7** 138–46

IOP Publishing

Soft Biological Shells in Bioengineering

Roustem N Miftahof and Nariman R Akhmadeev

Chapter 9

Pharmacological modulations

This chapter presents mathematical models to simulate the effects of different classes of drugs including reversible and competitive agonists and antagonists, allosteric interactions, and phosphodiesterase-5 inhibitors.

9.1 Biological preliminaries

Successful drug discovery requires a deep understanding not only of the mechanisms of diseases, but also of the full biological context of the drug target alongside the biochemical mechanisms of drug action. It involves creating a multilevel conceptual framework which allows the integration and variation of parameters and constants within the biological system to a high degree of precision. This can be achieved effectively by using the systems and computational biology approach as a thorough, quantitative, and qualitative interrogation of biological processes within the physiological milieu in which they function. It provides a new paradigm with which to study the combined behavior of interacting components.

The majority of pharmacological agents used in clinical practice act to alter the processes responsible for transmission by facilitating or inhibiting: (i) release of the neurotransmitter; (ii) enzymatic degradation of the neurotransmitter or modulator; (iii) the function of specific postsynaptic receptors; (iv) the second messenger system; or (v) the intracellular regulatory pathways. For example, N-type calcium ion channel blockers—derivatives of ω-conopeptides—interfere with the dynamics of cytosolic Ca_i^{2+} in the presynaptic nerve terminal. The decreased intracellular calcium concentration prevents activation of calmodulin protein and the movement of vesicles containing neurotransmitters towards the presynaptic membrane. Chemical agents that facilitate cholinergic and adrenergic neurotransmission can inhibit true and pseudo-acetylcholinesterase, monoamine oxidase, and catechol-*O*-methyl-transferase enzymes in the synaptic cleft.

There are more than 20 families of receptors that are present in the plasma membrane altogether, representing in total over 1000 proteins of the receptorome.

doi:10.1088/2053-2563/ab1a9ech9

Transmembrane and intracellular receptors, having a wide array of potential ligands, are being used as drug targets. To date only a small percentage of the receptorome has been characterized. The abilities of a ligand to react with a receptor depend on its specificity, affinity, and efficacy. Selectivity is determined by chemical structure and is related to physico-chemical association of the drug with a recognition (orthosteric) site on the receptor. The probability at which the ligand occupies the recognition site is referred to as affinity, and the degree to which the drug produces the physiological effect is defined as efficacy. Since different receptors are expressed differently in the human body, it is evident that disparate ligands acting alone or conjointly may elicit similar responses.

A given receptor may contain one or more binding sites for various ligands and can be linked to different second messenger systems. The interaction of a drug with a site that is topographically distinct from the orthosteric site is called allosteric. The essential features of an allosteric drug–receptor interaction are: (i) the binding sites do not overlap; (ii) interactions are reciprocal in nature; and (iii) the effect of an allosteric modulator could be either positive or negative with respect to association and/or function of the orthosteric ligand. Thus, the binding of a drug to the receptor changes its conformational state from an initial tense to a relaxed form. This either facilitates or inhibits the linking of the transmitter.

Drugs that act at receptors are broadly divided into agonists and antagonists. Ligands that interact with the orthosteric site of a receptor and trigger the maximum response are called full agonists. Related to them structurally are partial agonists, although these have lower biological efficacy. They are regarded as ligands with both agonistic and antagonistic effects, i.e. in the case of conjoint application of a full and partial agonist, the latter competes for receptor association causing a net decrease in its activation. In practice, partial agonists either induce or blunt a physiological effect, depending on whether an inadequate or excessive amount of endogenous transmitter is present, respectively.

Receptors that exhibit intrinsic basal activity that may initiate biological effects in the absence of a bound ligand are called constitutively active. Their function is blocked by application of inverse agonists, i.e. drugs that not only inhibit the association of an agonist with the receptor but also interfere with its activity. This pharmacokinetic characteristic distinguishes them from true competitive antagonists. Many drugs that have been previously classified as antagonists are being reclassified as inverse agonists.

A class of drugs that have selectivity and affinity, but no efficacy for their cognate receptor, are called antagonists. Antagonists that interact reversibly at the active site are known as competitive. Once bound, they block further association of an agonist with the receptor and thus prevent the development of a biological response. Ligands that react allosterically are called non-competitive. They stop the conformational changes in the receptor necessary for its activation. A subtype of non-competitive ligands that requires agonist–receptor binding prior to their association with a separate allosteric site is called uncompetitive. Their characteristic property is related to the effective blocking of higher, rather than lower, agonist concentrations.

Ligands that affect second messenger system function are classified according to the enzyme they act on. There are competitive selective and nonselective cAMP, PKA, PKC, PDE, DAG, Ca^{2+}-ATPase, etc, activators and inhibitors. Since a single enzyme is often involved in multiple regulatory pathways, drugs of this category have a narrow therapeutic index and many side effects.

All drugs, depending on the stability of the drug–acceptor complex that is being formed, show reversible or irreversible interaction. Reversible ligands have strong chemical affinity to a natural transmitter or modulator and normally form an unstable complex which quickly dissociates into a drug and a 'receptor'. By contrast, irreversible drugs are often chemically unrelated to the endogenous transmitter and covalently bind to the target creating a stable complex.

9.2 Modeling of competitive antagonist action

Let L_{At} be the competitive reversible antagonist. A part of the state diagram of signal transmission that describes ligand action is shown in figure 9.1, while other reactions in the general cycle remain unchanged.

Assuming that the reactions of association/dissociation of the antagonists (L_{At}) with the receptor (R) and the drug–receptor complex ($L_{\mathrm{At}} \cdot R$) formation satisfy the Michaelis–Menten kinetics, the governing system of equations is

$$d\mathbf{X}_{\mathrm{At}}/dt = \mathbf{D}_{\mathrm{At}}\mathbf{X}_{\mathrm{At}}(t) + \mathbf{C}_{0,\mathrm{At}}. \tag{9.1}$$

The matrix $\mathbf{D}_{\mathrm{At}}$ is the extension of the matrix $\mathbf{D}$

$$\mathbf{D}_{\mathrm{At}} = \begin{pmatrix} a_{ij} & \cdots & & 0 & 0 \\ & & b_{kl} & 0 & 0 \\ 0 & \cdots & 0 & c_{kl} & 0 \\ & & & d_{35,35} & d_{35,36} \\ 0 & \cdots & & d_{36,35} & d_{36,36} \end{pmatrix}, \quad \mathbf{X}_{\mathrm{At}}(t) = \begin{pmatrix} X_1 \\ \vdots \\ X \\ X_{29} \\ \vdots \\ X_{34} \\ X_{42} \\ X_{43} \end{pmatrix}, \quad \mathbf{C}_{0,\mathrm{At}} = \begin{pmatrix} 0 \\ \vdots \\ 0 \\ C_{30} \\ \vdots \\ C_{34} \\ 0 \\ 0 \end{pmatrix},$$

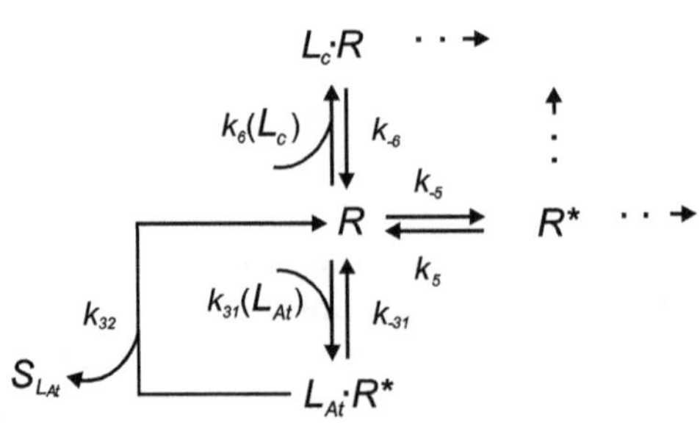

Figure 9.1. The state diagram of signal transduction in the presence of a reversible antagonist. Reprinted from Miftahof R N 2017 *Biomechanics of the Human Stomach* (Berlin: Springer) by permission of Springer Nature. Copyright 2017.

where the modified elements and new elements are given by

$$a_{5,21} = -k_{31}[X_5], \qquad a_{5,22} = k_{-31} + k_{32},$$
$$d_{35,35} = -k_{31}[X_5], \qquad d_{35,36} = k_{-31},$$
$$d_{36,35} = k_{31}[X_5], \qquad d_{36,36} = -(k_{-31} + k_{32}).$$

New components of the vector $\mathbf{X}_{\mathrm{At}}$ are defined by $X_{42} := L_{\mathrm{At}}$, $X_{43} := L_{\mathrm{At}} \cdot R$. To close the system, it should be complemented by initial values for L_{At} and $L_{\mathrm{At}} \cdot R$.

In the case of partial chemical equilibrium, which could be achieved after prolonged treatment with the antagonist, the dynamics of the receptor, drug, and drug–receptor complex conversions can be described by

$$\begin{aligned} \frac{d[X_{5(42)}]}{t} &= -k_{31}[X_5][\overline{X}_{42}] + k_{-31}[\overline{X}_{43}] \\ \frac{dd[X_{43}]}{t} &= k_{31}[X_5][\overline{X}_{42}] - k_{-31}[\overline{X}_{43}]. \end{aligned} \tag{9.2}$$

Here $[\bar{X}_{42}]$, $[\bar{X}_{43}]$ are equilibrium concentrations of the drug and the bounded complex, respectively. Summation of equations for $[X_5]$, $[X_{43}]$ yields

$$\frac{d[X_5]}{dt} + \frac{d[X_{43}]}{dt} = 0 \quad \text{or} \quad [X_5](t) + [\bar{X}_{43}](t) = \text{const}, \tag{9.3}$$

and from letting the concentration of total available receptors $[X_5]_0$ = constant, we obtain

$$[X_5](t) = [X_5]_0 - [\bar{X}_{43}](t). \tag{9.4}$$

Since $d(L_{\mathrm{At}} \cdot R)/dt = 0$, substituting equation (9.4) into the second equation of (9.2) and after simple algebra, we obtain

$$[\bar{X}_{43}](t) = \frac{K^*[X_5]_0}{K^* + [\bar{X}_{42}]^{-1}}. \tag{9.5}$$

Here $K^* = k_{31}/k_{-31}$ is the Michaelis–Menten equilibrium constant.

Finally, the dynamics of receptors in the presence of a competitive antagonist and a corresponding endogenous transmitter (L_c), e.g. ACh, adrenaline, is given by

$$[X_5](t) = [X_5]_0 - [\bar{X}_{43}](t) - [X_6](t) - [\bar{X}_8](t). \tag{9.6}$$

Here $[X_6](t)$ is the concentration of constitutively active receptors, and $[\bar{X}_8](t)$ is the equilibrium concentration of the $L_c \cdot R$-complex.

Substitution of equation (9.6) into (9.1) allows some simplifications in the governing system of equations.

9.3 Modeling of allosteric interaction

Two broad conceptual views underlie the majority of studies of allosterism. The first, developed initially in the field of enzymology, is based on the assumption that proteins possess more than one binding site that can react successively with more than one ligand. The second considers allosterism as the ability of receptors to undergo changes that eventually yield an alteration in the affinity of the orthosteric sites for endogenous transmitters.

Respectively, two types of mathematical models, i.e. concerted and sequential, along with their various expansions and modifications, have been proposed to simulate cooperative binding. The concerted model assumes that:

(i) enzyme (receptor) subunits in equilibrium attain an identical—tensed or relaxed—conformation;
(ii) it is affected by an allosteric effector;
(iii) a conformational change in one subunit is conferred equally to all other subunits.

In contrast, the sequential model does not require the satisfaction of conditions (i) and (iii) but dictates a fit binding of the ligand and a subsequent molding of the target instead.

Consider a modified part of the general state diagram of allosteric ligand–receptor interaction (figure 9.2). Positive non-competitive allosteric mechanism assumes binding of the ligand L_{AII} to the receptor in the R^{T} conformation. The $L_{\mathrm{AII}} \cdot R^{\mathrm{R}}$-complex further associates with the endogenous transmitter L_c and produces the active complex—$L_c \cdot R^{\mathrm{R}} \cdot L_{\mathrm{AII}}$. However, in the case of an uncompetitive positive allosteric mechanism, the transmitter L_c binds first to the R^{T}-receptor. Next it changes its configuration to the $L_c \cdot R^{\mathrm{R}}$ form and only then the ligand L_{AII} occupies the allosteric site. The $L_c \cdot R^{\mathrm{R}} \cdot L_{\mathrm{AII}}$-complex reacts with the G-protein system and enters the cascade of chemical transformations as described above.

A comparison of the unperturbed and current schemes gives $X_5 := R^{\mathrm{T}}$, $X_6 := L_{\mathrm{AII}} \cdot R^{\mathrm{R}}$, $X_7 := L_c \cdot R^{\mathrm{R}} \cdot L_{\mathrm{AII}}$, $X_8 := L_c \cdot R^{\mathrm{T}}$. Assuming that all reactions satisfy the Michaelis–Menten kinetics, the system of equations for allosteric interaction is given by

$$\mathrm{d}\mathbf{X}_{\mathrm{AII}}/\mathrm{d}t = \mathbf{D}_{\mathrm{AII}}\mathbf{X}_{\mathrm{AII}}(t) + \mathbf{C}_{0,\mathrm{AII}}. \tag{9.7}$$

Here $\mathbf{X}_{\mathrm{AII}}(t) = (X_1, \ldots, X_{34}, X_{44})^{\mathrm{T}}$, $\mathbf{C}_{0,\mathrm{At}} = (0, \ldots C_{30}, 0, \ldots 0, C_{34}, 0)^{\mathrm{T}}$, $X_{44} := L_{\mathrm{AII}}$.

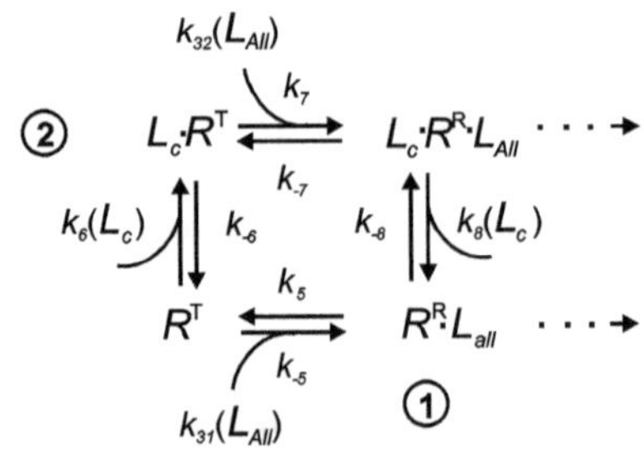

Figure 9.2. The state diagram of allosteric ligand–receptor interaction. Reprinted from Miftahof R N 2017 *Biomechanics of the Human Stomach* (Berlin: Springer) by permission of Springer Nature. Copyright 2017.

The matrix $\mathbf{D}_{\mathrm{All}}$ contains the modified matrix $\mathbf{D}$ and the additional new elements

$$a_{4,35} = k_{-6}[X_8] + k_{31}[X_5], \qquad a_{5,35} = k_{-6}[X_8] - k_{31}[X_5],$$
$$a_{6,35} = k_{31}[X_5], \qquad a_{7,35} = k_{32}[X_8],$$
$$a_{8,35} = -(k_{-6} + k_{32})[X_8], \qquad d_{35,4} = k_5[X_6] + k_6[X_5],$$
$$d_{35,7} = k_{-7}, \qquad d_{35,35} = -k_{31}[X_5](k_{-6} + k_{32})[X_8].$$

In contrast to competitive antagonists which cause a theoretically limitless rightward shift of the dose–occupancy and dose–effect curves for the endogenous transmitter, allosteric ligands attain a limit which is defined by the binding factor. Thus, allosteric agonists, applied conjointly with agonists and endogenous transmitters, can enhance their spatial and temporal selectivity at the given receptor's site.

9.4 Allosteric modulation of competitive agonist/antagonist action

One of the intriguing pharmacological properties of allosteric drugs is their potential ability to alter selectivity, affinity, and efficacy of bound and non-bound competitive agonists/antagonists by enhancing or inhibiting their cooperativity at receptor sites. During the last decade, the effect of different allosteric compounds has been studied extensively *in vivo* and *in vitro*. For example, it was found that gallamine diminishes the affinity of bound acetylcholine and inhibits its negative ionotropic and chronotropic effects in the myocardium, while alcuronium exerts positive allosteric modulation on the affinity of ACh. Radioligand binding studies with the human adenosine A_1 receptor revealed the diverse regulatory effects of the allosteric modulator (PD81,723) on the affinity of a partial agonist (LUF5831), a full agonist (N^6-cyclopentyl-adenosine (CPA)), and an inverse agonist/antagonist (8-cyclopentyl-1,3-dipropylxanthine—DPCPX), for the receptor. Results demonstrated that PD81,723 increased the affinity of CPA, slightly decreased the affinity of LUF5831, and significantly reduced the affinity of DPCPX. Therefore, allosteric ligands are capable of modifying signals carried by the exogenous and/or endogenous ligands in the system.

Let the tissue under consideration be exposed simultaneously to a competitive agonist (antagonist), $L_{\mathrm{Ag(ant)}}$, allosteric ligand, L_{All}, and the endogenous transmitter, L_c. The proposed state diagram of the interactions is shown in figure 9.3. It combines

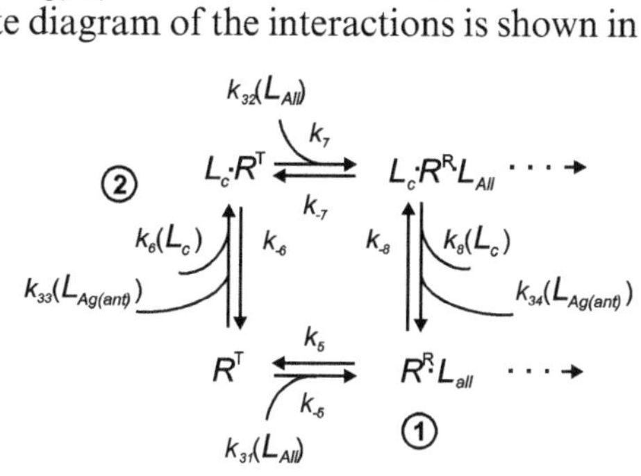

Figure 9.3. The state diagram of the effects of a competitive agonist/antagonist and allosteric ligand on the neurohormonal transmission. Reprinted from Miftahof R N 2017 *Biomechanics of the Human Stomach* (Berlin: Springer) by permission of Springer Nature. Copyright 2017.

non-competitive and uncompetitive allosteric mechanisms of action which involve: binding of $L_{\rm AII}$ to the receptor $R^{\rm T}$; the formation of the $L_{\rm AII}\cdot R^{\rm R}$-complex; the binding of the agonist (antagonist) $L_{\rm Ag(ant)}$ and the transmitter L_c to the newly formed complex; the binding of $L_{\rm Ag(ant)}$ and L_c to the receptor $R^{\rm T}$ with the subsequent addition of the ligand $L_{\rm AII}$. As a result of these reactions, the $L_c\cdot L_{\rm Ag(ant)}\cdot R^{\rm R}\cdot L_{\rm AII}$ active (inactive) complex is produced.

The governing system of equations for positive non-competitive allosteric modulation of the agonist (antagonist) action is

$$d\mathbf{X}_{\rm Am}/dt = \mathbf{D}_{\rm Am}\mathbf{X}_{\rm Am}(t) + \mathbf{C}_{0,\rm Am}. \tag{9.8}$$

The vector of reacting components is $\mathbf{X}_{\rm Am}(t) = (X_1, \ldots, X_{34}, X_{42}, \ldots, X_{46})^{\rm T}$, where $X_5 := R^{\rm T}$, $X_6 := L_{\rm AII}\cdot R^{\rm R}$, $X_7 := L_c\cdot R^{\rm R}\cdot L_{\rm AII}\cdot L_{\rm Ag}$, $X_8 := L_c\cdot R^{\rm T}\cdot L_{\rm Ag}$, $X_{42} := L_{\rm Ag}$, $X_{43} := L_{\rm Ag}\cdot R^{\rm T}$, $X_{44} := L_{\rm AII}$, $X_{45} := L_{\rm AII}\cdot R^{\rm R}\cdot L_{\rm Ag}$, $X_{46} := L_{\rm AII}\cdot R^{\rm R}\cdot L_c$. The meaning of other components is as described above. The vector of constant concentrations of substrates is $\mathbf{C}_{0,\rm Am} = (0, \ldots C_{30}, 0, \ldots 0, C_{34}, 0, \ldots 0)^{\rm T}$.

The matrix $\mathbf{D}_{\rm Am}$ is obtained from the general matrix $\mathbf{D}$ where the following elements are adjusted and new elements are introduced

$$\begin{aligned}
a_{44} &= k_2([E_0]-[X_8]) + k_6[X_5] + (k_{-8}+k_5+k_6)[X_6] \\
&\quad + k_{-11}[X_{10}] + (k_{-8}+k_8)[X_{45}], \\
a_{4,42} &= k_{34}[X_6] + k_{-6}[X_{46}], \quad a_{4,44} = k_{31}[X_5], \quad a_{5,42} = k_5[X_6], \\
a_{5,44} &= -k_{31}[X_5], \quad a_{64} = k_8[X_{45}] - k_6[X_6], \quad a_{65} = k_{31}[X_{44}], \\
a_{66} &= -k_{-8}[X_4] - (k_5 + k_{-10}k_{19}[X_{18}])[X_{12}] - k_5([X_{42}] + [X_4]), \\
a_{6,42} &= k_{-6}[X_{45}] - k_{34}[X_6], \quad a_{7,45} = k_{-8}[X_4] + k_3[X_{42}], \\
d_{42,4} &= (k_6+k_8)[X_{45}], \quad d_{42,5} = k_{31}[X_{44}], \quad d_{42,7} = k_{-6}, \\
d_{42,42} &= (k_5+k_{34})[X_6] + (k_{-6}+k_{34})[X_{46}], \quad d_{44,6} = k_5[X_{42}], \\
d_{44,44} &= k_5[X_6] - k_{31}[X_5], \quad d_{45,6} = k_{34}[X_{42}], \quad d_{45,7} = k_8, \\
d_{45,45} &= -(k_{-8}+k_8)[X_4], \quad d_{46,6} = k_6[X_4], \quad d_{46,7} = k_8, \\
d_{46,46} &= -(k_{-6}+k_{34})[X_{42}].
\end{aligned}$$

In the case of uncompetitive positive allosteric modulation the vector of reacting components is $\mathbf{X}_{\rm Am}(t) = (X_1, \ldots, X_{34}, X_{42}, \ldots, X_{47})^{\rm T}$, where $X_{47} := L_c\cdot R^{\rm T}$ and the meaning of other components is as described above. The vector of constant concentrations of substrates remains unchanged. The matrix $\mathbf{D}_{\rm Am}$ has new elements

$$
\begin{aligned}
a_{44} &= k_2([E_0] - [X_8]) + k_6[X_5] + (k_{-8} + k_5 + k_6)[X_6] \\
&\quad + k_{-11}[X_{10}] - k_{-6}[X_{43}], \\
a_{4,42} &= k_{-6}[X_{47}], \quad a_{4,44} = k_{-6}[X_8], \quad a_{54} = k_{-6}[X_{43}], \\
a_{55} &= (k_{-5} + k_6)[X_4] - k_{33}[X_{42}], \quad a_{5,42} = k_{-6}[X_{47}], \\
a_{7,44} &= k_{32}[X_8], \quad a_{88} = -k_{-6} - k_{-7} - (k_{-6} + k_{32})[X_{44}], \\
a_{8,42} &= k_{33}[X_4], \quad a_{8,43} = k_6[X_{44}], \\
d_{42,42} &= -k_{33}[X_5] + (k_{-6} + k_{33})[X_{47}], \\
d_{42,43} &= k_{-6}[X_4], \quad d_{42,44} = k_{-6}[X_8], \\
d_{43,42} &= k_3[X_5], \\
d_{44,43} &= -(k_{-6} + k_6)[X_4], \quad d_{43,44} = k_{-6}[X_8], \quad d_{44,7} = k_{-7}, \\
d_{44,42} &= k_{33}[X_{47}], \quad d_{44,44} = -(k_{-6} + k_{32})[X_8] + k_6[X_{43}].
\end{aligned}
$$

The initial concentrations of the reacting components close the system.

9.5 Modeling of a PDE-5 inhibitor

Cyclic nucleotide phosphodiesterases are the enzymes catalyzing the hydrolysis and inactivation of the second messengers, cAMP and cGMP. PDE inhibitors can also potentially increase signaling by inhibiting the cAMP enzyme breakdown.

Let L_{PDE5} be the specific reversible PDE-5 inhibitor. The proposed state diagram of its association with the enzyme is given in figure 9.4.

The corresponding system of equations of chemical reactions is

$$
d\mathbf{X}_{\mathrm{PDE}}/dt = \mathbf{D}_{\mathrm{PDE}}\mathbf{X}_{\mathrm{PDE}}(t) + \mathbf{C}_{0,\mathrm{PDE}}. \tag{9.9}
$$

Here $\mathbf{X}_{\mathrm{Am}}(t) = (X_1, \ldots, X_{26}, X_{28}, X_{29}, \ldots, X_{34}, X_{48})^{\mathrm{T}}$ where new components have been introduced: $X_{28} := \mathrm{PDE}$, $X_{48} := L_{\mathrm{PDE4}} \cdot \mathrm{PDE}$, $X_{49} := L_{\mathrm{PDE5}}$, and the vector $\mathbf{C}_{0,\mathrm{PDE}} = (0, \ldots, C_{28}, C_{30}, 0, \ldots 0, C_{34}, C_{48})^{\mathrm{T}}$, where $C_{28} = C_{48} = k_{-35}[X_{49}]_0$.

The matrix $\mathbf{D}_{\mathrm{PDE}}$ can be obtained from $\mathbf{D}$, where the following elements have been changed and added:

$$
\begin{aligned}
b_{33} &= -k_{23}[X_{48}], \quad b_{77} = -k_{35}[X_{48}] - k_{23}[X_{23}], \\
b_{7,36} &= -k_{-35}, \quad d_{36,36} = -k_{-35} - k_{35}[X_{28}].
\end{aligned}
$$

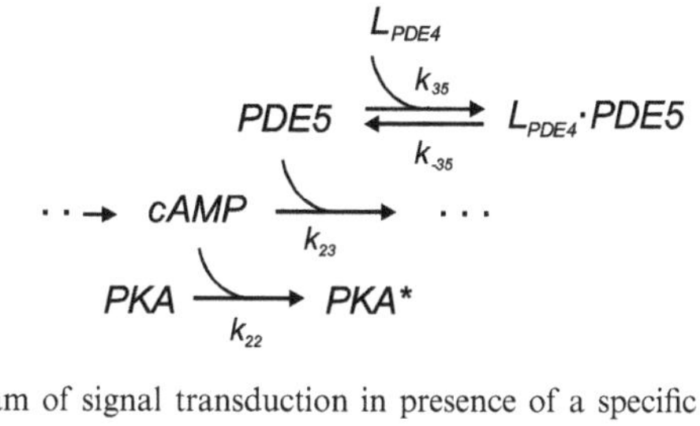

Figure 9.4. The state diagram of signal transduction in presence of a specific PDE-4 antagonist. Reprinted from Miftahof R N 2017 *Biomechanics of the Human Stomach* (Berlin: Springer) by permission of Springer Nature. Copyright 2017.

In the above derivations it has been assumed that the drug is always available, i.e. $[L_{PDE5}] = [X_{49}]_0$ = constant. Hence, the dynamics of its conversion in the system can be calculated from an algebraic equation

$$[X_{49}](t) = [X_{49}]_0 - [X_{48}](t). \tag{9.10}$$

Initial concentrations of the reacting substrates should be provided to close the problem.

Further reading

Kitano H 2007 *Nature Rev. Drug Disc.* **6** 202–10

Miftahof R N, Nam H G and Wingate D L 2009 *Mathematical Modeling and Simulation in Enteric Neurobiology* (Singapore: World Scientific)

Monod J, Wyman J and Changeux J P 1965 *J. Mol. Biol.* **12** 88–118

Stachan R T, Ferrara G and Roth B L 2006 Screening the receptorome: an efficient approach for drug discovery and target validation *Drug Disc. Today* **11** 708–16

Part II

Applications

IOP Publishing

Soft Biological Shells in Bioengineering

Roustem N Miftahof and Nariman R Akhmadeev

Chapter 10

The stomach

A one-dimensional functional element of the stomach, an SIP unit, is introduced and its behavior investigated under various physiological conditions. These results are expanded to model the whole stomach as a soft biological shell and used to study computationally the accommodation reflex, gastric tone, the dynamic response to feeding, and the role of the intrinsic control system in both coordination and synchronization of the organ's myoelectrical activity.

10.1 Anatomical considerations

The human stomach is an organ of the gastrointestinal tract located in the left upper quadrant of the abdomen. Its primary role is to accommodate and digest food. The shape of the stomach is greatly modified by changes within itself and in the surrounding viscera such that no one form can be described as typical. The existing classification of anatomical variants of the human stomach is based on radiological data. Four main types are proposed: J-shaped, hourglass (fish-hook), steer-horn, and cascade (figure 10.1). The chief configurations under normal physiological conditions are determined by the amount of contents, the stage of the digestive process, the degree of development of the gastric musculature, the condition of the adjacent organs, the loops of the small and large intestines, body habitus, sex, and age.

The human stomach is more or less concave on its right side and convex on its left. The concave border is called the lesser curvature; the convex border, the greater curvature. The region that connects the lower esophagus with the upper part of the organ is called the cardia. The uppermost adjacent part to it is the fundus. The fundus adapts to the varying volume of ingested food and frequently contains a gas bubble, especially after a meal. The largest part of the stomach is known simply as the body (corpus). The antrum, the lowermost part, is usually funnel-shaped, with its narrow end connecting with the pyloric region. The latter empties into the duodenum, the upper division of the small intestine. The pyloric portion tends to curve to the right, slightly upward and backward.

doi:10.1088/2053-2563/ab1a9ech10

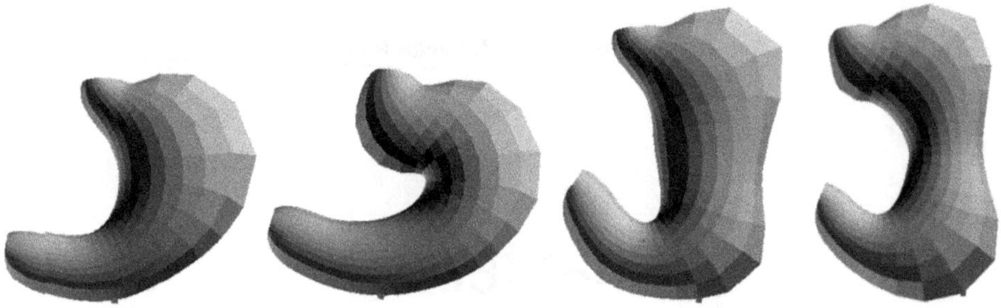

Figure 10.1. Radiologically defined common anatomical shapes of the human stomach. From left to right: steer-horn, cascade, J-shape, and hourglass (fish-hook). Reprinted from Miftahof R N 2017 *Biomechanics of the Human Stomach* (Berlin: Springer) by permission of Springer Nature. Copyright 2017.

The stomach functions as: (i) an expansile reservoir which allows the rapid consumption of large meals—the process is facilitated by relaxation of the stomach in response to food and is called gastric accommodation; (ii) a digestive and absorptive organ that breaks down large protein and carbohydrate molecules facilitating their absorption; (iii) a part of the endocrine and immune system—it secretes multiple hormones and neurotransmitters, e.g. gastrin, histamine, endorphins, somatostatin, serotonin, and intrinsic factor; and (iv) a biomechanical system that grinds, mixes, forms, and periodically discharges the preformed chyme into the duodenum as the physical and chemical condition of the mixture is rendered suitable for the next phase of digestion. The muscle tissue of the stomach wall is made of three distinct layers. The external longitudinal muscle layer continues from the esophagus into the duodenum. The middle uniform circular layer is the strongest and completely covers the stomach whilst the circular fibers are best developed in the antrum and pylorus. At the pyloric end, the circular muscle layer greatly thickens to form the pyloric sphincter. The innermost oblique muscular layer is limited chiefly to the cardiac region. Although syncytia within the tissue are morphologically distinct, there are intermediate muscle bundles that pass from one layer to the other.

The distinctive anatomical configuration of the human stomach correlates with its structural advantages. The organ contains optimal space both within itself and outside, exhibits a high degree of reserved strength and structural integrity along with efficient biomechanical functionality, has an optimal strength-to-weight ratio, and is ideal for resisting (supporting) internal pressure and external loads. The results of contrast-enhanced CT scans of stomachs of average-normal subjects demonstrate smooth thickening of the distal antrum $h \approx 3.5–6.6$ mm compared to the anterior wall of the body of the organ, $h \approx 1.6–2.4$ mm. The mean thickness h varies greatly with the distension of the stomach. The longitudinal (subscript l) length, from the pole of the fundus towards the sinus of the organ, measures $L_l \approx$ 20–30 cm and the circumferential (subscript c) length, taken from the lesser curvature to the greater curvature, $L_c \approx 10–15$ cm. Regardless of the small thickness of the gastric wall and its characteristic dimensions, it is capable of holding 2–5 l of mixed content without increasing intraluminal pressure.

10.2 Mechanical properties

The mechanical properties of the wall of the stomach are highly specific and depend on the topographical site. They are greatly influenced by food, environmental factors and age. To describe it quantitatively, the total force in the tissue can be decoupled into the passive and active component:

$$T = T^p(\lambda_1, \lambda_2, c_0, \dots, c_6) + T^a(\lambda_1, \lambda_2, Z_{mn}^{(*)}, [\mathrm{Ca}^{2+}], c_7, \dots, c_{11}), \quad (10.1)$$

where $c_0, \dots, c_{11}$ are empirically estimated material constants of the tissue, $Z_{mn}^{(*)}$ is the 'biofactor', and $[\mathrm{Ca}^{2+}]$ is the concentration of intracellular calcium.

In vitro uniaxial tension tests, conducted in the directions of three structurally anisotropic axis, i.e. along the orientation of the longitudinal, circumferential, and oblique smooth muscle layers, on specimens collected from different regions of the organ of males age 20–50 years, convincingly demonstrate that the tissue has nonlinear, viscoelastic properties (figure 10.2). Since the experiments were performed on segments removed from the host, it was assumed that the muscle fibers were fully relaxed and the mechanical contribution was attributed to mechanochemically inert components of smooth muscle cells along with elastin and collagen fibers.

Assuming the homogeneity of the stress and strain field and the incompressibility of the tissue, the force and stretch ratios can be calculated. Analysis of the force–stretch ratio curves (T^p–λ) show that the tissue is compliant at low levels of stretching, $1.0 < \lambda \leqslant 1.2$, with the force values varying $T^p \sim 0$–3.8×10 mN cm^{-1}, followed by a highly nonlinear transitory state, $1.2 < \lambda \leqslant 1.6$ and $T^p \sim 3.8 \times 10$–3.77×10^2 mN cm^{-1}. At greater levels of stretching $1.6 < \lambda \leqslant 2.4$ specimens demonstrate pure linear elastic behavior. The response remains characteristic for the tissue of the anterior and posterior walls of the stomach across all age groups. It should be noted that the posterior wall is the more compliant throughout the entire range of stretching. This is more prominent for $1.0 < \lambda \leqslant 1.2$ when the force T_{ant}^p exceeds the values of T_{post}^p by 40%–50%.

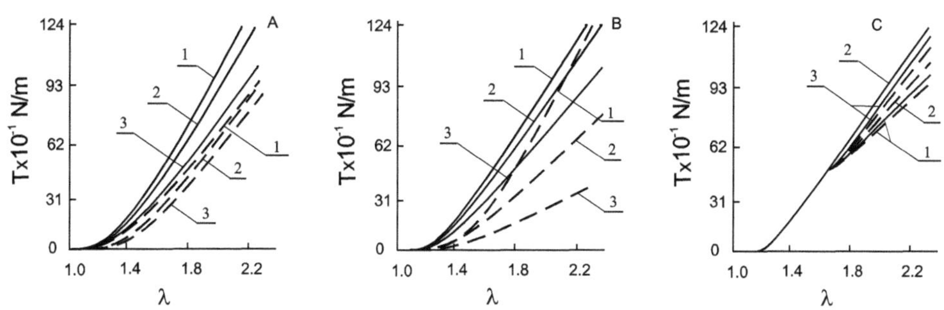

Figure 10.2. Experimental force–stretch ratio curves of the human gastric tissue under uniaxial loading along the morphostructural axis of anisotropy. 1: longitudinal, $T_l(\lambda_l)$; 2: circumferential, $T_c(\lambda_c)$; 3: oblique, $T_o(\lambda_o)$. A: specimens from the age group of 20–29 years; B: 30–39 years; C: 40–49 years. Solid lines refer to the anterior and dashed to the posterior wall of the organ. Reprinted from Miftahof R N 2017 *Biomechanics of the Human Stomach* (Berlin: Springer) by permission of Springer Nature. Copyright 2017.

Comparison of experimental curves obtained from different regions of the organ confirms the property of transverse curvilinear anisotropy. Age related changes of mechanical properties along the axis of anisotropy are uneven. Thus, the tissue is stiff longitudinally in the age group 20–29 years, while in the older group, 40–49 years, the wall becomes stiffer circumferentially. It is worth noting that while insignificant differences between the loading and unloading curves were present due to 'biological hysteresis', the force–stretch ration responses were independent of the stretching rate.

In general the wall of the stomach is stronger and more compliant longitudinally and obliquely rather than circumferentially. Thus, the maximum loads the tissue can withstand in the longitudinal and circumferential directions before rupture are: max $T_l^p = 1.434 \times 10^3 \pm 5.34 \times 10^2$ mN cm^{-1}, max $T_c^p = 1.176 \times 10^3 \pm 1.81 \times 10^2$ mN cm^{-1} for the posterior and anterior wall, respectively, and max $T_o^p = 1.29 \times 10^3 \pm 1.81 \times 10^2$ mN cm^{-1} for the anterior wall. These values decrease by 29% with age. Interestingly, the posterior wall is weaker compared to the anterior wall.

In both directions the ultimate stretch ratios are similar: max $\lambda \simeq 2.4 \pm 0.1$.

The uniaxial force–stretch ratio approximation of experimental data in the preferred axes of structural anisotropy yields

$$T_{c,l}^p = \begin{cases} 0, & \lambda_{c,l} \leqslant 1.2 \\ c_0\left[c_1 + c_2(\lambda_{c,l}^{\alpha} - 1)\right] & \lambda_{c,l} > 1.2 \end{cases}. \tag{10.2}$$

The biaxial tests conducted on square-shaped tissue specimens collected from different regions of the human stomach reveal the full in-plane mechanical properties of the wall of the organ. The edges of the specimens were aligned parallel and perpendicular to the orientation of the longitudinal and circular smooth muscle fibers which define the principal axis of transverse anisotropy. The experimental protocol to obtain quasistatic force–stretch ratio curves uses constant stretch ratios of $\lambda_l : \lambda_c$. The tissue under biaxial loading exhibits a complex response including nonlinear elasticity, transverse anisotropy, and finite deformability, with no dependence on the stretch rate (figure 10.3). The curves $T_{c,l}^p(\lambda_c, \lambda_l)$ show that as the stretch ratio λ_c increases gradually from 1 to 1.4, the extensibility along λ_l decreases from 1.9 to 1.5. The biomaterial is stiffer longitudinally: for $1.0 < \lambda_l < 1.3$ the intensity of $T_l(\lambda_l, 1.4) > T_l(\lambda_l, 1.2)$ by 50%–100%. For $\lambda_{c,l} > 1.4$ and $1 \leqslant \lambda_{l,c} \leqslant 1.6$ the force–stretch ratio curves display linear relationships. The maximum force the tissue bears during the biaxial tests is max $T_{c,l}(\lambda_c, \lambda_l) = 2200 \pm 180$ mN cm^{-1} and max $\lambda_{c,l} = 1.5$–2.3 which depends on the ratio $\lambda_l : \lambda_c$. The tissue of the posterior wall of the organ is more compliant and withstands lower maximal forces of rupture when compared with the anterior wall. Experiments show that the shear force applied to specimens is less than (max $T_{c,l}^p$) $\times 10^{-2}$ relative to the axial stretch force.

The results show an overall decrease in deformability and max $T_{c,l}^p$ with age on average by 50%.

The in-plane passive T_i^p forces under biaxial loading are approximated by

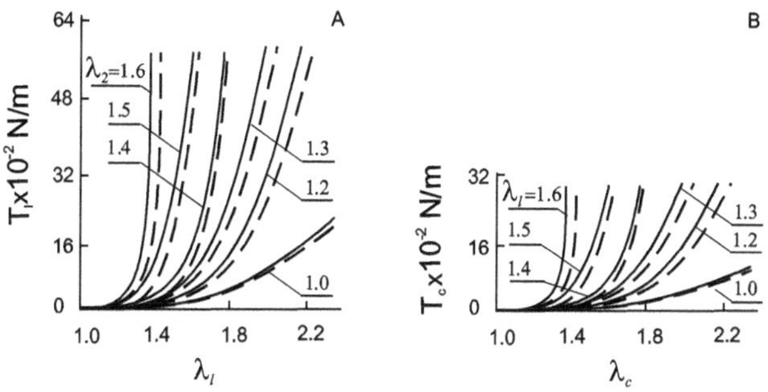

Figure 10.3. Characteristic experimental biaxial force–stretch ratio curves $T(\lambda_l, \lambda_c)$ of the human gastric tissue for the age group 20–29 years. A: $1.0 \leqslant \lambda_l \leqslant 1.6$, λ_c = const; B: $1.0 \leqslant \lambda_c \leqslant 1.6$, λ_l = const. Solid lines refer to the anterior and dashed to the posterior wall of the organ. Reprinted from Miftahof R N 2017 *Biomechanics of the Human Stomach* (Berlin: Springer) by permission of Springer Nature. Copyright 2017.

$$T^p_{l(c)} = \lambda_l^{\alpha 1} \lambda_c^{\alpha 2} \tilde{c}_0 \exp(c_3 + c_4\lambda_l^2 + c_5\lambda_c^2 + c_6\lambda_l\lambda_c). \tag{10.3}$$

Investigations into uniaxial and biaxial mechanical properties of actively contracting tissue remain a challenging area in biomechanics. At the time of writing, there are no experimental data available on in-plane active behavior of the wall of the human stomach. The main problem is to keep specimens physiologically viable and stable, i.e. for *in vitro* samples to reproduce myoelectrical patterns that are consistent with those observed *in vivo*. Thus, it is practically impossible to simultaneously sustain and control the slow wave, spiking, and contractile activity of smooth muscle syncytia.

10.3 Electromechanical phenomena

Current theories of motility of the gastrointestinal tract suggest that there are reciprocal mechanical relationships between the longitudinal and circular muscle syncytia. Such coordination leads to the generation of propagating peristaltic waves, in contrast to non-propagating spastic-type activity resulting from the simultaneous contraction of both muscle syncytia. This fact, together with the fine fibrillar structure of the smooth muscle, suggests that active forces are produced only in preferred directions, longitudinal or circumferential, and as such can be characterized in full by uniaxial tests. Furthermore, constructive modeling requires formulation of the excitation–contraction coupling phenomenon to provide the link between electrical events and muscle mechanics.

The electrical repertoire, i.e. rhythmic low amplitude depolarizations (slow waves) and the generation of action potentials (spikes) by gastrointestinal smooth muscle cells depend on the balanced function of transmembrane ion channels, namely: voltage-dependent L- and T-type Ca^{2+}, large conductance Ca^{2+}-activated K^+, voltage-gated K^+, and Cl^- channels. L-type Ca^{2+} channels in the human stomach are formed of five distinct subunits: $\alpha 1$, $\alpha 2$, $\beta 2/3$, δ, and γ. The $\alpha 1$C-subunit contains the channel pore, voltage sensor, and drug binding sites, while the α_2, β, δ, and γ-subunits modulate the channel's permeability. The channels possess characteristics of long-lasting, high-voltage dependence and ensure the main influx of extracellular calcium ions during depolarization.

Three subfamilies of T-type Ca^{2+} channels, which differ in α-subunits, have been identified by cloning techniques in human myocytes. They have distinct activation/deactivation kinetics being activated at low voltage and remain open for a short period of time. Experimental data suggest that T-type channels are responsible for the generation of spikes and pacemaker activity, playing a key role in regulating the frequency of phasic contractions.

Potassium channels constitute a superfamily of four channels: the large conductance Ca^{2+}-activated K^+ (BK_{Ca}), small conductance (SK_{Ca}), voltage-gated (K_v), and ATP-sensitive (K_{ATP}) potassium channels. The BK_{Ca} channel constitutes six transmembrane proteins. The channel's sensitivity to calcium and activity is regulated by phosphorylation of the pore-forming α-subunit. This offers a mechanism whereby cyclic nucleotides and protein kinase C modulate channel function. Two types of K_v channels are identified: delayed rectifying and rapidly inactivating. They are formed by a single unit of six transmembrane proteins and the pore–hairpin loop. The channels remain uncoupled at a low level $[Ca_i^{2+}]$ but switch to a calcium sensor mode with an increase in intracellular calcium. Together with SK_{Ca}, they determine the resting membrane potential, action potential repolarization, excitability, and muscle contractility.

The role of Ca^{2+} activated Cl^- channels has been implicated in the origin of slow waves in gastrointestinal smooth muscle. They have distinctive biophysical properties and their activity is triggered by oscillations in cytosolic Ca_i^{2+}. However, until the structure and electrophysiology of these channels are identified, their functionality remains the subject of speculation.

10.4 General model postulates

Biological and mechanical data on the human stomach can be summarized by the following biological postulates which are used in further modeling of the organ:

(i) The organ is a thin, soft biological shell. Its wall is composed chiefly of two smooth muscle layers embedded in the ECM—smooth muscle fibers in the outer layer are orientated longitudinally and in the inner layer circumferentially with respect to the cardia-pyloric axis of the stomach.

(ii) Smooth muscle (SM) fibers form two-dimensional electromechanical bisyncytia (layers) through gap junctions. SM layers have nonlinear viscoelastic mechanical properties which are non-uniform along the stomach, being compliant in the fundus and stiff in the antrum. The longitudinal layer also has anisotropic electrical characteristics whilst those of the circular layer are isotropic.

(iii) Contained within smooth muscle bisyncytia are clusters of widely dispersed ICC and PDGFRα^+ cells, firmly linked via electrical synapses and ionic conductances including L- and T-type Ca^{2+}, BK_{Ca}, and Cl^- channels, this ensures the electrogenic self-oscillatory activity of the SIP. SIPs are then divided into pools according to their firing frequencies.

(iv) The intrinsic regulatory system is comprised of Auerbach's and ICC/PDGFRα^+–MY(IM) plexi. The intramural Auerbach's nervous plexus is a regular two-dimensional network of spatially distributed interconnected ganglia, each ganglion being formed of primary sensory, motor, and interneurons. The neurons may co-localize and co-release neurotransmitters on demand.

(v) The separate networks of ICC/PDGFRα^+–MY(IM) serve the role of pacemakers, discharging action potentials continuously at their natural frequencies. The oscillators are arranged in pools according to their natural frequencies. Two oscillators communicate weakly if they have nearly equal frequencies, such that the phase of one is sensitive to the phase of the other, two oscillators are strongly connected if they have equal frequencies, and two oscillators are disconnected if they have essentially different frequencies.

(vi) Auerbach's and ICC/PDGFRα^+–MY(IM) plexi are interconnected via chemical synapses. There are low resistance electrical synapses and gap junctions between ICC–IM and SMCs. Mechanoreceptors on the primary sensory neurons and ICC serve as a feedback signal to the plexi.

(vii) Electromechanical coupling and mechanical responses by SMCs are a result of the evolution of slow waves and spikes; the slow wave and spiking activity represents the integrated function of: voltage-dependent L- and T-type Ca^{2+}; voltage-dependent K^+; Ca^{2+}-activated K^+ and leak Cl^- ion channels on smooth muscle membrane; ICC/PDGFRα^+–MY(IM); and the myenteric nervous plexus.

(viii) The generation of active forces involve a multi-cascade process with the activation of intracellular contractile proteins. Free intracellular Ca^{2+} is the key player in the dynamics of the transformation of microscopic properties of electrical excitatory events into macroscopic contractions. As an approximation it can be adopted that the experimental active force–intracellular Ca^{2+} relationship is

$$T^a_{c,l} = \begin{cases} 0, & [Ca_i^{2+}] \leqslant 0.1\ \mu M \\ c_7 + c_8[Ca_i^{2+}]^4 + c_9[Ca_i^{2+}]^3 + c_{10}[Ca_i^{2+}]^2 + c_{11}[Ca_i^{2+}], & \\ & 0.1 < [Ca_i^{2+}] \leqslant 1\ \mu M \\ \max T^a, & [Ca_i^{2+}] > 1\ \mu M \end{cases} \tag{10.4}$$

where $[Ca_i^{2+}]$ is the intracellular concentration of calcium ions.

(ix) Passive forces are explained by the biomechanics of viscoelastic ECM.

10.5 A functional unit

Interstitial cells of Cajal and PDGFRα^+ form a sheath around and also send branches within muscle bundles thus giving rise to a three-dimensional network within the SM thickness. Firmly connected through gap junctions with SMCs, they create a multicellular SM/ICC/PDGFRα^+ syncytium (SIP)—a functional unit of the human stomach. Within an SIP, SMC and ICC (i) associate closely with nerve bundles and varicosities of myenteric neurons, (ii) express receptors for various neurotransmitters, and (iii) receive extensive input from vagal efferent tracts. The nature of ICC–myenteric nerve connections is either a close contact of 20–200 nm or a synapse-like contact of 20 nm. The latter comes from immunohistochemical staining studies for synaptic specific molecules, e.g. soluble *N*-ethylmaleimide-sensitive factor attachment protein receptor and synaptosomal-associated protein-25. These synapses involve multiple excitatory and inhibitory neurotransmissions by ACh, NO, SP, VIP, and ATP and provide the functional integrity of SIP.

10.5.1 Mathematical model of SIP

Following the general principles of the Hodgkin–Huxley formalism, the system of equations of the dynamics of membrane potential $V_{c,l}$ generation in an SIP unit is described as

$$\tilde{\lambda} C_m \frac{dV_{c,l}}{dt} = -\sum_j \tilde{I}_j, \tag{10.5}$$

where $\tilde{\lambda}$ is the numerical parameter, C_m is the SIP membrane capacitance, and $\tilde{I}_j$ are the fast and slow inward Ca^{2+}, BK_{Ca}, voltage-dependent K^+, and leak Cl^- currents given by

$$\begin{aligned}
\tilde{I}^f_{Ca} &= \tilde{g}^f_{Ca}\tilde{m}^3_I\tilde{h}(V_{c,l} - \tilde{V}_{Ca}),\\
\tilde{I}^s_{Ca} &= \tilde{g}^s_{Ca}\tilde{x}_{Ca}(V_{c,l} - \tilde{V}_{Ca}),\\
\tilde{I}_K &= \tilde{g}_K\tilde{n}^4(V_{c,l} - \tilde{V}_{Ca}),\\
\tilde{I}_{Cl} &= \tilde{g}_{Cl}(V_{c,l} - \tilde{V}_{Ca})\\
\tilde{I}_{Ca-K} &= \tilde{g}^f_{Ca-K}[Ca^{2+}](V_{c,l} - \tilde{V}_{Ca})/(0.5 + [Ca^{2+}]).
\end{aligned} \tag{10.6}$$

Here $\tilde{V}_{Ca}$, $\tilde{V}_K$, $\tilde{V}_{Cl}$ are the reversal potentials and $\tilde{g}^f_{Ca}$, $\tilde{g}^s_{Ca}$, $\tilde{g}_K$, $\tilde{g}_{Ca-K}$, $\tilde{g}_{Cl}$ are the maximal conductances for the respective ion currents. $\tilde{m}$, $\tilde{h}$, $\tilde{n}$, and $\tilde{x}_{Ca}$ are dynamic variables described by

$$\begin{aligned}
&\tilde{m}_I = \tilde{\alpha}_m/(\tilde{\alpha}_m + \tilde{\beta}_m), \quad \tilde{\lambda}\hbar\frac{d\tilde{h}}{dt} = \tilde{\alpha}_h(1 - \tilde{h}) - \tilde{\beta}_h\tilde{h},\\
&\tilde{\lambda}\hbar\frac{d\tilde{n}}{dt} = \tilde{\alpha}_n(1 - \tilde{n}) - \tilde{\beta}_n\tilde{n}, \quad \tilde{\lambda}\tau_{xCa}\frac{d\tilde{x}_{Ca}}{dt} = \frac{1}{\exp(-0.15(V_{c,l} + 50))} - \tilde{x}_{Ca},\\
&\tilde{\lambda}\frac{d[Ca^{2+}]}{dt} = \wp_{Ca}\tilde{x}_{Ca}(\tilde{V}_{Ca} - V_{c,l}) - [Ca^{2+}],
\end{aligned} \tag{10.7}$$

where the activation $\tilde{\alpha}_y$ and deactivation $\tilde{\beta}_y$ ($y = m, n, h$) parameters of ion channels satisfy the following empirical relations

$$\begin{aligned}
\tilde{\alpha}_m &= 0.1(50 - \tilde{V}_{c,l})/(\exp(5 - 0.1\tilde{V}_{c,l}) - 1),\\
\tilde{\beta}_m &= 4\exp((25 - \tilde{V}_{c,l})/18),\\
\tilde{\alpha}_h &= 0.07\exp((25 - 0.1\tilde{V}_{c,l})/20),\\
\tilde{\beta}_h &= [1 + \exp(5.5 - 0.1\tilde{V}_{c,l})]^{-1},\\
\tilde{\alpha}_n &= 0.01(55 - \tilde{V}_{c,l})/(\exp(5.5 - 0.1\tilde{V}_{c,l}) - 1),\\
\tilde{\beta}_n &= 0.125\exp((45 - \tilde{V}_{c,l})/80).
\end{aligned} \tag{10.8}$$

Here $\tilde{V}_{c,l} = (127V_{c,l} + 8265)/105$, $\tau_{x\mathrm{Ca}}$ is the time constant and $\wp_{\mathrm{Ca}}$ is the parameter referring to the dynamics of calcium channels, $\hbar$ is the numerical constant.

The evolution of voltage-dependent Ca^{2+}-channels is defined by

$$\tilde{g}^s_{\mathrm{Ca}} = \delta(V_{c,l})\tilde{g}^s_{\mathrm{Ca}} \tag{10.9}$$

where

$$\delta(V_{c,l}) = \begin{cases} 1, & \text{for } V_{c,l} \geqslant V_{p(c,l)} \\ 0, & \text{otherwise} \end{cases}.$$

The discharge of the pacemaker, ICC–MY, initiates the electrical wave of depolarization V_l^s in the SIP syncytium. Electrophysiological extracellular recordings of the dynamics of the propagation of V_l^s revealed anisotropic electrical properties of the longitudinal SIP syncytium. The dynamics of V_l^s is described by equation (6.42),

$$C_m\frac{\partial V_l^s}{\partial t} = I_{m1}(\alpha_1, \alpha_2) + I_{m2}(\alpha_1 - \alpha'_1, \alpha_2 - \alpha'_2) + I_{\mathrm{ion}}, \tag{10.10}$$

where I_{m1}, I_{m2} are the transmembrane currents described by equations (6.38), (6.41). The intra- and extracellular conductivity $\hat{g}_{i(0)}$ of the syncytium is defined by

$$\hat{g}_{i(0)} := 1/R^m_{i(o)}, \tag{10.11}$$

where $R^m_{i(0)}$ is the intra- (subscript i) and extracellular (o) membrane resistance. According to Ohm's law

$$R^m_{i(0)} = \frac{R^{ms}_{i(0)}\lambda_{c,l}}{\tilde{S}_{s,l}}, \tag{10.12}$$

where $\lambda_{c,l}$ are the stretch ratios and $\tilde{S}_{c,l}$ are the cross-sectional areas of the SIP syncytium, $R^{ms}_{i(0)}$ is the specific resistance. Substituting equation (10.12) into (10.11) and assuming that $\tilde{S}_{c,l}$ is constant throughout deformation, we obtain

$$\hat{g}_{i(0)} = \frac{\tilde{S}_{c,l}}{R^m_{i(0)}\lambda_{c,l}} := \frac{\hat{g}^*_{i(0)}}{\lambda_{c,l}}, \tag{10.13}$$

where $\hat{g}^*_{i(0)}$ has the meaning of maximal intracellular and interstitial space conductivities. Substituting equation (10.13) into (6.38), (6.41), we find

$$I_{m1}(\alpha_1, \alpha_2) = M_{vs}\left\{\frac{2(\mu_{\alpha_2} - \mu_{\alpha_1})}{(1 + \mu_{\alpha_1})(1 + \mu_{\alpha_1})} \tan^{-1}\left(\frac{d\alpha_1}{d\alpha_2}\sqrt{\frac{G_{\alpha_2}}{G_{\alpha_1}}}\right) + \frac{\hat{g}^*_{0,\alpha_2}}{G_{\alpha_1}}\right\}$$
$$\times\left(\frac{\partial}{\partial\alpha_1}\left(\frac{\hat{g}^*_{0,\alpha_1}}{\lambda_c}\frac{\partial V_l^s}{\partial\alpha_1}\right) + \frac{\partial}{\partial\alpha_2}\left(\frac{\hat{g}^*_{0,\alpha_2}}{\lambda_l}\frac{\partial V_l^s}{\partial\alpha_2}\right)\right),$$
$$I_{m2}(\alpha_1, \alpha_2) = M_{vs}\iint_S \frac{(\mu_{\alpha_1} - \mu_{\alpha_2})}{2\pi(1 + \mu_{\alpha_1})(1 + \mu_{\alpha_1})}\frac{(\alpha_2 - \alpha'_2)/G_{\tilde{s}_2} - (\alpha_1 - \alpha'_1)/G\alpha_1}{[(\alpha_1 - \alpha'_1)/G_{\tilde{s}_1} - (\alpha_2 - \alpha'_2)/G\alpha_2]^2} \quad (10.14)$$
$$\times\left(\frac{\partial}{\partial\alpha_1}\left(\frac{\hat{g}^*_{0,\alpha_1}}{\lambda_c}\frac{\partial V_l^s}{\partial\alpha_1}\right)\frac{\partial}{\partial\alpha_2}\left(\frac{\hat{g}^*_{0,as_2}}{\lambda_l}\frac{\partial V_l^s}{\partial\alpha_2}\right)\right)d\alpha'_1 d\alpha'_2,$$
$$\mu_{\alpha_1} = \hat{g}^*_{0,\alpha_1}/\hat{g}^*_{i,\alpha_1}, \quad \mu_{\alpha_2} = \hat{g}^*_{0,\alpha_2}/\hat{g}^*_{i,\alpha_2},$$
$$G_{\alpha_1} = \frac{\hat{g}^*_{0,\alpha_1} + \hat{g}^*_{i,\alpha_1}}{\lambda_c}, \quad G_{\alpha_2} = \frac{\hat{g}^*_{0,\alpha_2} + \hat{g}^*_{i,\alpha_2}}{\lambda_l}, \quad G = \sqrt{G_{\alpha_1}G_{\alpha_2}},$$

where α_1, α_2 are Lagrange coordinates of the longitudinal and circular SIP syncytia, respectively, and the meaning of the other parameters is as described above.

The total ion current I_{ion} is given by

$$I_{\text{ion}} = \tilde{g}_{\text{Na}}\hat{m}^3\hat{h}(V_l^s - \tilde{V}_{\text{Na}}) + \tilde{g}_{\text{K}}\hat{n}^4(V_l^s - \tilde{V}_{\text{K}}) + \tilde{g}_{\text{Cl}}(V_l^s - \tilde{V}_{\text{Cl}}), \quad (10.15)$$

where $\tilde{g}_{\text{Na}}$, $\tilde{g}_{\text{K}}$, $\tilde{g}_{\text{Cl}}$ represent maximal conductances, and $\tilde{V}_{\text{Na}}$, $\tilde{V}_{\text{K}}$, $\tilde{V}_{\text{Cl}}$ are the reversal potentials of the Na^+, K^+, and Cl^- currents. The dynamics of change in the probability variables $\hat{m}$, $\hat{h}$, $\hat{n}$ of opening of the ion gates are obtained from

$$\frac{d\hat{y}}{dt} = \hat{\alpha}_{\hat{y}}(1 - \hat{y}) - \hat{\beta}_{\hat{y}}\hat{y} \quad (y = \hat{m}, \hat{h}, \hat{n}). \quad (10.16)$$

The activation $\hat{\alpha}_{\hat{y}}$ and deactivation $\hat{\beta}_{\hat{y}}$ parameters are given by

$$
\begin{aligned}
\tilde{\alpha}_m &= 0.005\left(V_l^s - \tilde{V}_m\right)/\left(\exp 0.1\left(V_l^s - \tilde{V}_m\right) - 1\right),\\
\hat{\beta}_m &= 0.2\exp\left(\left(V_l^s + \tilde{V}_m\right)/38\right)\\
\tilde{\alpha}_h &= 0.014\exp\left(-\left(\tilde{V}_h + V_l^s\right)/20\right),\\
\hat{\beta}_h &= 0.2/\left(1 + \exp 0.2\left(\tilde{V}_h - V_l^s\right)\right)\\
\tilde{\alpha}_n &= 0.006\left(V_l^s - \tilde{V}_n\right)/\left(\exp 0.1\left(V_l^s - \tilde{V}_n\right) - 1\right),\\
\hat{\beta}_n &= 0.75\exp\left(\tilde{V}_n - V_l^s\right).
\end{aligned}
\tag{10.17}
$$

In contrast the circular SIP syncytium possesses properties of electrical isotropy. The dynamics of the propagation of the electrical wave V_c^s along it satisfies equation (6.43),

$$
C_m\frac{\partial V_c^s}{\partial t} = \frac{M_{vs}}{1 + \mu_{\alpha_1}}\left\{\frac{\partial}{\partial\alpha_1}\left(\frac{\hat{g}^*_{0,\alpha_1}}{\lambda_c}\frac{\partial V_c^s}{\partial\alpha_1}\right) + \frac{\partial}{\partial\alpha_2}\left(\frac{\hat{g}^*_{0,\alpha_1}}{\lambda_l}\frac{\partial V_c^s}{\partial\alpha_2}\right)\right\} - I_{\text{ion}}, \tag{10.18}
$$

where equations (10.15)–(10.18) are used to calculate I_{ion}. In the above formulas V_l^s should be substituted by V_c^s.

The above system of equations, complemented by initial and boundary conditions, constitutes the mathematical model of coupled electromechanical syncytia of the human stomach and reproduces (i) the generation of slow waves, (ii) their propagation in the longitudinal and circumferential SIP syncytia, and (iii) production of action potentials.

The commonly used initial conditions assume that the electrical potentials of the circular and longitudinal SIP syncytia attain equilibrium values $V_{c,l}^r$; the concentrations of intracellular calcium ions in muscle cells are known,

$$
\text{at } t = 0: \quad V_{c,l} = V_{c,l}^r,\ V_{c,l}^s = 0,\ [\text{Ca}_i^{2+}] = [\text{Ca}_i^{02+}], \tag{10.19}
$$

and the dynamic variables of various ion channels are defined by

$$
\hat{m} = \hat{m}_\infty,\quad \hat{h} = \hat{h}_\infty,\quad \hat{n} = \hat{n}_\infty,\quad \tilde{h} = \tilde{h}_\infty,\quad \tilde{n} = \tilde{n}_\infty,\quad \tilde{x}_{\text{Ca}} - \tilde{x}_{\text{Ca}}^\infty. \tag{10.20}
$$

Boundary conditions should be specified depending on a particular problem.

10.5.2 Mathematical model of the SIP–ganglion unit

SIP linked to a ganglion represented by the afferent primary sensory and the effector motor neurons acts as a motor-sensory unit in the stomach and can operate independently with a certain degree of automaticity (figure 10.4). It generates: (i) non-propagating slow waves through ICC–IM and its myogenic component, (ii) spikes, (iii) contractions (deformations) of SMC, (iv) dendritic action potentials at the free nerve endings of the sensory neuron, (v) the propagating wave of depolarization in axons, (vi) action potentials at the somas of the sensory and motor neurons, and (vii) EPSP at chemical, axo-somatic, and electrical synapses. It is worth noting that the motor neuron makes direct synaptic-like contact with ICC–IM and SM of SIP.

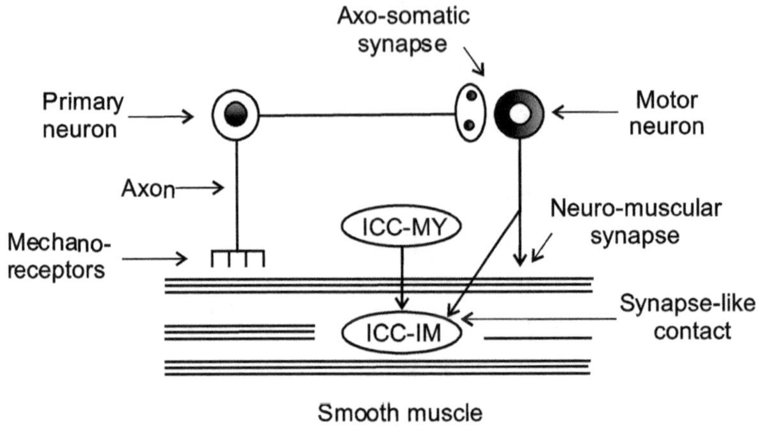

Figure 10.4. Cellular arrangements in the SIP–ganglion unit. Reprinted from Miftahof R N 2017 *Biomechanics of the Human Stomach* (Berlin: Springer) by permission of Springer Nature. Copyright 2017.

Let the SIP unit have a length L. The equation of its dynamics is given by

$$\rho\frac{\partial v}{\partial t} = \frac{\partial}{\partial \alpha}T, \quad (0 \leqslant \alpha \leqslant L), \tag{10.21}$$

where ρ represents density, v is velocity, T is force, α is the Lagrange coordinate of the unit, and t is time. Assuming that the unit possesses viscoelastic mechanical properties, for the total force T

$$T = k_v\frac{\partial(\lambda - 1)}{\partial t} + T^a([\mathrm{Ca}_i^{2+}]) + T^p(\lambda), \tag{10.22}$$

where T^a, T^p are the active and passive components that satisfy equations (10.2) and (10.4), λ is the stretch ratio, $[\mathrm{Ca}_i^{2+}]$ is the concentration of intracellular Ca^{2+}, and k_v is viscosity. Substituting equation (10.22) in (10.21) the following is obtained:

$$\rho\frac{\partial v}{\partial t} = \frac{\partial}{\partial \alpha}\left(k_v\frac{\partial(\lambda - 1)}{\partial t} + T^a([\mathrm{Ca}^{2+}]) + T^p(\lambda)T\right). \tag{10.23}$$

The myoelectrical cable properties of the unit are described by the modified Hodgkin–Huxley equations

$$C_m\frac{dV}{dt} = \frac{d_m}{R_s}\frac{\partial}{\partial \alpha}\left(\lambda(\alpha)\frac{\partial V}{\partial \alpha}\right) - \sum I_{\mathrm{ion}}, \tag{10.24}$$

where the dynamics of ion currents, I_{ion}, satisfy equations (10.11)–(10.13), d_m is the diameter, and R_s is the specific resistance of the unit. The meanings of the other parameters are as described above.

Myogenic electrical events are a result of activity of the autonomous oscillator and satisfy the system of equations (10.5)–(10.8), the dynamics of mechanoreceptor activity is given by equations (7.4)–(7.6), the propagation of electrical signal along the axons of neurons is described by equation (7.3), the processes of electrochemical coupling at the synapse with the generation of EPSP/IPSP are given by equations (8.1)–(8.12), and the production of the primary sensory and motor neuron soma action potentials are given by equations (7.8)–(7.13). When cAMP or PLC pathways are involved in the cascade of intracellular reactions, additional systems of equations should be considered.

It is assumed that the SIP unit is initially in the resting state and concentrations of chemical compounds are known. The excitation is provided by discharges of ICC–MY/MI. The ends of the unit are clamped and remain unexcitable throughout.

10.5.3 Self-oscillatory dynamics of SIP

ICC–MY/IM in the body (corpus) of the human stomach discharge high amplitude spikes at their natural frequency of $\nu = 0.1$ Hz. These pass to the gastric SM syncytium where they excite multiple transmembrane ion channels. Upon stimulation, L-type Ca^{2+} channels show nonlinear dynamics with the current $\tilde{I}^{s}_{\mathrm{Ca}}$ increasing at a rate of 4.6 nA s^{-1} to max $\tilde{I}^{s}_{\mathrm{Ca}} = -0.51$ nA. The channel remains fully open for the period of 3.2 s and returns to the unexcited state in the following 5.5 s (figure 10.5). There is a delay of 1.3 s after the excitation before T-type Ca^{2+} channels become active. The inward $\tilde{I}^{f}_{\mathrm{Ca}}$ current almost instantly reaches its maximum, −1.05 nA.

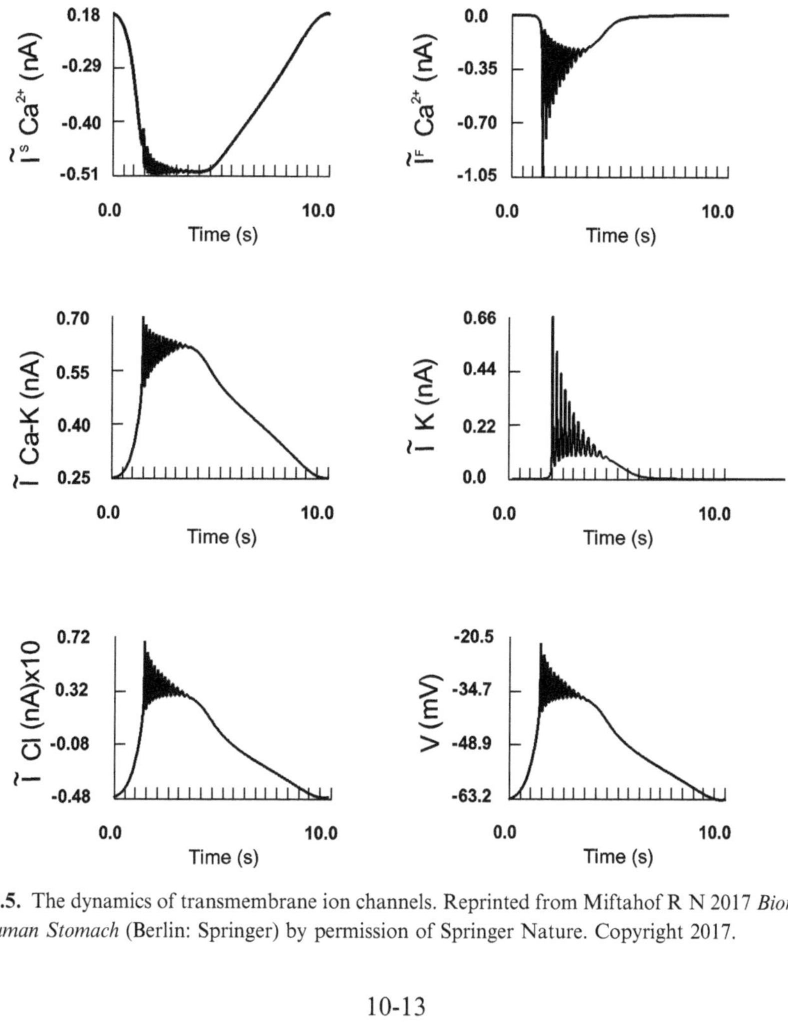

Figure 10.5. The dynamics of transmembrane ion channels. Reprinted from Miftahof R N 2017 *Biomechanics of the Human Stomach* (Berlin: Springer) by permission of Springer Nature. Copyright 2017.

It oscillates for 2 s and attains the intensity of 0.35 nA. The channel stays active for 8.5 s. The outward K^+ ion current is detectable for approximately 5 s and follows the dynamics of $\tilde{I}_{Ca}^{f}$. It reaches max $\tilde{I}_K$ = 0.66 nA and decays at an average rate of 0.13 nA s^{-1}. The Ca^{2+}-activated K^+ current achieves ~0.65 nA in 1.5 s and remains at this level for 2.8 s. It then decreases over 6 s to the unexcitable state, $\tilde{I}_K = 0.25$ nA at $d\tilde{I}_K/dt = 0.07$ nA s^{-1}. The alternating chloride current changes direction from an inward $\tilde{I}_{Cl} = -0.48$ nA to an outward max $\tilde{I}_{Cl} = 0.72$ nA. The Cl^- flux relates to the changes of the membrane potential V of the SM syncytium.

The ion channel activity triggers the production of slow waves of the amplitude $V = 39$ mV at the frequency 0.1 Hz. The wave rises exponentially from the resting value, $V^r = -69.8$ mV, to the maximum −28 mV. A few spikes of amplitude $V =$ 12 mV are generated on the crest of slow waves. The characteristic feature of the gastric slow wave is the presence of the plateau phase of depolarization ~−35.7 mV of a duration 3.8 s. It is followed by the slow decline of the membrane potential at a rate of 4.5 mV s^{-1} to the resting level (figure 10.6).

The concomitant intracellular processes are remarkable for fluctuations in free intracellular Ca^{2+} ion concentration. They are tightly linked to the voltage-dependent and independent selective transmembrane ion channels' dynamics and to the mechanisms of Ca^{2+} release from intracellular stores, i.e. the endoplasmic reticulum. The increase in calcium, $\max[Ca_i^{2+}] = 0.42\ \mu M$, leads to the activation of contractile proteins with the development of regular phasic contractions of amplitude $T^a =$ 9 mN cm^{-1} and a frequency of 0.1 Hz (figure 10.7). They are congruent with oscillations of Ca_i^{2+} and are preceded by slow waves. The degree of deformation of SIP is relatively small and insufficient to stimulate mechanoreceptors of the primary sensory neuron. As a result, the neurons of the ganglion remain idle.

The dynamics of intracellular calcium turnover in ICC and SMC plays a significant role in slow wave frequency. Thus a reduction in the activation of the IP_3—pathway, the release of Ca_i^{2+} from the IP_3—receptor operated cellular stores, and an influx of extracellular Ca^{2+} through transmembrane channels reduces the frequencies of ICC and slow waves to 0.084 Hz. This type of myoelectrical activity is characteristic of the fundus of the human stomach. Conversely, a rise in the Ca_i^{2+} turnover, which could be the case in the antral region, has the opposite effect. The number of cycles and the frequency increases to 0.13 Hz.

10.5.4 Dynamics of the SIP–ganglion unit

Let the unit in the antrum of the human stomach of length L be excited by discharges of (i) the pacemaker cell at a frequency, $\nu = 0.12$ Hz, and (ii) by five consecutive mechanical stretches of intensity $0.8L$ applied at different frequencies: $\nu_m = 0.132$; 0.21; 0.62 Hz. Each deformation initiates a unitary action potential of amplitude $V^e = 85$ mV and a duration of 1.8 s at the mechanoreceptors on SMCs. The spike propagates towards the soma of the sensory neuron where it triggers a rapid upstroke discharge of amplitude $V_p^s = 105.7$ mV. It subsides successively over 0.34 s to the stable level of −25 mV. These events produce a wave of depolarization of amplitude 75 mV which travels along the axon to the nerve terminal of the

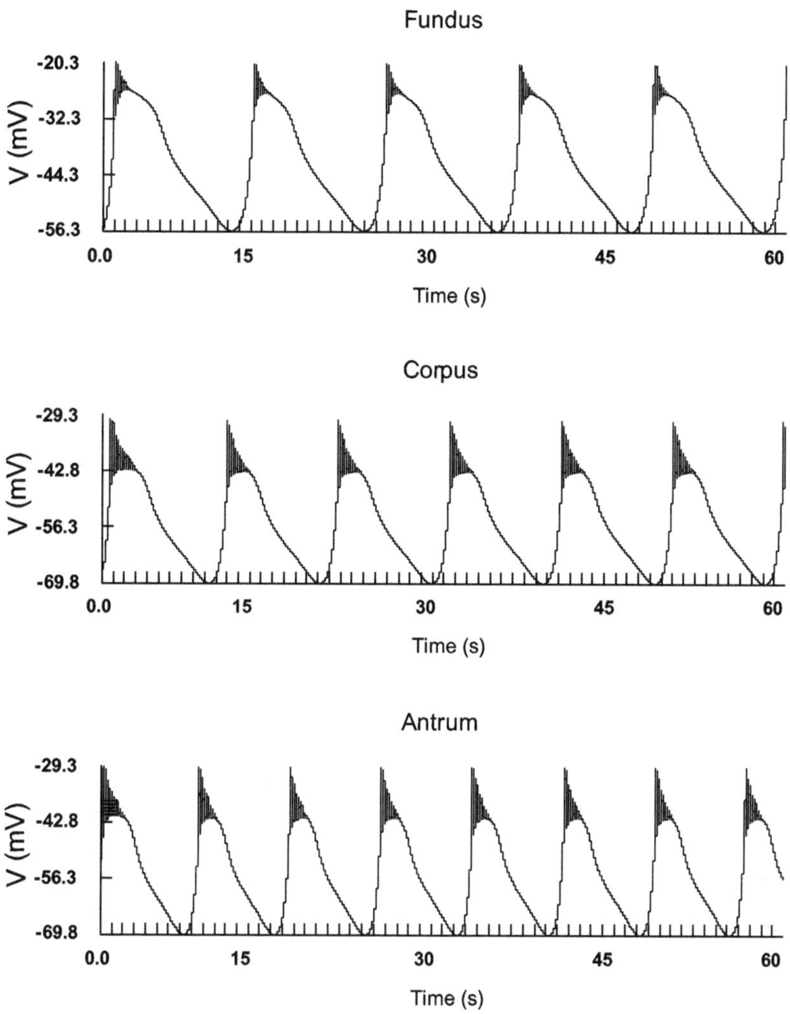

Figure 10.6. Regional frequency and configuration variations of slow waves. Reprinted from Miftahof R N 2017 *Biomechanics of the Human Stomach* (Berlin: Springer) by permission of Springer Nature. Copyright 2017.

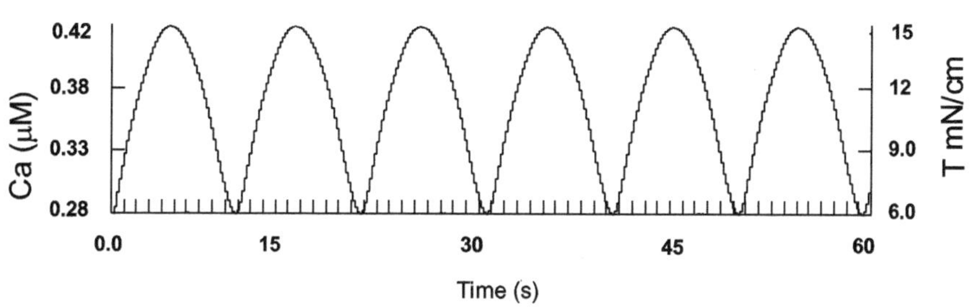

Figure 10.7. Changes in Ca_i^{2+} and force development in antral SIP. Reprinted from Miftahof R N 2017 *Biomechanics of the Human Stomach* (Berlin: Springer) by permission of Springer Nature. Copyright 2017.

axo-somatic cholinergic synapse on the soma of the motor neuron (figure 10.8). There it evokes a short-term influx of calcium ions through Ca^{2+} voltage-dependent channels. The amount of free cytosolic calcium quickly rises to attain a maximum of 19.4 μM. Some of the ions are immediately absorbed by the intracellular buffer system whilst others diffuse towards the ACh containing vesicles. Calcium ions bind to the active centers on vesicles and elicit the release of stored acetylcholine, ACh_v. Initially, the increase of the free fraction of acetylcholine, ACh_f, is slow at an average rate of 0.5 μM ms^{-1}, when the gush, ~10% of all ACh_v, is discharged at a max $d[ACh_v]/dt$ = 1.6 μM ms^{-1}. Half of the amount, ACh_f = 5.38 μM, diffuses into the synaptic cleft where it occupies 99.2% of postsynaptic receptors. As a result, the highly reactive (ACh_c–R)-complex, 0.11 μM, is formed. This leads to the generation of fEPSP of amplitude 87.1 mV. The complex is very unstable and quickly dissociates, releasing receptors.

The postsynaptic ACh undergoes further fission by the acetylcholine esterase enzyme with the formation of the (ACh_p–E)-complex. It rapidly breaks down into the enzyme and choline which is reabsorbed by the nerve terminal and is then drawn into a new cycle of ACh synthesis.

The fast excitatory postsynaptic potential (fEPSP) depolarizes the soma of the motor neuron. This fires high amplitude spikes of amplitude V_m^s = 96 mV at a constant frequency 12.2 Hz over a period of 1.9 s. Again, a wave of depolarization of amplitude 75 mV is generated which arrives at the presynaptic terminal of the nerve–ICC and nerve–SMC synapses. There the processes of electrochemical coupling with

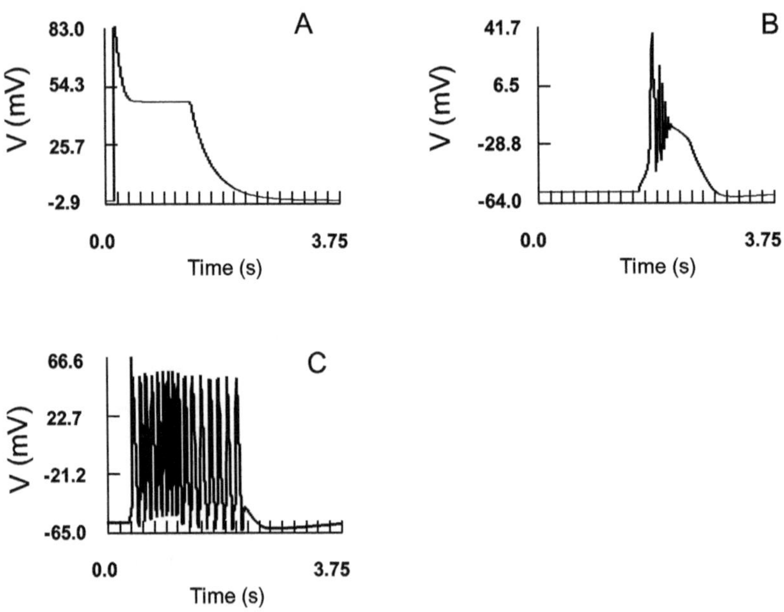

Figure 10.8. Action potentials in the SIP/ganglion unit. Dendritic (A), somatic primary (B), and motor (C) neuron potentials. Reprinted from Miftahof R N 2017 *Biomechanics of the Human Stomach* (Berlin: Springer) by permission of Springer Nature. Copyright 2017.

activation of muscarinic μ_2- and μ_3-type receptors on the smooth muscle cell and the generation of fEPSP repeat the processes as described above at the axo-somatic synapse.

If the frequency of mechanical deformation equals the firing frequency of ICC, $\nu_m = \nu = 0.12$ Hz, the unit produces unaltered slow waves with action potentials of amplitude, V = 35–46.6 mV, at a constant frequency 7.8 Hz (figure 10.9). These appear regularly on the crest of each slow wave with a duration of ~2.6 s. The smooth muscle syncytium responds with phasic contractions of max T^a = 16.5 mN cm^{-1}. The rate of contraction/relaxation is constant, dT^a/dt = 0.98 mN cm$^{-1}\cdot$s^{-1}.

An increase in ν_m to 0.62 Hz triggers the production of a continuous series of action potentials of an average amplitude V = 38.8 mV and a frequency 4.5 Hz. Each spike has a duration of 200 ms and shows an even upstroke and downstroke. The duration of slow waves increases to 34.1 s with their frequency decreasing to ν = 0.09 Hz. The unit responds with strong intensive contractions reaching maximum, T^a = 18.3 mN cm^{-1}, at a rate of 0.37 mN cm$^{-1}\cdot$s^{-1}. The process of relaxation of the unit proceeds faster at dT^a/dt = 1.11 mN cm$^{-1}\cdot$s^{-1}.

Irregular spiking behavior by SIP is observed when ν_m = 0.21 Hz, ν = 0.14 Hz. Thus short duration (5 s), high frequency (9.8 Hz) and amplitude (51.3 mV) action potentials are elicited in response to the ICC discharge, whilst spikes induced by mechanical stimuli have a lower frequency (4.5 Hz) and amplitude (45.8 mV). The frequency of slow waves also decreases to 0.11 Hz compared to the norm. The mechanical reaction of the unit becomes irregular. The duration and the rate

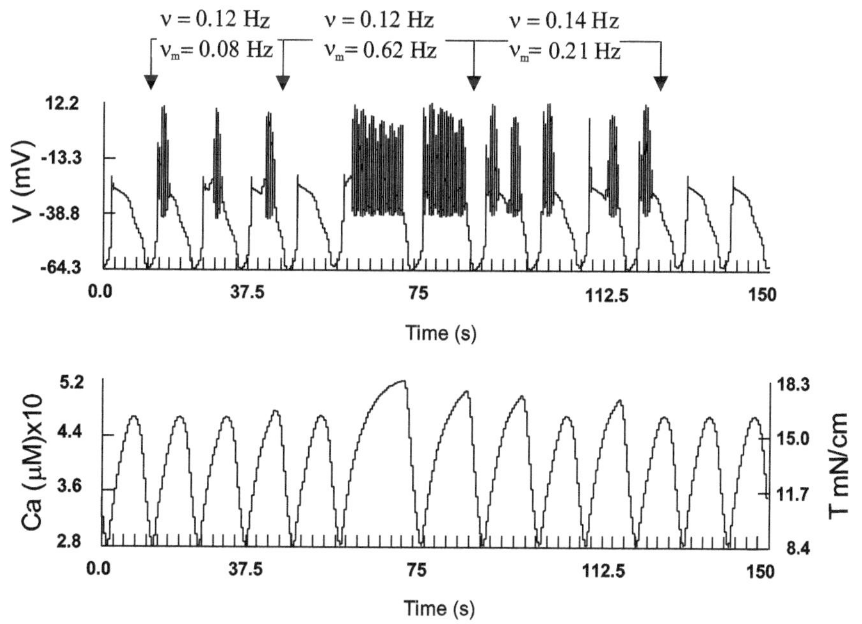

Figure 10.9. The effects of the firing frequency of ICC and mechanical stimuli on the electromechanical activity of the antral SIP–ganglion unit. Reprinted from Miftahof R N 2017 *Biomechanics of the Human Stomach* (Berlin: Springer) by permission of Springer Nature. Copyright 2017.

of the rise and decline of the active force of contraction is variable: t = 10–12.5 s; dT^a/dt = 0.53–0.67 mN cm^{-1}·s^{-1}; and 0.92–1.12 mN cm^{-1}·s^{-1}, respectively. The recorded maximum strength of T^a ranges between 16.1–17.2 mN.

The dynamics of intracellular calcium in SIP corresponds to the dynamics of active force development with max[Ca_i^{2+}] = 0.52 μM .

10.6 Co-transmission in the SIP–ganglion unit

10.6.1 ACh and SP

Cholinergic neurons are the most prominent in the ENS of the human stomach—only in the fundus of the organ they constitute (34.1 ± 6.1)%. At the time of writing no data were available to describe the density and spatial distribution of neurotransmitters in other parts of the organ such as the cardia, the body (corpus), and the antrum. Acetylcholine molecules are packed in vesicles at the presynaptic nerve terminals and are released upon stimulation by Ca^{2+}-dependent exocytosis. Postsynaptic metabotropic responses of ACh are mediated by muscarinic, μ_2 and μ_3–$G_{q/11}$, $G_{12/13}$–protein coupled receptors linked to the phospholipase C (PLC) intracellular signaling pathway. The ionotropic effect, on the other hand, is achieved through the activation of ligand gated voltage-dependent Ca^{2+}-channels. The electrophysiological outcome is normally characterized by the generation of fast excitatory postsynaptic potentials (fEPSPs) of 0.1–0.3 ms duration.

Tachykinins are a family of structurally related neuropeptides: SP, neurokinin A, and neurokinin B. A relatively small number of cells, (2.3 ± 1.1)%, in the fundus of the human stomach are immunoreactive to neuropeptide. Substance P exhibits a plethora of effects including the production of prolonged EPSP and contraction/relaxation of gastric smooth muscle, by binding selectively to two distinct ionotropic, NK_1 and metabotropic, NK_3, receptors. Both receptors are members of the G-protein coupled receptor family and employ the IP_3 as well as the adenylate cyclase—3′,5′ adenosine cyclic monophosphate (cAMP) and protein kinase C (PKC) signaling pathways. They enhance the release of Ca^{2+} from the sarcoplasmic reticulum through ryanodine receptor channels and its influx by opening L-type Ca^{2+} channels. Neurokinin A has a mainly neuronal action via NK_2 receptors.

Let ACh and SP be co-stored in the primary sensory and motor neurons. Assume that (i) ACh release precedes SP, (ii) ACh and SP interact synergistically, rather than additively, and (iii) in addition to muscranic type receptors distributed in the unit, as described above, there are NK_1 and NK_2 type receptors on SMCs, and NK_1, NK_3 receptors on the soma of the motor neuron and on ICC. These receptors are members of the G-protein coupled receptor family and employ the IP_3 signaling pathway in their signal transduction process.

The trigger in the release of SP is the rise of Ca_i^{2+}. This induces exocytosis of the neurotransmitter from the vesicular stores. The rate of SP release is not constant but rather depends on the [Ca_i^{2+}] and the frequency of applied stimuli. As a response to a single excitation 0.2 μM, SP is released and increases 14.5 times after a high frequency, 0.5 Hz, stimulation. The free fraction of SP diffuses further into the synaptic cleft where max[SP_c] = 0.056 μM is recorded. There, part of the SP is utilized by neutral endopeptidase, aminopeptidase, and angiotensin that convert enzymes whilst another part reaches the postsynaptic membrane. A general tachykinin conformer of the NK receptor binds to SP to form a complex, max[SP–NK] = 0.042 μM. The latter activates guanine-nucleotide G protein, [SP–NK–DAG] = 50 nM, which initiates the PLC signaling pathway. This cleaves phosphatidyl IP_3 to release IP_3 and DAG. IP_3 stimulates the release of Ca^{2+} from the endoplasmic reticulum. Four molecules of Ca_i^{2+} bind to calmodulin which serves as a co-factor in the DAG–PKC pathway. The final step in the cascade is the phosphorylation/dephosphorylation of intracellular proteins by protein-phosphatase. The quantity of active proteins rises to 166 nM and remains at this level for the duration of stimulation. They alter the permeability of transmembrane ion channels and cause the generation of long-lasting postsynaptic potentials of low amplitude, 20–40 mV.

SP acting alone has a profound effect on the firing rate of ICC and myoelectrical response of SIP. The frequency of pacemaker discharges increases nearly fourfold from the normal value. The smooth muscle syncytium becomes depolarized, V = −40.5 mV, and produces regular slow waves of average amplitude 26 mV at a ν = 4 Hz. The amount of [Ca_i^{2+}] quickly reaches 0.49 μM and stays at this level during the continued presence of reactive proteins. As a result, a long-lasting, tonic-type contraction of intensity max T^a = 25.4 mN cm^{-1} develops (figure 10.10).

Consider the conjoint effect of ACh and SP on the dynamics of the SIP/ganglion unit. Let the unit be subjected to a complex electrical stimulation by ICC and mechanical distension at frequencies of ν = 0.1 Hz and ν_m = 0.128 Hz, respectively. Fast excitatory postsynaptic action potentials triggered by ACh superimpose on the long-term potentiation curve elicited by SP. The maximum amplitude of depolarization reaches 55 mV. A further increase in ν_m to 0.16 Hz does not change the already set pattern of electrical response. A maximum concentration of free calcium ions, 0.53 μM, is attained. As a result, SMCs produce a tonic-type contraction of max T^a = 26.3 mN cm^{-1}.

10.6.2 NO and ACh

The inhibitory neurotransmission in the human stomach is mediated by NO and VIP. There are (24.2 ± 4.4)% of neurons positive for NOS in the fundus of the human stomach. NO is formed in the nerve terminals *de novo* on demand from the precursor, L-arginine, by the two classes of nitric oxide synthase (NOS) enzyme both constitutive and inductive. The former is calcium–calmodulin dependent and responsible for rapid biosynthesis of the transmitter, while the latter is activated under protective or pathological states showing a slow rate of synthetic activity. NO elicits inhibitory pre- and post-junctional effects on ganglionic neurons and SMCs. Intracellularly, NO activates soluble guanylate cyclase with the production of 3′, 5′-cyclic guanosine monophosphate (cGMP). This further upregulates protein kinase G which in turn phosphorylates phospholamban on the sarcoplasmic reticulum and increases the uptake of Ca_i^{2+}. The ionotropic effects of NO include the opening of large and small conductance K^+ channels, and the possible closure of Ca^{2+}-dependent Cl^- and L-type Ca^{2+} channels.

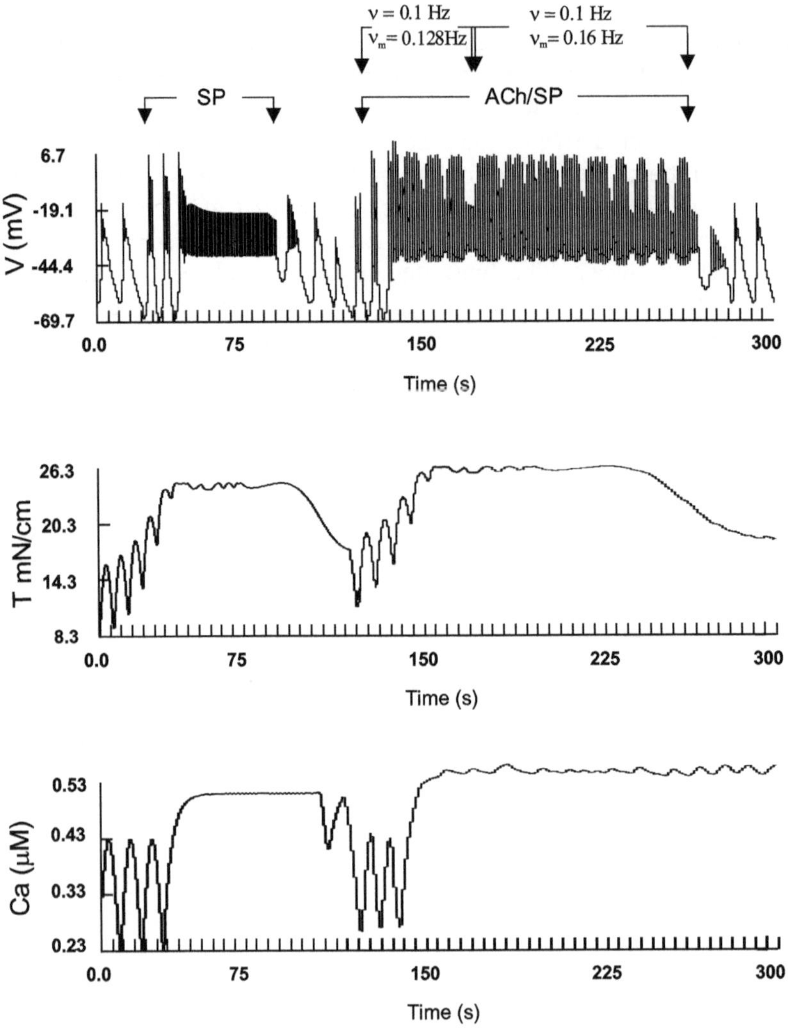

Figure 10.10. The effect of neurotransmission by ACh, SP, firings of ICC, and mechanical stimuli on the electromechanical activity of the antral SIP–ganglion unit. Reprinted from Miftahof R N 2017 *Biomechanics of the Human Stomach* (Berlin: Springer) by permission of Springer Nature. Copyright 2017.

Applied directly to gastric antral SIP at a low dose, NO hyperpolarizes the smooth muscle membrane by 6.5 mV, $V^r = -74.5$ mV. However, there are no changes in the dynamics of the upstroke potential of slow waves. An increase in the amount of NO reduces the frequency of ICC and the amplitude of slow waves, $\nu = 0.0.9$ Hz and $V =$ 14–30 mV, respectively (figure 10.11). These are linked to a decrease in Ca_i^{2+} to 0.13 μM. Subsequently, the smooth muscle relaxes to min $T^a = 0.5$ mN cm^{-1}. It is noteworthy that NO does not affect the rates of contraction/relaxation indicating that it does not impact the contractile apparatus of smooth muscle.

When SIP is exposed to ACh and NO conjointly, it responds with a production of triplets of action potentials at a frequency of 3 Hz and amplitude V = 53–60 mV. The smooth muscle produces transient rhythmic contractions of low intensity,

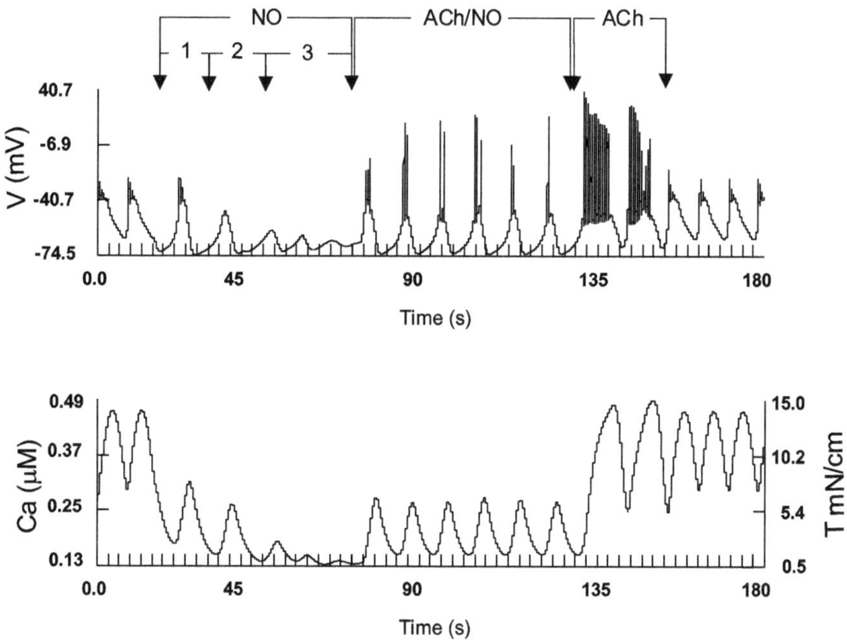

Figure 10.11. The conjoint effect of ACh and NO released at increasing doses (1–3) on the electromechanical activity of the antral SIP–ganglion unit. Reprinted from Miftahof R N 2017 *Biomechanics of the Human Stomach* (Berlin: Springer) by permission of Springer Nature. Copyright 2017.

T^a = 4.9 mN cm^{-1}. After NO is washed out, ICC recuperate their natural firing frequency and SMCs completely regain their basal muscle tone, 8.3 mN cm^{-1}. The addition of ACh elicits spikes of 65 mV on the crests of slow waves accompanied by strong phasic contractions of max T^a = 15 mN cm^{-1}.

Let the SIP/ganglion unit under consideration be influenced by nitroxidergic and cholinergic neurotransmitters. Assume that: (i) ACh and NO are released concurrently and are short acting; (ii) muscarinic μ_2- and μ_3-type receptors are located on the somas of the sensory and motor neurons, SMCs, and ICC; and (iii) NO is accessible to all ganglionic neurons. ICC discharge pacemaker potentials at a constant frequency of 0.12 Hz throughout and mechanical stretches are applied intermittently at variable frequencies: ν_m = 0.12; 0.08 Hz. Results of simulations show that under experimental conditions, NO does not affect the electrical activity of the sensory motor neurons which continue to fire action potentials of unaltered amplitudes and durations. Mechanical stimuli also do not alter the pattern of electromechanical responses observed earlier (figure 10.12).

10.6.3 VIP, SP, ACh, and NO

Vasoactive intestinal peptide (VIP) is widely distributed in the gastrointestinal tract and the human stomach. VIP is synthesized as a precursor molecule and cleaved further to the active peptide. It is stored in a vesicular form in presynaptic nerve terminals of myenteric neurons. Either brief high frequency (⩾10 Hz) or sustained low frequency (0.3–3 Hz) electrical stimuli trigger neuropeptide release into the

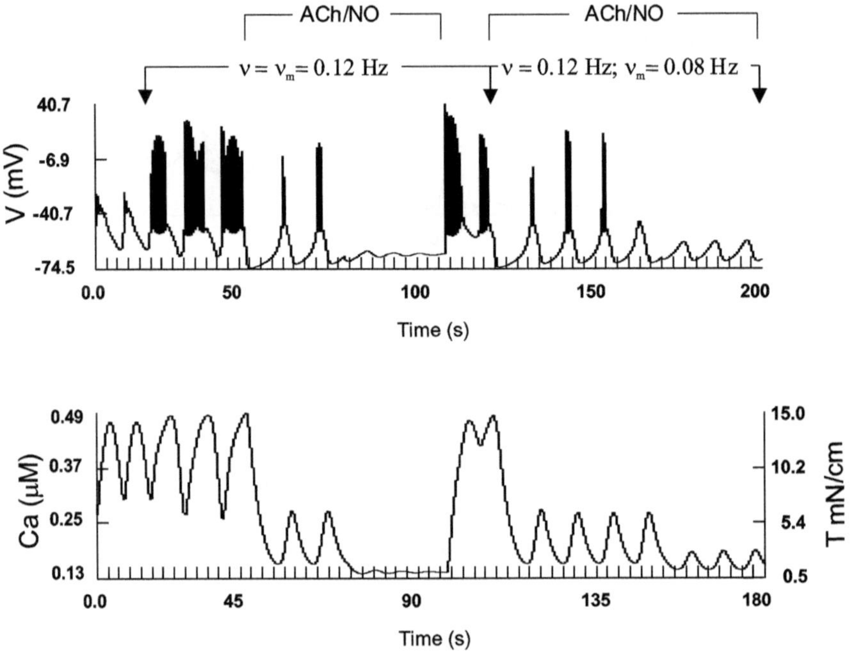

Figure 10.12. The effect of NO, ACh, firing of ICC and mechanical stimuli on the electromechanical activity of the antral SIP–ganglion unit. Reprinted from Miftahof R N 2017 *Biomechanics of the Human Stomach* (Berlin: Springer) by permission of Springer Nature. Copyright 2017.

synaptic cleft. Here it binds to $VPAC_2$ receptors and activates the cAMP/protein kinase A (PKA) transduction pathway. It is suggested that being a co-transmitter with NO (7.2% ± 6% of neurons in the fundus show NO/VIP co-localization), VIP stimulates intracellularly inducible NOS–NO–cGMP pathways and protein kinase G. This subsequently leads to: (i) the transient release of Ca^{2+} ions from the sarcoplasmic reticulum via ryanodine receptor channels, (ii) the opening of BK_{Ca} and SK_{Ca} channels, and (iii) the inhibition of L-type Ca^{2+} channels. NO in turn facilitates VIP release at the presynaptic nerve terminal.

Endogenously applied, VIP relaxes gastric antral SIP in a dose-dependent manner (figure 10.13). Thus, the rise in VIP from 3 nM to 100 nM decreases the resting muscle tone and the active force of contractions from 8.3 mN cm^{-1} to 0.2 mN cm^{-1} and 7.9 mN cm^{-1} to zero, respectively.

At frequencies ⩾10 Hz, relaxations of gastric SIP are mostly mediated by conjointly released NO and VIP. Consider the effect of a subsequent release of SP, NO, VIP, and ACh on the dynamics of the unit. SP evokes a long-lasting depolarization of SM with the development of a tonic-type contraction of max T^a = 26.3 mN cm^{-1}. An incremental increase in the added amount of NO and VIP from 30–100 nM, hyperpolarizes the smooth muscle membrane, V = −70.8 mV, and eliminates the production of slow waves. There is a concomitant reduction in free intracellular calcium and the intensity of contractions. Maximum active force T^a = 15 mN cm^{-1} recorded at VIP 30 nM, reduces to T^a = 3.7 mN cm^{-1} at VIP 100 nM (figure 10.14).

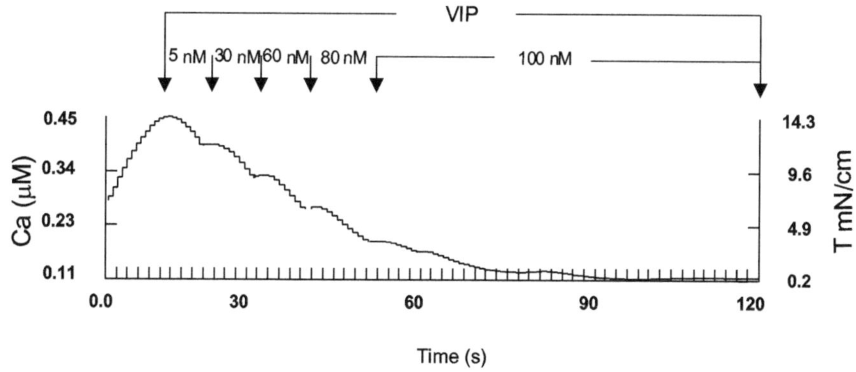

Figure 10.13. The dose-dependent effect of VIP on the mechanical activity of antral smooth muscle. Reprinted from Miftahof R N 2017 *Biomechanics of the Human Stomach* (Berlin: Springer) by permission of Springer Nature. Copyright 2017.

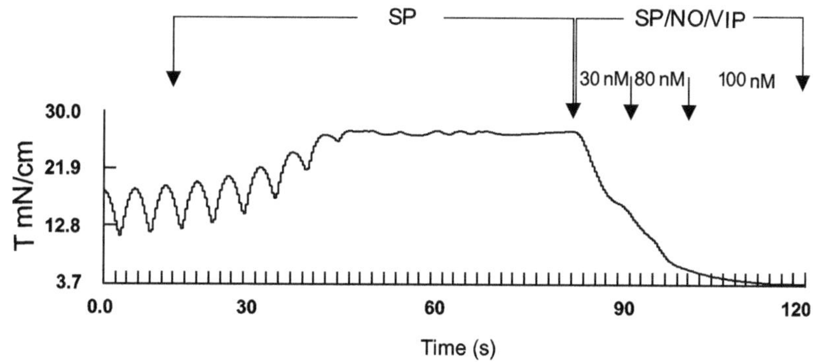

Figure 10.14. The effect of neurotransmission by SP, NO, and VIP, released at increasing doses, on the contractility of gastric smooth muscle. Reprinted from Miftahof R N 2017 *Biomechanics of the Human Stomach* (Berlin: Springer) by permission of Springer Nature. Copyright 2017.

Interestingly, the smooth muscle still maintains its basal tone due to the presence of SP. Since the effect of NO is short-lasting, it is masked by the longer-lasting and more potent action of VIP. ACh and extensive mechanical stimulation of the unit cannot reverse the inhibitory effects induced by NO and VIP.

10.6.4 ACh, 5-HT, and NO

The biogenic amine, serotonin (5-HT), is produced and stored in granules in the enterochromaffin cells and neurons of the myenteric plexus of the gut. The main factors leading to its exocytosis are mechanical or chemical stimuli. Serotonin acts as a neurotransmitter and a paracrine messenger with a wide range of physiological reactions. These are mediated through seven classes of 5-HT receptors. Their topographical distribution in the human stomach has not yet been precisely described and their description is based entirely on estimates obtained from animal and pharmacological studies. Thus, the presence of 5-HT_1 receptors in the organ is suggested from the experiments with sumatriptan and buspiron on fundal accommodation and gastric emptying of liquids. A gene cloning and physical mapping study has shown a low expression of 5-$HT_{3A/B}$ and a total lack of 5-$HT_{3D/E}$ receptor subunits in the human stomach. The confirmation of these findings comes from the inability of 5-HT_3 receptor antagonists to improve symptoms of gastroparesis in patients. Although *in vitro*, auto-radiographic, quantitative reverse transcription-polymerase chain reaction and *in vivo* clinical investigations suggest the existence of 5-HT_4 receptors on the nerve terminals and somas of motor neurons of Auerbach's plexus, their immunoreactivity has not yet been demonstrated. At the time of writing the physiological role of the other classes of receptors in the human stomach remains obscure.

Acknowledging the importance of 5-HT in the regulation of gastric motility and taking into account the uncertainties regarding the details of its mechanisms of action, consider the effects of serotonin and 5-HT_4 receptors on myoelectrical activity of the gastric SIP/ganglion unit. In addition to morphostructural arrangements in the unit, assume there are 5-HT_4 receptors on the soma of the motor neuron. These are positively linked to $G\alpha_s$ proteins and the adenyl cyclase second messenger—cAMP-signaling system. Their stimulation increases the conductivity of Na^+ and possibly, Ca^{2+} channels with a concurrent decrease in the permeability of BK_{Ca} and voltage-gated K^+ channels.

Let applied mechanical stretches be of intensity $0.8L$ and frequency of $\nu_{\mathrm{m}} = 0.137$ Hz. The conjoint release of ACh and 5-HT causes dose-dependent changes in the dynamics and the strength of ion channels on the soma of the motor neuron (figure 10.15). All channels reveal a beating oscillatory mode. Serotonin acting alone at 8 μM generates the inward Na^+ and Ca^{2+} currents of average amplitudes 1.8×10^3 nA and 3 nA, and the outward Ca^{2+}-activated K^+ and K^+ currents of 11.2 nA and 1.5×10^2 nA. An addition of ACh intensifies I_{Ca}, (max $I_{\mathrm{Ca}} = -9.7$ nA), and reduces two-fold the strength of Na^+ influx, max $I_{\mathrm{Na}} = -0.9$ nA. In the presence of serotonin, ACh does not affect the outward currents. However, it has a significant effect on the frequency of fluctuations of ion channels which rises to 9.9 Hz. As a result, the motor neuron produces spikes of high frequency and amplitude $V_m^s = 110$ mV over a period of 6.3 s.

A number of generated action potentials propagate along the axon to the nerve–SMC synapse. Here they cause a cascade of events including cholinergic transduction, the production of multiple fEPSPs and spikes on slow waves and, finally, contractions of SIP. Serotonin alone triggers a rhythmic mechanical reaction with max $T^a = 13.8$ mN cm^{-1}. Acting conjointly, ACh and 5-HT do not affect the phasic pattern of contractility. However, there is a dose-dependent increase in the strength and duration of generated active forces. Thus, max $T^a = 15.6$ mN cm^{-1} and 17 mN cm^{-1} are observed after the addition of serotonin 3 μM and 8 μM, respectively (figure 10.16). Intermittent releases of NO at different quantities induce short-term relaxations and the decline in the resting smooth muscle tone to 0.2 mN cm^{-1}.

10.6.5 Motilin, ACh, and NO

Motilin is a 22-amino-acid polypeptide produced primarily by endocrine 'M' mucosal cells of the duodenum and jejunum with a smaller quantity in the gastric antrum. It is stored mainly in cells found from the base to the neck of the oxyntic glands of the fundus and corpus with only a few in the antrum of the stomach.

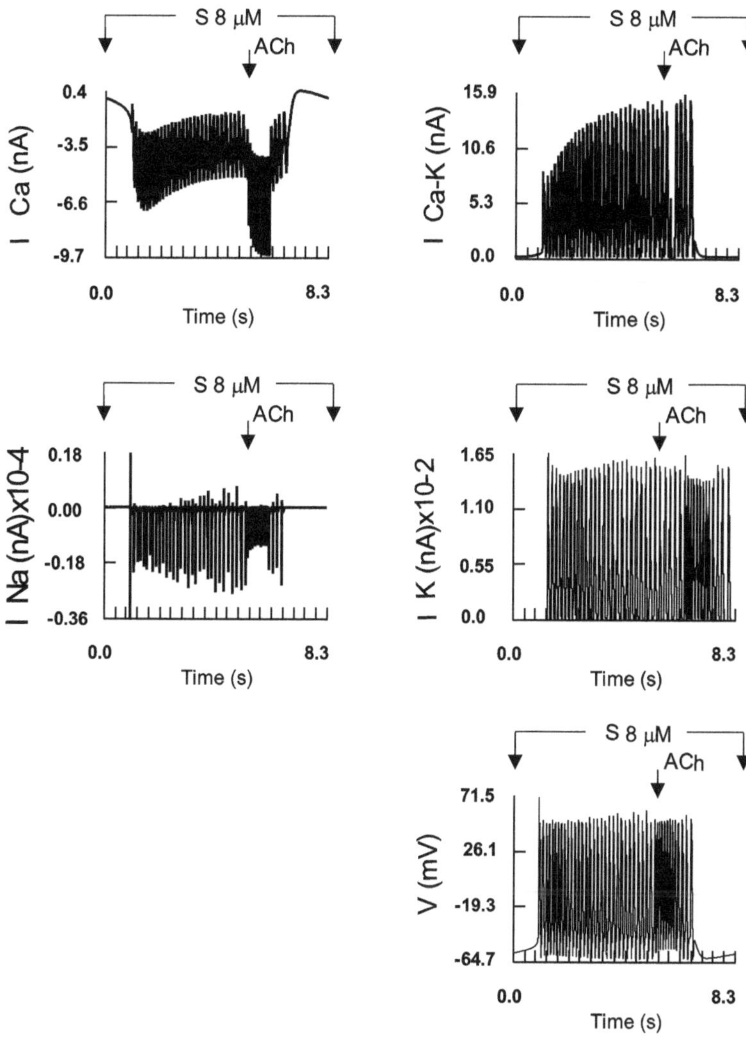

Figure 10.15. The dynamics of transmembrane ion channels and somatic action potential development on the soma of the motor neuron in response to endogenous release of 5-HT and ACh. Reprinted from Miftahof R N 2017 *Biomechanics of the Human Stomach* (Berlin: Springer) by permission of Springer Nature. Copyright 2017.

Motilin is released regularly every 90–120 min during fasting. The dynamics of intracellular Ca^{2+} tightly regulates the process. The peptide is unique in its ability to accelerate gastric emptying in the inter-digestive rather than in the postprandial state. It is believed that mechanical distension along with chemical changes in the microenvironment plays a part in this. Pharmacological, immunohistochemical, and transcription-polymerase chain reaction studies have provided compelling evidence regarding the distribution of motilin receptors—heterotrimeric guanosine triphosphate G-protein coupled receptor 38 (GPR38)—on SM cells and neurons of Auerbach's plexus right across the human stomach. However, there remain imponderables surrounding the complex transduction mechanisms of motilin. *In vivo* and *in vitro* experimental results point to an intracellular G_q-mediated

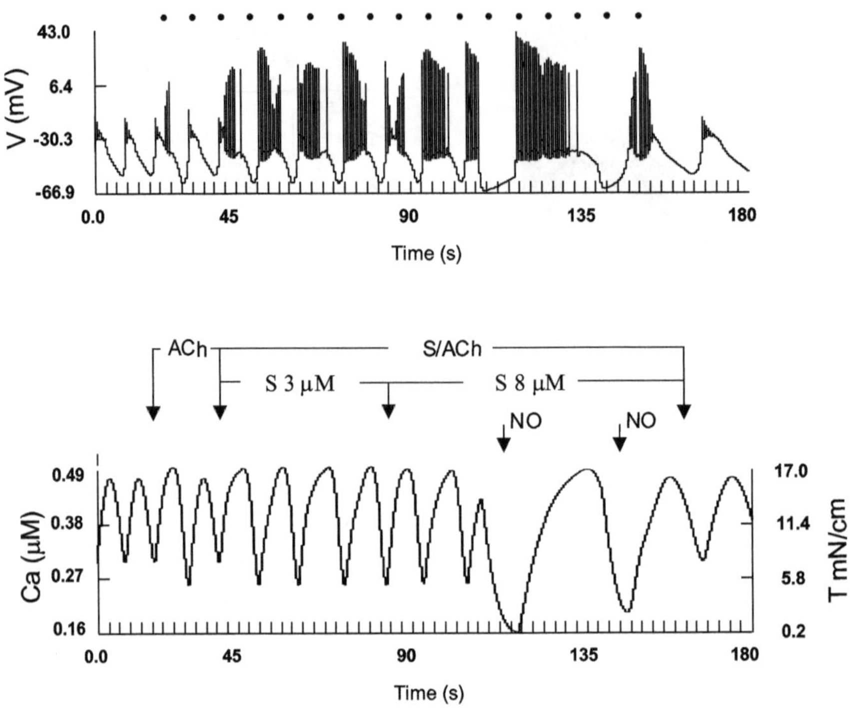

Figure 10.16. The electromechanical response of the antral SIP/ganglion unit to a complex stimulation: ICC fire at their natural regional frequency, $\nu = 0.13$ Hz throughout; mechanical stimuli applied at a regular frequency of $\nu_m = 0.137$ Hz (black dots); neurotransmitters including ACh, 5-HT, and NO released at the times indicated. Reprinted from Miftahof R N 2017 *Biomechanics of the Human Stomach* (Berlin: Springer) by permission of Springer Nature. Copyright 2017.

outflow of Ca^{2+} from the endoplasmic reticulum and an associated activation of transmembrane L-type Ca^{2+} channels. The effects of the hormone on gastric contractile activity is dose-dependent. Thus, at low concentrations, 0.03–10 nM, motilin affects myenteric cholinergic transduction by enhancing the prejunctional release of ACh, whilst at higher concentrations, 10–100 nM, it directly evokes the mechanical reaction of smooth muscle.

Consider the effects of the conjoint action of ACh, NO, and high concentrations of motilin on myoelectrical activity of the antral SIP/ganglion unit. The case of low dose peptide resembles the results discussed in the previous paragraph of cholinergic signaling amplification at the motor neuron level with the production of prolonged contractions. In addition to the modeling assumptions previously formulated, motilin GPR38 receptors are present on the smooth muscle syncytium. The unit is excited by discharges of pacemaker cells and external mechanical stretches.

Let ICC fire continuously at their natural frequency, $\nu = 0.13$ Hz. Acting alone at increasing doses, motilin steadily depolarizes the SMC membrane, $V = -54$ to -42 mV, reduces the amplitude and shortens the duration of slow waves (figure 10.17). These changes correspond to a significant rise in the basal muscle tone, 12–15 mN cm^{-1}, and a slight increase in the active force of contraction, max $T^a = 16.1$ mN cm^{-1}. The activation of the ganglion elements by applied deformations of

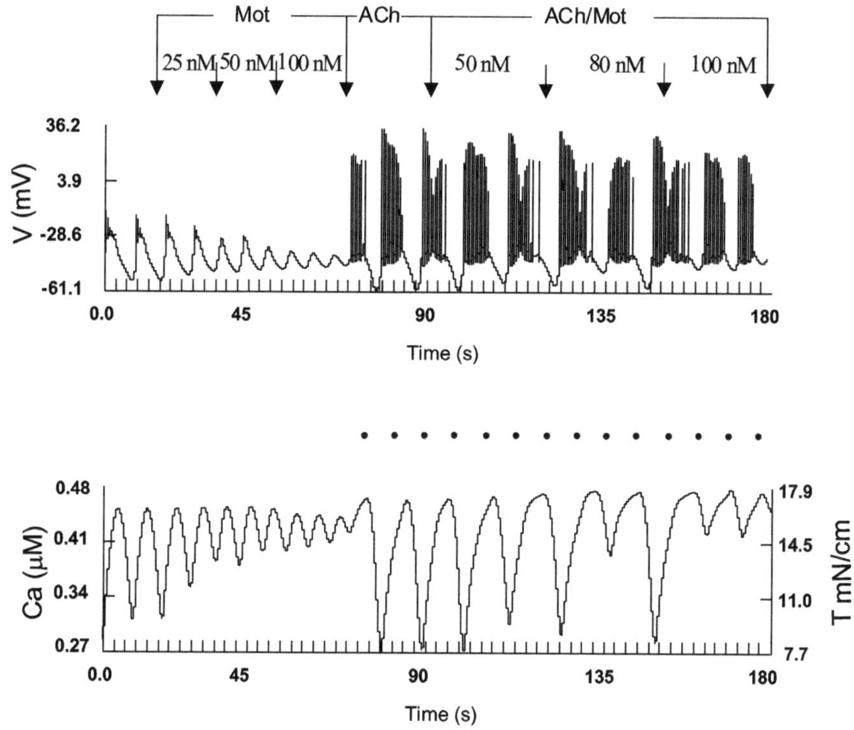

Figure 10.17. The effect of ACh, motilin, firings of ICC, and mechanical stimuli (black dots) on the electromechanical activity of the antral SIP–ganglion unit. Reprinted from Miftahof R N 2017 *Biomechanics of the Human Stomach* (Berlin: Springer) by permission of Springer Nature. Copyright 2017.

intensity $0.8L$ at a frequency of $\nu_m = 0.13$ Hz with the subsequent release of ACh at the motor neuron–SM syncytium synapse, results in the production of regular spikes on the crests of slow waves. The response of smooth muscle is strong phasic contractions of magnitude, $T^a = 8.3$ mN cm^{-1}. The concomitant application of motilin at 50–100 nM does not affect the cholinergically mediated myoelectrical activity of the syncytium. However, the peptide evokes contractions of inconsistent amplitudes ranging from 2.9 mN cm^{-1} to 8.3 mN cm^{-1}. The dynamics of intracellular calcium oscillations is closely related to that of SM.

Interestingly, the release of a 'puff' of NO on a unit exposed to the action of ACh and motilin fails to exert any inhibitory effect on smooth muscle (figure 10.18). Only when the addition of NO precedes ACh and motilin, are acute short-lasting relaxations with min $T^a = 7.7$ mN cm^{-1} achieved.

The asynchrony between the firing rate of ICC and cholinergic reactions mediated by the ganglion in the presence of a high level of motilin, 85 nM, causes the production of active forces of wavering strength. Thus, at $\nu_m = 0.22$ Hz and $\nu = 0.13$ Hz, short-lasting contractions of a duration 6.8 s and max $T^a =$ 17.9 mN cm^{-1} are generated. The muscle fails to relax completely. A minimum tension of 13.4–16 mN cm^{-1} is recorded. A lower frequency of ganglionic activity, $\nu_m = 0.09$ Hz, allows a greater degree of relaxation, min $T^a = 8$ mN cm^{-1}, and contractions of larger amplitude, 9.9 mN cm^{-1}. The observed inconsistency in the

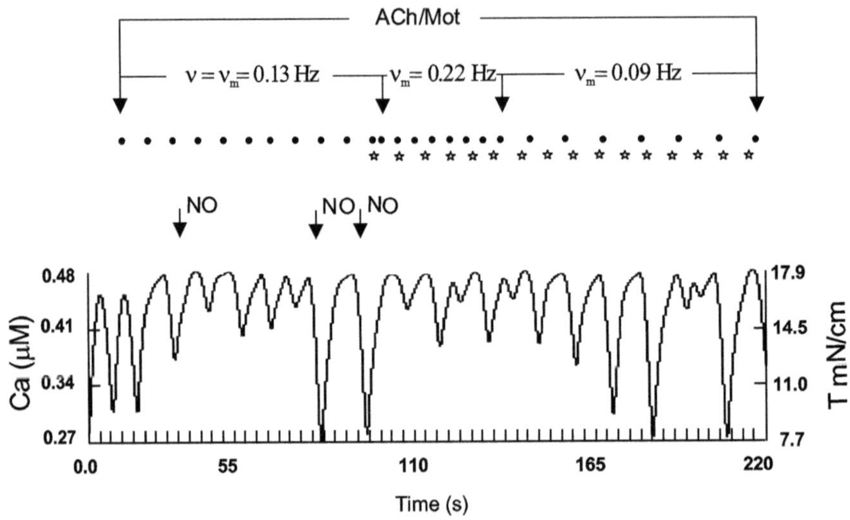

Figure 10.18. The effect of ACh, motilin, an intermittent release of NO, and irregular mechanical stimulation on the mechanical activity of the antral SIP/ganglion unit. ICC fire continuously at their natural regional frequency of ν = 0.13 Hz (open stars). Reprinted from Miftahof R N 2017 *Biomechanics of the Human Stomach* (Berlin: Springer) by permission of Springer Nature. Copyright 2017.

dynamics of $T^a(t)$ is due to the chronotropic allosteric interaction among the neurotransmitter, polypeptide, and ICC.

10.7 The stomach as a soft biological shell

Mathematical formulation of the electromechanical dynamics of the human stomach as a soft biological shell under complex loading makes up a system of equations: the dynamics of the soft shell—equation (5.102); myoelectrical activity in SIP—equations (10.5)–(10.8); the dynamics of signal transduction within Auerbach's nervous plexus including the primary sensory, motor and interneurons, and ICC—equations (7.8)–(7.13); the propagation of the wave of excitation within electrically anisotropic longitudinal and electrically isotropic circular smooth muscle syncytia, equations (10.6)–(10.14); electrochemical coupling at synapses, equations (8.10), (8.11); cAMP dependent pathway; PLC pathway; co-transmission by multiple neurotransmitters; and constitutive relations for the tissue, equations (10.2), (10.4).

In the following simulations it is assumed, unless specified, that the cardiac and pyloric ends of the stomach are clamped and remain unexcitable throughout. At the initial moment of time the organ is in a state of electromechanical equilibrium. It is excited by electrical discharges of ICC and/or mechanical deformations.

10.8 Gastric accommodation

Postprandial active expansion—the adjustment of the human stomach to the volume of the ingested meal—depends on: (i) the anatomical shape of the organ, (ii) the biomechanical properties of the wall, and (iii) the physiological response or accommodation reflex. The latter constitutes two separate chronotropically related, although clinically indistinguishable, receptive and adaptive relaxation phases. The first is of short duration and induced by swallowing and acute gastric distension, whilst the second is a prolonged neurohormonally mediated reaction to food. The reflex is associated with dilation of the organ, a non-rise in intraluminal pressure, and an isotonic decrease in smooth muscle tone. These are modulated externally and intramurally by the vago-vagal and myenteric plexus reflexes. Impaired gastric accommodation contributes to the pathogenesis of functional dyspepsia and is associated with diabetic vagal neuropathy, gastroesophageal reflux disease, achalasia, vagotomy, distal gastrectomy, and post-fundoplication among others.

10.8.1 Gastric tone

The average minimal intragastric distending pressure in a healthy subject is ~8 kPa, equivalent to $\check{V} \geqslant 30$ ml of content. To evaluate the gastric tone and the dynamics of stress–strain distribution in the four (steer-horn, cascade, J-shape, and fish-hook) radiologically distinct anatomical shapes of the human stomach during fasting, consider the inflation of the bioshell by intraluminal pressure $p(\check{V})$. Assume that Auerbach's plexus is inactive throughout.

The strain distribution in the steer-horn and fish-hook stomachs at $p = 8$ kPa in a state of dynamic equilibrium is shown in figure 10.19. The cascade and J-shapes show similar patterns of deformation but are not given here. Maximal longitudinal elongation, $\lambda_l = 1.28$ (1.36), is recorded in the cardio-fundal regions. Values in parentheses refer to the fish-hook shape. In contrast, the fundus and corpus along the greater and lesser curvatures, along with the antrum–pylorus experience extensive stretching circumferentially, $\lambda_c = 1.4$ (1.62). Most notably, the entire organ undergoes biaxial distension.

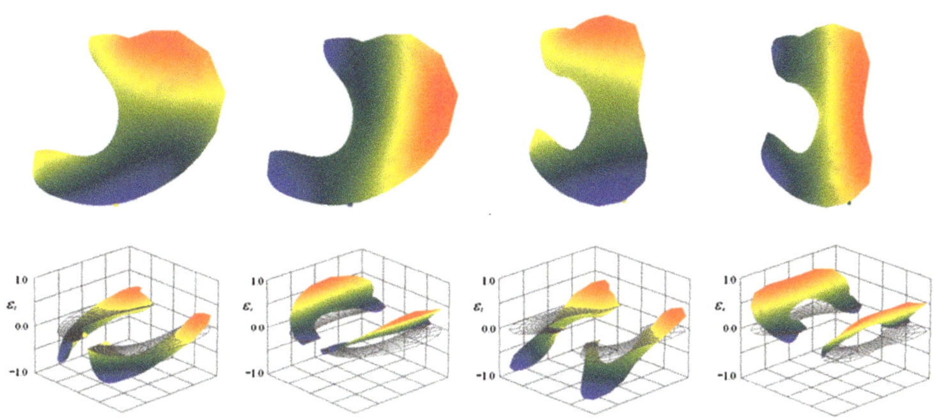

Figure 10.19. The circumferential and longitudinal rates of elongation in the steer-horn and fish-hook shaped stomachs at $p = 8$ kPa. Reprinted from Miftahof R N 2017 *Biomechanics of the Human Stomach* (Berlin: Springer) by permission of Springer Nature. Copyright 2017.

Stress distribution analysis reveals disparities among different anatomical configurations of the bioshell. In the fundus there is a deviation in the magnitude of maximal longitudinal membrane forces, max $T_l = 90.1$ (steer-horn), 78.2 (cascade), 89.0 (J-shape), and 93.7 (mN cm^{-1}) (fish-hook), with no significant variations in the circumferential direction, max $T_c = 15.7$, 15.3, 15.8, and 17.3 mN cm^{-1} (figure 10.20). The body of the J- and fish-hook stomachs is uniformly stressed along the axis of structural anisotropy with the average $T_l = 68.4\ \text{mN cm}^{-1}$, $T_c = 25.2\ \text{mN cm}^{-1}$, and $T_l = 52.3\ \text{mN cm}^{-1}$, $T_c = 18.5\ \text{mN cm}^{-1}$, respectively. The bulk of the body of the steer-horn and cascade stomachs encounter biaxial tension, $T_l = 62.3\ \text{mN cm}^{-1}$, $T_c = 15.3\ \text{mN cm}^{-1}$, with the exception of small areas at the greater curvature and at the anatomical flexure of cascade formation. Here, maxima of $T_l = 70\ \text{mN cm}^{-1}$, $T_c = 30.7\ \text{mN cm}^{-1}$, and $T_l = 83.6\ \text{mN cm}^{-1}$, $T_c = 61.8\ \text{mN cm}^{-1}$, are observed. In the antrum and pylorus, total forces of intensity $T_l \simeq 30\ \text{mN cm}^{-1}$, $T_c \simeq 14\ \text{mN cm}^{-1}$ are recorded. The circumferential tension of 15 mN cm^{-1} is registered across the antrum and pylorus of the J- and fish-hook stomachs. While these regions in

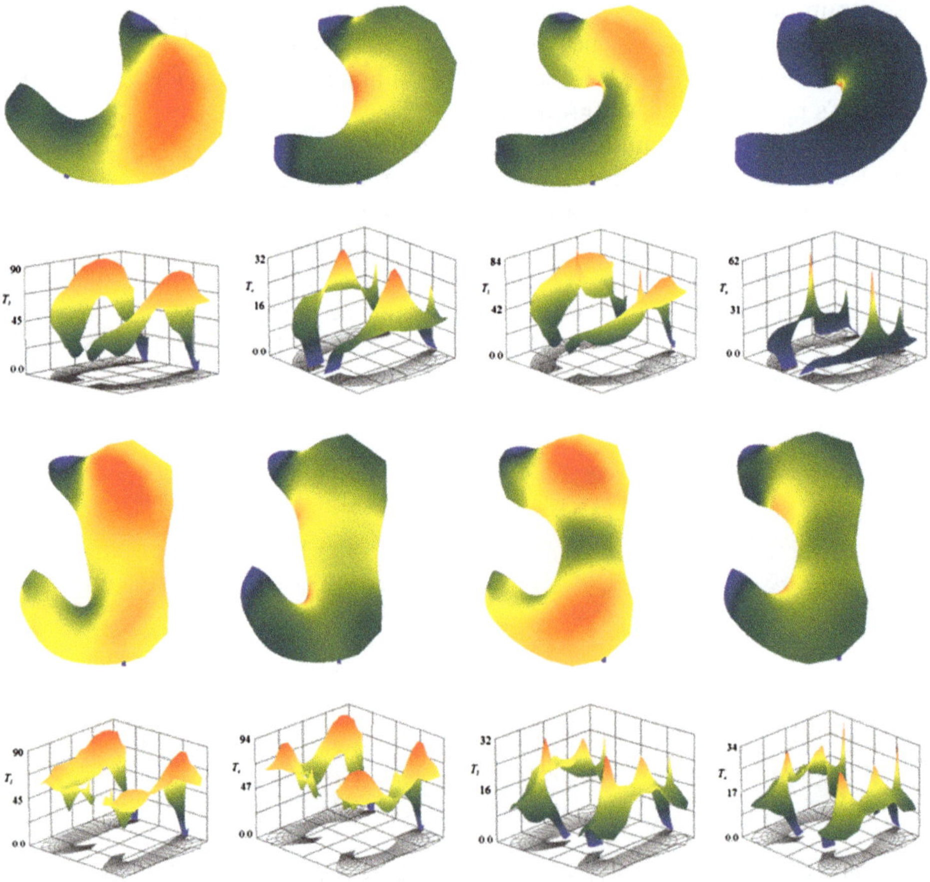

Figure 10.20. Comparative total force T_c and T_l distribution in various anatomical shapes of the human stomach at $p = 8$ kPa. Reprinted from Miftahof R N 2017 *Biomechanics of the Human Stomach* (Berlin: Springer) by permission of Springer Nature. Copyright 2017.

the J-shape bioshell are evenly stressed longitudinally, $T_l \simeq 73$ mN cm^{-1}, in the fish-hook stomach the magnitude of T_l in the antrum, $T_l \simeq 86$ mN cm^{-1}, appears greater compared with the pylorus, $T_l \simeq 65$ mN cm^{-1}.

It is worth noting that intraluminal pressure equivalent to mechanical stimulation does not trigger peristaltic activity in the bioshell. Despite the fact that SIPs continue generating action potentials and slow waves at their regular natural frequencies, there are no strong connections or synchronization in the firing of ICC–MY(IM). This is provided by the intramural Auerbach's plexus. Contractions produced across different regions of the organ are indiscriminate and jumbled causing irregular changes in the shape.

Stiffening of the gastric wall commonly seen in patients with diabetis, systemic sclerosis, *linitis plastica*, chronic gastritis, and normal aging, results in a decrease in deformability of the organ. For example, in the steer-horn stomach stretch ratios $\lambda_l = 1.2$, $\lambda_c = 1.12$ are recorded in the cardio-fundal region and the fundus, while in the body of the stomach at the greater curvature the distension attains $\lambda_l = 1.26$, $\lambda_c = 1.3$. There is a significant loss in deformability of the antrum–pylorus. As a result, the intragastric volume reduces to 18.5 ml. Maxima $T_l = 120.3$ mN cm^{-1}, $T_c = 22.5$ mN cm^{-1} are registered in the fundus and the body of the organ. In the antrum and the pylorus total forces of average intensity $T_l \simeq 52.8$ mN cm^{-1}, $T_c \simeq 28.7$ mN cm^{-1} are recorded. Analogous changes are also attributed to the cascade, J-, and fish-hook stomachs.

10.8.2 Response to 'feeding'

A gradual increase in intragastric volume to 700 ml through drinking a viscous and/ or nutrient saline solution (20 mPa·s) or tap water (1.002 mPa·s) raises intraluminal pressure to 21.3 and 30.1 kPa, respectively. The process of 'feeding' initiates the accommodation reflex. Although the details of the morpho-functional mechanisms remain elusive, it is conceivable, based on experimental evidence, that there is a decrease in cholinergic and an increase in nitrergic signaling at the SIP–ganglion unit. The former is due to noradrenaline (NA) acting via α_2-adrenoceptors at neurons of the myenteric plexus and α_1-adrenoceptors at SMCs. The latter is a direct post-junctional effect of NO on smooth muscle. Despite the extensive co-localization of VIP and NO, there is currently no affirmative physiological and pharmacological data exist to suggest the role of VIP as a co-transmitter.

Consider the intraganglionic circuit comprised of cholinergic (1) and adrenergic (2) neurons linked via the adrenergic axo-axonal synapse (figure 7.2). Let α_2- and α_1-adrenoceptors be on the axon and the nerve terminal of neuron 2, respectively. For mathematical formulation of the problem see chapter 7.

Electrical stimuli of a given strength and intensity applied at the somas of neurons induce action potentials of amplitude $V_1 = V_2 = 75$ mV which propagate along the unmyelinated axons. Upon arrival at the synapse, V_2 triggers the influx of Ca^{2+} and the exocytosis of NA from the 'releasable' store. The rate of release, although slow in the beginning, 0.66 μM ms^{-1}, accelerates towards the end of the process, 2.87 μM ms^{-1}. Free noradrenaline, $[NA_f] = 97$ μM, diffuses into the synaptic cleft where max $[NA_c]$ = 86.3 μM, is registered. A major part of NA_c is rapidly inactivated by the uptake-1 and the catechol-*O*-methyltransferase dependent uptake-2 mechanisms. The rest of the NA, 35.2 μM, binds to postsynaptic α_2-adrenoceptors. As a result, 8.53 μM of the reactive (NA_p–$R\alpha_2$)-complex is produced. This activates the intracellular second messenger system with the generation of an inhibitory postsynaptic potential of amplitude −76.2 mV and duration 2–3 ms.

To achieve inhibition of signal transduction along the axon, the amplitude, frequency, and duration of the excitatory potential V_1 and the locally generated IPSP have to be subtly synchronized. The time delay, Δt, of interaction between the two signals plays an important role in the dynamics of V_{sum}. Thus, for $\Delta t \geqslant 1.68$ ms the amplitude and the velocity of V_1 remain unaffected. It reaches the cholinergic synapse successfully and initiates nerve-pulse transmission (figure 10.21). With the shortening of Δt, the inhibitory effect becomes more prominent. For a delay of 0.6 ms and 0.39 ms, the amplitude of V_1 is reduced to 44.2 mV and 9.5 mV, respectively. Further decrease in Δt or earlier development of IPSP, results in a complete block of V_1. Similar dynamics are observed at the axo-somatic synapses but are not given here.

Assume that under normal conditions the stomach attains an anatomical and electrophysiological organization. Fine-tuning between the sympathetic and parasympathetic systems for the accommodation of a meal is required. Consider gastric response to feeding, i.e. an incremental increase in intragastric volume. The comparative analysis of electromechanical events during the dynamic process is carried out at representative points chosen in three areas of interest: the fundus, the corpus, and the antrum of the steer-horn, cascade, and fish-hook shape bioshells. Both qualitatively and quantitatively, results for the J-shape organ closely resemble those obtained for the fish-hook and are therefore not shown.

In the presence of ACh, the distension of the bioshell causes an increase in total forces from the baseline. There are configuration and region-dependent disparities in the stress–strain distribution. Thus, the fundus of the fish-hook shape stomach experiences maximal longitudinal tension, $T_l = 94$ mN cm^{-1}, whereas in the steer-horn organ, max $T_l = 62$ mN cm^{-1} is developed (figure 10.22). This pattern reverses

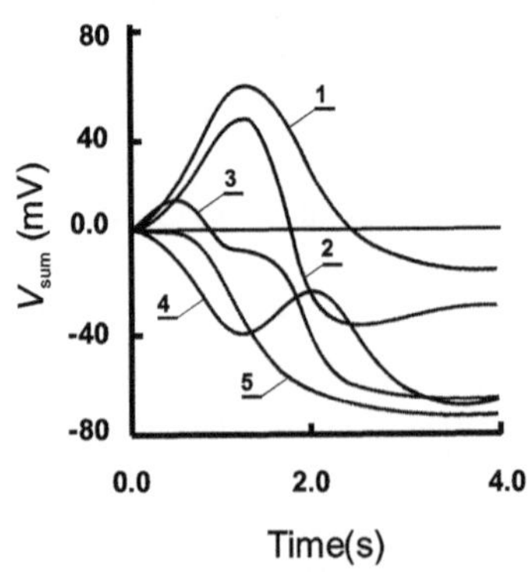

Figure 10.21. Resulting potentials at the axo-axonal synapse of the inhibitory circuit. 1: $\Delta t = 1.68$ ms; 2: $\Delta t =$ 0.6 ms; 3: $\Delta t = 0.39$ ms;. 4: $\Delta t = 0$ ms; 5: $\Delta t = -1.5$ ms. Reprinted from Miftahof R N 2017 *Biomechanics of the Human Stomach* (Berlin: Springer) by permission of Springer Nature. Copyright 2017.

in the body of the bioshells where max T_l = 115 and 95 mN cm^{-1} are recorded, respectively. In the case of the cascade stomach the intensity of T_l in the above regions attains intermediate values.

The strongest membrane forces are produced in the distal part of the stomach. The antrum of the steer-horn shape bioshell is maximally stressed, T_l = 155 mN cm^{-1}, and in the case of the cascade configuration the lowest level, T_l = 124 mN cm^{-1}, is recorded. In contrast, the fish-hook stomach appears equally stressed circumferentially

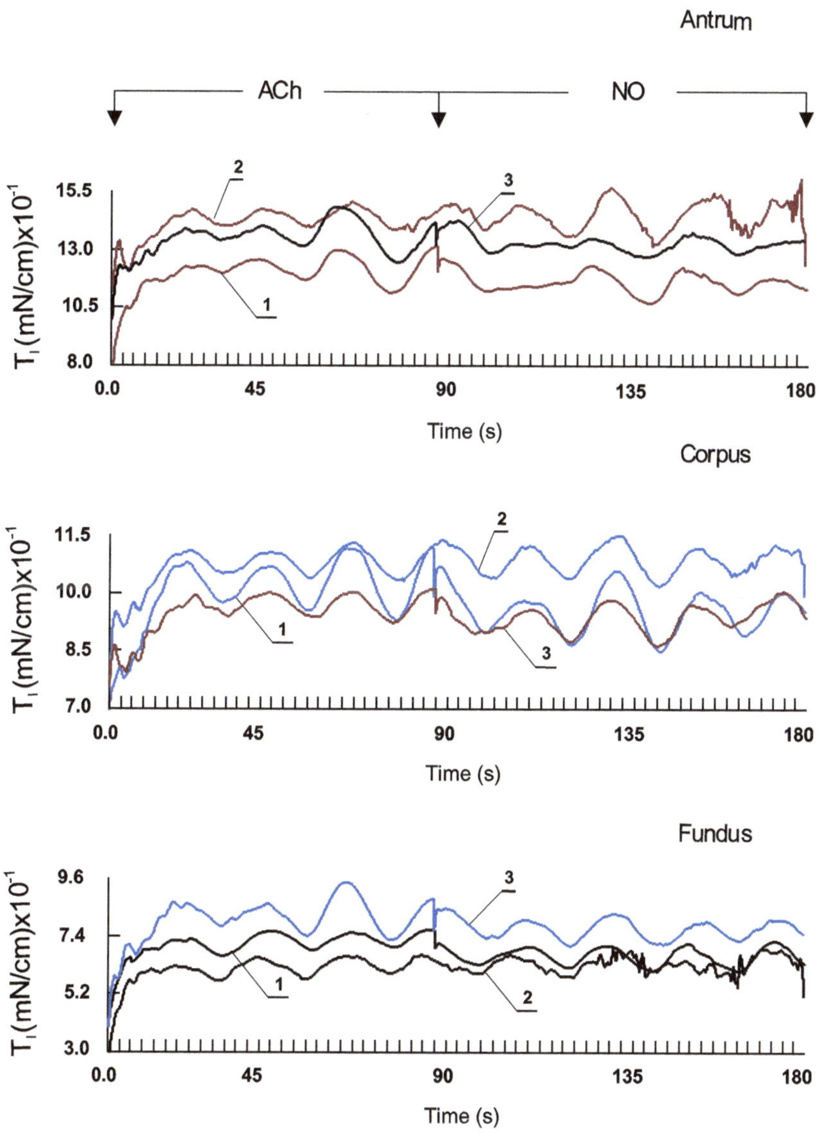

Figure 10.22. Changes in the total longitudinal force T_l in steer-horn (1), cascade (2), and fish-hook (3) shaped human stomachs during 'feeding'. Reprinted from Miftahof R N 2017 *Biomechanics of the Human Stomach* (Berlin: Springer) by permission of Springer Nature. Copyright 2017.

in the fundus and the corpus, T_c = 203.5, 215 mN cm^{-1}, respectively, with max T_c = 255 mN cm^{-1} observed in the antrum. A similar pattern of force distribution is observed in the steer-horn shape: T_c = 143 mN cm^{-1} in the fundus, 186 mN cm^{-1} in the body, and 219 mN cm^{-1} in the antral region (figure 10.23).

The firing of ICC–IM at their natural regional frequencies, the increase in gastric volume, the activation of mechanoreceptors, and the intraganglionic cholinergic signal transduction within the SIP/ganglion units initiate the contractile response in

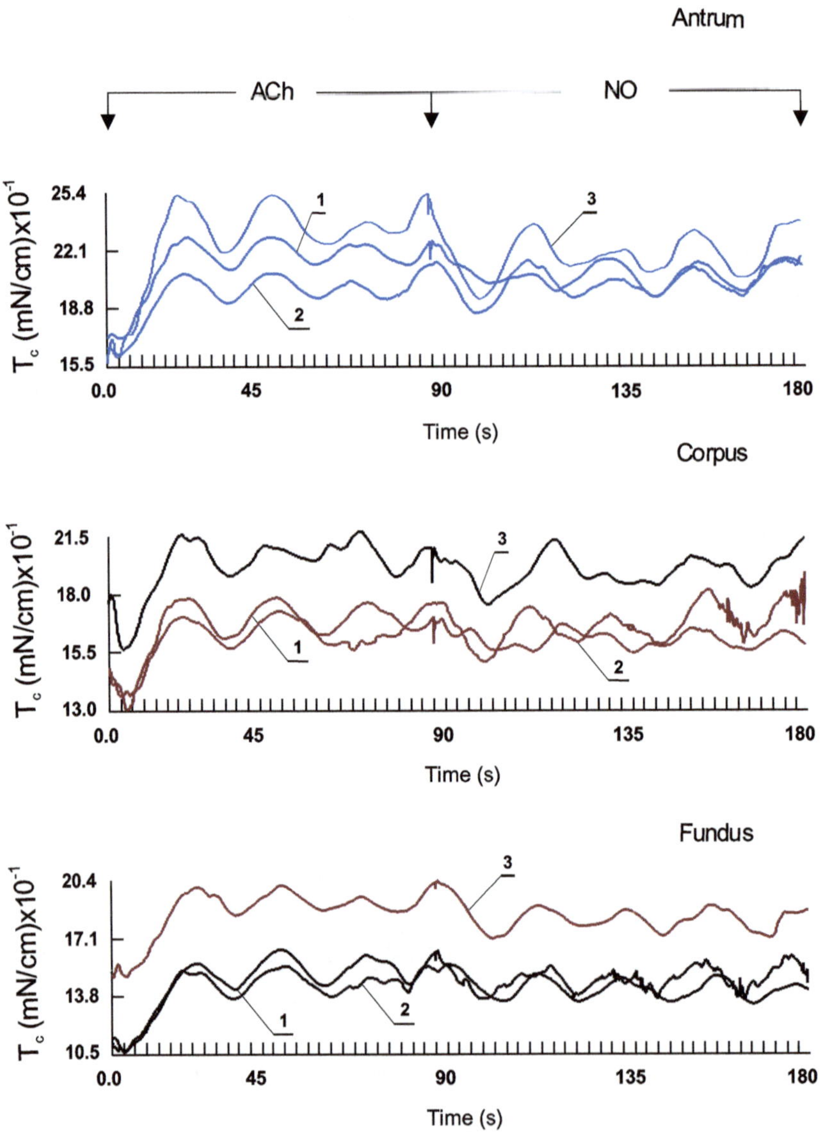

Figure 10.23. Changes in the total circumferential force T_c in steer-horn (1), cascade (2), and fish-hook (3) shaped human stomachs during 'feeding'. Reprinted from Miftahof R N 2017 *Biomechanics of the Human Stomach* (Berlin: Springer) by permission of Springer Nature. Copyright 2017.

the bioshell. Maximal active membrane forces are generated in the body and antrum of the steer-horn and fish-hook stomachs, T_l^a = 82.9 mN cm^{-1} and T_c^a = 106.5 mN cm^{-1}, but are significantly less in the fundus, T_l^a = 41.5 mN cm^{-1} and T_c^a = 52.8 mN cm^{-1}. The amplitude of contractions also varies across the organ from the smallest being recorded in the fundus, 8.5–11.8 mN cm^{-1}, to the greatest in the antrum, 19.6–35.3 mN cm^{-1}.

The dynamics of intragastric pressure reflects the combined effect of passive viscoelastic and active forces in the bioshell during an increase in $\breve{V}$. The baseline distending pressure for $\breve{V}$ = 650 ml varies between 25.8 kPa in the fish-hook, to 27.3 kPa in the cascade stomach. It undulates at an average amplitude of 7.3 kPa and frequencies which correspond to the oscillatory activity of SIPs (figure 10.24).

The elimination of the release of ACh at SIP–ganglia units and the application of NO directly to longitudinal and circumferential smooth muscle syncytia have a marked effect on gastric accommodation. There is a considerable reduction in the intensity of circumferential forces across all regions of the stomach: T_c = 192 mN cm^{-1} (fundus), 200 mN cm^{-1} (corpus), and 240 mN cm^{-1} (antrum) for the fish-hook and T_c = 137 mN cm^{-1} (fundus), 170 mN cm^{-1} (corpus), and 210 mN cm^{-1} (antrum) for the cascade shape organ. The gastric wall produces weak, low amplitude contractions ranging from 7–10 mN cm^{-1} in the distal to 20–26 mN cm^{-1} in the proximal parts. Notably, there are no discernable changes in the magnitude and dynamics of T_l. The circumferential smooth muscle layer is more responsive to relaxation by endogenous NO as compared to the longitudinal layer. This allows the organ to expand circumferentially rather than longitudinally as one might expect. As a result, there is a concomitant fall in intraluminal pressure against the initial distending pressure.

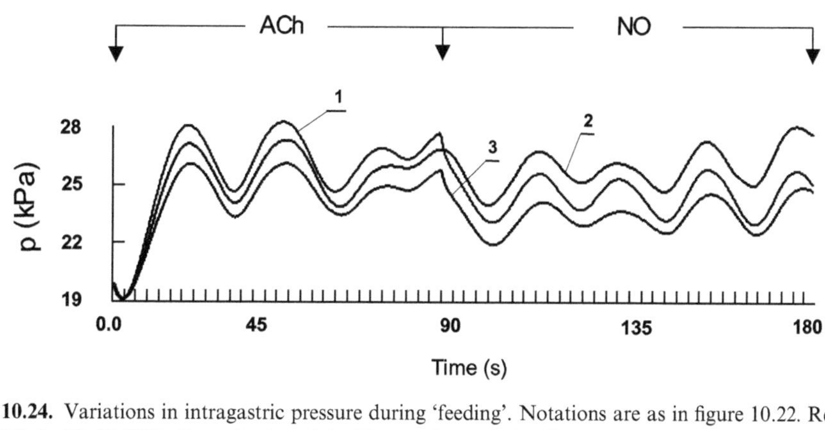

Figure 10.24. Variations in intragastric pressure during 'feeding'. Notations are as in figure 10.22. Reprinted from Miftahof R N 2017 *Biomechanics of the Human Stomach* (Berlin: Springer) by permission of Springer Nature. Copyright 2017.

10.9 The intrinsic regulatory system

10.9.1 The ICC/PDGFRα^+–MY(IM) network

Pacemaker activity and the subsequent production of slow waves in the human stomach can be offered by both ICC/PDGFRα^+–MY and IM plexi. These are non-homogenous and demonstrate subtle region-dependent morpho-functional differences including shape, distribution, and electrophysiological characteristics of ICC. The greatest number of cells are present in the fundus, 31.7 ± 1.8 (per area of 0.12 mm^2), with a lesser amount found in the corpus, 19.6 ± 1.8, and the antrum. Their density across the gastric wall is also uneven with the largest number of ICC located (i) in the submucous layer of the fundus, 8 ± 0.7, and the corpus, 4.1 ± 0.7, and (ii) along the myenteric border, 6.3 ± 0.5 (fundus) and 4.3 ± 0.6 (corpus). The cell distribution in the circular and longitudinal smooth muscles in the proximal part of the organ is relatively homogenous and varies from 3.4 to 6.1 per 0.12 mm^2. Cytological analyses reveal small fusiform bodies of ICC with two long slender processes and a few ramifications in the fundus. Larger cells with three or more processes and multiple thin ramifications rich in protrusions are found in the corpus and antrum. Interconnected via gap junctions (electrical synapses), they form a polygonal multi-dimensional network. The ICC of different regions have ascribed well-defined electrical properties, i.e. the amplitude of generated spikes is ~90–100 mV, their natural frequencies being 0.08–0.09 Hz (fundus), 0.09–0.1 Hz (corpus), and 0.12–0.13 Hz (antrum).

The nature of gap junctions along with a structural symmetry of connections are essential for reciprocal synchronization as well as a feed-forward propagation of excitation in the network. Discharging sporadically at random, regions weakly connected ICC generate nuclei of transient depolarizations of maximum amplitude 80 mV and duration ~0.5 s (figure 10.25). These make the signal transmission incoherent. The time- and cluster firing lock helps establish some degree of organization among cells, i.e. even weakly coupled neurons firing at their own frequencies when depolarized simultaneously start firing in near synchrony. These confluence to create spatio-temporal patterns of electrical activity of various intensities in the fundus, corpus, and antrum. Despite the synaptic symmetry, the excitation in the proximal and central part of the stomach propagates more efficiently longitudinally, and circumferentially in the antrum. In the body close to the lesser curvature, signals evolve into a target pattern which is, however, short-lived and thus cannot sustain signal transmission. The network becomes desynchronized with firing occurring at random locations.

The effect of synchronization and stabilization of firing activity in the network can be attributed to the presence of a dominant pacemaker (DP) which establishes and sustains the required strong connectivity among cells. In the human stomach, it is considered conventionally to be a group of specialized ICC found along the greater curvature in the corpus. Recent clinical evidence indicates the possible existence and occurrence of multiple pacemakers in different parts of the organ. At the time of writing, information on the origin and defining oscillatory properties of DPs was not available. Proposed mechanisms including group-cluster, voltage-

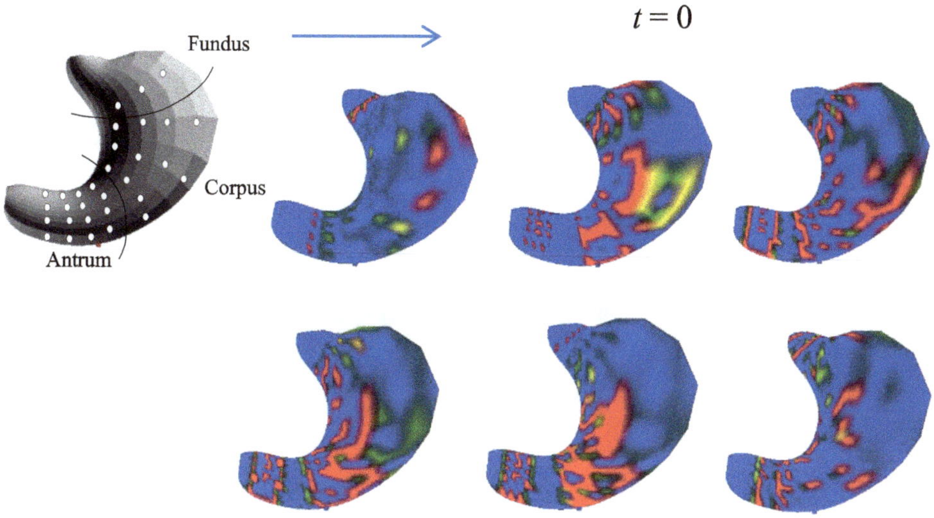

Figure 10.25. Self-synchronization of myoelectrical activity in the ICC/PDGFRα^+–MY(IM) (open circles) network. Reprinted from Miftahof R N 2017 *Biomechanics of the Human Stomach* (Berlin: Springer) by permission of Springer Nature. Copyright 2017.

dependent, and intracellular Ca^{2+} transients are speculative and do not support the essentials of observable dynamics.

Let the dominant pacemaker be in the corpus along the greater curvature of the stomach. Spontaneous signals of high amplitude, 100 mV, and frequency, 0.12 Hz, are produced which precede the time-scale of discharges of neighboring cells. Assume that a time- and frequency-lock condition is imposed on ICC of the fundus, corpus, and antrum, i.e. they oscillate harmoniously at their natural region-specific frequencies. The DP offers the pacing and coordinated spread of excitation across the network even when action potentials produced by a cell are of subthreshold levels. Simultaneous activity of ICC in the vicinity can result in an amplified potential that is above the required threshold.

There is less nucleation within the fundus where most of the body and the proximal part of the antrum form target patterns of electrical activity (figure 10.26). These sweep across the entire organ during the following 0.7 s. With the cessation of the DP, the network regains its original state with ICC discharging incoherently.

10.9.2 MP–ICC/PDGFRα^+–MY(IM) interactions

Immunolabeling, ultrastructural, *c-Kit* mutation, gene modulation, mechanical, and electrophysiological studies provide compelling evidence that the ICC/PDGFRα^+–MY(IM) plexus functions cooperatively with, and serves as, an intermediary for signal transduction between the myenteric nervous plexus and SIP syncytia in the stomach. The dynamics of the SIP–ganglion unit has been extensively studied in the previous chapter. Here the main focus is on analyzing synchronization of electrical activity between the two networks, the MP and ICC/PDGFRα^+–MY(IM). Despite similarities in architecture, they differ in (i) morphology (a homogeneous pool of

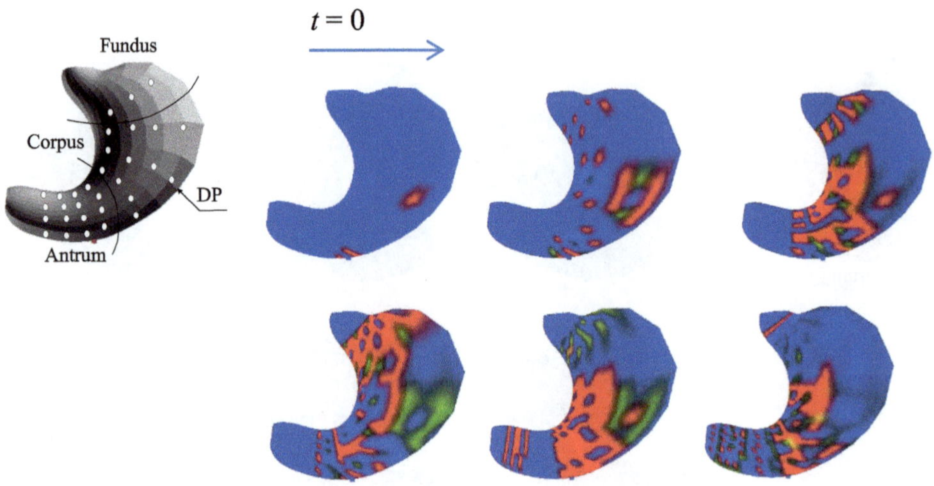

Figure 10.26. Synchronization of myoelectrical activity in the ICC/PDGFRα^+–MY(IM) network by the dominant pacemaker (DP). Reprinted from Miftahof R N 2017 *Biomechanics of the Human Stomach* (Berlin: Springer) by permission of Springer Nature. Copyright 2017.

identical cells versus various neurons), (ii) density (3583 ± 500 cells cm^{-2} versus 46 260 ± 3289 neurons/cm^2), (iii) functional unit (a single cell versus interconnected ganglia of 3–5 neurons), (iv) synapses (homotypic electrical, excitatory only versus chemical, both excitatory and inhibitory, with multiple neurotransmitters and polymodal receptors), (v) dynamic pattern (continuous self-oscillatory type versus organization of electromechanical processes into coherent physiological responses), and (vi) propagation (spatio-temporal synchronization of sporadically occurring nuclei of excitation versus quiescent, or wave of depolarization and/or hyper-polarization formation).

The myenteric plexus is non-uniformly distributed in a space between the longitudinal and circumferential smooth muscle layers of the stomach. It is sparse in the proximal and dense in the distal part of the organ. Neuronal ganglia are entwined through direct, bypass, divergent, convergent, and backward inhibitory dendro-somatic and axo-somatic synaptic connections in a rectangular two-dimensional neuronal network. Its cytoarchitectural mesh measures ~200–500 μm.

The MP and ICC/PDGFRα^+–MY(IM) plexi coupled together via synapse-like structures, form a large-scale dynamic system. Their exact nature, density, and distribution are not known. Two biologically feasible but mutually exclusive theories can be offered at this stage: a homogeneous even distribution versus a cluster-type arrangement. The former supports the notion of random occurrence whilst the latter favors the presence of morpho-functionally distinct areas of pacemaker activity. The duplicity is overcome due to excessive plasticity and adaptability, wherein the synapse-like structures ensure the leading role of the MP in producing not only the requisite signaling patterns but also a high degree of flexibility. The release of a balanced combination of neurotransmitters adds a large number of tuneable parameters to the system, e.g. the concentration of chemical substances and receptors, association and dissociation rates of chemical reactions, etc. This enables the desired modulations of intensity, shape, phase lags, and frequency of ICC discharges.

Assume there are two neurotransmitters, ACh and NA, involved in signal transduction dynamics within the MP. This rather restricted assumption is used as proof of concept only, but can be expanded to include other transmitters if and when required. Suppose that the generated fast excitatory and inhibitory postsynaptic potentials summate linearly on the somas of neurons, with the resultant potential triggering of spikes when a defined threshold value is exceeded. Otherwise, the neuron remains unexcited.

At rest, the MP remains quiescent while ICC demonstrate sporadic oscillatory activity. Multiple scattered nuclei of discharges are produced over the entire gastric surface. In the fundus and distal part of the corpus, cell clusters firing at nearly equal frequencies undergo self-synchronization.

Let mechanical stretch stimuli, $n = 5$, of intensity $\varepsilon(t) = 0.6L$, and a frequency of $\nu_m = 0.114$ Hz be applied at a single ganglion in the proximal part of the corpus along the greater curvature of the stomach. These generate regular action potentials at the free nerve endings that travel towards the sensory neuron and on further to the inter- and motor neurons. Dispersed interneuron axonal projections support the spread of excitation among myenteric ganglia (figure 10.27). The frequency of discharges by interneurons is irregular and depends on the intensity of synaptic activity, the release of neurotransmitters and binding to postsynaptic receptors. The detailed quantitative analysis of electrical and chemical processes involved has been given previously. Bursts of action potentials of amplitude 76.4 mV are produced. These form a wave of depolarization which propagates at a velocity of ~3.3 mm s^{-1} in a longitudinal and ~2.95 mm s^{-1} in a circumferential direction. Experimental

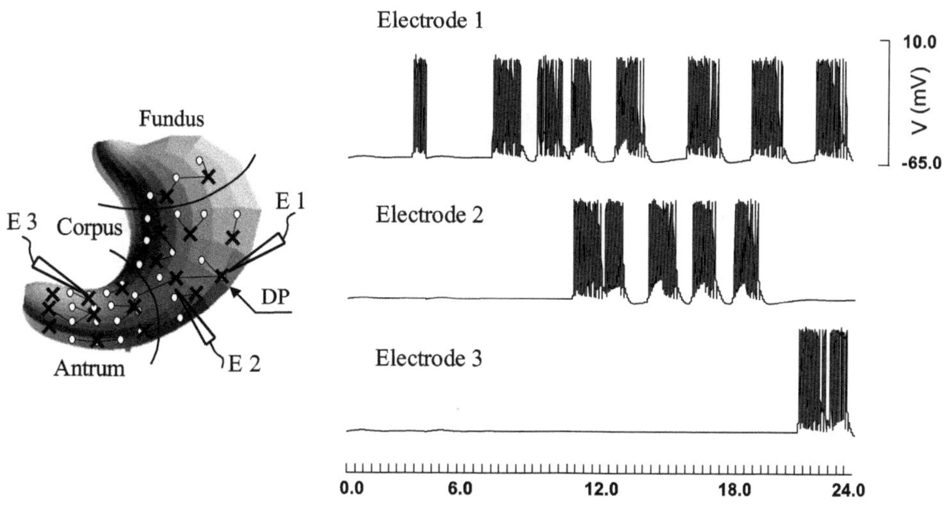

Figure 10.27. Myoelectrical activity in the MP–ICC/PDGFRα^+–MY(IM) network. Crosses refer to the myenteric nervous plexus ganglia; open circles represent ICC/PDGFRα^+–MY(IM). Reprinted from Miftahof R N 2017 *Biomechanics of the Human Stomach* (Berlin: Springer) by permission of Springer Nature. Copyright 2017.

measurements conducted on healthy volunteers using a novel noninvasive high resolution electrogastrogram give similar results.

The wave of excitation reorganizes and enhances the motor-neuron–synapse-like associations between the two networks at each ganglionic site. These provide an essential signaling input to realize time-, space-, and frequency-dependent firing synchronization of ICC. Strong connections are achieved in the cellular ensemble and a coherent traveling wave is successfully formed (figure 10.28). Over a period of subsequent neuronal stimulations, the global intercellular and oscillatory coupling in the ICC/PDGFRα^+–MY(IM) network is attained. With the cessation of neuronal activity in the MP, ICC/PDGFRα^+–MY(IM) become desynchronized and resume random oscillations.

10.9.3 Slow wave and electromechanical activity

The fundamental motor functions of the human stomach are closely related to electrical wave processes. A large repertoire of movements is a result of intricately regulated signal exchanges between the MP–ICC/PDGFRα^+–MY(IM) plexi (control system) and electromyogenic gastric smooth muscle syncytia. Intercellular structural arrangements and responsible transduction mechanisms remain controversial. There is compelling experimental evidence for and against the existence of gap junctions between ICC–MY and SMCs. In contrast, there is a strong consensus, supported by ultrastructural studies, that there is low resistance electrical connectivity between intramuscular ICC and SMCs. Based on close morphological

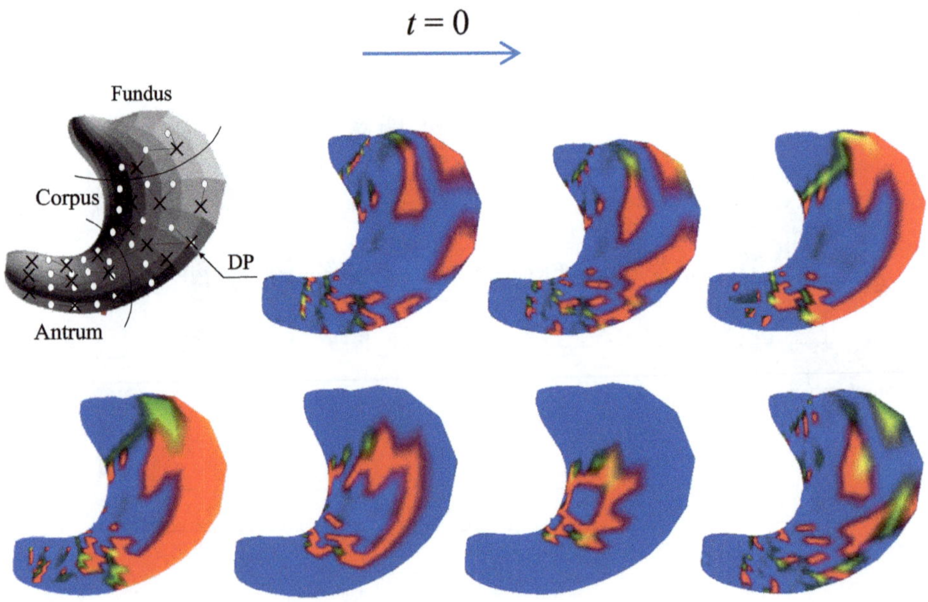

Figure 10.28. The spatio-temporal organization and propagation of myoelectrical patterns in the MP–ICC/PDGFRα^+–MY(IM) network. Notations are as in figure 10.27. Reprinted from Miftahof R N 2017 *Biomechanics of the Human Stomach* (Berlin: Springer) by permission of Springer Nature. Copyright 2017.

associations to motor neurons and the expression of multiple receptors for neurotransmitters, it is speculated that ICC–IM, along with myenteric motor neurons, function as mediators of neural inputs to smooth muscle.

Pacemaker signals from neuro-interstitial plexi are reflected as prolonged, low amplitude (slow wave) and short, high amplitude (spike) membrane potential changes of SMCs. Their highest frequency, as recorded during surgeries using flexible printed circuit board arrays from the serosa of the anterior wall of the body (corpus) of the intact human organ, is 0.06 Hz, whilst the lowest is 0.04 Hz, recorded in the antro-pyloric region. A more recent thorough investigation of slow wave dynamics in excised longitudinal and circular smooth muscle strips using intracellular microelectrodes has revealed the highest frequency in the antrum region, 0.12–0.13 Hz, an intermediate frequency in the corpus, 0.087–0.1 Hz, and the lowest in the fundus, 0.08–0.09 Hz. It is worth noting that, although slow waves are ubiquitous across the stomach, spikes are predominantly generated in the distal corpus, antrum, and pylorus.

Despite smooth muscle possessing well developed cell-to-cell connections through gap junctions, its passive membrane properties—the corresponding values of internal resistance, time, and length constants 125–300 Ω·cm, 100–250 ms, and 1.34 ± 0.21 mm, respectively—does not favor the propagation of slow waves. The process is orchestrated by the control system which guarantees stabilization and sustainability of slow wave dynamics.

Assume that at the initial moment of time, SM syncytia are in a stable state. The excitation from the MP–ICC/PDGFRα^+–MY(IM) plexi is conveyed to SMCs at the sites of their direct contacts defined by the topography of chemical and electrical synapses. These trigger the generation of slow waves ($0 < t < 37$ s) which undulate at characteristic frequencies of corresponding ICC–MY(IM). Simulated electromyogenic traces recorded from the circular smooth muscle layer in the fundus, proximal body, and antrum of the human stomach are shown in figure 10.29. For $50 < t < 60$ s, the propagating wave of electrical activity in the control system synchronizes in space and time SM membrane potential oscillations. The three areas under consideration become time-, phase-, and frequency-interlocked and produce, what appears to be, the front of a spreading slow wave (figure 10.30). Spikes occurring on the crests of slow waves are a result of cholinergic inputs from the myenteric motor neurons. The independent concurrent effect of the latter is through activation of muscarinic receptors on SMCs. In the absence of coordinative signaling, syncytia continue to be desynchronized for 22 s. With the next wave of excitation, $80 < t < 90$ s, strong connectivity is re-established and a new slow wave front is formed.

Slow waves, *per se*, induce mechanical responses in the fundus but not in the distal regions of the stomach where high amplitude action potentials are required. These activate voltage-dependent calcium channels on the smooth muscle membrane and cause a rapid influx of extracellular calcium inside cells. A rise in the free cytosolic calcium ion concentration triggers the cascade of intracellular reactions with the generation of active forces of contraction. These are concomitant in phase and time with Ca^{2+} oscillations. The active forces in the fundus and the body of the steer-horn type stomach are $T_l^a = 61.4$ mN cm^{-1} and $T_c^a = 74.3$ mN cm^{-1}. The cardia and the antrum–

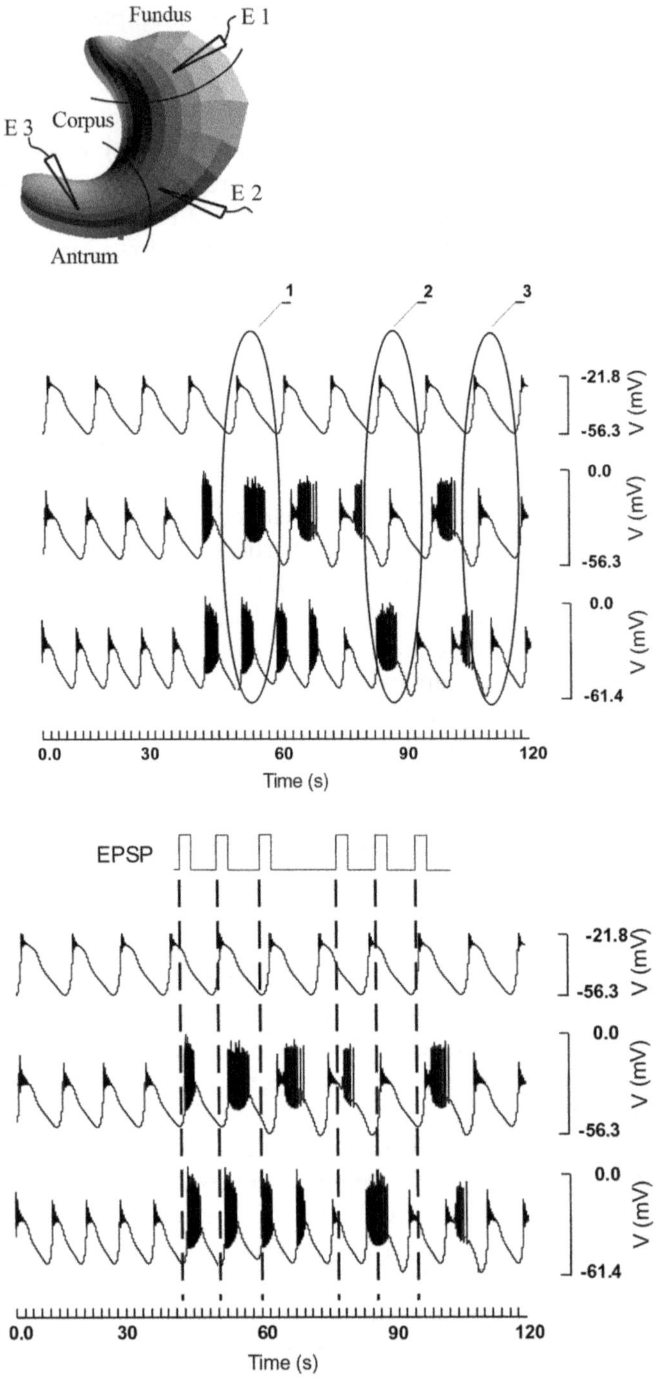

Figure 10.29. The proposed mechanism of slow wave organization in the human stomach. EPSPs represent cholinergic inputs from motor neurons. Reprinted from Miftahof R N 2017 *Biomechanics of the Human Stomach* (Berlin: Springer) by permission of Springer Nature. Copyright 2017.

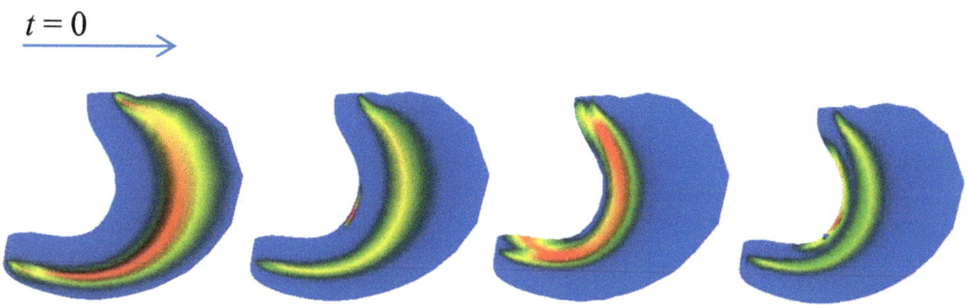

Figure 10.30. The spatial propagation of an organized slow wave. Reprinted from Miftahof R N 2017 *Biomechanics of the Human Stomach* (Berlin: Springer) by permission of Springer Nature. Copyright 2017.

pylorus experience fewer stresses T_l^a = 3.0–3.6 mN cm^{-1} and T_c^a = 3.7–4.4 mN cm^{-1}. The most intense contractions are produced by the longitudinal syncytium in the corpus, max T_l^a = 79.2 mN cm^{-1}. There is a small zone at the lesser curvature where max T_c^a = 105.3 mN cm^{-1}. The fundus undergoes uniform contractions in both smooth muscle layers: T_l^a = 69.1 mN cm^{-1}, T_c^a = 84.7 mN cm^{-1}.

Wrinkles that originate in the antrum–pylorus extend along the greater curvature to the distal part of the body of the organ. Uniaxial longitudinal stretching persists also in the cardia. Additionally, there are wrinkles along the longitudinal axis at the lesser curvature of the bioshell.

The pattern of total force distribution is similar to that reported earlier. Greater tension is consistent with the generation of active forces by muscle syncytia. Maxima T_l = 151 mN cm^{-1}, T_c = 224 mN cm^{-1} are recorded in the body, and max T_l = 27 mN cm^{-1}, max T_c = 53 mN cm^{-1} in the cardia and the pylorus of the stomach.

The stretching of ICC–IM and activation of mechanoreceptors of the primary sensory neurons, produce signals that are transferred to the control system to generate an inhibitory response. The effect is attained through the nitrergic and 'vipergic' neuro-modulatory mechanisms according to the dynamics discussed in the previous paragraphs.

Before closing the chapter, the reader is reminded that the considerations above rely on data obtained mainly from animal investigations. This information, if correct and applicable to the human stomach, could help in answering fundamental questions regarding the normal physiology of the pacemaker, the diversity of its behavior, its variability in frequencies, space-cyclic meandering, MP–ICC/PDGFRα^+–MY synchronization, and slow wave formation and propagation, amongst others.

Further reading

El-Sharkawy T Y, Morgan K G and Szurszewski J H 1978 *J. Physiol.* **279** 291–307

Gharibans A A, Kim S, Kunkel D C and Coleman T P 2017 *IEEE Trans. Biomed. Eng.* **64** 807–15

Knowles C H *et al* 2011 *Neurogastroent. Mot.* **23** 115–24

Mandić P, Filipović T, Gašić M, Djukić-Macut N, Filipović M and Bogosavljević I 2016 *Vojnosanitetski Pregled* 46–53

Metzger M 2010 *Arch. Ital. Biol.* 14873–83

Miftahof R N 2017 *Biomechanics of the Human Stomach* (Cham: Springer)
Miftahof R N and Nam H G 2010 *Mathematical Foundations and Biomechanics of the Digestive System* (Cambridge: Cambridge University Press)
Sanders K M, Koh S D, Ro S and Ward S M 2012 *Nat. Rev. Gastroent. Hep.* **9** 633–45
Sanders K M, Ward S M and Koh S D 2014 *Physiol. Rev.* **94** 859–907
Yun H-Y *et al* 2010 *Korean J. Physiol. Pharm.* **14** 317–24
Zhang R-X, Wang X Y, Chen D and Huizinga J D 2011 *Neurogastroent. Mot.* **23** e356–71

Chapter 11

The small intestine

The concept of the functional unit of the small intestine as a myoelectrically active soft cylindrical bioshell is introduced. The latter is employed to simulate various stereotypical motor patterns in the small intestine including pendular movements, segmentation, peristalsis, and self-sustained periodic activity, under physiological conditions and after pharmacological modulations.

11.1 Anatomical and physiological considerations

The small intestine is a long cylindrical tube that extends from the stomach to the caecum of the colon. The absolute length of the small bowel in general makes up between 80% and 90% of the entire length of the gut. In the abdomen most of the intestine is loosely suspended by the mesentery and is being looped upon itself. The diameter of the intestine is not constant but gradually decreases from the proximal to the distal part. For example, the diameter of the duodenum is 25–35 mm, the jejunum is ~30 mm, but the ileum it is 20–25 mm.

The intestinal wall is a biological composite formed of four layers: the mucosa, submucosa, muscular, and serosa. The mucosa is the innermost layer and its primary function is to digest and absorb nutrients.

The submucosa consists mainly of connective tissue and serves a purely mechanical function. Septa of connective tissue fibers carrying nerves, blood, and lymphatic vessels penetrate into the muscle layer to form a fibrillary three-dimensional network. This maintains the stable organization of the wall and allows the intestine to undergo reversible changes in length and diameter, offering remarkable properties of both stiffness and elasticity.

The muscle coat is made of two smooth muscle layers—a thick (inner) layer of circumferentially orientated smooth muscle cells, and a thin (outer) layer of longitudinally orientated muscle elements. The two layers are distinct and separate although there are intermediate bundles that pass from one layer to the other. The smooth muscle cells form planes and run orthogonal to one another. They form

doi:10.1088/2053-2563/ab1a9ech11

cell–stroma junctions that are of mechanical significance, i.e. equivocal stress–strain distribution during the reaction of contraction–relaxation. The thickness (h) of the muscle layers varies greatly between individuals and the anatomical part of the organ ($h \approx 0.5$–0.7 mm).

Serosa is composed of a thin sheet of epithelial cells and connective tissue.

Electromechanical processes in the small intestine have similar basic physiological principles to the stomach. However, the smooth muscle layers of the small intestine are electrically isolated. Therefore, it is to be expected that these organs have a few electrophysiological differences, e.g. the frequency of slow waves is higher in the small intestine, $\nu = 0.15$–0.2 Hz, when compared to the stomach, lasting ~2 s, with an amplitude that varies from 15 to 30 mV. The slow wave recorded from the small intestine has a sinusoidal configuration with a rapid depolarization and a slow repolarization phase. Their occurrence is essential for the development of contractions.

The variety of mechanical activity of the small intestine—pendular movements, segmentations, peristalsis—is regulated by intrinsic reflexes originating in the enteric nervous system. A basic neuroanatomical circuit is morphologically and functionally uniform and thus can be viewed as a functional unit. The minimum length of a functional unit in which a local contraction can be visualized and recorded is 1–2 cm. Structurally combined together and arranged by gating mechanisms, the functional units respond as an entity. Gating mechanisms are provided by the enteric nervous system which determine the distance, velocity, and intensity of propagation of electromechanical waves.

Contractile events in the fasting intestine reveal a three-phase stereotypic motor pattern repeated every 90 min. Phase 1 has spiking and motor quiescence, followed by a phase 2 with irregular spiking activity and intermittent contractions. The third and final phase of the cycle consists of high frequency action potential production and powerful regular contractions occurring at the frequency of slow waves. The cardinal element of the fasting motor complex is its migratory nature. The velocity of its propagation depends on the anatomical region of the intestine and the phase. Thus, in the duodenum the velocity is maximal during phase 3 (8.5 ± 2.4 cm s^{-1}), while in the ileum—the terminal part of the small intestine—it is only 4.0 ± 1.0 cm s^{-1}.

The role of pacemaker cells and intermediaries in signal transduction between the enteric nervous plexus and smooth muscle layers is played by ICC. The leading role in pacemaker activity belongs to the cells located in the enteric nervous plexus, ICC–MY. These discharge action potentials $V_i = 90-100$ mV with durations of 2–3 s. The ICC distributed throughout the circular and longitudinal smooth muscle layers also produce high amplitude, $V_i = 70-85$ mV, and short duration, 2–4 s, action potentials but at a lower frequency when compared to ICC–MY.

11.2 General model postulates

Anatomical and physiological data concerning the small intestine can be specified by the following modeling assumptions:

(i) The small intestine is a soft cylindrical shell formed of identical overlapping myogenic functional units (loci). Each locus is of a given length L, and radius r (figure 11.1).
(ii) The wall of the bioshell is composed of two smooth muscle layers embedded in the ECM network. The muscle fibers in the outer layers are orientated longitudinal to the anatomical axis of the locus, whilst in the inner layer they run in a circumferential direction.
(iii) Both muscle layers are electrogenic two-dimensional bisyncytia with cable electrical properties. The longitudinal layer has anisotropic, and the circular layer has isotropic electrical properties.
(iv) Self-oscillatory activity of syncytia, V_l, V_c, is a result of spatially distributed oscillators. The oscillators are divided into pools according to their natural frequencies.
(v) The slow wave and spiking activity of the functional unit represents the integrated function of voltage-dependent L- and T-type Ca^{2+}, potential sensitive K^+, Ca^{2+} activated K^+, and leak Cl^- ion channels.
(vi) The role of pacemaker cells belongs to ICC. Their discharges, V_i, generate the propagating excitatory waves in the longitudinal and circular muscle syncytia, V_l^s and V_c^s, while V_l^s, V_c^s modulate the permeability of L-type Ca^{2+} channels. The effect is mainly chronotropic with an increase in the time of opening of the channel.
(vii) Electromechanical coupling in the SM and the generation of forces of contraction–relaxation are a result of the evolution of the excitatory waves. Active forces of contraction, $T_{l,c}^a$, result from a multicascade process on the activation of the contractile protein system. Passive forces, $T_{l,c}^p$, are explained by the mechanics of viscoelastic connective tissue stroma formed from the collagen and elastin fibers arranged in a regular orthogonal net.
(viii) The bioshell is supported by intraluminal pressure p.

11.3 Investigations into intestinal smooth muscle

We shall start our analysis of biomechanical phenomena in the small intestine with a one-dimensional model of intestinal SM fiber. All considerations will be based on the approach previously developed for the stomach. Mathematically, the problem

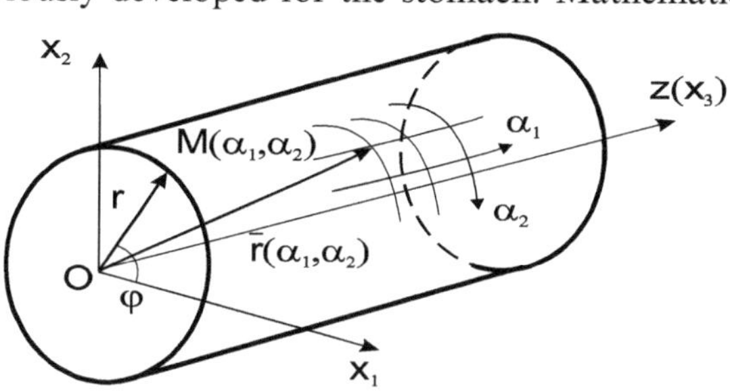

Figure 11.1. A segment of the small intestine as a soft biological shell. Reproduced from Miftahof R M and Nam H 2010 *Mathematical Foundations and Biomechanics of the Digestive System* (Cambridge: Cambridge University Press) with permission of the Licensor through PLSclear. Copyright R Miftahof and H Nam 2010.

leads to the governing system of equations that describe the electromechanical wave processes in the smooth muscle fiber, supplementary equations for the dynamics of ion currents, the propagation of the wave of depolarization within the fiber, and the dynamics of pacemaker activity, ICC–MY. The intestinal muscle fiber is initially in the resting state. It is excited by the discharge from ICC–MY. The ends of the fiber are clamped and remain unexcitable throughout.

11.3.1 Myoelectrical phenomena

Changes in the permeability of the T-type Ca^{2+} channels induce alterations in the dynamics of membrane potential oscillations (figure 11.2). At first, slow waves have a constant amplitude $V^s = 25$ mV and a frequency of 0.18 Hz. The depolarization phase lasts 1.6 s to be followed by a short plateau of duration 0.4 s, with a slow

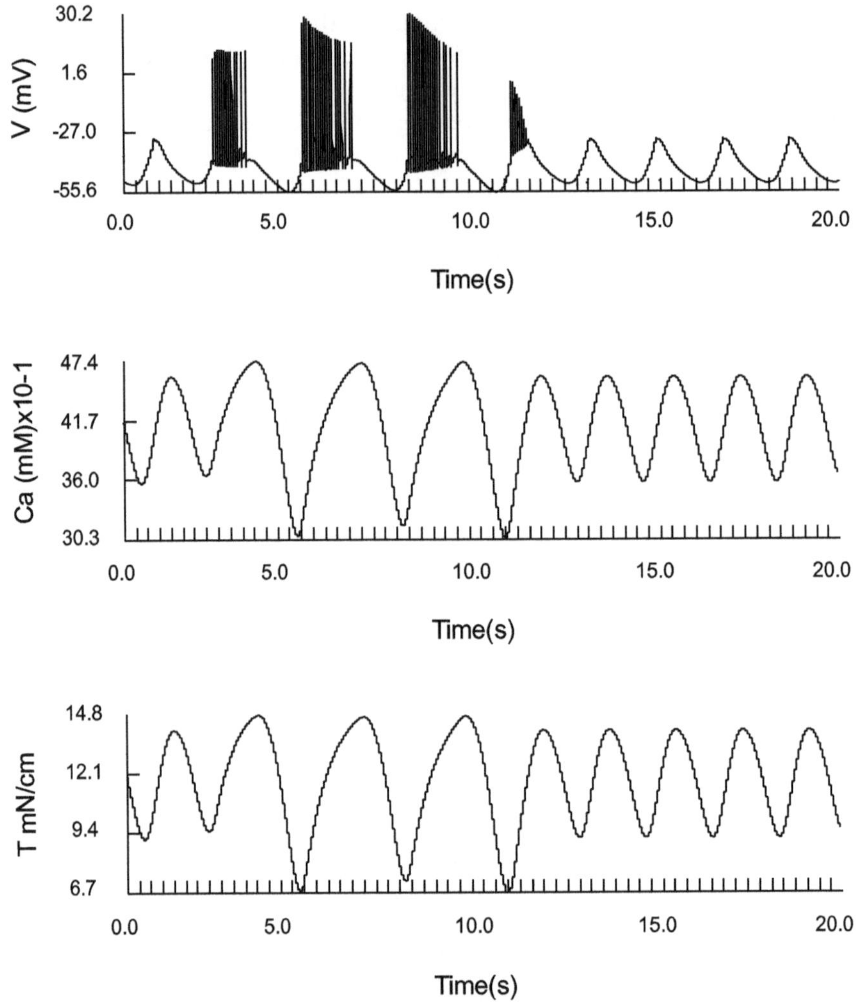

Figure 11.2. Myoelectrical activity in a normal intestinal smooth muscle 'fiber'. Reproduced from Miftahof R M and Nam H 2010 *Mathematical Foundations and Biomechanics of the Digestive System* (Cambridge: Cambridge University Press) with permission of the Licensor through PLSclear. Copyright R Miftahof and H Nam 2010.

decrease to a final resting value of $V_r^s = -51$ mV. The flux of Ca^{2+} ions (max[Ca^{2+}] = 0.49 μM) triggers regular rhythmic contractions of intensity, $T^a = 4.8$ mN cm^{-1}. The maximum total force generated by the muscle fiber is $T = 14$ mN cm^{-1}.

Over a period of time, the smooth muscle begins to fire action potentials $V^s = 56-72$ mV at a frequency $\simeq$17 Hz. The dynamics of Ca^{2+} ion influx coincides in phase with the depolarization process, i.e. the concentration of intracellular calcium rises concomitantly with the production of spikes. It achieves a max[Ca^{2+}] = 0.47 μM immediately after the firing ends. As a result, phasic contractions with a maximum total force $T = 15.1$ mN cm^{-1} are generated by the intestinal muscle fiber.

With a decrease in $\tilde{g}_{\mathrm{Ca}}^f \leqslant 0.65$ mSm cm^{-2}, the system transforms to irregular bursting mode and later reverts to a slow wave regime.

11.3.2 Effects of a non-selective Ca^{2+} channel agonist

Consider the effect of metoclopramide—a non-selective T- and L-type Ca^{2+} channel agonist—on the biomechanics of the intestinal fiber. The pharmacological action of the drug is simulated by a simultaneous increase in maximal conductances of $\tilde{g}_{\mathrm{Ca}}^s$ and $\tilde{g}_{\mathrm{Ca}}^f$. Application of the drug induces a beating type of myoelectrical activity (figure 11.3). High frequency, ~4 Hz, and amplitude, $V^s = 60$ mV, action potentials are produced.

The intracellular concentration of calcium ions attains 0.48–0.5 μM and remains constant. As a result, the smooth muscle fiber produces a tonic contraction of T = 15.6 mN cm^{-1}.

11.3.3 Effects of a Ca^{2+}–K^+ channel agonist

Consider the pharmacological effect of forskolin, a Ca^{2+}-activated K^+ channel agonist. Its effect in the model is achieved by varying the parameter $\tilde{g}_{\mathrm{Ca-K}}$. Results of simulations show that a gradual increase in the conductivity of Ca^{2+}-activated K^+-channels has a dose-dependent hyperpolarizing effect on the smooth muscle fiber. 'Low' concentrations of the drug reduce the resting membrane potential to $V_r^s = -62.5$ mV. 'High' concentrations of forskolin hyperpolarizes further the muscle membrane to $V_r^s = -67.6$ mV (figure 11.4). Forskolin abolishes slow wave electrical activity in the muscle fiber.

Conjoint application of ACh and forskolin fails to induce action potentials in the smooth muscle. There is a significant decrease in the concentration of free intracellular Ca^{2+} ions, max[Ca^{2+}] = 0.048–0.09 μM. As a result, the fiber remains hyperpolarized and mechanically inactive throughout.

A simultaneous treatment of the muscle fiber with forskolin and a concurrent increase in the concentration of extracellular potassium ions shows a strong depolarizing effect during which the membrane potential V^s rises to −21.5 mV. The depolarization leads to an influx of extracellular calcium and activation of the contractile proteins with the generation of the force of intensity $T = 16.4$ mN cm^{-1}. After the excess extracellular K^+ is removed, the fiber returns to the hyperpolarized state.

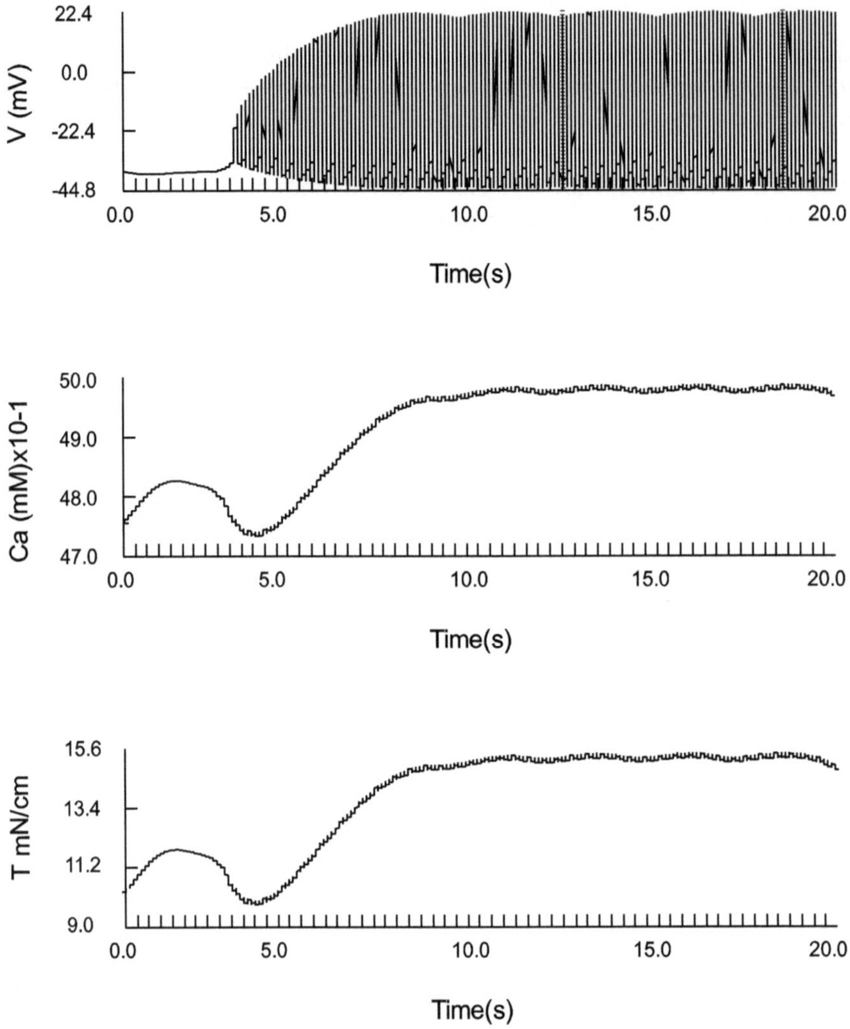

Figure 11.3. Effect of metoclopramide on electromechanical activity of the intestinal 'fiber'. Reproduced from Miftahof R M and Nam H 2010 *Mathematical Foundations and Biomechanics of the Digestive System* (Cambridge: Cambridge University Press) with permission of the Licensor through PLSclear. Copyright R Miftahof and H Nam 2010.

11.3.4 Effects of a selective K^+ channel agonist

Lemakalim is a selective K^+-channel agonist. The action of the drug in the model is achieved by varying the parameter $\tilde{g}_K$. Results show that an increase in conductivity of K^+-channels depolarizes the membrane, $V^s = -19.2$ mV, which remains at this level throughout (figure 11.5).

The dynamics of cytosolic Ca^{2+} changes and active force production corresponds to the dynamics of $V^s(t)$. Lemakalim abolishes phasic contractile activity in the fiber and tonic type contractions with $T = 17.2$ mN cm^{-1} generated instead.

The addition of lemakalim to muscle fiber pre-exposed to high extracellular potassium ion concentration causes its slight hyperpolarization. The concentration

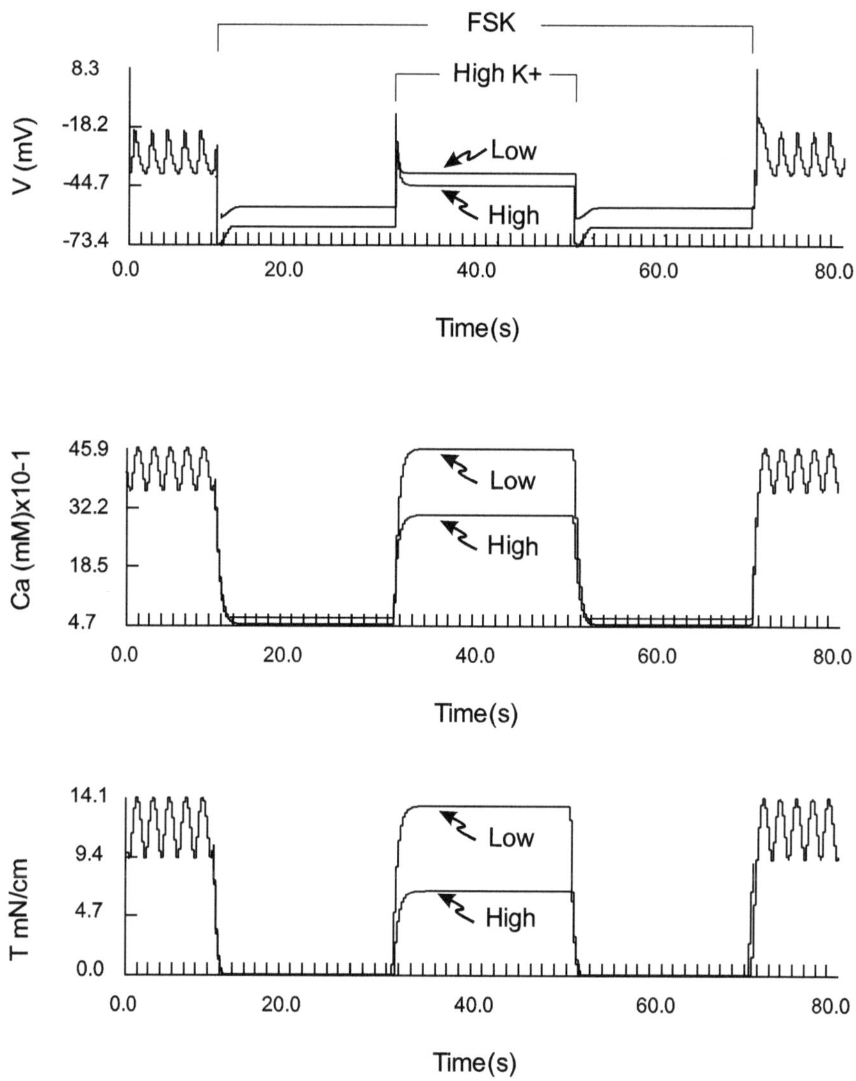

Figure 11.4. Effect of forskolin and changes in extracellular K^+ concentration on electromechanical responses of the intestinal muscle 'fiber'. Reproduced from Miftahof R M and Nam H 2010 *Mathematical Foundations and Biomechanics of the Digestive System* (Cambridge: Cambridge University Press) with permission of the Licensor through PLSclear. Copyright R Miftahof and H Nam 2010.

of free intracellular calcium and the magnitude of total force rise to 0.52 μM and 17 mN cm^{-1}, respectively.

The conjoint application of lemakalim and external ACh induces bursting in the intestinal muscle fiber. It generates high amplitude action potentials V^s = 68–72 mV of high frequency ν = 6–8 Hz. The subsequent introduction of forskolin hyperpolarizes the syncytium and abolishes its electromechanical activity.

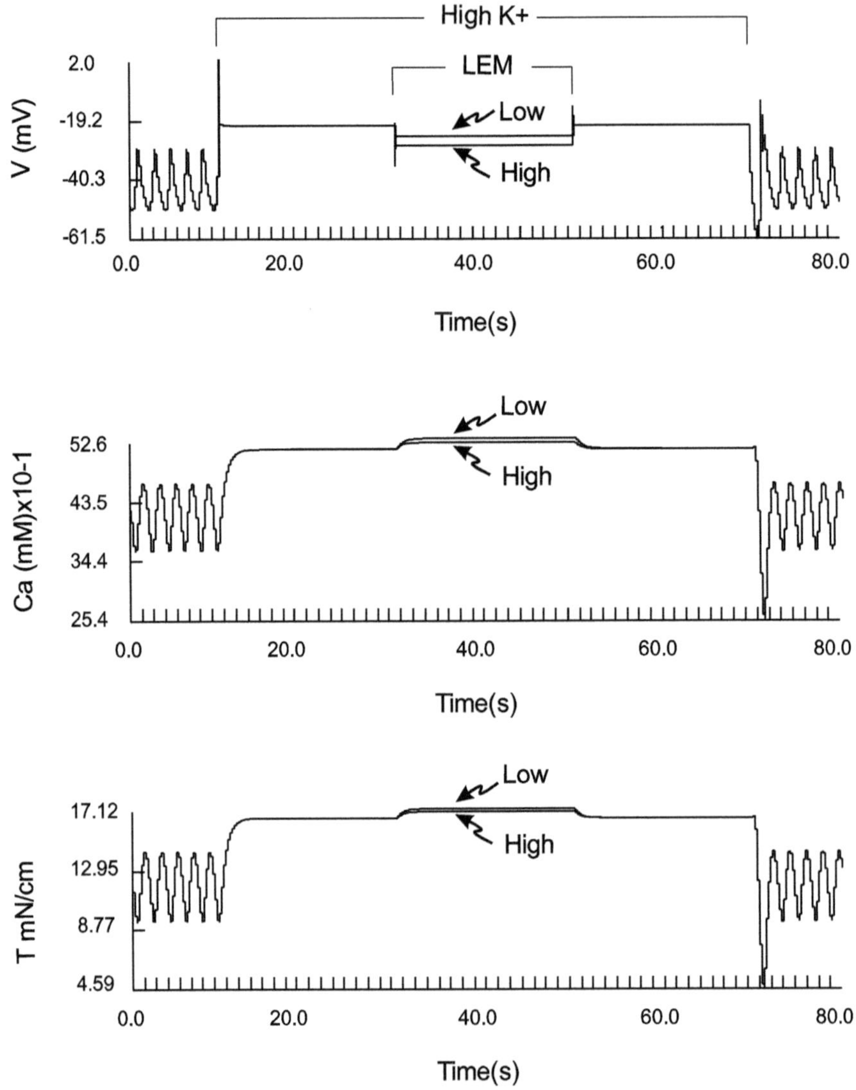

Figure 11.5. Dose-dependent effects of lemakalim and extracellular K^+ on the biomechanics of the intestinal smooth muscle 'fiber'. Reproduced from Miftahof R M and Nam H 2010 *Mathematical Foundations and Biomechanics of the Digestive System* (Cambridge: Cambridge University Press) with permission of the Licensor through PLSclear. Copyright R Miftahof and H Nam 2010.

11.3.5 Effect of a selective K^+ channel antagonist

Consider the pharmacological effects of phencyclidine—a selective K^+-channel antagonist—on the myoelectrical activity of the muscle fiber. The pharmacological effect of the compound in the model is simulated by setting $\tilde{g}_K = 0$. Phencyclidine abolishes slow waves and depolarizes the smooth muscle membrane, $V^s = -16.9$ mV. The depolarization process is accompanied by an increase in free intracellular Ca^{2+} (max$[Ca^{2+}] = 0.48\ \mu$M) and the development of a tonic contraction of intensity $T = 15.4$ mN cm^{-1}.

11.3.6 Effects of changes in Ca^{2+} and K^+ dynamics

Consider the conjoint effect of a high extracellular concentration of Ca^{2+} and K^+ ions, thapsigargin, a sarcoplasmic calcium storage inhibitor, and methoxyverapamil, a selective L-type Ca^{2+} channel antagonist, on the biomechanics of isolated intestinal smooth muscle fiber. Their actions are simulated by varying the parameters $\tilde{V}_{Ca}$, $\tilde{V}_K$, ρ, K_c, and $\tilde{g}^s_{Ca}$, respectively. Let the concentration of extracellular calcium be constantly elevated, $\tilde{V}_{Ca} = 150$ mV. An incremental increase in the concentration of external potassium, $[K^+]_0$ leads to stable depolarization of the muscle membrane. Slow waves and phasic contractions are abolished. The fiber undergoes a sustained tonic contraction, $T = 24.6$ mN cm^{-1} (figure 11.6).

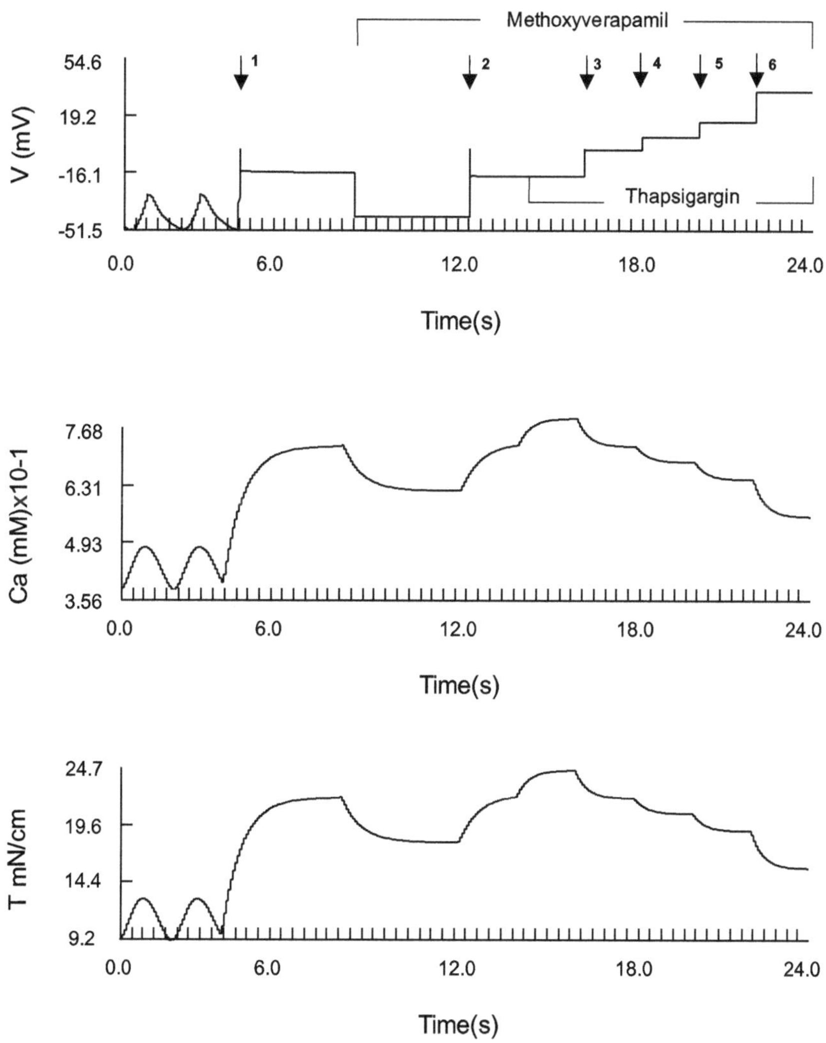

Figure 11.6. Myoelectrical activity of the intestinal wall in the presence of high $[Ca^{2+}]_0$ and $[K^+]_0$ ions, methoxyverapamil and thapsigargin. Reproduced from Miftahof R M and Nam H 2010 *Mathematical Foundations and Biomechanics of the Digestive System* (Cambridge: Cambridge University Press) with permission of the Licensor through PLSclear. Copyright R Miftahof and H Nam 2010.

Subsequent application of methoxyverapamil further hyperpolarizes the fiber, $V^s = -43.6$ mV. It also decreases the inward calcium current. As a result, there is a fall in $[Ca^{2+}] = 0.53$ μM and in the total force $T = 17.5$ mN cm^{-1}.

The addition of thapsigargin with a concurrent gradual increase in $[K^+]_0$ reverses the effect of methoxyverapamil. The muscle becomes depolarized. The level of depolarization depends on $[K^+]_0$. The total force dynamics are nonlinear and depend on the concentration of thapsigargin present. Thus, at 'low' concentrations of the compound there is an increase in intracellular calcium concentration, $[Ca^{2+}] = 0.76$ μM, and the intensity of contraction, $T = 24.7$ mN cm^{-1}. As the concentration of thapsigargin continues to rise, the concentration of Ca^{2+} begins to decline and the muscle fiber relaxes, min $T = 15$ mN cm^{-1}.

11.4 The intestine as a soft biological shell

The system of equations that describes the electromechanical processes in the bioshell, a segment of the small intestine, includes: the equations of motion of the soft cylindrical bioshell equation (5.102); equations (10.5)–(10.9) that describe the myoelectrical activity and the dynamics of ICC; equations (10.10)–(10.18) that model the process of propagation of the wave of excitation within electrically anisotropic longitudinal, and electrically isotropic circular smooth muscle syncytia; constitutive relations in the form equations (10.1), (10.2); initial and boundary conditions (in simulations it is always assumed that the ends of the bioshell are clamped and the right boundary remains electrically unexcitable throughout); and an additional equation that describes the dynamics of intraluminal pressure.

11.4.1 Pendular movements

Pendular movements of the small intestine are a result of electromechanical activity of the longitudinal muscle layer. The circular smooth muscle remains electrically and mechanically idle. Pendular movements are classified as local contractions and propagate over relatively short distances, 3–9 mm. Their physiological significance is to facilitate stirring and mixing of intestinal content.

Assume that the longitudinal muscle layer is excited by a single discharge of the pacemaker of amplitude $\overset{0}{V_i} = 100$ mV and duration 1.5 s. Immediately following excitation, a wave of depolarization, $V_l^s = 5$ mV, is generated. Its anterior front has the shape of an ellipse with the main axis oriented in the direction of electrical anisotropy (figure 11.7). The maximum amplitude $V_l^s = 68.2$ mV is seen in the vicinity of the left boundary of the unit. The wave V_l^s has a constant length of 0.5–0.55 cm and propagates along the smooth syncytium at a velocity of $\approx$2.5 cm s^{-1}. The eccentricity of the wave profile is sustained throughout the dynamics process. As the wave V_l^s reaches the right boundary, it splits into two waves that propagate circumferentially. A short unsustainable increase in amplitude to 78.8 mV is observed in the zone where the two fronts interact.

As a result of excitation, a short-term relaxation is produced by the syncytium. A mechanical wave of amplitude $T_l^p = 11.7$ mN cm^{-1} and length 0.4–0.5 cm is recorded (figure 11.8). As it propagates along the surface of the bioshell, its

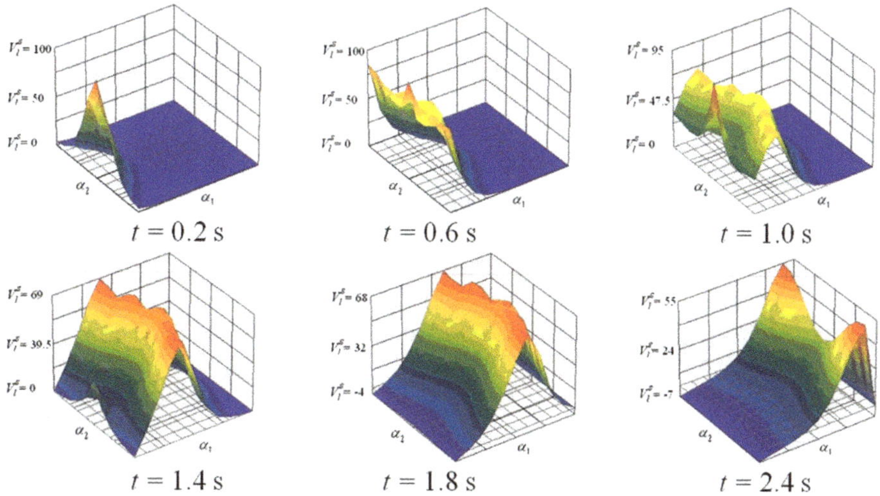

Figure 11.7. Propagation of the mechanical wave V_l^s within the longitudinal smooth muscle syncytium of the bioshell (intestine). Reproduced from Miftahof R M and Nam H 2010 *Mathematical Foundations and Biomechanics of the Digestive System* (Cambridge: Cambridge University Press) with permission of the Licensor through PLSclear. Copyright R Miftahof and H Nam 2010.

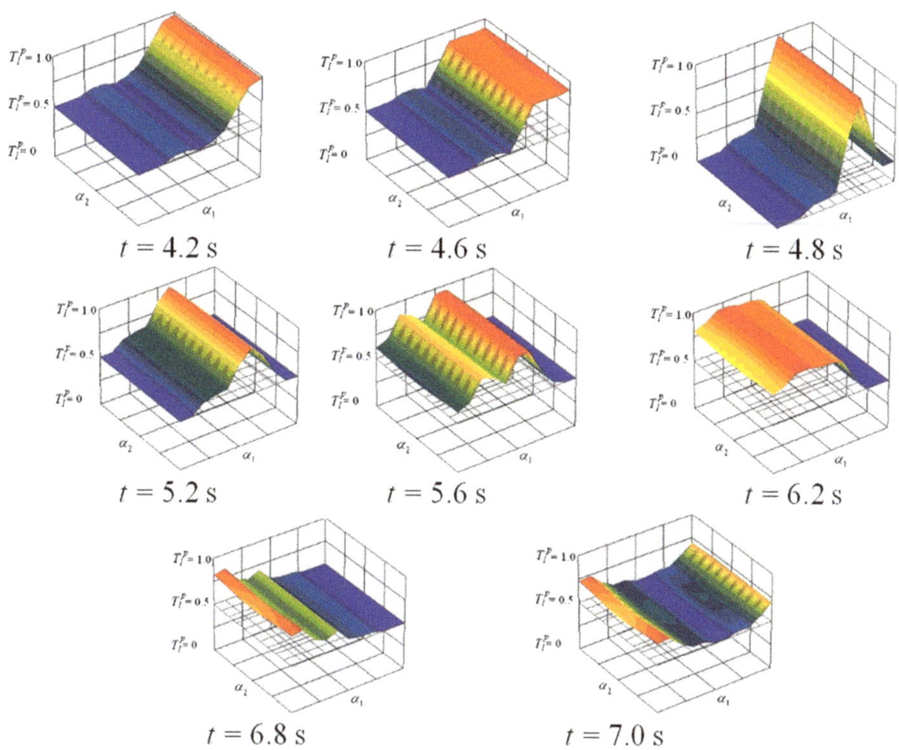

Figure 11.8. Propagation of the mechanical wave T_l^p in the bioshell during pendular movements. Reproduced from Miftahof R M and Nam H 2010 *Mathematical Foundations and Biomechanics of the Digestive System* (Cambridge: Cambridge University Press) with permission of the Licensor through PLSclear. Copyright R Miftahof and H Nam 2010.

amplitude decreases to 5.5 mN cm^{-1}. The bioshell experiences a biaxial stress-stretched state with max $T_l^p = 7.6$ mN cm^{-1} at the distal end. There is a slight increase in amplitude to 8.4 mN cm^{-1} following the reflection of the wave T_l^p from the right boundary.

The propagation of this reflected wave T_l^p is blocked by the developing contraction with the amplitude of the wave $T_l^a = 14.8$ mN cm^{-1} propagating at a constant velocity of 2.5 cm s^{-1}. Initial phasic contractions are followed by tonic contractions of amplitude $T_l^a = 10.5$ mN cm^{-1}. More than half of the bioshell undergoes a biaxial stress-stretched state with max $T_l^a = 10.2$ mN cm^{-1} (figure 11.9).

The dynamics of the total force T_l coincides with the dynamics of the electrical wave V_l^s. The initial concentric circular wave T_l has an amplitude of 16.2 mN cm^{-1} (figure 11.10) and propagates at a velocity of 2.4 cm s^{-1}. It achieves a maximum value of $T_l = 19.1$ mN cm^{-1}. The central region of the intestinal segment experiences a prolonged depolarization. With repolarization of the muscle syncytium the bioshell returns to the initial undeformed state.

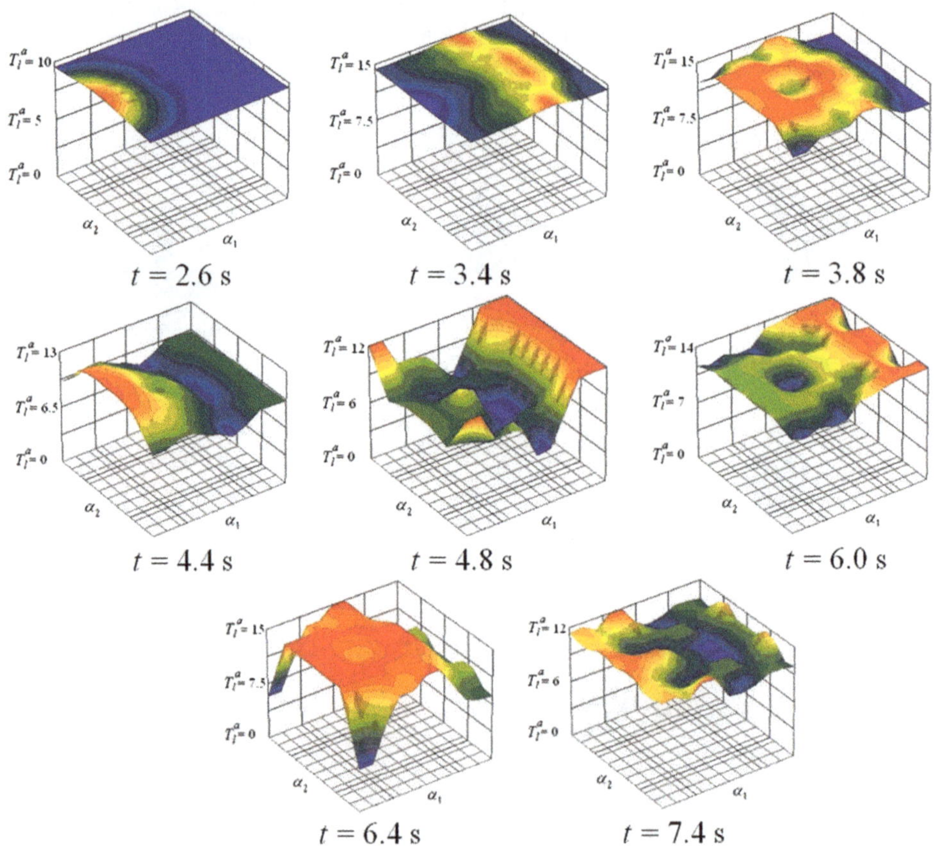

Figure 11.9. Dynamics of the wave T_l^a in the bioshell. Reproduced from Miftahof R M and Nam H 2010 *Mathematical Foundations and Biomechanics of the Digestive System* (Cambridge: Cambridge University Press) with permission of the Licensor through PLSclear. Copyright R Miftahof and H Nam 2010.

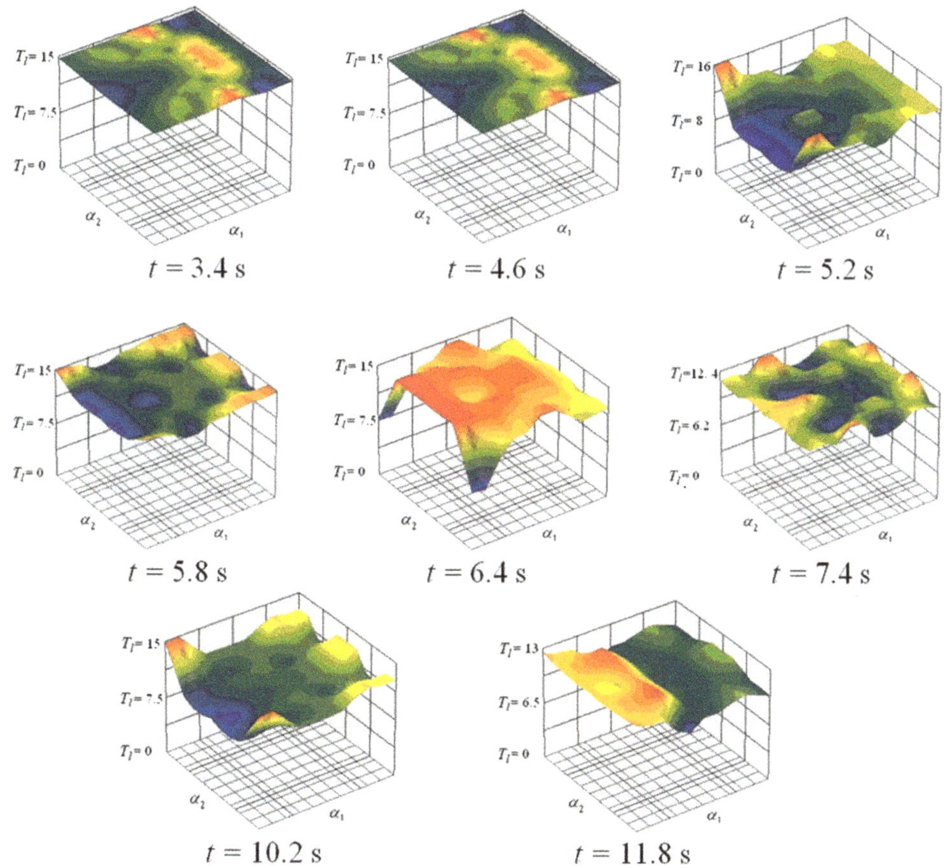

Figure 11.10. Total force T_l dynamics during pendular movements. Reproduced from Miftahof R M and Nam H 2010 *Mathematical Foundations and Biomechanics of the Digestive System* (Cambridge: Cambridge University Press) with permission of the Licensor through PLSclear. Copyright R Miftahof and H Nam 2010.

11.4.2 Segmentation

Segmentations of the small intestine are a result of electromechanical activity of the circular muscle layer only. These contractions are normally focal and non-propagating. However, there are experimental data indicating the possibility of their aboral propagation.

Assume that the circular muscle syncytium is excited by the discharge from pacemaker of amplitude V_i = 100 mV and duration 1.5 s. The syncytium responds with the generation of a wave of depolarization, V_c^s = 62–72 mV, that propagates at a velocity of 1.9–2.0 cm s^{-1} along the bioshell. Its anterior front takes the shape of a circle (figure 11.11). As in the case of pendular movements, an unsustainable increase in amplitude of V_c^s to 82 mV is observed in the vicinity of the right boundary. This is the result of interaction between the waves V_c^s as they propagate towards each other in a circumferential direction. Owing to a slower conduction

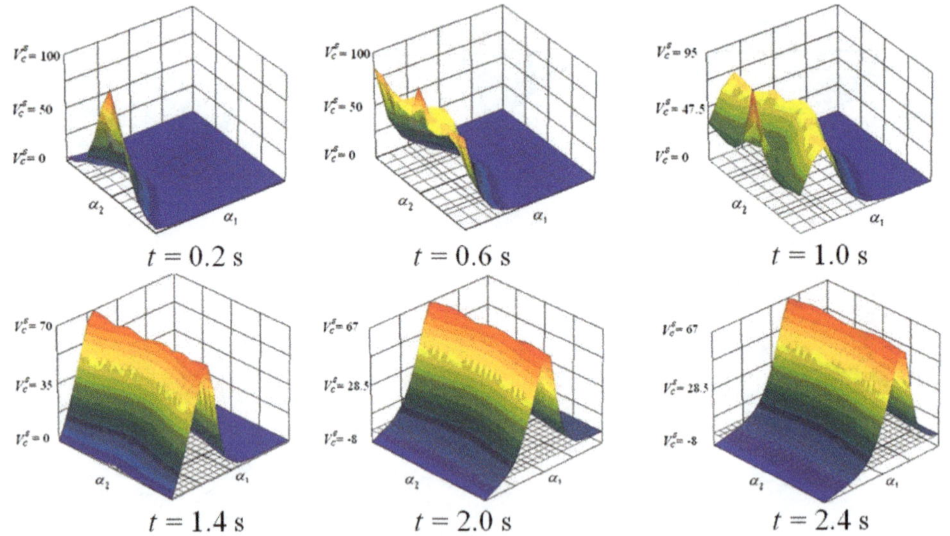

Figure 11.11. Propagation of the wave of depolarization V_c^s within the circular smooth muscle syncytium. Reproduced from Miftahof R M and Nam H 2010 *Mathematical Foundations and Biomechanics of the Digestive System* (Cambridge: Cambridge University Press) with permission of the Licensor through PLSclear. Copyright R Miftahof and H Nam 2010.

velocity, the circular muscle syncytium experiences depolarization for a longer period when compared to the longitudinal muscle layer.

The wave of the active forces of contraction T_c^a = 12.2 mN cm^{-1} is produced propagating at a velocity of 1.8–1.9 cm s^{-1} (figure 11.12). With the development of a tonic contraction, more than half of the bioshell experiences a uniform biaxial stretching with max T_c^a = 18.6 mN cm^{-1}.

The wave T_c of amplitude 28–32 mN cm^{-1} propagates in the aboral direction at a velocity of 0.5 cm s^{-1} (figure 11.13). The wave T_c maintains a constant length of 0.6 cm. As the wave reaches the right boundary, the wave T_c^p reflects from the boundary and begins to propagate backwards. However, it is stopped by the contraction of the muscle syncytium and the wave T_c^a = 17.8 mN cm^{-1}.

Changes in configurations of the bioshell show asymmetry during the first (phasic) stage of segmental contractions. Only with the development of tonic contractions is the symmetry in deformation of the proximal part of the bioshell observable.

11.4.3 Peristalsis

Reciprocal relations between the longitudinal and circular smooth muscle layers are essential in the development of peristalsis. The first contraction normally starts in the longitudinal syncytium. When the total force in the layer reaches a maximum, an activation of the circular muscle layer begins. This coincides with simultaneous relaxation of the longitudinal layer and *vice versa*.

Let two identical pacemaker cells be located at the longitudinal and circular smooth muscle syncytia. These discharge electrical impulses of amplitude V_i = 100 mV

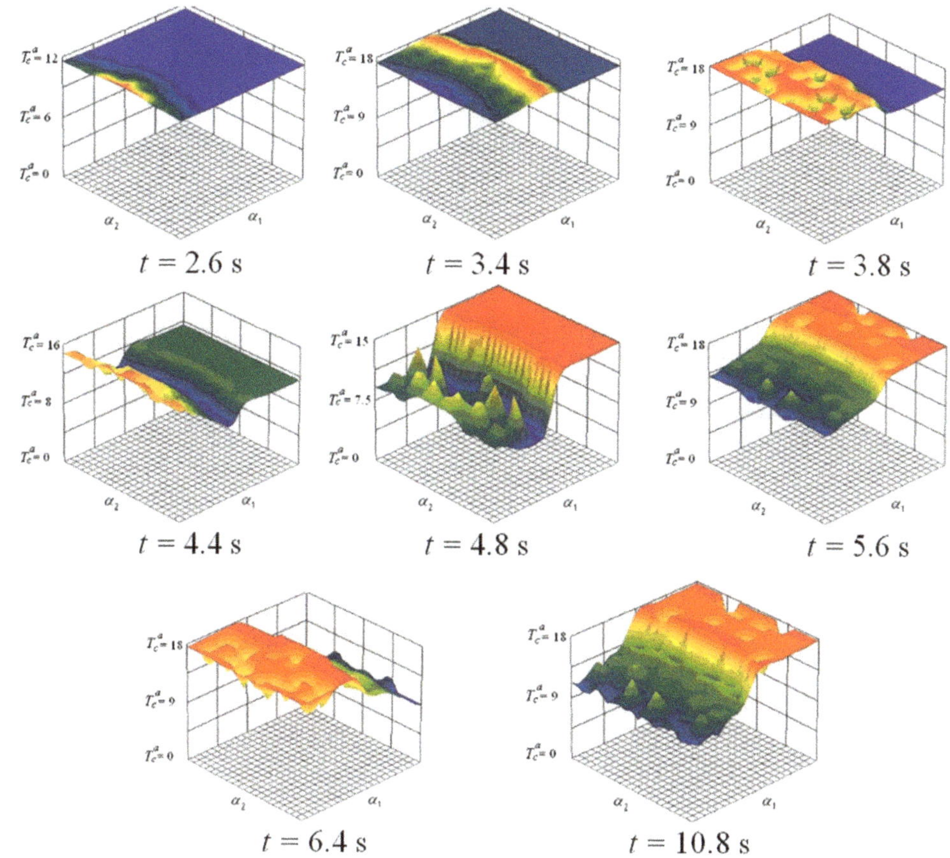

Figure 11.12. Dynamics of the wave T_c^a in the bioshell. Reproduced from Miftahof R M and Nam H 2010 *Mathematical Foundations and Biomechanics of the Digestive System* (Cambridge: Cambridge University Press) with permission of the Licensor through PLSclear. Copyright R Miftahof and H Nam 2010.

and duration 1.5 s. The time lag between discharges is specified by the dynamics of the total force, T_l, development. The discharge of the pacemaker cell on the outer muscle layer of the bioshell initiates the excitatory wave of depolarization $V_l^s = 69$ mV. The characteristics of the wave V_l^s and the induced mechanical wave T_l, i.e. their dynamics, are similar to those described above. Once the maximum force of contraction is achieved, the ICC–MY discharges action potentials on the circular muscle syncytium to generate an electromechanical wave in the circular smooth muscle syncytium. The pattern of movements of the wall along with the force dynamics resemble processes observed during pendular movements and segmentation (figure 11.14).

11.4.4 Self-sustained periodic activity

The frequency in discharges of ICC–MY and the electrical properties of the intestinal wall play a dominant role in the development of self-sustained periodic myoelectrical activity in the intestine.

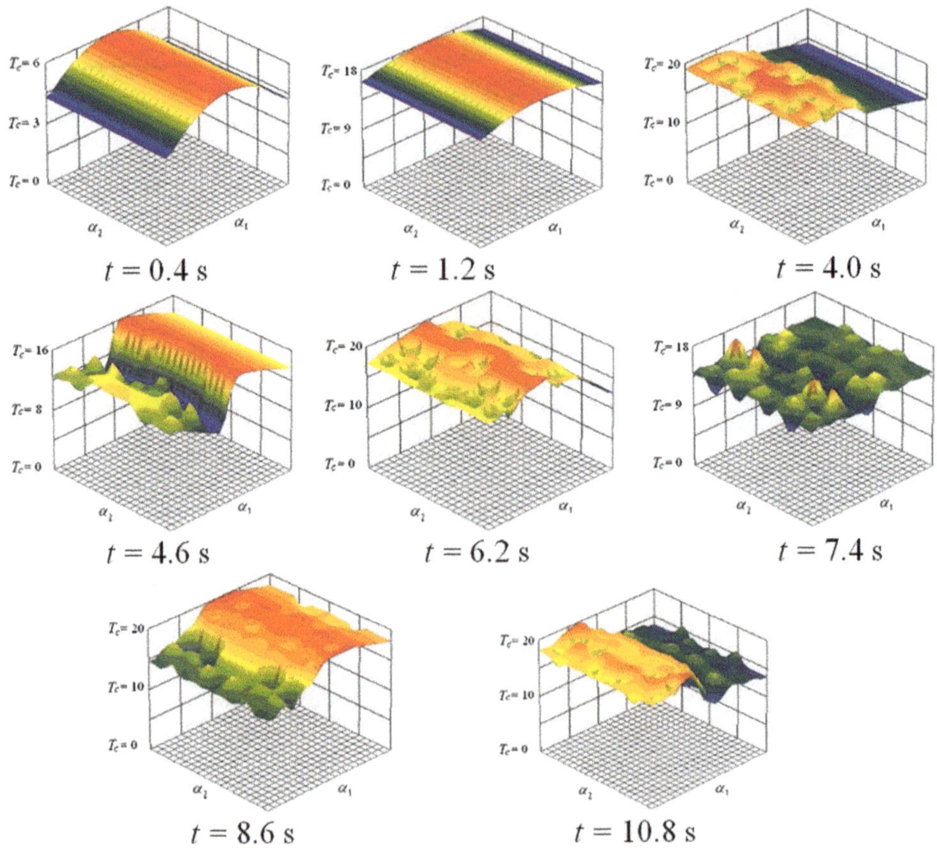

Figure 11.13. Total force T_c dynamics during segmental contractions. Reproduced from Miftahof R M and Nam H 2010 *Mathematical Foundations and Biomechanics of the Digestive System* (Cambridge: Cambridge University Press) with permission of the Licensor through PLSclear. Copyright R Miftahof and H Nam 2010.

Let the frequency of firing be $\nu = 0.16$ Hz. Following discharges of the longitudinal and circular smooth muscle syncytia, the bioshell produces peristaltic movements as described above. At $t = 13.3$ s of the dynamic process, the middle part of the bioshell experiences the biaxial stress-stretch state, $\lambda_l = 1.35$, $\lambda_c = 1.42$. Stretching of the syncytia causes an increase in membrane resistance resulting in a reduction in the maximum amplitude of depolarization waves, $V_l^s \approx V_c^s \approx 55.7$ mV.

This has a detrimental effect on the connectivity among myogenic oscillators in that region and on the dynamics of the propagation of succeeding waves V_l^s. These split into two separate waves in the 'affected' part (figure 11.15). As the two separate waves reach the right boundary of the bioshell, their tails collide with the generation of a new solitary wave $V_l^s = 70.8$ mV. This is strong enough to self-sustain its propagation backwards, i.e. from the electrically unexcitable right boundary towards the left boundary. As the reflected wave reaches the distended part of the bioshell it splits into two separate waves thus producing a spiral wave of amplitude 65 mV which continues to circulate over the surface of the intestinal segment. The spiral waves provide strong connections among the spatially distributed myogenic

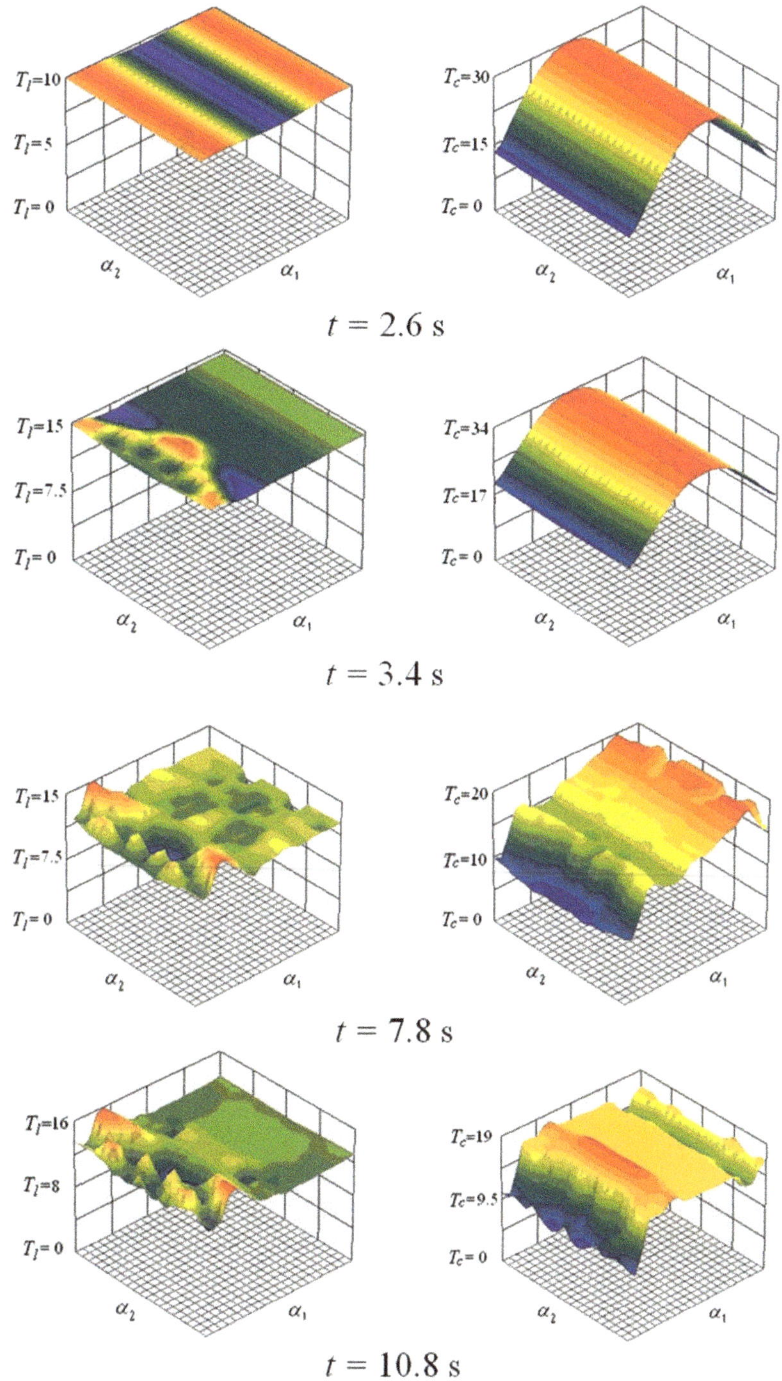

Figure 11.14. Total force T_l and T_c distributions in the bioshell during peristalsis. Reproduced from Miftahof R M and Nam H 2010 *Mathematical Foundations and Biomechanics of the Digestive System* (Cambridge: Cambridge University Press) with permission of the Licensor through PLSclear. Copyright R Miftahof and H Nam 2010.

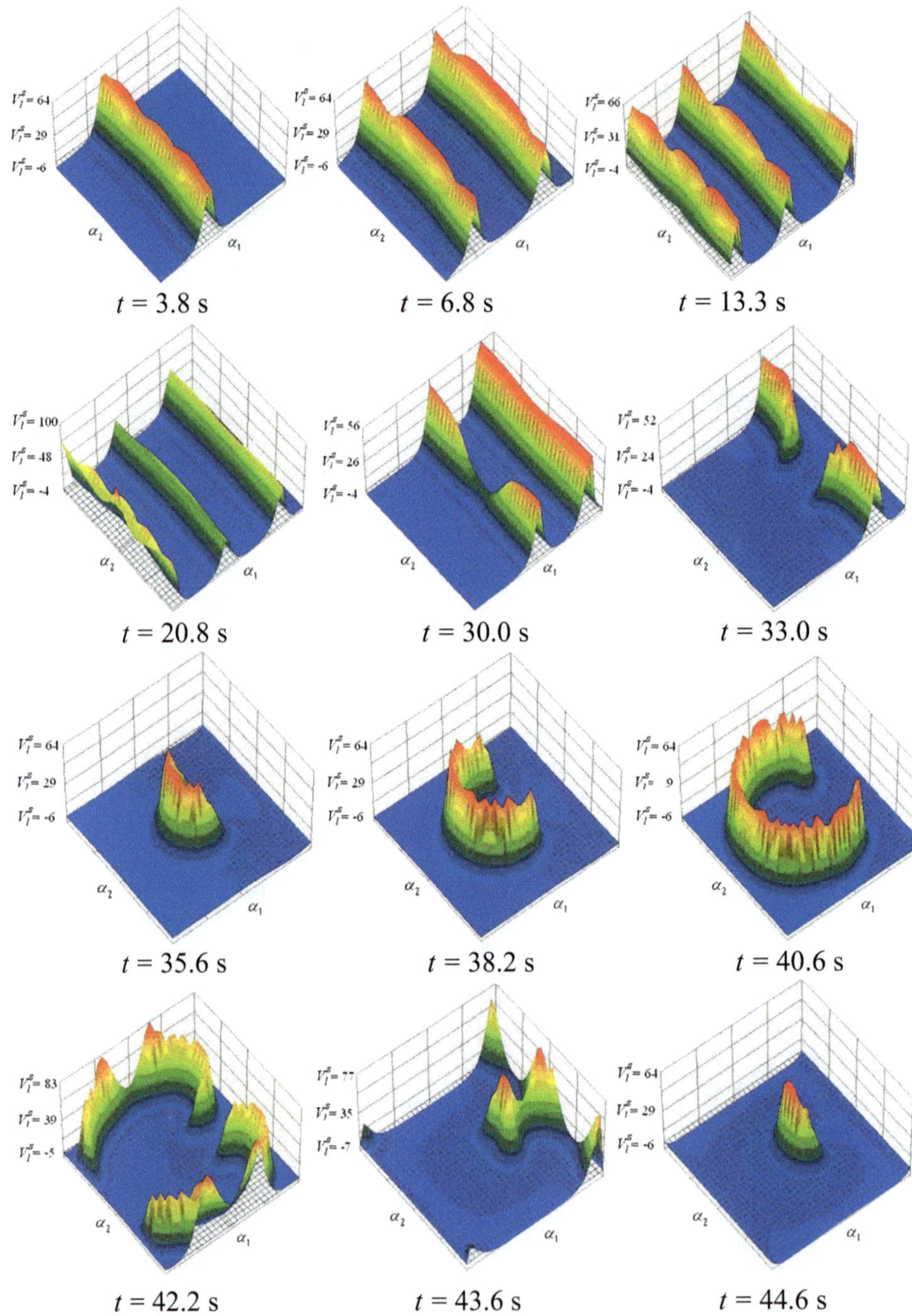

Figure 11.15. Dynamics of self-sustained myoelectrical activity and spiral wave formation in the longitudinal smooth muscle syncytium. Reproduced from Miftahof R M and Nam H 2010 *Mathematical Foundations and Biomechanics of the Digestive System* (Cambridge: Cambridge University Press) with permission of the Licensor through PLSclear. Copyright R Miftahof and H Nam 2010.

oscillators and, therefore, support mechanical wave activity in the longitudinal syncytium.

The self-sustained spiral wave phenomenon is produced only by the electrically anisotropic longitudinal smooth muscle syncytium. It can never be simulated by the electrically isotropic circular smooth muscle syncytium. Waves V_c^s propagate without disruption along the surface of the bioshell and afterwards vanish at the right boundary.

11.5 Pharmacology of intestinal motility

11.5.1 Effect of lidocaine

The spiral wave phenomenon, as described above, could be a physiological mechanism of intestinal dysrhythmia—a medical condition associated with the altered motility of the small intestine. In an attempt to abort the spiral wave formation and to restore the system to normal, consider the effect of lidocaine, a drug that blocks both fast sodium-dependent action potentials and voltage-dependent, non-inactivating Na^+ conductance. Its pharmacological action in the model is achieved by decreasing the maximal conductance $\tilde{g}_{Na}$. At 'high' concentrations lidocaine abolishes spiral waves and mechanical activity in the bioshell with the intestinal segment returning to a resting state.

Although lidocaine 'successfully reversed' dysrhythmia in the model, its clinical application is limited because of its narrow therapeutic index and possible high-dose induced cardiotoxicity.

Further reading

Du P, Paskaranandavadivel N, Timothy R, Angeli T R, Cheng L K and O'Grady G 2016 *Wiley Interdiscip. Rev. Syst. Biol. Med.* **8** 69–85

Miftahof R N, Nam H G and Wingate D L 2009 *Mathematical Modeling and Simulation in Enteric Neurobiology* (Singapore: World Scientific)

Sokolis D P 2017 *J. Mech. Behav. Biomed. Mater.* **74** 93–105

Tadakada Y (ed) 2009 *Textbook of Gastroenterology* (Hoboken, NJ: Blackwell)

Chapter 12

The large intestine (colon)

This chapter presents a mathematical model of a segment of the large intestine (colon) with an enclosed solid non-deformable pellet. The model is used to reproduce haustral churning, peristalsis, and propulsive movements of the pellet under physiological conditions and after application of Lotronex® and Zelnorm®.

12.1 Anatomical and physiological considerations

The human large intestine (colon) is a visceral organ that lies with loops and flexures in varying configurations around the abdomen. The length of the organ is 125–154 cm and its diameter is approximately 4.5 cm. Functionally the colon is divided into two parts, the right and left colon. The right colon extends from the caecum and ascending colon to the mid transverse colon, and the left colon from the mid transverse colon through the descending colon and sigmoid to the rectum.

The wall of the organ consists of four layers—the mucosa, submucosa, circular and longitudinal muscle layers, and serosa. The wall thickness of the large intestine is relatively constant, $h \approx 0.4$–0.5 mm. Cells lining the mucosa and submucosa resemble those found in the small intestine. However, they contain a significantly greater numbers of goblet cells. These secrete viscous mucus into the lumen and thus moisturize and lubricate the passage of the waste. The layers play a major role in the digestion and absorption of food, water, and electrolytes. It is the absorption of fluids and bacterial processing that transforms the intraluminal effluent into solid stool.

The longitudinal muscle is organized in three bands—teniae coli. These run from the caecum to the rectum where they fuse together to form a uniform outer muscular layer. The circular muscle layer is homogenous and uniformly covers the entire colon.

The serosa is composed of a thin sheet of epithelial cells and connective tissue.

The innervation of the colon is a complex interaction between the enteric nervous and autonomic nervous system. The cell bodies of neurons in the enteric nervous

doi:10.1088/2053-2563/ab1a9ech12

system are organized into spatially distributed ganglia with inter-connecting fiber tracts. They form the submucosal and myenteric plexi that contain local neural reflex circuits which modulate multiple functions of the organ. The autonomic nervous system is comprised of sensory, motor, sympathetic, and parasympathetic nerves. Autonomic nerves modulate the intramural enteric neural circuits and provide neural reflexes at the higher organizational levels including the autonomic ganglia, spinal cord, and brain.

Although it is generally accepted that colon movements are regulated by ICC, the exact mechanisms of coordinated motility are not known. A subpopulation of cells distributed along the submucosal border of the circular smooth muscle layer, the ICC–IM is responsible for myoelectrical activity of the large intestine and plays a key role in its pacemaker activity.

Five types of motor patterns are observed in the organ: (i) haustral churning, (ii) peristalsis, (iii) propulsive movements, (iv) defecation reflex, and (v) cooperative abdominal effort. Haustral churning is a combined simultaneous shallow contraction of the longitudinal and circular smooth muscles. Its significance is to stir up the liquid intraluminal content as fluids are extracted until the stool is formed. The contractions propagate over short distances upstream and downstream from their point of origin. The coordinated reciprocal electromechanical activity of the muscle layers is known as peristalsis. This gently moves the soft content along through the right colon to the rectum from where it is evacuated. A modified type of peristalsis is propulsive movement. This is characterized by extensive clustered contractions of the colon separated by short dilated regions and *en masse* propulsion of the fecal material. Defecation reflex and cooperative abdominal effort represent the final stage in the expulsion of stools from the rectum.

The molecular and electrophysiological processes underlying colonic functions are similar to those described in the stomach and small intestine. The migrating motor complex is a fundamental motility phenomenon and is tightly controlled by the enteric reflex pathways. Evoked by chemical or mechanical stimulation of intrinsic primary afferent neurons, its blockade with tetrodotoxin abolishes all types of myoelectrical activity. In contrast, stimulation of nicotinic ganglionic and muscarinic receptors with ACh along with SP and 5-HT induces rapid excitatory responses. The major inhibitory neurotransmitter is assumed to be NO. In the case of a congenital absence of NO containing neurons, the colon fails to relax and remains constricted at all times.

The migrating motor complexes have patterns typical of periodic oscillatory activity. Phases of rapid contractions and action potential production are separated by periods of quiescence. The patterns are reproduced in all parts of the colon at a constant frequency. However, their duration and amplitude vary significantly along the length of the organ. The longest complexes of the highest amplitude are recorded in the right colon, $\approx$3–4 min, and the shortest of small amplitude in the left colon, $\approx$0.7–1.2 min. The high amplitude action potentials are produced in the caecum and the ascending part of the colon whilst the lowest are in the recto-sigmoid region. It is worth noting that migrating motor complexes are intimately related to the dynamics of pressure waves produced in the intraluminal content.

A common condition associated with altered motility of the colon is constipation. The underlying mechanisms are poorly understood and may vary between different groups of patients. Some cases result from systemic diseases, others from abnormalities within the colonic wall itself. Transit through different regions of the large bowel can be measured using a variety of techniques including colonic scintigraphy, magnetic resonance imaging, radio-labeled markers (pellets), and video mapping. The plastic or metallic pellets used usually take the shape of a sphere or ellipsoid. Reported physiological transit times are 7–24 h for the right colon, 9–30 h for the left colon, and 12–44 h for the recto-sigmoid. Although the methods allow scientists to appreciate gross variations in motility patterns, they do not offer: (i) the desired resolution to establish the relationship between spatiotemporal distribution of migrating motor complexes or (ii) sufficient depth of accessibility to a combined analysis of the system's intricate mechanisms of function.

Over the last decade considerable effort has been directed towards investigating peristaltic propulsion of mainly Newtonian and non-Newtonian fluids in the intestine. There are large numbers of original publications and excellent reviews on the subject which the reader should consult for details. In contrast, the research into the propulsion of solids and biologically active chyme is very limited. In their pioneering work, Bertuzzi *et al* (1983), formulated a mathematical model to study the dynamics of non-deformable bolus propulsion in a viscoelastic tube—a segment of the small bowel. Working under severe biological naïveté and the limiting assumption of axial symmetric deformation, they reproduced the propagation of a ring-like electromechanical wave to simulate *en masse* movement of a solid sphere and to calculate the average velocity of transit. Recently Miftahof *et al* studied the general physiological principles of peristaltic transport of a solid bolus in a segment of the gut. The authors analyzed the dynamics of propulsion as the result of electromechanical wave dynamics in the smooth muscle syncytia and explored the motion of the bolus both under normal physiological conditions and after the application of drugs that affect peristaltic activity of the organ.

12.2 The colon as a soft biological shell

A segment of the large intestine can be viewed as a hollow muscular tube—a bioshell of length L, and radius $R(\alpha_1, \alpha_2)$, where α_1, α_2 are the orthogonal curvilinear coordinates on the undeformed surface of the bioshell (figure 12.1).

Let the bioshell contain a solid non-deformable sphere of radius R_{sp} = const. Based on the anatomical and physiological characteristics of the large intestine assume that:

(i) The tissue possesses the property of nonlinear viscoelastic orthotropy (no reliable experimental data on the uniaxial and biaxial mechanical characteristics of either the animal or human colon currently exist so the modeling assumptions are based on a comparative histomorphological and biomechanical analysis of the small and large intestine).

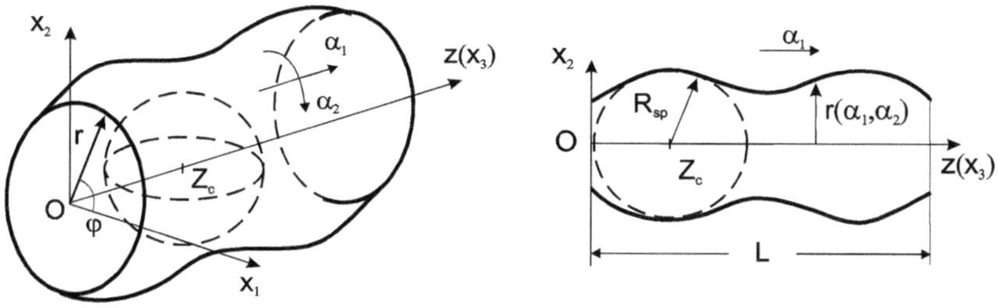

Figure 12.1. A segment of the colon as a soft biological shell. Reproduced from Miftahof R M and Nam H 2010 *Mathematical Foundations and Biomechanics of the Digestive System* (Cambridge: Cambridge University Press) with permission of the Licensor through PLSclear. Copyright R Miftahof and H Nam 2010.

(ii) The teniae coli and circular smooth muscle layer are excitable syncytia, the teniae have anisotropic properties and the circular layer has isotropic electrical properties.
(iii) The role of pacemaker cells belongs to the subpopulation of interstitial ICC–IM. They discharge action potentials V_i at a known frequency, amplitude, and duration.
(iv) The generation and propagation of the waves of depolarization, V_l^s, V_c^s, along the syncytia are a result of the integrated function of voltage-dependent L- and T-type Ca^{2+}, potential sensitive K^+, Ca^{2+} activated K^+, and leak Cl^- ion channels. The waves V_l^s, V_c^s modulate the permeability of L-type Ca^{2+} channels on the smooth muscle membrane.
(v) On the activation of intracellular contractile proteins, multicascade processes lead to the production of active forces, $T_{l,c}^a$. Passive forces, $T_{l,c}^p$, are the result of the deformation of the viscoelastic ECM stroma.
(vi) The bioshell contains a solid spherical pellet supported by intraluminal pressure p. The pellet is subjected to dry and viscous friction. The contact forces act at the perpendicular to the surface of the pellet.

Mathematical formulation of the problem of peristaltic propulsion of a solid non-deformable sphere by a segment of the colon includes: the equations of motion of the soft myoelectrically active bioshell (5.102), (10.5)–(10.9); equation (9.9) for the dynamics of ICC–IM; equations (10.10)–(10.18) for propagation of the wave of excitation within the electrically anisotropic and isotropic smooth muscle syncytia; constitutive relation equations (10.1), (10.2); and the equation of the motion of the pellet,

$$\eta_{sp}\frac{dZ_c}{dt} + F_d = \int_{z_1}^{z_2}\int_{r_0}^{r} F_c dz d\zeta, \tag{12.1}$$

where F_c, F_d are the contact force and the force of dry friction, η_{sp} is the coefficient of viscous friction. Assuming that at all stages of propulsion the wall makes contact with the surface of the sphere, we have

$$K_{sp} = \{(Z_c - u_1)^2 + (r_0 - u_2)^2 + (r_0 - \omega)^2 - R_{sp}^2 < 0\}, \quad z \in [z_1, z_2]. \tag{12.2}$$

Here u_1, u_2, ω are components of the displacement vector, Z_c is the position of the center of the pellet at time t, z_1, z_2 are the boundary points of contact of the pellet with the bioshell. In all simulations the initial position of the pellet is assumed to be known *a priori*.

The initial conditions assume that the bioshell is in the resting state. It is excited by a series of electrical discharges of pacemaker cells located at the left boundary. The impulses have a constant amplitude of $V_i = 100$ mV, a duration of $t_d = 1.5$ s, and a frequency of $\nu = 0.016$ Hz. Depending on the type of movement, different smooth muscle layers that make up the wall of the shell are excited. In peristalsis, a reciprocal relation is ascertained in contraction–relaxation between the teniae coli and circular muscle syncytium. The first contractions start in the longitudinal layer to be followed by the activation of the circular layer.

The left boundary of the bioshell is clamped throughout:

$$\begin{aligned} &r(\alpha_1, 0) = r_0, \quad \varphi(\alpha_1, 0) = z(\alpha_1, 0) = 0, \\ &v_r(\alpha_1, 0) = v_\varphi(\alpha_1, 0) = v_z(\alpha_1, 0) = 0, \end{aligned} \tag{12.3}$$

where $v_r = dr/dt$, $v_\varphi = d\varphi/dt$, $v_z = dz/dt$ are the components of the velocity vector. On the right boundary the following types of conditions are considered:

(i) clamped end

$$\begin{aligned} &r(\alpha_1, L) = \varphi(\alpha_1, L) = 0, \quad z(\alpha_1, L) = L, \\ &v_r(\alpha_1, L) = v_\varphi(\alpha_1, L) = v_z(\alpha_1, L) = 0; \end{aligned} \tag{12.4}$$

(ii) expanding end by the propagating pellet

$$\begin{aligned} &r(\alpha_1, L) = K_{sp}(t), \quad \varphi(\alpha_1, L) = K_{sp}(t), \quad z(\alpha_1, L) = L, \\ &v_r(\alpha_1, L) = v_\varphi(\alpha_1, L) = dK_{sp}(t)/dt, \quad v_z(\alpha_1, L) = 0; \end{aligned} \tag{12.5}$$

(iii) dilated end

$$\begin{aligned} &r(\alpha_1, L) = R_{sp}, \quad \varphi(\alpha_1, L) = 0, \quad z(\alpha_1, L) = L, \\ &v_r(\alpha_1, L) = v_\varphi(\alpha_1, L) = v_z(\alpha_1, L) = 0. \end{aligned} \tag{12.6}$$

12.2.1 Haustral churning

In the event of haustral churning the pacemaker cells located in the teniae coli and the circular smooth muscle layer fire simultaneously. Action potentials of amplitude $V_i = 100$ mV and frequency $\nu = 0.33$ Hz are produced. This induces the excitation and propagation of waves of depolarization V_l^s, V_c^s (subscript t refers to the teniae coli) within the wall of the bioshell.

As a result of electromechanical coupling, active forces of contraction develop. An initial wave T_c^a of intensity 10 mN cm^{-1} and wavelength 0.5 cm is produced (figure 12.2). This encases the entire segment with average $T_c^a = 12$ mN cm^{-1}. The bioshell experiences a uniform biaxial stress state throughout.

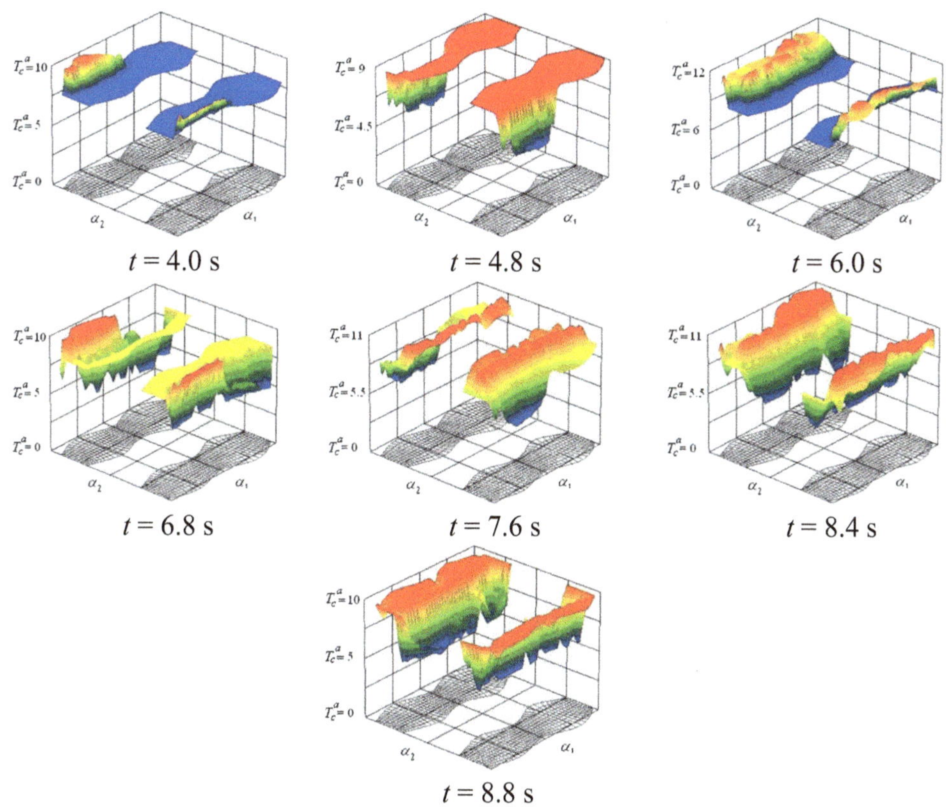

Figure 12.2. Active force T_c^a development in a colonic segment during haustral churning. Reproduced from Miftahof R M and Nam H 2010 *Mathematical Foundations and Biomechanics of the Digestive System* (Cambridge: Cambridge University Press) with permission of the Licensor through PLSclear. Copyright R Miftahof and H Nam 2010.

The total force $T_c = 35$ mN cm^{-1} is registered in the bioshell upon the excitation of the circular smooth muscle layer (figure 12.3). In the area of contact with the pellet, a maximum $T_c = 41$ mN cm^{-1} is produced. Since the wave T_c does not propagate, the pellet does not move but rather undergoes small librations around the initial point $Z_c = 0.35$ cm. It is open to speculation that, were the pellet deformable, the strong occluding contractions similar to those produced during haustral churning could break the content into parts with the subsequent displacement of the fragments along the colonic segment. This event has been observed experimentally. However, from the point of view of the mechanics of solids, this problem poses a considerable mathematical challenge and is not considered here.

12.2.2 Contractions of the teniae coli

Assume that only the teniae coli are myoelectrically active. As a result of excitation a wave T_t^a of average intensity 7.0 mN cm^{-1} is produced (figure 12.4). It has a length

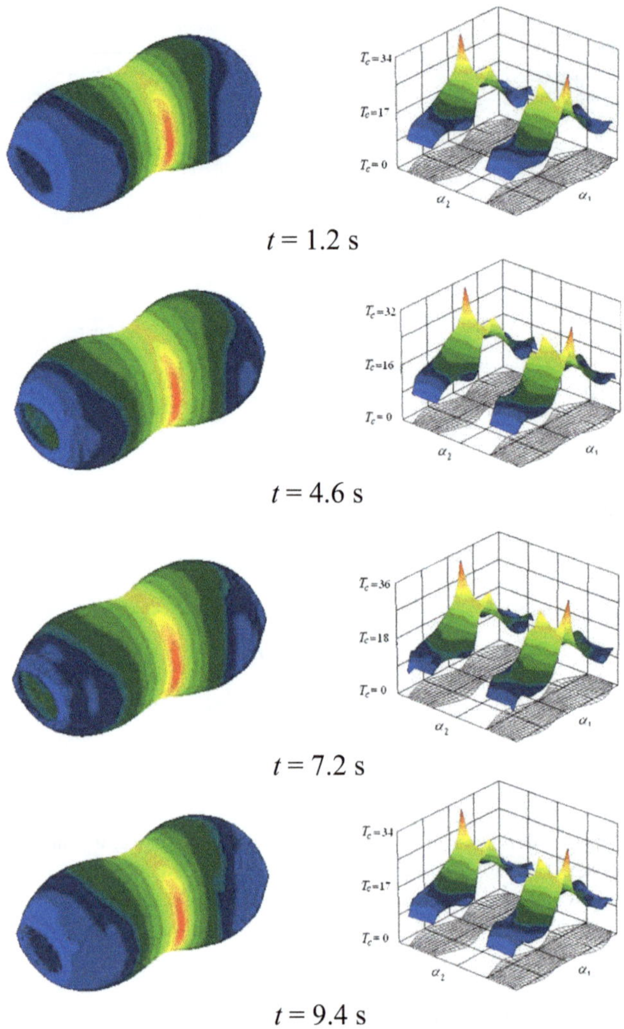

Figure 12.3. Total force T_c dynamics during haustral churning. Results are presented for a segment of the colon and its surface envelope. Reproduced from Miftahof R M and Nam H 2010 *Mathematical Foundations and Biomechanics of the Digestive System* (Cambridge: Cambridge University Press) with permission of the Licensor through PLSclear. Copyright R Miftahof and H Nam 2010.

of 0.6 cm and propagates at a velocity of 0.35 cm s^{-1} in the aboral direction along the surface of the bioshell. It increases in strength generating a maximum force T_t^a = 10.5 mN cm^{-1} in the contact zone between the pellet and the colon wall.

The dynamics of the total force T_t corresponds to the dynamics of the development of wave T_t^a. At the beginning of the process its magnitude is influenced mainly by the intensity of the active force (figure 12.5). With the development of forces in the connective tissue network, a uniform stress distribution in the colon is achieved. A maximum total force of 12.5 mN cm^{-1} develops in the contact zone and is

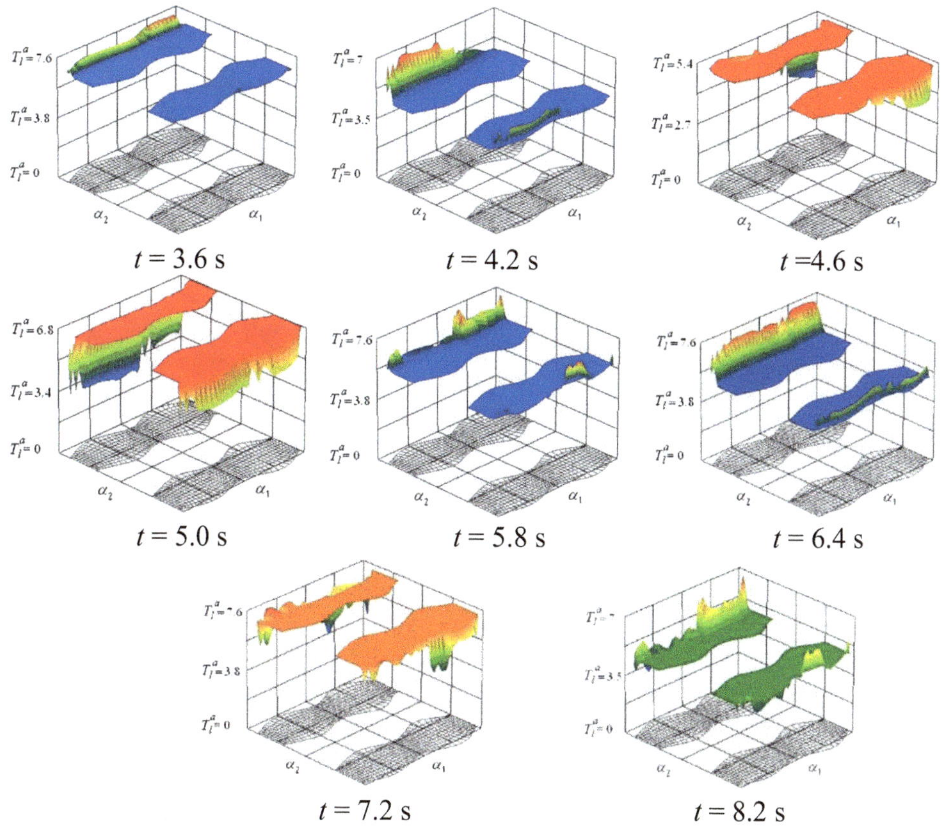

Figure 12.4. Active force T_t^a development in a colonic segment during contractions of the teniae coli. Reproduced from Miftahof R M and Nam H 2010 *Mathematical Foundations and Biomechanics of the Digestive System* (Cambridge: Cambridge University Press) with permission of the Licensor through PLSclear. Copyright R Miftahof and H Nam 2010.

associated with the intensive propulsion of the pellet. Initially it moves backwards by 0.06 cm to be followed by incessant propulsion during which the pellet is pushed forward by 0.25 cm at an average velocity of 0.01 cm s^{-1}. For $t \geqslant 25.6$ s the wave T_t pushes the pellet backwards. From $t > 38$ s the pellet experiences small displacements of ≈0.03 cm about the point $Z_c = 0.41$ cm. The transit velocity of the pellet varies from 1.05 to −1.1 cm s^{-1}.

Note that separate activation of the teniae coli and the associated movements of colonic content are analogous to the gradual reflex described in the small intestine. It is during this preliminary phase of propulsive activity that the most intensive mixing of the intraluminal content takes place.

12.2.3 Peristalsis and propulsive movements

Let both the teniae coli and the circular smooth muscle layer of the colon segment be reciprocally activated. The mechanical waves T_t and T_c propagate at a constant

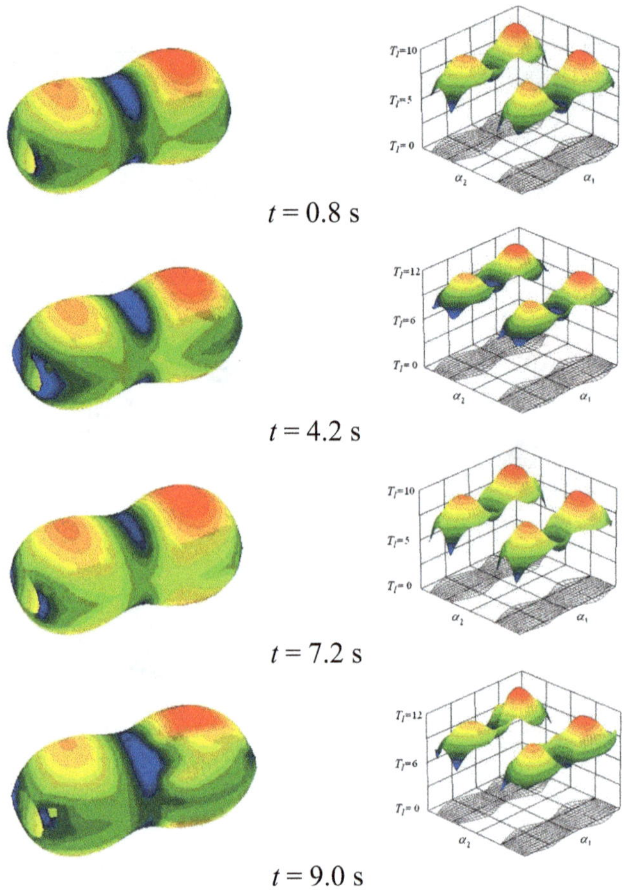

Figure 12.5. Total force T_t dynamics during contractions of the teniae coli. Reproduced from Miftahof R M and Nam H 2010 *Mathematical Foundations and Biomechanics of the Digestive System* (Cambridge: Cambridge University Press) with permission of the Licensor through PLSclear. Copyright R Miftahof and H Nam 2010.

velocity of 0.35 cm s^{-1} towards the right boundary. Maximal total forces, T_t = 13.2 mN cm^{-1} and T_c = 35.5 mN cm^{-1} are generated in the zone of contact of the bioshell with the pellet. For $t > 21.2$ s the intensity of the wave T_c begins to exceed the value of T_t. The pattern of force distribution in the bioshell is similar to that observed during haustral churning and isolated contractions of the teniae coli.

During peristalsis, the pellet moves forward at an average velocity of 0.01 cm s^{-1}. At t = 21.2 s its center is positioned at Z_c = 0.57 cm. A rapid, squeezing-type movement followed by a period of librations about the point Z_c = 0.68 cm is observed leading to the final propulsion of the pellet towards the left boundary. Analysis of the velocity profile shows that the maximum velocity of downward propulsion is 0.125 cm s^{-1}.

In the case of the pliable right end of the bioshell the movement of the pellet concurs with the dynamics of the propagation of electromechanical waves along the syncytia. Once again there is a mixing-type of back-and-forth movement with the preferred movement being towards the left end. The average velocity of propulsion is 0.8 cm s^{-1} (figure 12.6).

The pattern of propulsion of the pellet changes if the right end is constantly dilated. A brisk short length movement is observed at the beginning of the process after which the motion of the pellet slows down to achieve a relatively constant velocity of 0.44 cm s^{-1}. In this case more intense forces are generated by smooth muscle syncytia exceeding those recorded in the flexible end of the bioshell by a factor of two.

12.3 Pharmacology of colonic motility

12.3.1 Effect of Lotronex® on colonic propulsion

Consider the effects of Lotronex® (GSK), a selective 5-HT type 3 receptor antagonist, on the biomechanics of pellet propulsion. The mechanism of action of the drug is a decrease in the permeability of the Ca^{2+}, K^+, and Na^+ channels. In the model its pharmacological effect is achieved by altering the parameters $\tilde{g}_{Ca-K}$, $\tilde{g}_K$, and $\tilde{g}_{Na}$.

Results of simulations show that treatment of the colon segment with the drug causes an increase in the frequency of slow waves and abolishes the production of spikes. The smooth muscle syncytia become hyperpolarized, $V_{t,c}^s = -68.2$ mV. There is a significant reduction in the strength of the active forces of contraction in the teniae coli, $T_t^a = 7.2$ mN cm^{-1}, and the circular smooth muscle layer, $T_c^a =$ 9.1 mN cm^{-1}. As a result, there is a slowdown in propulsion. The average velocity of transit of the pellet is reduced to 0.23 cm s^{-1}.

The subsequent application of ACh restores the normal dynamics of the colon. High amplitude spikes of average amplitude $V_{t,c}^s = 67.4$ mV are produced. Tonic-type contractions, $T_c^a = 25$ mN cm^{-1}, are recorded in smooth muscle syncytia. These are non-propagating in nature and have a detrimental effect on propulsion bringing the pellet to a standstill. Only after removal of ACh does the segment regain its propulsive activity in the presence of Lotronex®.

12.3.2 Effect of Zelnorm®

Zelnorm® (Novartis, AB) is a 5-HT type 4 receptor agonist. The 5-HT type 4 receptors belong to the family of G-protein coupled receptors and involves the second messenger transduction mechanism. The drug increases the permeability of Ca^{2+}-activated K^+ and Na^+ channels. The pharmacological effect of Zelnorm® in the model is simulated by varying the parameters $\tilde{g}_{Ca-K}$ and $\tilde{g}_{Na}$.

Throughout simulations, smooth muscle layers sustain a reciprocal relationship in contraction–relaxation in the presence of the drug. Zelnorm® has no effect on the dynamics of propagation of the wave of depolarization within muscle syncytia. There is an increase in tone in the teniae coli, $T_t = 18$ mN cm^{-1}, with no significant changes in strength in the circular smooth muscle layer, $T_c = 35$ mN cm^{-1}. The bioshell experiences biaxial stress–strain states preserving propagation of

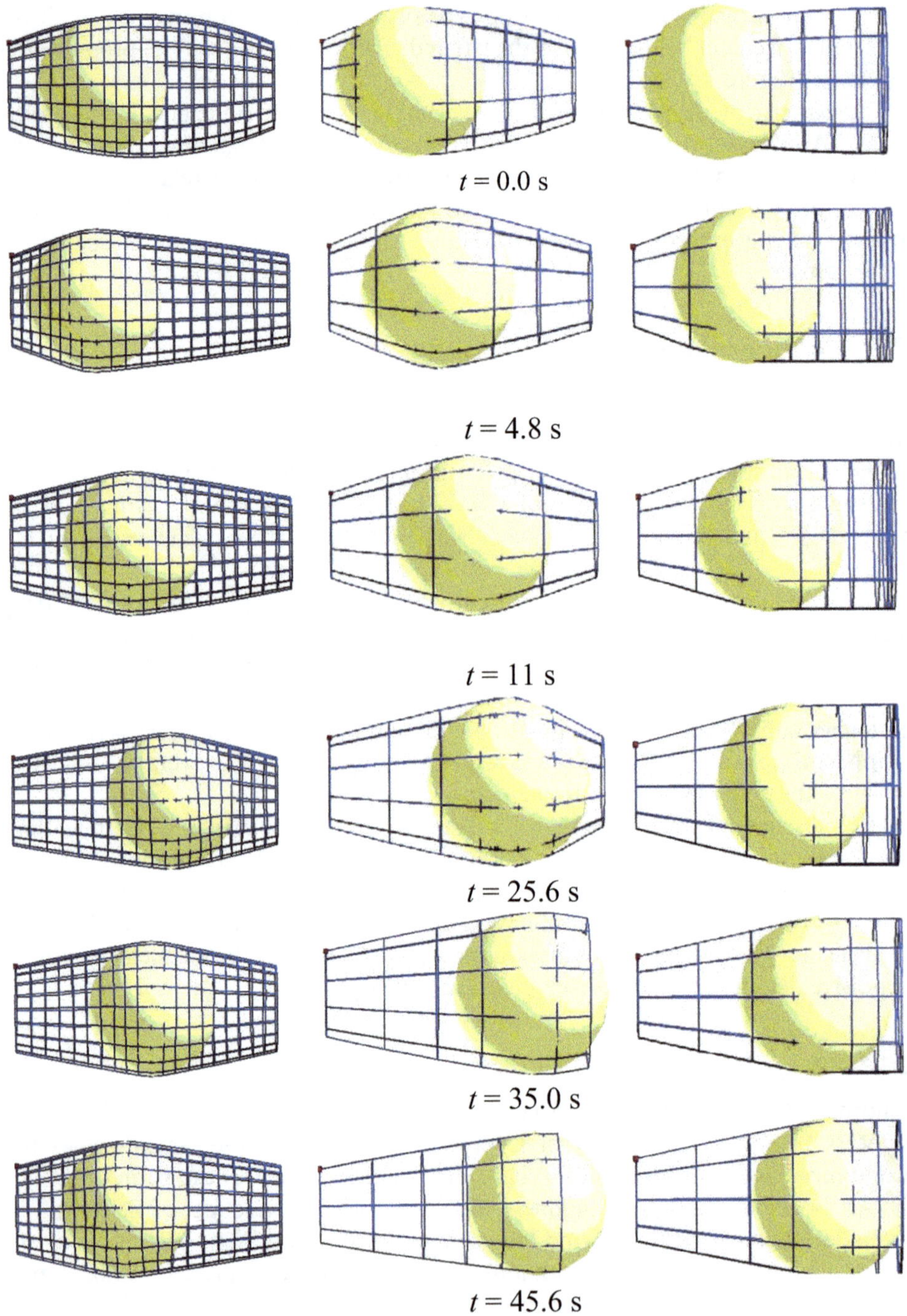

Figure 12.6. Pellet propulsion in a colonic segment in cases of a clamped (left column), pliable (middle column), and a dilated (right column) end. Reproduced from Miftahof R M and Nam H 2010 *Mathematical Foundations and Biomechanics of the Digestive System* (Cambridge: Cambridge University Press) with permission of the Licensor through PLSclear. Copyright R Miftahof and H Nam 2010.

electromechanical waves along its surface. The pellet moves along the segment at velocity ~0.4 cm s^{-1}. However, no mixing component of intraluminal content is present.

Further reading

Bertuzzi A, Marcinelli R, Ronzoni G and Salinari S 1983 *J. Biomech.* **16** 459–64

D'Antona G, Hennig G W, Costa M, Humphreys C M and Brookes S J H 2001 *Neurogastroent Mot.* **13** 483–92

Miftahof R and Akhmadeev N 2007 *J. Theor. Biol.* **246** 377–93

Sinnott M D, Clearly P W, Arkwright J W and Dinning P G 2012 *Comput. Biol. Med.* **42** 492–503

Roustem N Miftahof and Nariman R Akhmadeev

Chapter 13

The gravid uterus

A mathematical formulation of a one-dimensional model of the myometrial fiber, a functional unit of the uterus, is given followed by a numerical investigation into its biomechanics, looking at the effects of changes in the extracellular/intracellular ion environment, pharmacological interventions, and co-transmission by multiple neurotransmitters. The gravid uterus is then modeled as a soft biological shell which is used to study the stress–strain distribution in the organ close to term and during the first and second stages of labor. The chapter closes with a numerical simulation of pathological conditions including constriction ring, uterine dystocia, and hyper- and hypotonic uterine inertia.

13.1 Anatomical considerations

The non-pregnant human uterus is a hollow, thick-walled organ situated deep in the pelvic cavity. At its upper part it measures on average 7.5 cm in length, 5 cm in breadth and has a thickness of nearly 2.5–4 cm (figure 13.1). Anatomically the organ is divided into: the fundus, the body, the uterotubal angles, and the cervix. The region between the body and the cervix is called the isthmus. The cervix of the uterus is conical or cylindrical in shape with a truncated apex.

The uterus is supported by anterior, posterior, dual lateral, uterosacral, and round ligaments. The anterior and posterior ligaments consist of the vesicouterine and the rectovaginal folds of the peritoneum and contain a considerable amount of fibrous tissue and non-striped muscular fibers. At one end they are attached to the sacrum and constitute the uterosacral ligaments. These two broad ligaments pass from the sides of the uterus to the lateral walls of the pelvis. The round ligaments are two flattened bands situated between the layers of the broad ligament in front of and below the uterine tubes. They consist principally of muscular tissue prolonged from the uterus and also of some fibrous tissue. The ligaments contain blood and lymph vessels along with nerves. Additionally, there are fibrous tissue bands on either side of the cervix uteri known as the ligamentum transversalis coli. These are attached

doi:10.1088/2053-2563/ab1a9ech13

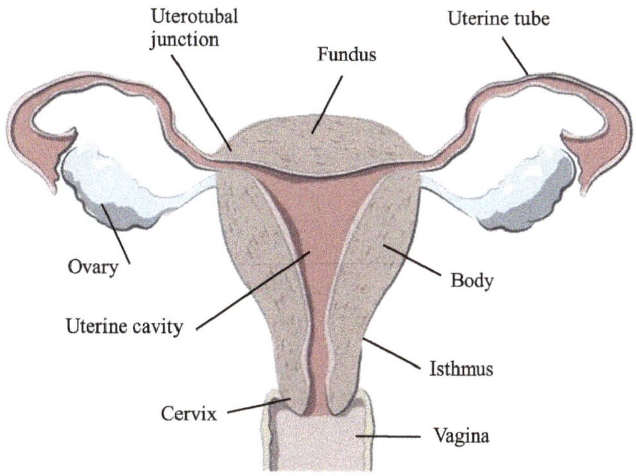

Figure 13.1. Anatomy of the non-pregnant human uterus. Reprinted from Miftahof R M and Nam H G 2011 *Biomechanics of the Gravid Human Uterus* (Berlin: Springer) by permission from Springer Nature. Copyright 2011.

not only to the side of the cervix uteri, but also to the lateral walls of the pelvis and to a part of the vagina.

The arterial supply to the uterus is mainly from the hypogastric artery. The arteries are remarkable for their tortuous course and frequent anastomoses within the wall of the organ. The venous return corresponds to the course of the arteries and drains in the uterine plexi. In the pregnant uterus the arteries carry the blood to the intervillous space of the placenta whilst the veins convey it away from the same.

The nerves are derived from both the hypogastric and ovarian plexi and from the third and fourth sacral nerves. It should be noted that there is afferent but no efferent innervation to the uterus.

The actual position of the body of the uterus in the adult is liable to considerable variation. It depends chiefly on the condition of the nearby organs, namely the urinary bladder and rectum. When the bladder is empty the uterus is bent on itself at the junction of the body with the cervix lying upon the bladder. As the urinary bladder fills, the uterus becomes more ‘erect’. Once the bladder is fully distended, the fundus of the uterus may face the sacrum. Movements of the cervix, however, are very restricted.

The cavity of the non-pregnant womb resembles a mere flattened slit. It is triangular in shape, with the base being formed by the internal surface of the fundus and the apex. The uterine tubes are connected on either side of the fundus thus allowing the ova to enter the uterine cavity. If an ovum is fertilized it imbeds itself in the uterine wall and is normally retained there until prenatal development is completed.

13.2 A functional unit

The human uterus is a multi-component system with optimal spatiotemporal arrangements among morphological elements. It is composed of three histologically distinct layers (from inside out): the endometrium, the myometrium, and the perimetrium. The endometrium of the womb is lined with a surface epithelium and has three types of cells: secretory, ciliated, and basal. The main function of the endometrium is to provide for the implantation of a fertilized ovum and to support the growth of a fetus. The uttermost perimetrium is composed of a thin layer of connective tissue—collagen and elastin fibers.

The most prominent layer, the myometrium, is divided into three poorly delineated self-embedded layers (strata)—the strata supravasculare, vasculare, and subvasculare. The morphostructural functional unit of the muscle tissue of the uterus is the uterine smooth muscle cell (myocyte). Its morphoanatomical structure and contractile apparatus are similar to those of SMCs, as described above (chapter 6).

Multiple pore structures between myometrial cells allow cell-to-cell communication via diffusible intracellular components—gap junctions. Immunofluorescent studies have shown that these are formed predominantly of the connexin-43 protein with varying degrees of connexins 40 and 45. Gap junctions provide the structural basis for electrical and metabolic communications, support synchronization, and long-range integration in myocytes. These ensure the property of myogenic syncytia necessary for the coordinated phasic contractions of labor. Immunohistochemical labeling studies have demonstrated that the expression of connexin-43 is not even in the pregnant uterus. There is a significant increase in the protein content in the fundus as compared to the lower segment of the organ. This fact has been suggested as pivotal to electrogenic coupling asymmetry and conductance anisotropy.

Myometrial cells adjust their structure and function acutely by reorganizing the cytoskeleton and altering signaling pathways. Thus, hypertrophic changes in the pregnant uterus are associated with the remodeling of ECM from a fibrillar to a sponge-like architecture. Activation of integrin and fibronectin proteins promotes the development of new cell-matrix contacts and the formation of a mesh-like fine fibrillar matrix on the cell surface with their cytoplasmic domains attached to cytoskeletal proteins (figure 13.2). Such changes ensure myometrial homogeneity and affirm even stress–strain distribution in the tissue.

13.3 Electrophysiological properties

Myometrial contractions are driven by waves of electrical activity. The resting membrane potential of freshly isolated human uterine smooth muscle cells varies between $V^r \simeq -70$ to -45 mV. The level depends on their gestational status, i.e. cells become more depolarized towards full term and delivery. Direct measurements have revealed that the specific membrane resistance of myocytes is $R_{\mathrm{m}} \simeq 6$ k$\Omega\cdot$cm^2 and the capacitance $C_{\mathrm{m}} \simeq 1.6$ μF cm^{-2}.

The myometrium is spontaneously excitable and produces low amplitude (~10–20 mV) slow waves with a frequency of ~0.008–0.1 Hz, and high frequency (~17–25 Hz) action potentials (spikes) with an amplitude of ~40–50 mV. Although the existence of slow waves in the myometrium is debated, *in vivo* and *in vitro* recordings from pregnant human uteri clearly demonstrate long-period, ~1.5–2 min, oscillations of

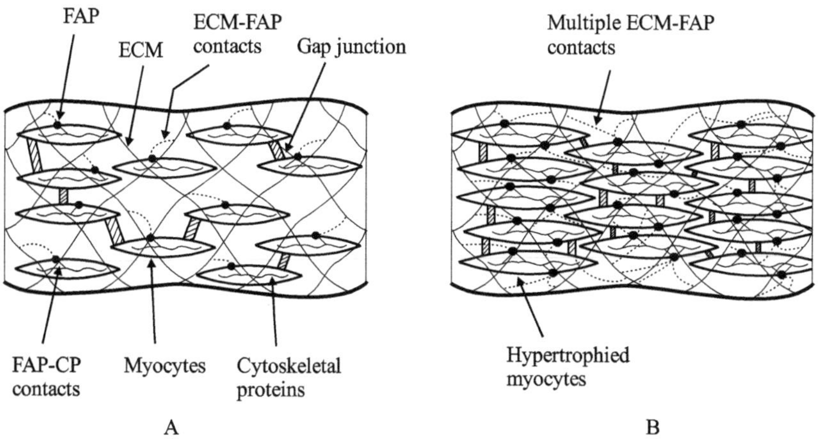

Figure 13.2. Structure of myometrium in non-pregnant (A) and pregnant (B) uteri. Reprinted from Miftahof R M and Nam H G 2011 *Biomechanics of the Gravid Human Uterus* (Berlin: Springer) by permission from Springer Nature. Copyright 2011.

membrane potentials. The dynamics of action potentials is greatly influenced by neurohormonal factors. Spikes are almost absent during the entire pregnancy and are generated only at late-term, labor, and delivery. Their duration varies between 100–250 ms. The velocity of the propagation of excitation in the myometrium is 1.0–9.0 cm s^{-1} and depends on the anatomical site and physiological status of the uterus. The excitatory waves both synchronize myoelectrical activity in the organ and organize contractions. Non-invasive myographic and electrohysterographic studies have revealed a preferred propagation of excitation from the fundus towards the cervix in pregnant human uteri.

Pacemaker cells have not yet been found in the uterus. Ultrastructural and immunohistochemical studies have helped to identify interstitial Cajal-like cells (IC) in the myometrium and fallopian tubes. This is based mainly on morphological similarities with ICC found in the gastrointestinal tract, where their role as pacemakers has been ‘firmly’ established. Extrapolations have been made to associate them with uterine pacemaker cells. In contrast, electrophysiological recordings of spontaneous spiking activity from impaled myocytes suggest a concept of variable wandering pacemakers or, in other words, any myometrial muscle cell or a group of cells is capable of acting as either a pacemaker or pace-follower.

13.4 Neuroendocrine modulators

Although electrical waves of depolarization induce spontaneous contractions of the myometrium, fine-tuning of its mechanical reactivity during gestation and parturition is provided by the fetal–maternal hypothalamic–pituitary–adrenal–placental axis. This involves a number of multiple neuropeptides and hormones. Their effects are spatiotemporally integrated at the synaptic level, quantifying the amount of chemically coded information required to be passed into the cell. The concept of neuroendocrine modulation of uterine activity includes: intricate signal transduction mechanisms of synthesis; storage, release, and utilization of transmitters; their binding to and activation of receptors; and enzymatic degradation with subsequent initiation of a variety of cellular events.

Neuroendocrine modulators are broadly divided into contractors (uterotonics), amongst which the most powerful are oxytocin (OT), prostaglandins $F_{2\alpha}$ and E_2 ($PGF_{2\alpha}$, PGE_2), ACh, and relaxants (tocolytics)—progesterone (PR) and adrenaline/noradrenaline. They exert their effects through a number of specific and G-protein coupled receptors. The expression and sensitivity of receptors depend on the gestational status. Moreover, the receptor co-localization allows the myocyte to respond to more than one neuroendocrine modulator at a time thereby assuring its highly adaptive properties.

Acetylcholine acts via transmembrane muscarinic type 2 (μ_2) $G\alpha_{i(1-3)}$ coupled receptors located at the myocytes. The ACh–receptor complex generates a postsynaptic response, i.e. the inhibition of the intracellular cAMP pathway. This involves the inactivation of adenylyl cyclase enzyme, cyclic adenosine monophosphate production from adenosine 5′-triphosphate, and the protein kinase A pathway. The result is a suppression of phosphorylation of myosin light chain kinase, and potentiation of myometrial SM contractility. cAMP decomposition into adenosine monophosphate is catalyzed by the enzyme phosphodiesterase 4–2B (PDE4–2B).

The neurohypophysial hormone oxytocin is a potent and specific stimulant of uterine contractions. The peptide is synthesized as an inactive precursor protein from the OT gene and progressively hydrolyzed by a series of enzymes to form the active oxytocin nonapeptide. OT is packaged in large, dense-core vesicles of the corpus luteum and placental cells and is secreted upon stimulation by exocytosis. Myometrial OT receptors are functionally coupled to $G\alpha_{q/11}$ proteins. Their expression and sensitivity to OT increases 12-fold towards late pregnancy and during labor. Activation of the receptor together with $G\beta\gamma$ stimulates the phospholipase C pathway. Additionally, OT activates the c-Src and focal adhesion kinases adding to the production of inositol-1,4,5-triphosphate. It has been demonstrated experimentally that OT directly increases the calcium influx through voltage-gated or ligand-operated channels. The effect is to be nifedipine insensitive. Oxytocin is metabolized predominantly in the placenta and, to a lesser extent, in the myometrium and decidua by two major enzymes: aminopeptidase and post-proline endopeptidase.

Prostaglandins $F_{2\alpha}$ and E_2 are prostanoids and belong to the eicosanoid family of biologically active lipids. They are synthesized from arachidonic acid through a combination of cyclooxygenases (COX-1 and -2) and specific synthase enzymes in the decidua, the chorion laeve, and the amnion. PG levels depend on the presence and activity of the principle metabolizing enzyme, 15-hydroxy-prostaglandin dehydrogenase. Released into the bloodstream, they exert their paracrine effect on the myometrium. It is accepted that $PGF_{2\alpha}$ mediates its actions via FP–$G\alpha_{q/11}$ protein coupled receptors and the activation of the PLC pathway. Experiments on isolated myometrial cells have led to the notion that its primary effect is to promote Ca^{2+} entry through L-type Ca^{2+} channels. PGE_2 transmits signals in the human myometrium by binding to the four distinct $G\alpha_i$ coupled receptors ($EP_{1-3A,D}$). EP_1- and EP_{3D}-type receptors cause an elevation in intracellular calcium and increase contractility through the activation of L-type Ca^{2+} channels, whilst stimulation of the EP_2 receptor increases cAMP production. Activation of EP_{3A} augments mitogen-activated protein kinase—serine/threonine-specific protein kinase—activity and impedes the cAMP pathway. Additionally, stimulation of the EP_{3D} receptor enhances the phosphatidyl–inositol turnover via the PLC pathway thereby adding to a rise in cellular calcium. Prostaglandins are deactivated in the placenta by 15-hydroxyprostaglandin dehydrogenase and 13,14-prostaglandin reductase.

Adrenaline, also known as epinephrine, is both a hormone and a neurotransmitter. An intracellular rise of Ca^{2+} triggers its release from chromaffin granules by exocytosis. AD acts via two main groups of G-protein coupled adrenoceptors, α and β. Subtypes α_1, α_2, β_1, β_2, and β_3 adrenoceptors, $AR_{\alpha i,\beta i}$, are present in the human uterus. The excitatory α_1-AR is coupled to $G\alpha_{q/11}$ protein and, upon activation, stimulates the PLC signaling pathway. The α_2-$AR_{\alpha 2}$ is linked to $G\alpha_i$ protein and decreases cAMP production. β_1 and β_3 $AR_{\beta i}$ are coupled to $G\alpha_s$, and β_2 type to $G\alpha_s$ and $G\alpha_{i(1-3)}$ proteins. Their function is associated with activation of the cAMP-dependent pathway. Adrenaline exerts negative feedback to down-regulate its own synthesis at the presynaptic α_2 adrenoceptors. Excess adrenalin is removed by two mechanisms: uptake-1 and uptake-2. The uptake-1 mechanism involves deamination of AD by monoamine oxidase whilst the uptake-2 mechanism involves its degradation by catechol-*O*-methyltransferase enzyme to metabolic products.

Progesterone belongs to a class of hormones called progestogens and is the major naturally occurring human progestogen. It is synthesized from cholesterol to form pregnenolone which is further converted to progesterone in the presence of 3β-hydroxysteroid dehydrogenase/$\Delta(5)$–$\Delta(4)$ isomerase. PR exerts its action through the G-protein bound membrane (mPR) and nuclear (nPR) ligand-activated transcription factor receptors. Three isoforms, PR-A, PR-B, and PR-C, all of which differ in their molecular weight, affinity, and functionality, have been identified in the human uterus. The mPRs are coupled to $G\alpha_i$ proteins, their activation resulting in a decline in cAMP levels. Activation of mPR receptors leads to transactivation of nPR-B. The PR–nPR-B receptor complex undergoes dimerization and enters the nucleus where it binds to DNA. The following transcription leads to the formation of messenger ribonucleic acid (mRNA) and the production of specific proteins. 17α and 21α hydroxylases are responsible for the enzymatic conversion of progesterones to mineralocorticoid, cortisol, and androstenedione.

There is accumulating evidence that inflammatory cytokines, IL-1β, IL-6, and IL-8 and the tumor necrosis factor are involved in normal term labor. For example, IL-1β is produced by macrophages, monocytes, fibroblasts, and dendritic cells as a proprotein. It is proteolytically converted to its active form by caspase 1. This cytokine is a powerful pro-labor mediator through the stimulation of the PLC pathway, the induction of Ca^{2+} ion release from the sarcoplasmic reticulum, the activation of p38MAPK, and the enhanced production of COX-2 enzyme and prostaglandins. IL-8 expression in the myometrium is maximal at term. The chemokine contributes to cervical maturation by stimulating extravasation of neutrophils. The latter release matrix metalloproteinases that denature the collagen within ECM, whilst also increasing cervical compliance and uterine contractility.

The list of potential uterotonics can be extended to include estrogen, tachykinins, adenosine 5′-triphosphate, endothelin-1, platelet activating factor A_2, thrombin, as well as tocolytics—human chorionic gonadotrophin (hCG), relaxin, calcitonin-gene-related peptide. It is apparent, however, that electrical, neuroendocrine, and mechanical stimuli can initiate and regulate mechanical activity in the pregnant myometrium at term. However, operating alone or conjointly they cannot sustain the required strength, frequency, and duration of the contractions needed to expel the products of conception. To be robust they must be organized and integrated in time and space. Failure to achieve dynamic coordination results in pathological conditions such as dystocia and impediment of labor.

13.5 Coupling phenomena

Individual myocytes require the presence of flexible dynamic links among intrinsic electrical, chemical (neurohormonal), and mechanical processes to perform as a physiological entity. These complex forward–feedback interactions modulate the function of extra- and intracellular protein pathways, the expression and distribution of gap junctions, ion channels, surface membrane, and nuclear receptors in the organ.

Electro-chemo-mechanical coupling is a sequence of events heralded by myometrial contractions preceded by a wave of depolarization of the cell membrane and/or ligand–receptor complex formation. The main functional link in the cascade of processes is Ca_i^{2+}. Two major sources for it are: (i) the flux of extracellular calcium inside the cell and (ii) its release from the internal store—sarcoplasmic reticulum (SR). The influx is enabled by voltage-gated L- and T-type, and ligand-operated L-type Ca^{2+} channels. Depolarization as well as the binding of OT, $PGF_{2\alpha}$, and PGE_2 to the membrane receptors increases the channels' open state probability, with a resulting rise in $[Ca_i^{2+}]$. Recent studies have highlighted a possible direct activation of L-type Ca^{2+} channels by DAG although the exact mechanism is unclear. The blockade of L-type Ca^{2+} channels with selective antagonists, nifedipine and verapamil, abolishes cytosolic calcium transience and reduces both spontaneous and induced mechanical activity. The release of Ca^{2+} from the SR is accomplished by stimulation of the ryanodine and IP_3 receptors on its membrane. However, the amount of Ca_i^{2+} released is small compared to that entering the cell through Ca^{2+} channels. Free cytosolic calcium binds to calmodulin protein to form the Ca^{2+}–calmodulin complex. It further induces a cascade of downstream reactions with subsequent inhibition in phosphorylation of MLCK, and activation of *h*-caldesmon, calponin, and the light chain myosin. Active light myosin interacts with actin to form actin–myosin crossbridges and, hence, contraction.

Experiments with wortmannin, a myosin light chain kinase inhibitor, have demonstrated that myocytes continue to produce an active force in the presence of the drug, albeit of lower strength and intensity. It has been suggested that other intracellular pathways dependent on the Ca_0^{2+} influx might be involved in myometrial contractility. Thus, membrane dense plaque proteins serve as molecular signaling platforms to mechanochemical coupling. An externally applied stretch induces phosphorylation of tyrosine dependent focal adhesion proteins, c-Src, and intracellular kinases to promote the interaction of structural proteins, mainly paxillin, vinculin, and talin. The formation of a focal adhesion proteins complex and its association with phosphorylated *h*-caldesmon leads to contraction. It is worth noting that tyrosine kinase directly modulates the L-type Ca^{2+} channel.

The myometrium produces two types of contractions, namely tonic and phasic. Tonic contractions prevail during the late phase of labor and immediately after delivery whilst intensive phasic contractions are observed chiefly during delivery. Although the actin–myosin complex formation is universally accepted as the only mechanism responsible for force development by SM, *in vitro* studies have recorded active contractions of the myometrial extracellular matrix as well. The exact mechanism remains unclear but actin polymerization and its remodeling have been offered as an explanation for contractility.

Relaxation of the myometrium is brought about by the processes of hyperpolarization, reduction in $[Ca_i^{2+}]$, and activation of the cAMP-dependent inhibitory pathway. Activation of the BK_{Ca}, K_v, and Cl^- channels is the major regulatory feedback element that causes hyperpolarization of the cell membrane. Two mechanisms have been identified, namely extrusion by the Na^+/Ca^{2+} exchanger and active re-uptake of Ca_i^{2+} into the SR control cytosolic calcium at the necessary levels. Progesterone and adrenaline stimulate PKA via the cAMP-dependent pathway. PKA further phosphorylates MLCK thereby attenuating its affinity for the Ca^{2+}–calmodulin complex. This results in the dissociation of the actin–myosin complexes. In addition, the protein promotes desensitization of $G\alpha_q$ receptors, decreases gap junction permeability, and inhibits the phospholipase C pathway with a cumulative effect of myometrial relaxation.

13.6 Crosstalk phenomena

Over the years, the physiological function of different modulators has been studied and analyzed independently. However, there is an important factor which has been overlooked, namely the co-transmission by multiple signaling molecules and their integrated effect on myometrial contractility. Positive crosstalk between caveolae co-localized β_2-ARs, BK_{Ca}, and K_v channels facilitates hyperpolarization of the membrane and uterine relaxation. Activation of β adrenoceptors has also been shown to exert negative regulation on the PLC pathway by reducing IP_3 production through the cAMP-dependent mechanism. Co-localization of α_1-adrenoceptors with the OT receptor permits the adrenaline modulation of myometrial activity. However, the number of α_1- and β_1-ARs in the human myometrium is relatively small, making their role in relaxation insignificant.

Immunoprecipitation and matrix-assisted laser desorption 'time-of-flight' mass spectrometry studies have revealed a strong association of BK_{Ca} channels with α- and γ-actin cytoskeletal filaments. It has been postulated that mechanical stretch can modulate channel activity and *vice versa*. The stretching of uterine myocytes has also been shown to increase the expression of contraction-associated proteins, and the up-regulation of COX-2 mRNA, p38MAPK, and the chemokine IL-8. The induction of labor by prostaglandins is associated with greater expression of IL-8, suggesting an interaction between PRs and the chemokine.

Although OT and PGE_2 stimulate IP_3 accumulation and Ca^{2+} release from the SR via the IP_3-sensitive mechanism, only OT-induced high frequency Ca^{2+} oscillations are ryanodine-sensitive. Inhibition of the $G\beta\gamma$ subunit stimulates PLCβ2 and PLCβ3 through phosphorylation of the cAMP-dependent PKA indicating the possible combined regulatory effects of acetylcholine, adrenaline, and progesterone. The secretion of PGE_2 is controlled by human chorionic gonadotrophin through the expression of COX-2 messenger ribonucleic acid. The stimulant effects of $PGF_{2\alpha}$ on uterine contractility are also augmented by ATP via activation of $P2X_{1,3}$ receptors. Chemokines have been shown to increase (IL-1β) or decrease (IL-6) $PGF_{2\alpha}$ levels in cultures of human uterine myocytes. The effects are mediated in part by protein kinase C, but are independent of MAPK, PLC, and IP_3 kinases. Interestingly, mechanical stretch has no effect on $PGF_{2\alpha}$ mRNA expression.

Extensive crosstalk exists among progesterone receptors. PR-B receptors are antagonized by PR-A receptors which are dominant repressors of transcription. Therefore, it has been suggested that an increase in their expression during labor causes 'functional' progesterone withdrawal and induction of delivery. nPR-C receptors reside mainly in the cytosol of myocytes and have high affinity for progesterone. Their activation diminishes the concentration of PR–nPR-B complexes thus promoting contractions. Additionally, progesterone represses connexin-43 levels and gap junction density in myocytes at term. Hence, PR can attenuate electrical coupling and disrupt the process that leads to the propagation of the wave of excitation in the myometrium.

Human chorionic gonadotrophin plays an essential role in establishing pregnancy and its continuation. There is convincing experimental evidence that it promotes uterine quiescence by binding positively to hCG–$G\alpha_s$ protein coupled receptors and stimulating the cAMP/PKA pathway. Currently, it is not clear what specific targets are phosphorylated downstream by PKA. The available data suggest that the hormone interferes with OT signaling. Moreover, hCG down-regulates gap junction formation, directly activates BK_{Ca} channels, impedes Ca_i^{2+} availability by the inactivation of voltage-gated Ca_i^{2+} channels, and inhibits the PDE5 enzyme.

Net myometrial contractile activity is determined by the balance of receptors present. To date, no detailed quantitative studies have been conducted to analyze the pattern of either receptor distribution or receptor types in human uteri. It remains of utmost importance to establish receptor topography and its expression throughout the fundus to the cervix both during gestation and labor. Ligand binding studies have revealed heterogeneous ratios of EP_1, EP_3, and $PGF_{2\alpha}$ receptors in the organ with the highest concentration in the fundus. The lower segment of the uterus at term has been demonstrated to respond more to relaxatory (EP_2) rather than to excitatory (EP_3) receptor activation. Myometrial oxytocin receptor levels have been found in greater abundance in the fundus and the corpus rather than in the lower uterine segment where their concentration is at its lowest.

Functional binding, Western blot, and polymerase chain reaction experiments have shown the predominance of β_3-adrenoceptors over the β_2-AR type in the myometrium. There is also a gradual increase in the total number of α_1-ARs during pregnancy although little is known about their hormonal modulation. Elevation of 17β-estradiol has been demonstrated to increase the myometrial response to a selective β_3-AR agonist. Tachykinin NK_2, purinergic $P2X_1$, serotonergic $5HT_{2A}$, and histamine H_2 receptors have been identified recently in the pregnant human myometrium. Sadly, however, data on their distribution, co-localization, and co-transmission are currently lacking.

13.7 Biological changes in the gravid uterus

During pregnancy the uterus evolves considerably with dynamic changes related to both special and temporal processes—an overall process controlled by intrinsic and extrinsic regulatory mechanisms. The gravid organ extends from the pelvis to occupy the lower and middle abdomen. It undergoes changes in size and structure to accommodate itself to meet the needs of the growing embryo—'uterine conversion'. The pregnant human uterus exhibits marked differences in its morphology and protein expression patterns when compared to the non-pregnant organ, collectively referred to as 'phenotypic modulation'. The latter includes four distinct phenotypes (phases): (i) early proliferative, (ii) intermediate synthetic, (iii) contractile phase, and (iv) highly active labor.

During the first stage uterine myocytes proliferate rapidly, predominantly in the longitudinal layer. The following synthetic phase is remarkable for myometrial cell hypertrophy associated with increased synthesis and deposition of an interstitial matrix. As pregnancy progresses, the uterus advances into a contractile phenotype. At this stage the rate of cellular hypertrophy remains constant. There is a continuous increase in the γ-smooth muscle actin, the expression of L-, T-type Ca^{2+} and Ca^{2+}-activated K^+ ion channels, receptors for oxytocin and prostaglandins, gap junction proteins, connexin-43, contraction-associated proteins, and the stabilization of focal adhesions. The reinforcement of ligand–integrin interaction guarantees tight intercellular cohesion and electromechanical syncytial properties of the myometrium. Significant changes are also seen in the interstitial matrix with an increased production of collagen type IV, fibronectin, and laminin $\beta 2$. These grow into a regular fibrillar stroma providing additional mechanical support to myocytes.

At the full term of gestation through phenotypic modulation and fetal growth the human uterus measures 40–42 cm in the axial (the fundal height) and 35–37 cm in the transverse directions. Ultrasonographic data show that the thickness of the wall varies in different regions between 0.45 and 0.7 cm, whilst the radius of curvature changes within a range of 8–14 cm. The fundal height reflects fetal growth and the increasing development of amniotic fluid in the amniotic sac, a two-layered membrane that surrounds the fetus. Amniotic fluid is primarily produced by the mother in the first trimester of pregnancy and after this period by the fetus. It provides nourishment, allows free fetal movements inside the womb and cushions the baby from external 'blows'. The amount of fluid is greatest at 34 weeks gestation, $\check{V} \simeq 800$ ml, reducing to $\check{V} \simeq 600$ ml over the following 6–7 weeks. Smaller or excessive amounts of amniotic fluid are called oligo- and polyhydramnios, respectively, and are usually manifestations of various medical conditions.

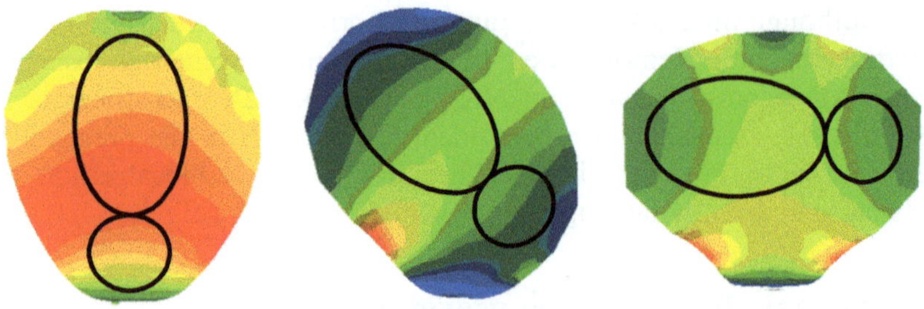

Figure 13.3. Anatomical configurations of the pregnant uterus with the fetus in: (a) cephalic, (b) oblique, and (c) transverse presentation. Reprinted from Miftahof R M and Nam H G 2011 *Biomechanics of the Gravid Human Uterus* (Berlin: Springer) by permission from Springer Nature. Copyright 2011.

Stress–strain curves of uniaxial stretching *in vitro* experiments of myometrial strips obtained from different parts of the non-gravid and gravid uteri have shown their high nonlinearity and large deformability, 40%–100%.

In the resting state amniotic fluid generates intrauterine pressure, p, of 2–12 mmHg. During labor intrauterine pressure rises to 60–100 mmHg and is concurrent with the contractile activity of the myometrium. The pattern of changes in p serves as an important predictor of normal delivery.

The shape of the pregnant human womb is pear-like. Its actual configuration before labor, however, greatly depends on the position of the fetus and the amount of amniotic fluid. The most common presentation is vertex or head downwards, whilst less common presentations are oblique and transverse in which the baby lies either obliquely or crosswise in the uterus, respectively (figure 13.3). The head downwards position is normally delivered vaginally, whilst babies in the oblique and transverse positions are delivered by Cesarean section.

After parturition the uterus gradually returns to close to its usual size, although certain traces of its enlargement remain. Its cavity is now larger than in the pre-pregnant state with its vessels tortuous and muscular layers more prominent.

13.8 Modeling of the gravid uterus

13.8.1 Biomechanical models

In recent years the biomedical research on reproduction has been focused mainly on molecular, neuroendocrine, and pharmacological aspects of uterine activity. A relatively small amount of work has been dedicated to modeling the uterus *per se*. Knowledge of the mechanical properties of the myometrium is crucial for the integration of motor functions into a biologically plausible biomechanical model of the organ. Experiments on quasi-static uniaxial stretching of linear human myometrial strips have revealed nonlinear viscoelastic properties of the tissue. Thus, the maximum deformability and tension recorded from the non-pregnant myometrium are $\varepsilon = 0.4$, $\sigma = 22$ mN mm^{-2}, and at term, $\varepsilon = 0.8$, $\sigma = 41.6$ mN mm^{-2}. Mechanical characteristics show a high degree of regional variability and hormonal dependency.

A large number of studies on isolated uterine tissue have been carried out by recording electrically induced contractions. However, these results do not allow the reconstruction of active, $T^a(\lambda)$, and passive, $T^p(\lambda)$, force–stretch ratio relationships which are of prime importance. To date no experimental data are available on active uniaxial and biaxial stress–strain characteristics of the wall of the human uterus. Therefore, it is not surprising that biophysically credible models of the tissue as a mechanical continuum have not yet been constructed.

Under the assumptions of general isotropy and the zero stress–strain initial state, the constitutive equation for the passive myometrium yields

$$\begin{aligned}\sigma_s^r = &\left[\left(-c_1 + \frac{c_3}{c_2}\right) - \frac{c_3}{c_2}\frac{1 + \mathrm{I} - \mathrm{II}}{1 + \mathrm{I} - \mathrm{II} + \mathrm{III}}\right]\delta_s^r \\ &- \left[\frac{c_3}{c_2}\frac{1 + \mathrm{I}}{1 + \mathrm{I} - \mathrm{II} + \mathrm{III}}\right]\dot{\varepsilon}_s^r \\ &+ \left[\frac{c_3}{c_2^3}\frac{1}{1 + \mathrm{I} - \mathrm{II} + \mathrm{III}}\right]\dot{\varepsilon}_\alpha^r\dot{\varepsilon}_s^\alpha,\end{aligned} \tag{13.1}$$

where σ_s^r is the stress tensor, $\dot{\varepsilon}_s^r$ is the strain-rate tensor, δ_s^r is the Kronecker delta, I, II, III are the principal invariants of the ratio $\dot{\varepsilon}_s^r/c_2$, and c_i $(i = \overline{1, 3})$ are empirical constants. However, the relevance and validity of this model has never been examined. It is sufficient to note that in previous research the authors have demonstrated that it is only during the first short stage of labor that the myometrium exhibits isotropic characteristics. In advanced labor and during delivery it behaves as a material with properties of curvilinear anisotropy.

Various approaches have been developed for the modeling of uterine mechanics during parturition, the majority relying on assumptions of geometrical and physical linearity. In phenomenological models the 'uterus' is composed of N identical cells. At any given time, t, they are either in an active, $N_1(t)$, refractory, $N_2(t)$, or quiescent, $N_3(t)$, state. The system of differential equations is

$$\begin{aligned}\frac{dN_1(t)}{dt} &= \alpha N_3(t) - \frac{N_1(t)}{\tau} \\ \frac{dN_2(t)}{dt} &= \frac{N_1(t)}{\tau} - \frac{N_1(t - t_r)}{\tau} \\ \frac{dN_3(t)}{dt} &= \frac{N_1(t - t_r)}{\tau} - \alpha N_3(t), \quad t \geqslant 0 \\ 0 \leqslant N_i(t),\ N_i(t) &\leqslant N, \quad \text{where } i = 1, 2, 3 \\ N &= N_1(t) + N_2(t) + N_3(t).\end{aligned} \tag{13.2}$$

Here α is the excitability of the myocytes, τ is the natural lifetime of the active state, and t_r is the duration of the refractory state.

Results of numerical simulations obtained for different values of parameters and constants resemble the patterns of spontaneous contractility observed during normal labor. For large t, $t \gg 1/\alpha$, τ and t_r, the population of cells attain constant values

$$
\begin{aligned}
n_1(\lim) &= \frac{\alpha\tau N}{1+\alpha(\tau+t_r)}, \quad n_2(\lim) = \frac{\alpha t_r N}{1+\alpha(\tau+t_r)}, \\
n_3(\lim) &= \frac{N}{1+\alpha(\tau+t_r)},
\end{aligned}
\tag{13.3}
$$

where the amplitude of oscillations decreases and the 'uterus' succumbs to tonic contraction.

In a model of excitation with the contraction coupling in a single uterine smooth muscle cell, the calcium current accounts for the activity of voltage-gated Ca^{2+} channels

$$
I_{Ca} = \frac{g_{Ca}(V^s - V_{Ca})}{1 + \exp(V_{Ca,1/2} - V/S_{Ca,1/2})}, \tag{13.4}
$$

where I_{Ca} is the Ca^{2+} current, V^s is the transmembrane potential, $V_{Ca,1/2}$ is the half-activation potential, $S_{Ca,1/2}$ is the slope factor for the Ca^{2+} current, and g_{Ca} is the maximal conductance of the channel. The net $[Ca_i^{2+}]$ is defined by

$$
\frac{d[Ca_i^{2+}]}{dt} = I_{Ca} - I_{Ca,pump} + I_{Na/Ca}, \tag{13.5}
$$

where the efflux of Ca^{2+} through pumps was given by

$$
I_{Ca,pump} = V_{p,max} \frac{[Ca_i^{2+}]^{n_M}}{[Ca_i^{2+}]_{1/2}^{n_M} + [Ca_i^{2+}]^{n_M}}, \tag{13.6}
$$

and the Na^+/Ca^{2+} exchanger as

$$
I_{Na/Ca} = g_{Na/Ca} \frac{[Ca_i^{2+}]}{[Ca_i^{2+}]_{Na/Ca} + [Ca_i^{2+}]}(V^s - V_{Na/Ca}). \tag{13.7}
$$

In the above $[Ca_i^{2+}]_{1/2}^{n_M}$, $[Ca_i^{2+}]_{Na/Ca}$ are concentrations of Ca^{2+} for half-activation of the pump and the exchanger, respectively, $V_{Na/Ca}$ is the reversal potential of the Na^+/Ca^{2+} exchanger, $V_{p,max}$ is the maximal velocity of ion extraction by the Ca^{2+} pump, $g_{Na/Ca}$ is the conductance, and n_M is the Hill coefficient.

The four-state cross-bridge model relies on the dynamics of myosin light chain phosphorylation

$$\begin{aligned}\frac{dF_M}{dt} &= -k_1(t)F_M + k_2F_{Mp} + k_7F_{AM}\\ \frac{dF_{Mp}}{dt} &= k_4F_{AMp} + k_1(t)F_M - (k_2 + k_3)F_{Mp}\\ \frac{dF_{AMp}}{dt} &= k_3F_{Mp} + k_6(t)F_{AM} - (k_4 + k_5)F_{AMp}\\ \frac{dF_{AM}}{dt} &= k_5F_{AMp} - (k_7 + k_6(t))F_{AM},\end{aligned} \tag{13.8}$$

with the constraint

$$F_M(t) + F_{Mp}(t) + F_{AMp}(t) + F_{AM}(t) = 1. \tag{13.9}$$

The stress, σ, in the myocyte was calculated as

$$\sigma = \sigma_{\max}(F_{AM}(t) + F_{AMp}(t)). \tag{13.10}$$

Here F_M, F_{Mp}, F_{AMp}, F_{AM} are the fractional amounts of free unphosphorylated, phosphorylated (subscript p), attached phosphorylated, and attached dephosphorylated crossbridges, respectively, and k_{1-7} are the rates of chemical reactions.

The excitation–contraction coupling is ensured by the dependence of the rate parameter of MLCK phosphorylation $k_1(t)$ and $[\mathrm{Ca}_i^{2+}]$

$$k_1(t) = \frac{[\mathrm{Ca}_i^{2+}]^{n_\mathrm{M}}}{[\mathrm{Ca}_{\mathrm{MLCK}}^{2+}]_{1/2}^{n_\mathrm{M}} + [\mathrm{Ca}_i^{2+}]^{n_\mathrm{M}}}, \tag{13.11}$$

where $[\mathrm{Ca}_{\mathrm{MLCK}}^{2+}]_{1/2}^{n_\mathrm{M}}$ is the concentration of intracellular calcium required for half-activation of MLCK by Ca^{2+}–calmodulin.

Model simulations have reproduced voltage-clamp traces recorded experimentally on pregnant rats and human non-pregnant myometrial cells.

In their pioneering work Mizrahi and Karni (1975, 1978) modeled the gravid uterus as a thin axisymmetric elastic shell. The myometrium was treated as a homogeneous isotropic biomaterial with the general characteristics of smooth muscle tissue. The uterus was subjected to inner amniotic fluid pressure and its internal volume remained constant throughout. Deformations and displacements of the shell were small and only a single contraction was evaluated. The following kinematic relations were obtained

$$
\begin{aligned}
\varepsilon_{11}^{z} &= \frac{1}{\left(1+G_{31}^{1}x^{3}\right)}\left[\varepsilon_{11} + x^{3}\frac{\partial}{\partial\alpha^{1}}\left(2\frac{g_{12}\varepsilon_{23}-\varepsilon_{13}}{H^{2}}\right)\right.\\
&\quad \left. + \frac{\partial}{\partial\alpha^{1}}\left(2\frac{g_{12}\varepsilon_{13}-\varepsilon_{23}}{H^{2}}\right)g_{12} + \left(2\frac{g_{12}\varepsilon_{13}-\varepsilon_{23}}{H^{2}}\right)G_{211}\right]\\
\varepsilon_{22}^{z} &= \frac{1}{\left(1+G_{32}^{2}x^{3}\right)}\left[\varepsilon_{22} + x^{3}\frac{\partial}{\partial\alpha^{1}}\left(2\frac{g_{12}\varepsilon_{13}-\varepsilon_{23}}{H^{2}}\right)\right.\\
&\quad \left. + \frac{\partial}{\partial\alpha^{2}}\left(2\frac{g_{12}\varepsilon_{23}-\varepsilon_{13}}{H^{2}}\right)g_{12} + \left(2\frac{g_{12}\varepsilon_{23}-\varepsilon_{13}}{H^{2}}\right)G_{122}\right]\\
2\varepsilon_{12}^{z} &= \frac{1}{\left(1+G_{32}^{2}x^{3}\right)}\left[\omega_{2} + x^{3}\frac{\partial}{\partial\alpha^{2}}\left(2\frac{g_{12}\varepsilon_{23}-\varepsilon_{13}}{H^{2}}\right)\right.\\
&\quad \left. + \frac{\partial}{\partial\alpha^{2}}\left(2\frac{g_{12}\varepsilon_{13}-\varepsilon_{23}}{H^{2}}\right)g_{12} + \left(2\frac{g_{12}\varepsilon_{13}-\varepsilon_{23}}{H^{2}}\right)G_{212}\right]\\
&\quad + \frac{1}{\left(1+G_{31}^{1}x^{3}\right)}\left[\omega_{1} + x^{3}\frac{\partial}{\partial\alpha^{1}}\left(2\frac{g_{12}\varepsilon_{13}-\varepsilon_{23}}{H^{2}}\right)\right.\\
&\quad \left. + \frac{\partial}{\partial\alpha^{1}}\left(2\frac{g_{12}\varepsilon_{23}-\varepsilon_{13}}{H^{2}}\right)g_{12} + \left(2\frac{g_{12}\varepsilon_{23}-\varepsilon_{13}}{H^{2}}\right)G_{121}\right],
\end{aligned}
\tag{13.12}
$$

where (α^1, α^2) are the coordinate lines on the middle surface (S) of the shell, x^3 is the normal coordinate to S, g_{12} is the mixed component of the metric tensor, ε_{ij}, ε_{ij}^{z} $(i, j = 1, 2)$ are the strain tensors defined on the middle and equidistant, S_z, surfaces, respectively, ω_i $(i = 1, 2)$ is the rotation vector, G_{jk}^{i} is the geodesic torsion, and G_{iji}, G_{ii}^{j} $(i, j, k = 1, 2, 3)$ are the normal and geodesic curvatures, respectively.

The initial strain values at four distinct points on S_z were defined from measurements recorded from the abdominal surface of pregnant women in labor. The system of equation (13.12) was solved numerically. Time variations of the radii of curvature and torsions along the longitudinal and circular fibers were assessed. The results revealed that during the most intense contraction the curvature in the longitudinal direction increased by 200%, but in the circumferential direction by only 20%. These changes were associated with the transformation of the uterus from a pear-like to a more spherical shape.

A model of the uterus as a thin ellipsoid of revolution has been formulated and investigated. The myometrium was treated as a homogeneous, isotropic, and incompressible material. Deformations and displacements were finite. The equilibrium equations of the shell in terms of the undeformed reference configuration $(\bar{r}_1,\ \bar{r}_2,\ \phi)$ are given as

$$
\begin{aligned}
\frac{d\psi}{d\phi} &= \frac{P_n r_1 \lambda_\theta \lambda_\phi}{N_\theta} - \frac{N_\theta r_1}{N_\phi r} \sin\psi \\
\frac{d\lambda_\phi}{d\phi} &= \left(\frac{dN_\phi}{d\phi}\right)^{-1} \left(N_\theta \cos\phi - N_\phi \frac{r_1}{r} \cos\psi\right) - \frac{dN_\phi}{d\theta}\left(\frac{dN_\theta}{d\phi}\right)^{-1} \frac{d\lambda_\phi}{d\phi} \\
\frac{d\lambda_\theta}{d\phi} &= \frac{r_1}{r}(\lambda_\phi \cos\psi - \lambda_\theta \cos\phi),
\end{aligned}
\tag{13.13}
$$

where P_n is the internal amniotic fluid pressure, $\bar{r}_1$, $\bar{r}_2$, ϕ, ψ are geometric parameters, λ_ϕ, λ_θ are the stretch ratios, and N_ϕ, N_θ are the in-plane forces per unit length in the longitudinal and circumferential directions, respectively. Two types of constitutive relationships have been considered, i.e. Mooney–Rivlin

$$
\begin{aligned}
N_\phi &= \frac{2}{\lambda_\phi}(\lambda_\phi^2 - \lambda_\theta^{-2}\lambda_\phi^{-2})(1 + \underline{\alpha}\lambda_\theta^2) \\
N_\theta &= \frac{2}{\lambda_\theta}(\lambda_\theta^2 - \lambda_\theta^{-2}\lambda_\phi^{-2})(1 + \underline{\alpha}\lambda_\phi^2), \qquad \underline{\alpha} - \text{const}
\end{aligned}
\tag{13.14}
$$

and neo-Hookean ($\underline{\alpha} = 0$)

$$
\begin{aligned}
N_\phi &= \frac{2}{\lambda_\phi}(\lambda_\phi^2 - \lambda_\theta^{-2}\lambda_\phi^{-2}) \\
N_\theta &= \frac{2}{\lambda_\theta}(\lambda_\theta^2 - \lambda_\theta^{-2}\lambda_\phi^{-2}).
\end{aligned}
\tag{13.15}
$$

The lower segment and apex of the uterus were clamped and the organ maintained axial symmetry throughout. The effect of physical nonlinearities and the initial configuration on intrauterine pressure and volume were analyzed.

The stress–strain distribution in the organ under static conditions with regard to internal amniotic pressure was investigated on a three-dimensional finite element model of the uterus. An agreement between theoretical results and *in vivo* clinical measurements was achieved through multiple numerical experiments and adjustments of input parametric data.

Studies have been conducted to analyze the process of cervix opening during the first short stage of labor. The cervix was modeled as an axisymmetric orthotropic thin membrane. The tissue was assumed to be a homogeneous, incompressible biocomposite with exponentially elastic and viscoelastic properties. Deformations were small but displacements were finite. The head was in the vertex position and exerted dilatational constant pressure on the membrane. No friction condition was imposed between the head and the cervix. The axial load was defined *a priori* as a function of time.

The four degrees-of-freedom linear element approximation was solved for deflection confined by sliding curved restraints. The results of the model predicted an elastic stretch and a small viscous strain during a single contraction, a monotonic relationship between internal pressure and dilatation, and continuous opening of the cervix following unimpeded fetal descent. However, no comparison to real experimental data was made.

The biomechanics of cervical insufficiency, a medically worrisome condition related to a dilatation of the cervix in the absence of myometrial contractions, has been investigated experimentally and studied theoretically. The cervix constitutes a viscoelastic two compartmental continuum. The first compartment is comprised of connective tissue, i.e. collagen and elastin fibers, embedded into the hydrated ground substance of glycosaminoglycans and proteoglycans. The second is represented by interstitial fluid. Diffusion of interstitial fluid between the two compartments satisfies Darcy's law. The constitutive model both accounts for the mechanics of the individual components and captures tissue growth and remodeling. It takes the form

$$\sigma = \frac{1}{J}(f_1^0 J_1\sigma_1 + f_2^0 J_2\sigma_2) + \sigma_{el} + \Delta p, \tag{13.16}$$

where

$$\sigma_1 = \sigma_c + \sigma_{\mathrm{BG}} + \sigma_{\mathrm{IC}}, \qquad \sigma_2 = \sigma_{\mathrm{FG}}.$$

Here σ is the macroscopic Cauchy stress in the cervical stroma, f_i^0 is the volume fractions, J, J_i are the total and compartmental volumetric stretches, ($i = 1, 2$ indicates compartments), and p is hydrostatic pressure. Macroscopic stresses in the collagen and elastin networks, σ_c, σ_{el}, stresses produced by bound, σ_{BG}, and free, σ_{FG}, aminoglycans, and inter-compartmental pressure, σ_{IC}, are given by

$$\begin{aligned}
\sigma_c &= \frac{\mu\lambda_L}{\xi^3 J_1}\left[\frac{1}{\lambda_c}\beta\left(\frac{\lambda_L}{\lambda_c}\right)\mathbf{B}_c - \beta_0\mathbf{I}\right] \\
\sigma_{el} &= B_{el}(J - 1)\mathbf{I} \\
\sigma_j &= B_{\mathrm{GAG}}\ln(J_j)\ (j = \mathrm{BG, FG}) \\
\sigma_{\mathrm{IC}} &= \sigma_0\sqrt[m]{\dot{\varepsilon}_v/\dot{\varepsilon}_v^0}\,.
\end{aligned} \tag{13.17}$$

Here $\mathbf{B}_c$, $\mathbf{I}$ are the left Cauchy–Green and identity tensors, respectively, of the gradient of deformation, μ is the initial collagen modulus, λ_L, λ_c are the maximal (L) and current (c) stretch ratios of a collagen fibril, B_{el}, B_{GAG} are the bulk moduli of elastin and glycosaminoglycans, σ_0 is the flow strength, $\dot{\varepsilon}_v^0$, $\dot{\varepsilon}_v$ are the initial and current volumetric flow rates, and ξ, m, β, β_0 are structural parameters.

The configurations of the uterus and surrounding anatomical structures have been reconstructed digitally from a set of magnetic resonance images obtained from gravid women. It was assumed that the uterus underwent axisymmetric deformations throughout. Contractions of the myometrium were mimicked by varying the amniotic pressure versus time. Stress–strain distribution in the organ was analyzed using a commercial finite element solver. Continuum four-node tetrahedron elements were adopted to model the uterus and three-node triangular general-purpose shell elements were chosen to simulate the amniotic membrane. Mechanical parameters were estimated from *in vitro* experiments on samples excised from pregnant human uteri. The 'missing' data were amended during numerical simulations. Results have provided an insight into the stress–strain distribution in the cervical region and the 'dynamics' of dilatation at quasi-static states.

13.8.2 Models of myoelectrical activity

A plausible model of electrical activity of a myocyte employs the general principles of the Hodgkin–Huxley formalism

$$C_m \frac{dV^s}{dt} = -(I_{\mathrm{Na}} + I_{\mathrm{Ca}} + I_{\mathrm{K}_v} + I_{\mathrm{Ca-K}} + I_{\mathrm{Cl}}) + I_{\mathrm{stim}}. \tag{13.18}$$

Here I_{Na}, I_{Ca}, I_{K_v}, I_{Ca-K}, I_{Cl} are the voltage-gated Na^+, Ca^{2+}, $\mathrm{K_v}$ (a mix of three different types of potassium), Ca^{2+}-activated K^+ and Cl^- currents, respectively, I_{stim} is the stimulus current, and C_m is the specific membrane capacitance. Each current was related to the membrane voltage, reversal potentials, V_i, for $i = \mathrm{Na}^+$, Ca^{2+}, K^+ and Cl^- ions, the specific conductance, g_i, and gating variables m_i, n_i, and h_i as

$$\begin{aligned}
I_{\mathrm{Na}} &= g_{\mathrm{Na}} m_{\mathrm{Na}}^2 h_{\mathrm{Na}} (V^s - V_{\mathrm{Na}}) \\
I_{\mathrm{Ca-K}} &= g_{\mathrm{K(Ca)}} \left(\frac{[\mathrm{Ca}_i^{2+}]^n}{[\mathrm{Ca}_i^{2+}]_{1/2}^n + [\mathrm{Ca}_i^{2+}]^n} \right) (V^s - V_{\mathrm{Na}}) \\
I_{\mathrm{Ca}} &= g_{\mathrm{Ca}} m_{\mathrm{Ca}}^2 h_{1\mathrm{Ca}} h_{2\mathrm{Ca}} (V^s - V_{\mathrm{Ca}}) \\
I_{\mathrm{K}} &= g_{\mathrm{K}} n_{\mathrm{K1}} n_{\mathrm{K2}} h_{\mathrm{K1}} (V^s - V_{\mathrm{K}}) \\
I_{\mathrm{Cl}} &= g_{\mathrm{Cl}} (V^s - V_{\mathrm{Cl}}).
\end{aligned} \tag{13.19}$$

The dynamics of intracellular calcium are described by

$$\frac{d[\mathrm{Ca}_i^{2+}]}{dt} = f_c (\alpha I_{\mathrm{Ca}} - K_{\mathrm{Ca}} [\mathrm{Ca}_i^{2+}]). \tag{13.20}$$

Here f_c is the probability of the influx of Ca^{2+}, α is the conversion factor, and K_{Ca} represents the sequestration, extrusion, and buffering processes of calcium by intracellular compartments.

The variation of m_i, n_i, and h_i satisfy the first order differential equations

$$\begin{aligned}
\frac{dm_{\mathrm{Na}}}{dt} &= \frac{1}{\tau_{m\mathrm{Na}}}(m_{\mathrm{Na}\infty} - m_{\mathrm{Na}}), & \frac{dh_{\mathrm{Na}}}{dt} &= \frac{1}{\tau_{h\mathrm{Na}}}(h_{\mathrm{Na}\infty} - h_{\mathrm{Na}}), \\
\frac{dm_{\mathrm{Ca}}}{dt} &= \frac{1}{\tau_{m\mathrm{Ca}}}(m_{\mathrm{Ca}\infty} - m_{\mathrm{Ca}}), & \frac{dh_{1\mathrm{Ca}}}{dt} &= \frac{1}{\tau_{h1\mathrm{Ca}}}(h_{1\mathrm{Ca}\infty} - h_{1\mathrm{Ca}}), \\
\frac{dh_{2\mathrm{Ca}}}{dt} &= \frac{1}{\tau_{h1\mathrm{Ca}}}(h_{2\mathrm{Ca}\infty} - h_{2\mathrm{Ca}}), & \frac{dn_{\mathrm{K1}}}{dt} &= \frac{1}{\tau_{\mathrm{K1}}}(n_{\mathrm{K1}\infty} - n_{\mathrm{K1}}), \\
\frac{dn_{\mathrm{K2}}}{dt} &= \frac{1}{\tau_{\mathrm{K2}}}(n_{\mathrm{K2}\infty} - n_{\mathrm{K2}}), & \frac{dh_{\mathrm{K1}}}{dt} &= \frac{1}{\tau_{h1}}(h_{\mathrm{K1}\infty} - h_{\mathrm{K1}}),
\end{aligned} \tag{13.21}$$

where

$$
\begin{aligned}
m_{\mathrm{Na}\infty} &= 1\bigg/\left(1 + \exp\frac{(V^s + 21)}{-5}\right),\\
h_{\mathrm{Na}\infty} &= 1\bigg/\left(1 + \exp\frac{(V^s + 58.9)}{8.7}\right),\\
m_{\mathrm{Ca}\infty} &= 1\bigg/\left(1 + \exp\frac{(V^s + V_{\mathrm{Ca},1/2})}{S_{\mathrm{Ca}}}\right),\\
h_{1\mathrm{Ca}\infty} &= 1\bigg/\left(1 + \exp\frac{(V^s + 34)}{5.4}\right),\\
n_{\mathrm{K}j\infty} &= 1\bigg/\left(1 + \exp\frac{(V^s + V_{\mathrm{K}j,1/2}}{S_{\mathrm{K}j}}\right),\\
h_{\mathrm{K}1\infty} &= 1\bigg/\left(1 + \exp\frac{(V^s + V_{h\mathrm{K}1,1/2})}{S_{h\mathrm{K}1}}\right).
\end{aligned}
\tag{13.22}
$$

Here $V_{\mathrm{Ca},1/2}$, $V_{\mathrm{K}j,1/2}$, $V_{h\mathrm{K}1,1/2}$ are the half-activation potentials, and S_{Ca}, $S_{\mathrm{K}j}$, $S_{h\mathrm{K}1}$ $(j = 1, 2)$ are the slope factors for specific currents. Time constants

$$
\begin{aligned}
\tau_{m\mathrm{Na}} &= 0.25\exp(-0.02V^s)\\
\tau_{h\mathrm{Na}} &= 0.22\exp(-0.06V^s) + 0.366\\
\tau_{m\mathrm{Ca}} &= 0.64\exp(-0.04V^s) + 1.188\\
\tau_{h1\mathrm{Ca}}, \tau_{\mathrm{K}j}, \tau_{h1} &= \text{const},
\end{aligned}
\tag{13.23}
$$

are adjusted during simulations.

The model reproduces a variety of electrical patterns, i.e. slow wave and bursting with action potential generation, recorded in the myometrium at term.

In a model of the propagation of the wave of excitation, $V^s = V^s(x, y)$, in a two-dimensional electrically isotropic uterine syncytium, only three ion currents are retained:

$$
C_m\frac{\partial V^s}{\partial t} = \frac{1}{R_a}\nabla V^s - (I_{\mathrm{Ca}} + I_{\mathrm{K}_v} + I_{\mathrm{Ca-K}}) + I_{\mathrm{stim}}. \tag{13.24}
$$

Here $\nabla(\nabla = \frac{\partial}{\partial x}\bar{i} + \frac{\partial}{\partial y}\bar{j})$ is the spatial gradient operator, R_a is the axial syncytial resistance, and the meanings of the other parameters are as described above. The dynamics of I_{Ca}, I_{K_v}, $I_{\mathrm{Ca-K}}$ currents are given by equations (13.19)–(13.24).

The results of numerical simulations have revealed the preferred axial spread of excitation. The amplitude of V decreases away from the pacemaker whilst the predicted conduction velocity corresponds to the value obtained experimentally from the rat myometrium at term.

A bidomain model of the abdomen with an enclosed uterus has been proposed. This aims to study the propagation of the wave of depolarization, $V^s = V^s V(\bar{r}, t)$, in the myometrium, and the induced magnetic field, $\vec{B}$, on the abdominal surface. The model formulation is given by

$$C_m \frac{\partial V^s}{\partial t} = \left(G_i - \frac{G_i}{G_i + G_e} \right) \nabla^2 V^s - I_{\text{ion}} + I_{\text{stim}}$$
$$\nabla \times \vec{B} = - G_i(\mu_A + \sigma_A) \nabla V^s. \qquad (13.25)$$

Here G_i, G_e are the intracellular and extracellular conductivities and μ_A, σ_A are the permeability and conductivity constants of the abdominal space. The uterus has been considered as an electrically anisotropic sphere of radius $\bar{r}$, with the pacemaker cell located in the polar region. A modified form of the Fitzhugh–Nagumo equations has been employed to describe the ion current dynamics

$$I_{\text{ion}} = k(V^s - V_a)(V^s - 1)V^s - v^*$$
$$\frac{dv^*}{dt} = \underline{\varepsilon}(V^s - \gamma v^*), \qquad (13.26)$$

where v^* is the recovery variable and k, V_a, $\underline{\varepsilon}$, γ are empirical parameters.

The model supposedly reproduces electromyograms and magnetograms recorded from the pregnant uterus. However, the results of numerical simulations are inconclusive.

Investigations into the conditions and morphostructural principles for autorhythmicity have proved that the organization of the myometrium is of fundamental importance to the generation, maintenance, and propagation of the wave of excitation within it. Multiple components of interconnected signaling pathways play various roles in the temporal features of the oscillation phenomenon. Assuming a linear coupling by gap junctions, their evolution is governed by

$$C_{mi} \frac{dV_i^s}{dt} = -I_{\text{ion},i} + (-1)^i g(V_1 - V_2) \quad i = 1, 2 \qquad (13.27)$$

and clearly demonstrates the possibility of bursting activity. In the above, $i = 1$ is referred to as a group of excitable cells, $i = 2$ is a group of non-excitable cells, and g is the coupling conductance. The ion current $I_{\text{ion},1}$ is defined by equation (13.18), and $I_{\text{ion},2} = g_m(V_2 - V_r)$, where g_m is the membrane conductance and V_r is the resting membrane potential. A sensitivity analysis reveals that ion channels with fast activation/deactivation dynamics are responsible for spike production. Essential elements for the existence and sustainability of pacemaker activity are: relative uncoupling of the pacemaker from the surrounding tissue, the presence of a gradual transition zone, and distributed tissue anisotropy.

A model analysis of synchronization and bursting in the uterine muscle in late pregnancy reveal four types of spatial automaticity: (i) sparse, with reduced amplitude of spikes; (ii) clustered, wherein a group of cells act as an independent local pacemaker; (iii) uniform, with constant depolarization or small amplitude spike oscillations; and (iv) coherent, with a synchronous discharge of spatially distributed pacemakers. The specific pattern depends entirely on the strength of cellular coupling.

The existing models of the gravid human uterus, as described above, are based on the application of the general principles of solid mechanics and the theory of thin elastic shells. They incorporate some morphological data on the structure and function of the organ giving hope that the principles of biomechanics can be applied to the uterus during labor and delivery. Although these models are of limited biomedical value, they do serve as a platform for the further development of integrative and biologically plausible models.

13.9 General model postulates

Based on experimental data and clinical observations obtained during pregnancy and delivery (section 13.7), it becomes clear that the pregnant uterus satisfies all the hypotheses and assumptions of the theory of soft shells.

Myometrial contractions in the gravid uterus are triggered by underlying electrical events in myocytes. The principle electrophysiological phenomena assume that:

(i) The human myometrium is composed of two interspersed muscle strata, longitudinal and circumferential, with fasciculi running orthogonally within them.

(ii) The myometrium at term endows the properties of weak electrical anisotropy (longitudinal layer) and isotropy (circumferential layer) with multiple gap junctions composed of connexin proteins of types 40, 43, and 45, providing a low electrical resistance gating among myocytes.

(iii) The electrical activity of either single spikes or bursts of spikes represents the integrated function of the following ion channels: voltage-dependent Ca^{2+} channels of L- and T-types, large Ca^{2+}-activated K^+ channels (BK_{Ca}), potential sensitive K^+ channels, and Cl^- channels, (the expression of the two voltage-gated Na^+ channels has been reported in the human uterus although their role in gestation and labor is still a matter of debate). The properties of the channels are neurohormonally modulated; the effect is mainly chronotropic with an increase in the time of permeability for specific ions.

(iv) Pacemaker cells *per se* have not been found in the uterus, although there are localized functional pacemaker zones near the uterotubal junctions responsible for the generation of electrical signals and the coordinated rhythmic contractions of labor.

(v) Contractions are involuntary and, for the most part, independent of external control; internal regulation is provided by multiple neurotransmitters and hormones. All chemical reactions of substrate transformation satisfy first order Michaelis–Menten kinetics.

(vi) The active force T^a–Ca_i^{2+} activity relationship is a generalized approximation of the experimental curves characteristic of SM given by equation (10.4).

(vii) The total force $T_{c,l}$ generated by the myometrial layers is the result of deformation of its passive elements, T^p (λ_c, λ_l, c_i), i.e. collagen and elastin fibers, and active contraction–relaxation of SMCs, T^a ($\lambda_{c,l}$, $Z_{mn}^{(*)}$, $[Ca_i^{2+}]$, c_i).

Electrochemical and chemoelectrical coupling in the system is guaranteed by separate and/or conjoint activation of multiple intracellular pathways along with ligand-dependent transmembrane ion channels as previously described.

13.10 Investigations into the myometrium

13.10.1 Mathematical model of the myometrium

Smooth muscle cells in the fasciculus are connected by tight junctions to form a homogeneous electromechanical biological continuum that is treated as a soft fiber thread. Let the fasciculus of length L be referred to a local Lagrange coordinate system. Its equation of motion is given by equation (10.23), while the force–stretch ratio and the active-force–intracellular Ca_i^{2+} relationship for the myometrium yields equations (10.2) and (10.4), respectively. The system of equations for the oscillatory activity of the membrane potential V yields the system of equations (10.5)–(10.9).

The evolution of L- and T-type Ca^{2+}-channels depends on the wave of depolarization, V^s, and is defined by

$$\begin{aligned} g_{Ca}^{s}(t) &= [\delta(V) + (\lambda(t) - 1)](\max g_{Ca}^{s}), \\ g_{Ca}^{f}(t) &= (\lambda(t) - 1)g_{Ca}^{f}, \end{aligned} \tag{13.28}$$

where

$$\lambda(t) \geqslant 1.0, \quad \delta(V) = \begin{cases} 1, & \text{for } V \geqslant V_p^s \\ 0, & \text{otherwise} \end{cases}.$$

Here V_p^s is the threshold value for V^s.

The propagation of the wave of excitation V^s is described by

$$C_m = \frac{\partial V^s}{\partial t} = \frac{d_m}{R_s}\frac{\partial}{\partial \alpha}\left(\lambda(\alpha)\frac{\partial V^s}{\partial \alpha}\right) - (I_{Na} + I_{K2} + I_{Cl}), \tag{13.29}$$

where d_m is the diameter, R_s is the specific resistance of the fasciculus, and

$$\begin{aligned} I_{Na} &= g_{Na}\hat{m}^3\hat{h}(V^s - V_{Na}) \\ I_{K2} &= g_{K2}\hat{n}^4(V^s - V_{K2}) \\ I_{Cl} &= g_{Cl}(V^s - V_{Cl}). \end{aligned} \tag{13.30}$$

Here g_{Na}, g_{K2}, g_{Cl} are the maximal conductances, and V_{Na}, V_{K2}, V_{Cl} are the reversal potentials of the membrane currents Na^+, K_{v2}^+, and Cl^-, respectively. The dynamics of the variables $\hat{m}$, $\hat{h}$, $\hat{n}$ are described by

$$\frac{d\hat{m}}{dt} = \hat{\alpha}_m(1 - \hat{m}) - \hat{\beta}_m\hat{m}$$
$$\frac{d\hat{h}}{dt} = \hat{\alpha}_h(1 - \hat{h}) - \hat{\beta}_h\hat{h} \qquad (13.31)$$
$$\frac{d\hat{n}}{dt} = \hat{\alpha}_n(1 - \hat{n}) - \hat{\beta}_n\hat{n}$$

with the activation $\hat{\alpha}_y$ and deactivation $\hat{\beta}_y$ $(y = \hat{m}, \hat{h}, \hat{n})$ parameters given by

$$\hat{\alpha}_m = \frac{0.005(V^s - V_m)}{\exp 0.1(V^s - V_m) - 1}, \quad \hat{\beta}_m = 0.2\exp\frac{(V^s + V_m)}{38},$$
$$\hat{\alpha}_h = 0.014\exp\frac{-(V_h + V^s)}{20}, \quad \hat{\beta}_h = \frac{0.2}{1 + \exp 0.2(V_h - V^s)}, \qquad (13.32)$$
$$\hat{\alpha}_n = \frac{0.006(V^s - V_n)}{\exp 0.1(V^s - V_n) - 1}, \quad \hat{\beta}_n = 0.75\exp(V^n - V^s).$$

Here V_m, V_h, V_n are the reversal potentials for activation and inactivation of Na^+ and $K_{v2}{}^+$ ion currents of the myometrium.

It has been assumed that at the initial moment the fasciculus is in an unexcitable state

$$V^s(\alpha, 0) = 0, \quad v(\alpha, 0) = 0, \quad [Ca_i^{2+}] = [\overset{0}{Ca}{}_i^{2+}],$$
$$\hat{m} = \hat{m}_\infty, \quad \hat{h} = \hat{h}_\infty, \quad \hat{n} = \hat{n}_\infty, \quad \tilde{h} = \tilde{h}_\infty, \quad \tilde{n} = \tilde{n}_\infty, \quad \tilde{x}_{Ca} = \tilde{x}_{Ca}^\infty. \qquad (13.33)$$

It is activated by a series of discharges of action potentials

$$V^s(0, t) = \begin{cases} \overset{0}{V^s}, & 0 < t < t^d \\ 0, & t \geqslant t^d \end{cases}, \quad V^s(0, t) = V(t). \qquad (13.34)$$

The ends of the myofiber are clamped and remain unexcitable throughout

$$V^s(0, t) = V^s(L, t) = 0, \quad v(0, t) = v(L, t) = 0. \qquad (13.35)$$

The mathematical formulation as above describes: (i) the self-oscillatory behavior and/or myometrial electrical activity of the myofiber induced by discharges of a 'pacemaker' cell; (ii) the generation and propagation of the wave of depolarization along the myofiber; (iii) the coupling of spatially distributed oscillators; (iv) the generation of action potentials; (v) the dynamics of the cytosolic Ca^{2+} transients; (vi) active and passive force generation; and (vii) the deformation of the fasciculus and the following excitation of the cell membrane with contractions.

The parameters and constants used in simulations have been derived from the published literature. Values not found have been adjusted during the experiments in order to closely mimic the behavior of the biological prototype.

13.10.2 Physiological responses

The resting membrane potential of the fasciculus is $V^r = -59$ mV. Continuous fluctuations are at a low rate with amplitudes of L-type (0.08 nA) and T-type Ca^{2+} (0.48 nA), respectively. The outward K^+ (0.03 nA), BK_{Ca} (0.62 nA), and small chloride (0.04 nA) currents result in oscillations of the membrane potential V known as slow waves. Their frequency, $\nu = 0.02$ Hz, and amplitude, $V = 27$ mV, remain constant. The maximum rate of depolarization is calculated as 9 mV s^{-1} and for repolarization, 7.5 mV s^{-1}.

The slow wave induces the flux of Ca^{2+} ions inside the cell at a rate of 0.057 μM s^{-1}. There is a 20 s time delay in the intracellular calcium transients when compared to the wave of depolarization. Free cytosolic calcium at $\max[Ca_i^{2+}] = 0.44$ μM activates the contractile protein system with the production of spontaneous contractions, $T^a = 13.6$ mN cm^{-1} (figure 13.4). In both phase and time these follow the dynamics of calcium oscillations and are normally preceded by slow waves.

High frequency discharges of an intrinsic pacemaker initiate high magnitude ion currents: $\tilde{I}^s_{Ca} = 0.4$, $\tilde{I}^f_{Ca} = 0.51$, $\tilde{I}_{K1} = 0.2$, $\tilde{I}_{Ca-K} = 1.0$, and $\tilde{I}_{Cl} = 0.5$ nA, respectively, and the generation of action potentials of amplitudes 38–45 mV at a frequency of 2.7 Hz. A concomitant rise in intracellular calcium to 0.51 μM causes the development of active force, 16.6 mN cm^{-1}. Once electrical discharges are terminated, the myofiber returns to its unexcited state.

13.10.3 Effects of changes in Ca_0^{2+}

A gradual increase in extracellular calcium leads to depolarization of the membrane. Concentrations of Ca_0^{2+} that are between three and five times above normal cause the up-shift of the resting potential to −34 mV and −31 mV, respectively (figure 13.5). This is associated with an exponential rise in free intracellular calcium to 0.72 μM. The myometrium undergoes a tonic contraction, $T^a = 23.75$ mN cm^{-1}.

A concurrent electrical stimulation of the myofiber evokes ion currents of intensities $\tilde{I}^s_{Ca} = 1.3$, $\tilde{I}^f_{Ca} = 0.61$, $\tilde{I}_{K1} = 0.62$, $\tilde{I}_{Ca-K} = 1.63$, and $\tilde{I}_{Cl} = 1.89$ nA, and the transient production of a burst of high frequency, $\nu = 6$ Hz, with action potentials of amplitude 53 mV. The fast T-type Ca^{2+} current provides the main influx of intracellular calcium during which $\max[Ca_i^{2+}] = 0.62$ μM is recorded. The fasciculus generates the active force, $T^a = 20.7$ mN cm^{-1}. The reversal of extracellular calcium to its physiological level brings the myofiber back to its original electromechanical activity.

Slow wave oscillations cease in a calcium free environment. The fasciculus becomes hyperpolarized at a constant level, $V = -50$ mV. The concentration of intracellular calcium decreases to 0.1 μM and is now insufficient to sustain mechanical contractions. The myofiber remains relaxed.

13.10.4 Effects of changes in K_0^+

A two-fold increase in the concentration of extracellular potassium depolarizes the membrane, $V^r = -30$ mV, and abolishes slow waves (figure 13.6). The ion currents

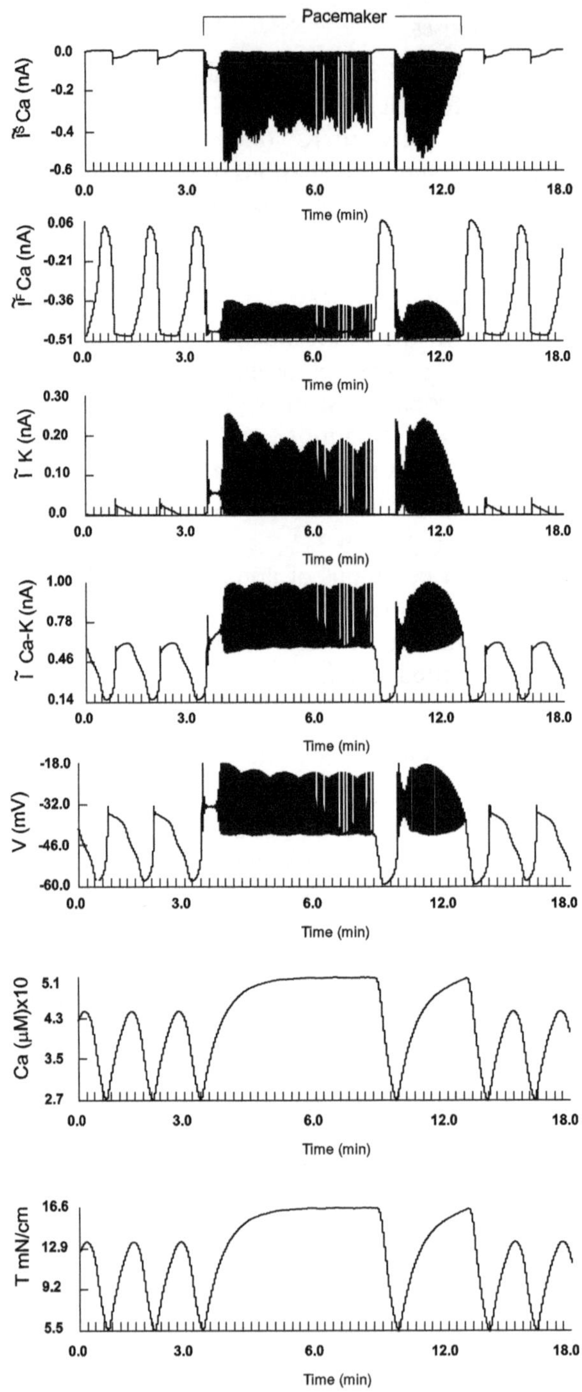

Figure 13.4. Normal electromechanical activity of the myometrial fasciculus. Traces from top to bottom indicate: ion currents, depolarization wave dynamics, intracellular calcium changes, and total force. Reprinted from Miftahof R M and Nam H G 2011 *Biomechanics of the Gravid Human Uterus* (Berlin: Springer) by permission from Springer Nature. Copyright 2011.

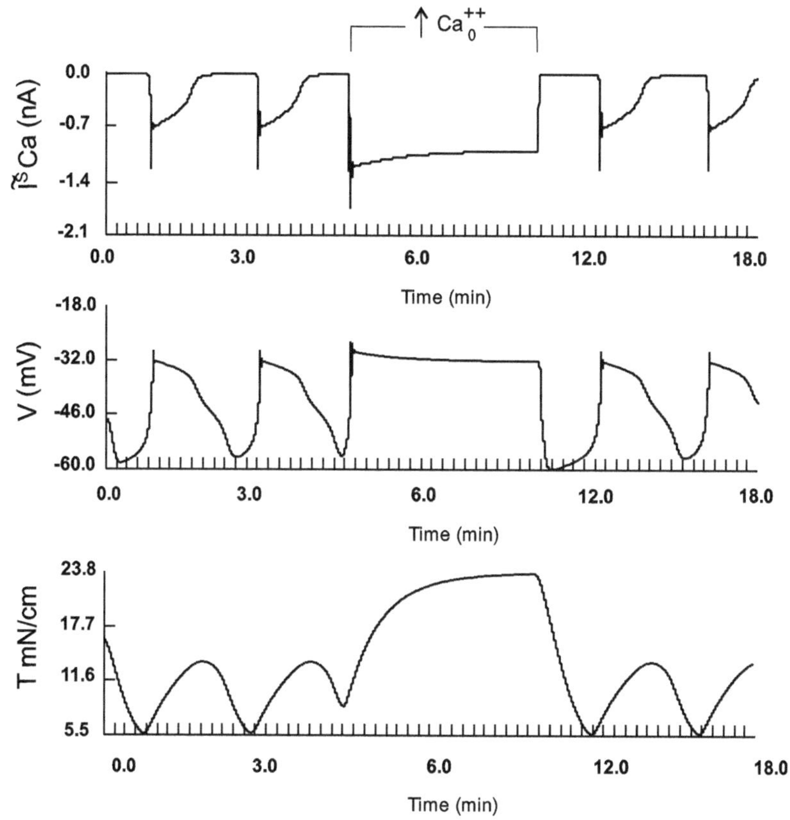

Figure 13.5. Response of the myofiber to changes in external Ca^{2+} concentration. Reprinted from Miftahof R M and Nam H G 2011 *Biomechanics of the Gravid Human Uterus* (Berlin: Springer) by permission from Springer Nature. Copyright 2011.

display constant dynamics: $\tilde{I}^s_{Ca} = 0.04$, $\tilde{I}^f_{Ca} = 0.48$, $\tilde{I}_{K1} = 0.42$, and $\tilde{I}_{Ca-K} = 0.51$ nA. The L- and T-type Ca^{2+} currents contribute equally to a rise in the intracellular calcium level, $[Ca_i^{2+}] = 0.5$ μM, and the contraction of the myofiber, $T^a = 15$ mN cm^{-1}.

The following four-fold increase in $[K_0^+]$ further depolarizes the membrane, $V^r = -20$ mV. The intensity of the outward potassium current increases to 0.52 nA with a concomitant attenuation of the respective currents: $\tilde{I}^s_{Ca} = 0.032$, $\tilde{I}^f_{Ca} = 0.39$, and $\tilde{I}_{Ca-K} = 0.14$ nA. There is an exponential decline in $[Ca_i^{2+}]$ to 0.44 μM and in the intensity of force, $T^a = 13.6$ mN cm^{-1}.

A superimposed electrical excitation leads to a burst of high amplitude, $V = 30$ mV, and frequency, $\nu = 7.3$ Hz, action potentials. The intracellular calcium content rises to 0.52 μM, and the fasciculus produces an active force of 16.8 mN cm^{-1}.

A simultaneous elevation in the concentration of extracellular potassium and calcium ions stabilizes the membrane potential at -18 mV. The intracellular calcium, $[Ca_i^{2+}] = 0.65$ μM, triggers a strong contraction of the myofiber, max $T^a = 21.8$ mN cm^{-1} (figure 13.7).

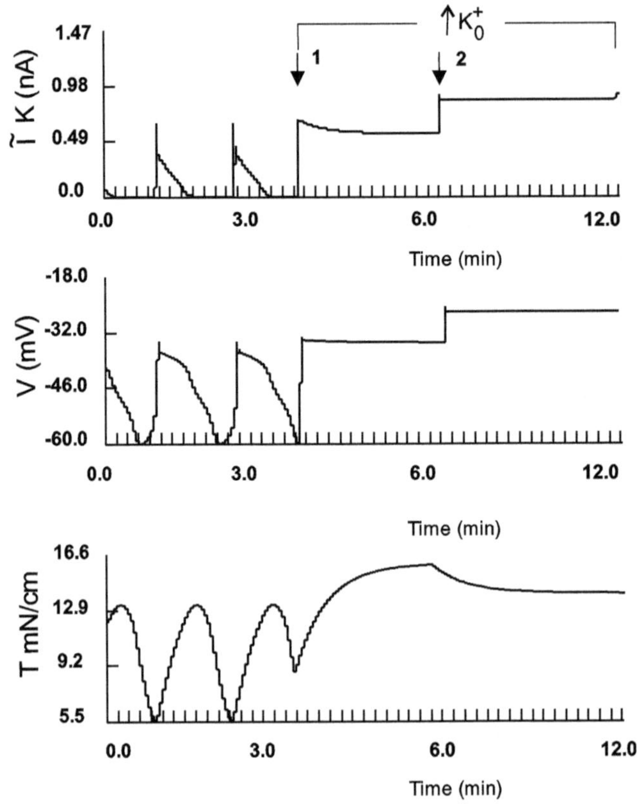

Figure 13.6. Dose-dependent responses of the 'fiber' to changes in external K^+ concentration. Reprinted from Miftahof R M and Nam H G 2011 *Biomechanics of the Gravid Human Uterus* (Berlin: Springer) by permission from Springer Nature. Copyright 2011.

A gradual reduction of $[K_0^+]$ hyperpolarizes the fasciculus, $V^r = -70$ and -88 mV (figure 13.8). The slow wave amplitude and frequency increase to 40 mV, $\nu = 0.032$ Hz and 58 mV, $\nu = 0.037$ Hz. Concurrent multiple discharges of a pacemaker bring about the production of spikes of average amplitude 60 mV at a frequency of ~6 Hz. There is a weakening of the calcium influx, $\max[Ca_i^{2+}] = 0.25$ and $0.18\ \mu$M, and tension, $T^a = 4.5$ and 2.2 mN cm^{-1}. Interestingly, the electrical stimulation further reduces the strength of contraction, $T^a = 1.1$ mN cm^{-1}, whilst the duration of contractions also decreases.

13.10.5 Effects of changes in Cl_0^-

A decrease in the chloride extracellular concentration at 1.5 times above the normal rate lowers the resting membrane potential of the myometrium to -68 mV. Slow waves are generated at a frequency of 0.027 Hz and an amplitude of 35 mV. There is a decrease in intracellular calcium, 0.33 μM, and an associated fall in the strength of tension, $T^a = 10$ mN cm^{-1}. A two-fold decrease in $[Cl_0^-]$ hyperpolarizes the fasciculus to -75 mV, causing its oscillatory activity to cease. The concentration of

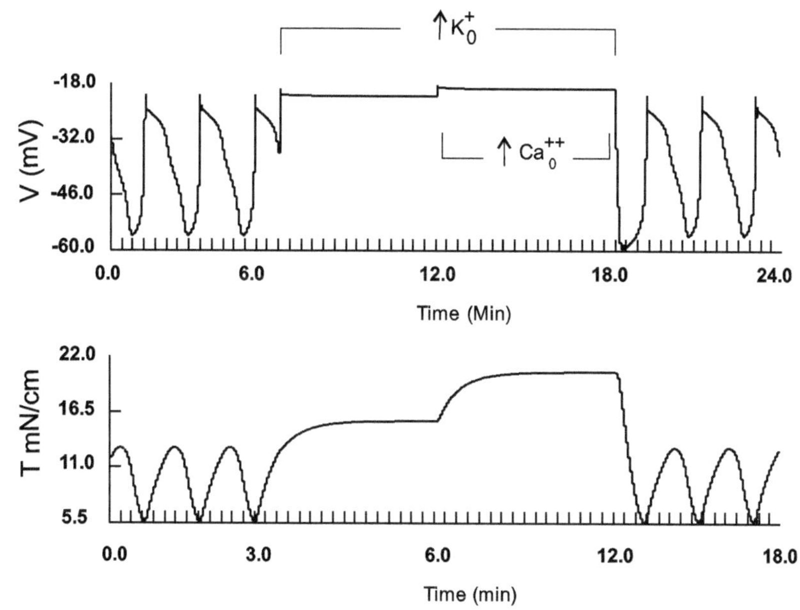

Figure 13.7. Effect of conjoint changes in extracellular K^+ and Ca^{2+} concentrations on electromechanical responses of the myofiber. Reprinted from Miftahof R M and Nam H G 2011 *Biomechanics of the Gravid Human Uterus* (Berlin: Springer) by permission from Springer Nature. Copyright 2011.

intracellular calcium drops to 0.03 μM and thus spontaneous mechanical contractility cannot be induced (figure 13.8).

The subsequent elevation of the extracellular chloride concentration abolishes slow waves and depolarizes the membrane at −35 mV. It is associated with a rise in cytosolic calcium to 0.48 μM and the development of tonic contraction, $T^a = 16.5$ mN cm^{-1}.

13.10.6 Effects of a T-type Ca^{2+} channel antagonist

The cumulative addition of a selective T-type Ca^{2+} channel blocker, mibefradil, produces a concentration-dependent reduction not only of the fast inward calcium current, but also in the amplitude and frequency of slow waves, calcium transients, and the intensity of contractions of the myometrium (figure 13.9). Thus, immediately following application of the drug there is a decrease in the amplitude of the fast T-type Ca^{2+} to 0.2 nA. The amplitude and frequency of slow waves diminish to 10 mV and 0.015 Hz, respectively. The concentration of intracellular calcium drops to 0.3 μM, and the strength of the active force falls to 12.1 mN cm^{-1}. At 'high' concentrations mibefradil abolishes oscillatory electrical and inhibits phasic spontaneous contractions. The membrane becomes depolarized, $V^r = -44$ mV, and the myofiber produces a spastic, tonic-type contraction, $T^a = 11.6$ mN cm^{-1}.

Conjoint application of mibefradil and electrical stimulation of the myometrium induces a high frequency and low amplitude transient T-type Ca^{2+} current of strength 0.13 nA. There is an increase in $[Ca_i^{2+}] = 0.5$ μM and an intensity of contraction, max $T^a = 16.7$ mN cm^{-1}. After washout of the drug, however, the fasciculus does regain its normal physiological activity (figure 13.10).

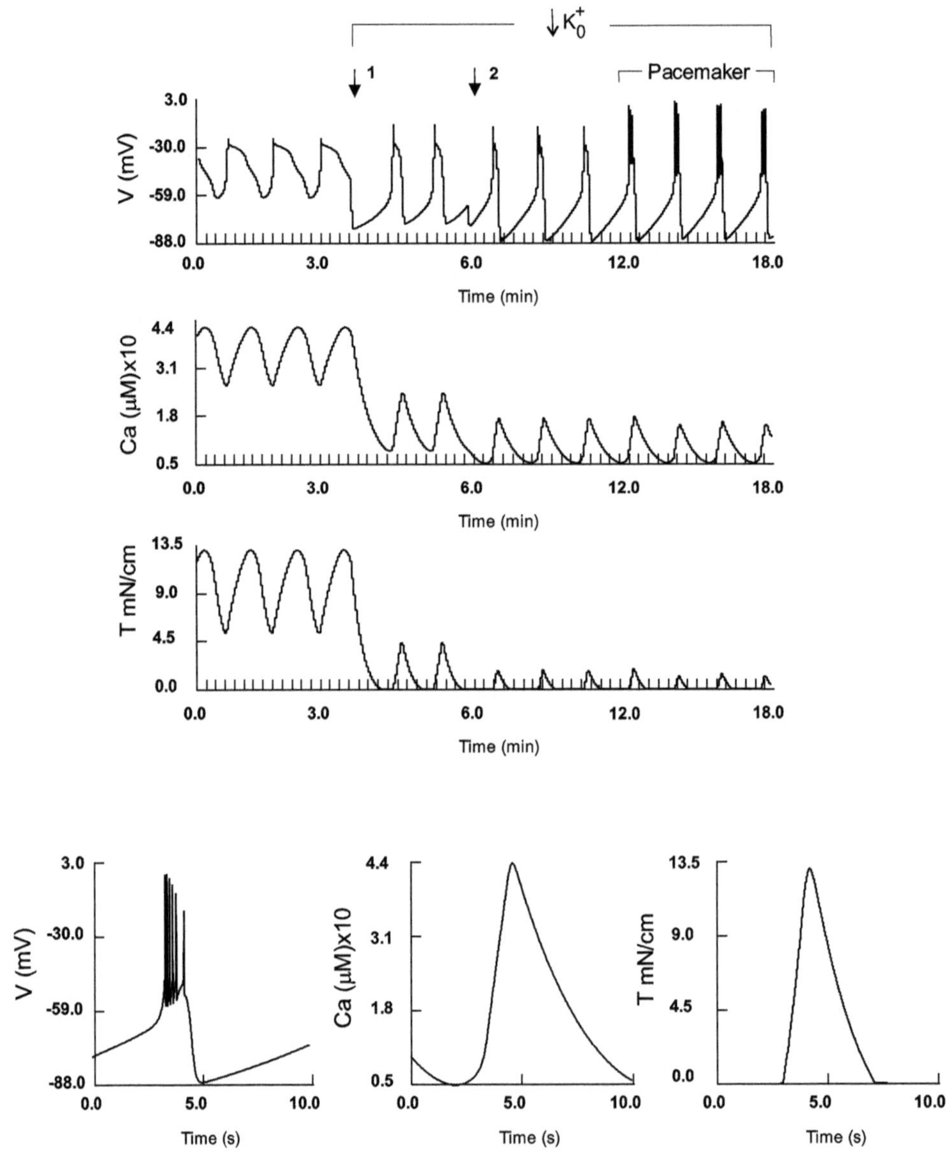

Figure 13.8. Dose-dependent responses of the fasciculus to gradual changes in external K^+ concentration and high frequency electrical stimulation. Reprinted from Miftahof R M and Nam H G 2011 *Biomechanics of the Gravid Human Uterus* (Berlin: Springer) by permission from Springer Nature. Copyright 2011.

13.10.7 Effects of L-type Ca^{2+} channel antagonists

At low doses, nimodipine, a selective L-type Ca^{2+} channel blocker, slightly increases the frequency but decreases the amplitude of slow waves, $V = 19.3$ mV (figure 13.11). A reduction in the intensity of the slow inward calcium current to 0.02 nA results in a decrease in free cytosolic calcium, $[Ca_i^{2+}] = 0.31$ μM. The strength of contractions also diminishes, $T^a = 7.2$ mN cm^{-1}. An increase in the concentration of the drug

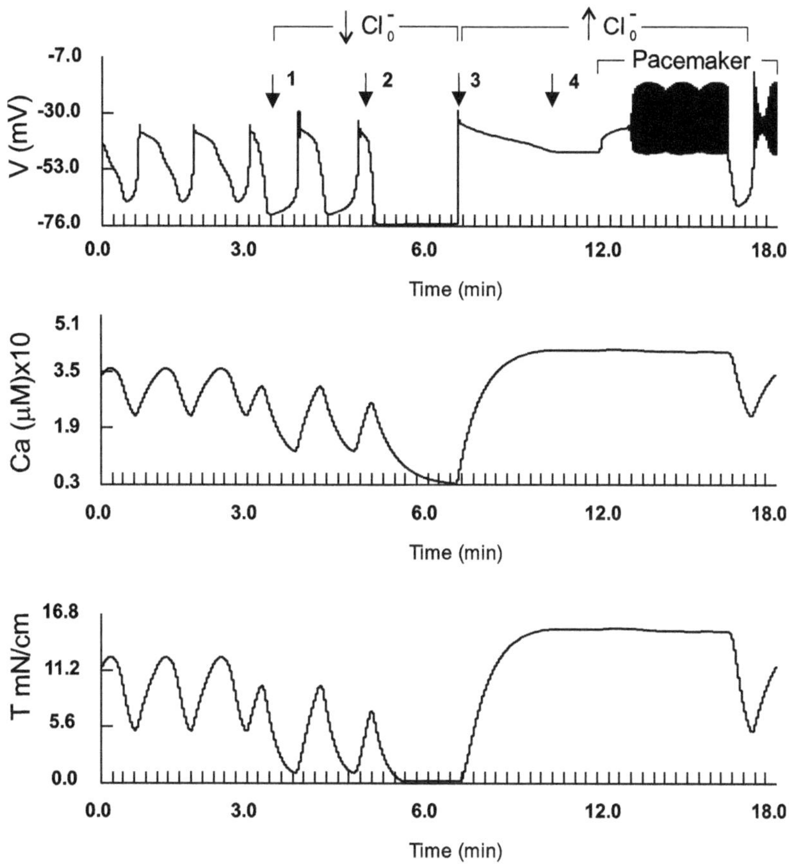

Figure 13.9. Effects of altered external Cl^- ion concentration and pacemaker discharges on electromechanical activity of the fasciculus. Reprinted from Miftahof R M and Nam H G 2011 *Biomechanics of the Gravid Human Uterus* (Berlin: Springer) by permission from Springer Nature. Copyright 2011.

practically abolishes the influx of extracellular calcium, $\tilde{I}_{Ca}^{s} \simeq 0$ nA, and attenuates further the amplitude of slow waves, $V = 12$ mV. However, the myofiber continues to generate phasic contractions of 4.4 mN cm^{-1}.

Conjoint electrical discharges of the pacemaker cell in the presence of nimodipine induce high amplitude action potentials, $V = 38$ mV, on the crests of slow waves. The myometrium contracts with $T^a = 10$ mN cm^{-1}. A 'high' dose of the drug inhibits spiking but not mechanical activity of the fasciculus which continues to generate an active force of amplitude 4.4 mN cm^{-1}.

Nimodipine in a Ca_0^{2+} free medium inhibits electrical activity in the myofiber totally. It remains relaxed and depolarized, $V = -56$ mV.

The application of nifedipine, a non-selective T- and L-type Ca^{2+} channel antagonist, or a combination of nifedipine and mibefradil, inhibits spontaneous electrical and mechanical contractile activity. The intracellular calcium level decreases to 0.03 μM and no contractions are produced.

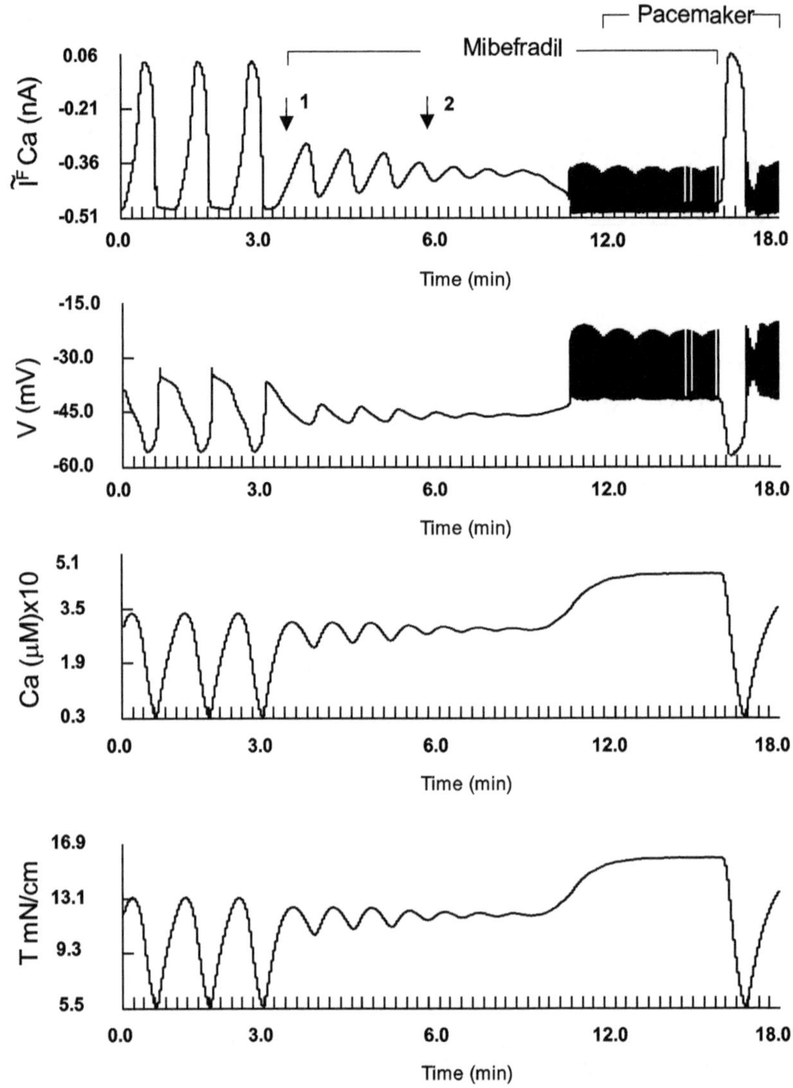

Figure 13.10. Changes in electromechanical activity of the fasciculus after application of mibefradil and conjoint electrical stimulation. Reprinted from Miftahof R M and Nam H G 2011 *Biomechanics of the Gravid Human Uterus* (Berlin: Springer) by permission from Springer Nature. Copyright 2011.

The response of the myofiber to treatment with Bay K 8644, a weakly selective L-type Ca^{2+} channel agonist, is dose-dependent. At 'low' concentration, the drug has a depolarizing effect on the myometrium, $V^r = -33$ mV, without attenuating its excitability. Multiple discharges of the pacemaker evoke high frequency, $\nu \simeq 6$ Hz, spikes of average amplitude, $V = 35$ mV. The concentration of intracellular calcium rises exponentially to 0.5 μM and is associated with active force production, max $T^a = 16.5$ mN cm^{-1} (figure 13.12). Bay K 8644 at 'high' dose inhibits slow waves totally. The myofiber becomes depolarized and undergoes tonic contraction.

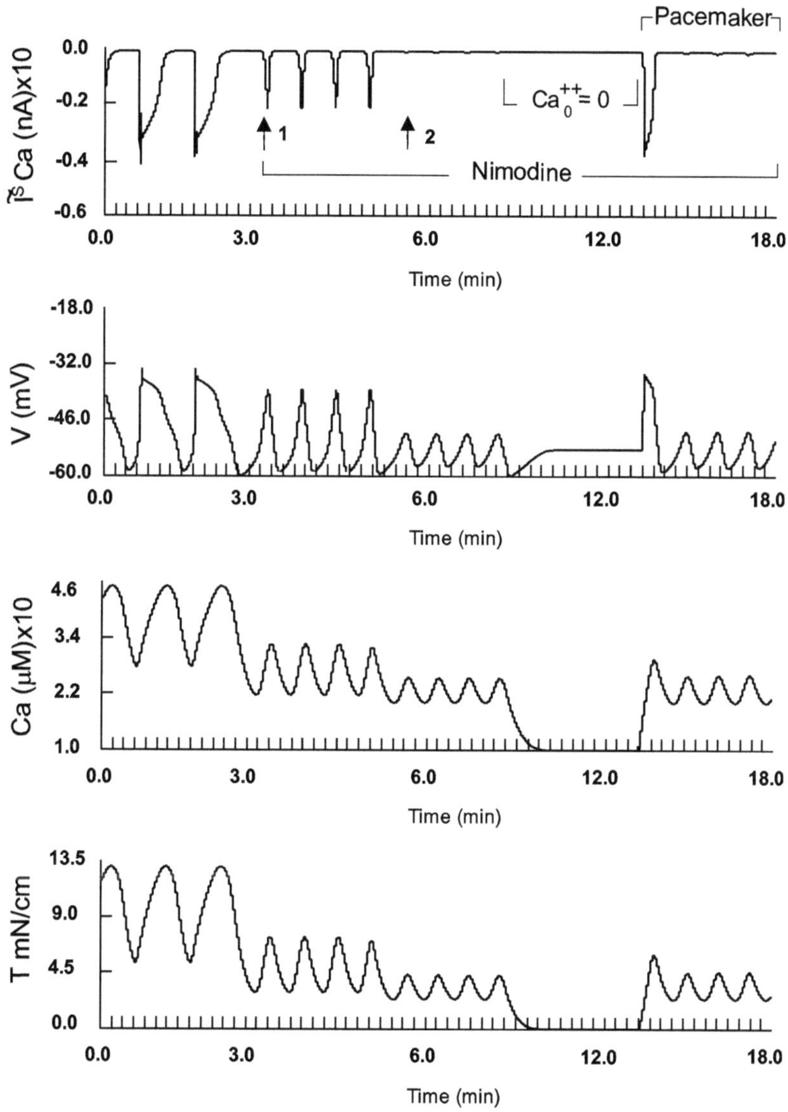

Figure 13.11. Electromechanical response of the fasciculus to nimodipine, a selective L-type Ca^{2+} channel antagonist, $[Ca_0^{2+}] = 0$ and pacemaker discharges. Reprinted from Miftahof R M and Nam H G 2011 *Biomechanics of the Gravid Human Uterus* (Berlin: Springer) by permission from Springer Nature. Copyright 2011.

13.10.8 Effects of BK_{Ca} channel antagonists

Treatment of the electrically stimulated myometrium with iberiotoxin, a selective Ca^{2+}-activated K^+ channel blocker, exerts a strong excitatory effect on its myoelectrical activity. There is a slight increase in the amplitude of action potentials, $V =$ 48–50 mV with a frequency, $\nu = 3.2$ Hz. The level of free intracellular calcium rises to a maximum of 0.51 μM and the myofiber generates a tonic contraction, max $T^a =$ 16.2 mN cm^{-1} (figure 13.13).

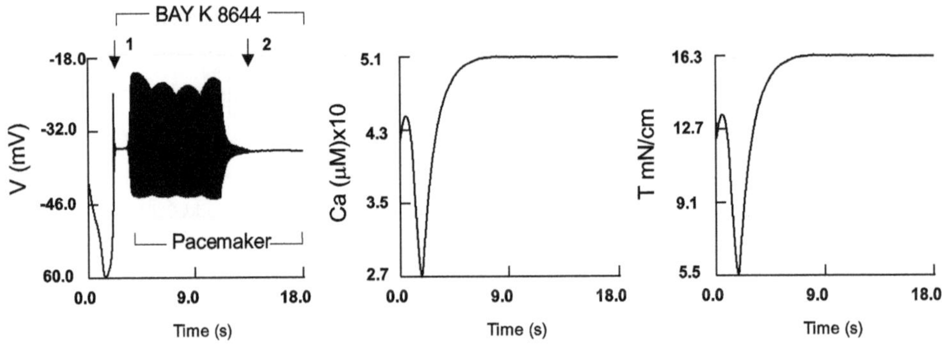

Figure 13.12. Effect of Bay K 8644 on biomechanics of the fasciculus. Reprinted from Miftahof R M and Nam H G 2011 *Biomechanics of the Gravid Human Uterus* (Berlin: Springer) by permission from Springer Nature. Copyright 2011.

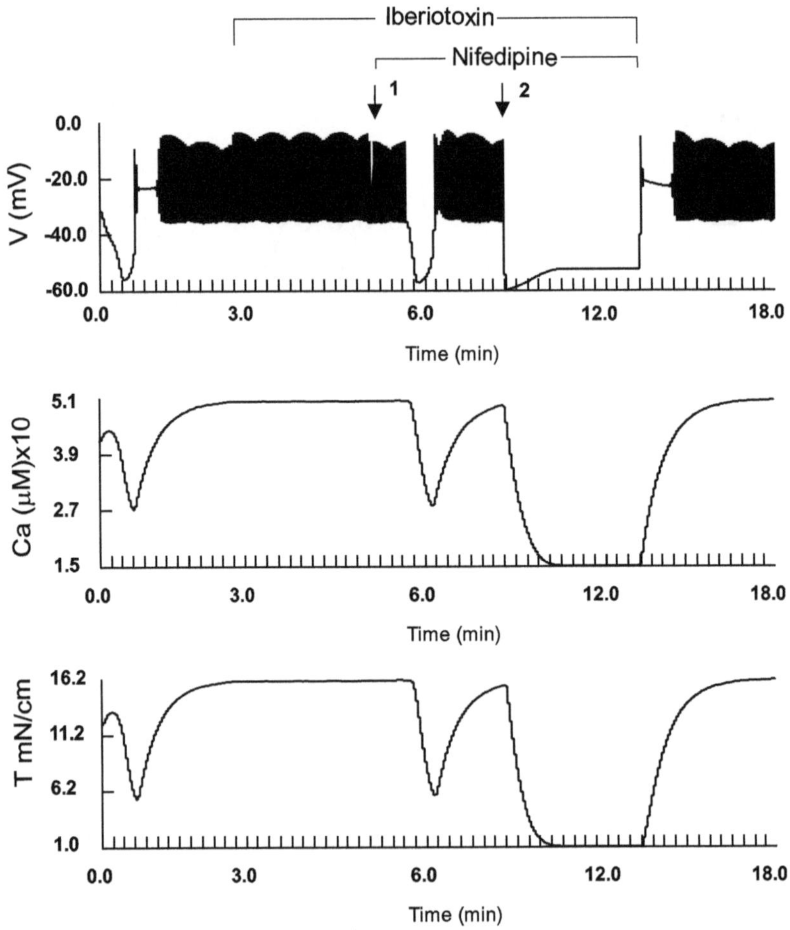

Figure 13.13. Myoelectrical activity of the fasciculus in the presence of iberiotoxin and nifedipine. Reprinted from Miftahof R M and Nam H G 2011 *Biomechanics of the Gravid Human Uterus* (Berlin: Springer) by permission from Springer Nature. Copyright 2011.

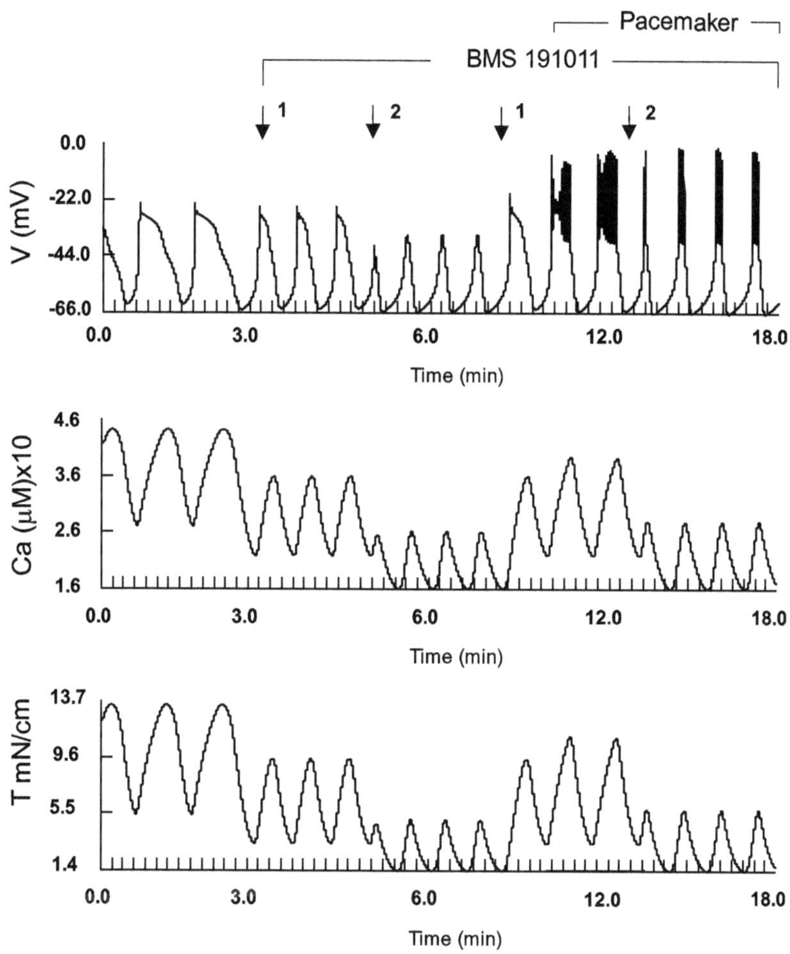

Figure 13.14. Dose-dependent effects of BMS 191011 and high frequency electrical stimulation on biomechanics of the fasciculus. Reprinted from Miftahof R M and Nam H G 2011 *Biomechanics of the Gravid Human Uterus* (Berlin: Springer) by permission from Springer Nature. Copyright 2011.

The addition of a 'low' dose of nifedipine disrupts the continuous pattern of activity. The myofiber generates regular bursts of spikes with a duration of two minutes at normal amplitude. The contractility pattern changes from tonic to phasic-type. An increase in the concentration of the drug hyperpolarizes the cell membrane, $V^r = -52$ mV, and abolishes its oscillatory activity. Free intracellular calcium of 0.15 μM triggers the active force development of intensity 1 mN cm^{-1}. After the washout of iberiotoxin and nifedipine, the fasciculus regains its physiological myoelectrical activity.

At a 'low' concentration, BMS 191011, a potent selective BK_{Ca} channel agonist, causes a slight increase in the frequency of slow waves without changes in their amplitude. It has a distinct effect on the dynamics of both intracellular calcium and contractility. The maximum $[Ca_i^{2+}]$ declines to 0.35 μM, and the active force to

9.6 mN cm^{-1} (figure 13.14). At 'high' concentrations, the compound hyperpolarizes the membrane, $V^r = -66$ mV, and causes a decrease in the amplitude of V to 24 mV. The myofiber continues to produce phasic contractions of strength, T^a = 6.4 mN cm^{-1}.

BMS 191011 does not inhibit the excitability of the myometrium. It generates bursts of action potentials of 50 mV in response to discharges of the intrinsic pacemaker. However, the duration of action potentials decreases when the concentration of the added compound is increased.

13.10.9 Effects of a K$^+$ channel antagonist

The addition of tetraethylammonium chloride (TEA), a non-selective voltage-gated K^+_{v1}-channel antagonist, prolongs the plateau membrane potential duration and

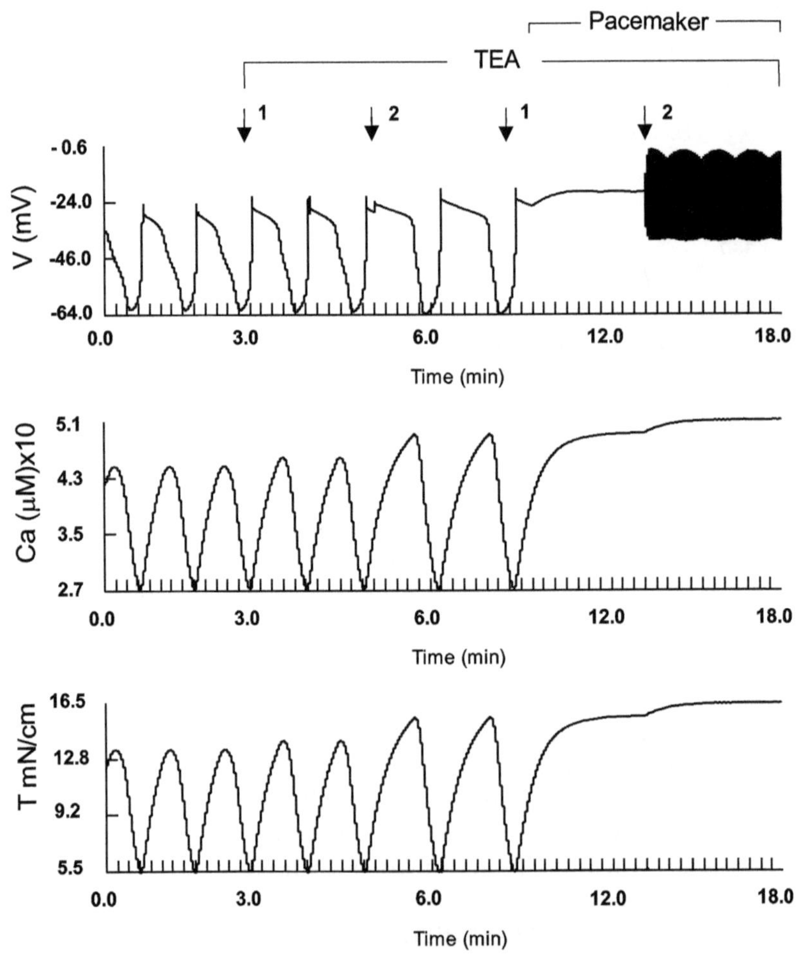

Figure 13.15. Effects of TEA applied in gradually increased concentrations on biomechanics of the fasciculus. Reprinted from Miftahof R M and Nam H G 2011 *Biomechanics of the Gravid Human Uterus* (Berlin: Springer) by permission from Springer Nature. Copyright 2011.

increases its amplitude, $V = 28$–30 mV. There is an increase in the influx of calcium ions inside the cell, $[Ca_i^{2+}] = 0.35$ μM, and a rise in the tension of contractions, $T^a = 16$ mN cm^{-1}. These effects are dose-dependent (figure 13.15).

Electrical stimulation of the fasciculus in the presence of the drug at 'low' concentration inhibits slow waves and depolarizes the membrane, $V = -26$ mV. These events coincide with an increase in cytosolic calcium $[Ca_i^{2+}] = 0.48$ μM and the production of tonic contraction. At 'high' concentrations TEA evokes long-lasting bursts of regular action potentials, $V = 25$–27 mV. The myometrium generates an active force of maximum 16.5 mN cm^{-1}.

13.10.10 Effects of a Cl^- channel antagonist

At 'low' concentrations, niflumic acid, a non-selective Cl^--channel antagonist and a potent stimulator of the BK_{Ca} channel, reduces the strength of the leak chloride current to 0.4 nA without significant changes in the intensities of other ion currents (figure 13.16). At 'high' doses, the drug causes a rise in amplitudes of slow inward calcium and potassium currents to 0.2 nA and 0.11 nA, respectively, while the amplitude of the chloride current diminishes to 0.15 nA. The membrane becomes hyperpolarized, $V^r = -70$ mV. However, the myometrium continues to generate slow waves of amplitude ~40 mV at a frequency of 0.44 Hz. Electrical stimuli induce action potentials, $V = -10$ mV, on the crests of slow waves.

A gradual increase in the concentration of niflumic acid causes a decrease in the intracellular concentration of free calcium to 3 μM at 'low' doses, and to 2.2 μM at 'high' doses, respectively. At 'high' doses the drug causes a further decline in cytosolic calcium, $[Ca_i^{2+}] = 0.08$ μM. This significantly weakens the contractility of the myofiber which generates an active force of 4.3 mN cm^{-1}. High intensity electrical stimulation does not have any positive effect on the dynamics of contractions.

13.11 Co-transmission in the myometrium

13.11.1 ACh and OT

Consider the effect of co-transmission by ACh and OT on the dynamics of the myometrial fasciculus. The combined system of equations (7.4)–(7.7), (8.1)–(8.8), (8.9)–(8.12), (8.24), (8.25), (10.2), (10.4), and (10.23)–(10.24), in which $p \propto$ T-Ca_i^{2+}, $q \propto$ OTR*, provides the mathematical formulation of the problem. This system describes: (i) the excitation and release of the transmitters/modulators, (ii) the electrochemical coupling at the synapse, (iii) intracellular processes of transduction, and (iv) myometrial responses.

It should be noted that the role of the stimulatory signal, V^s, in the boundary condition could be replaced by the synaptic potential, V_{syn}.

The conjoint effects of ACh and OT are studied numerically. The amount of neurotransmitter released depends on the strength of depolarization of the nerve terminal, V^f. The effects of different concentrations of oxytocin have been modeled by varying the conductivity parameter for the fast Ca^{2+} channel, g_{Ca}^f.

The results of simulations show that the depolarization of the presynaptic membrane activates a short-term influx of extracellular calcium ions into the

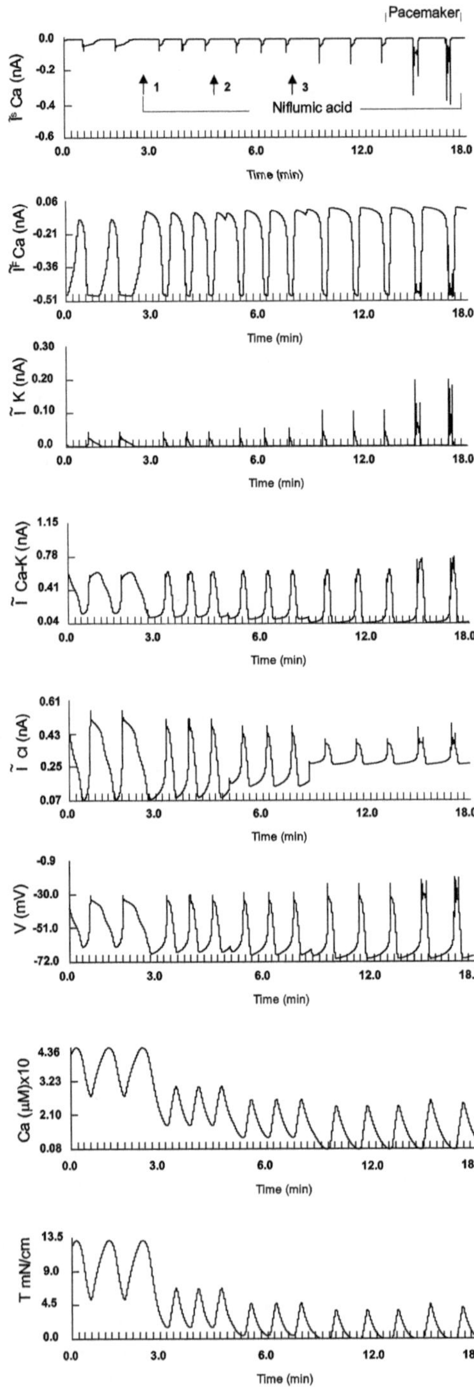

Figure 13.16. Dose-dependent responses of the fasciculus to niflumic acid at different concentrations and pacemaker discharges. Reprinted from Miftahof R M and Nam H G 2011 *Biomechanics of the Gravid Human Uterus* (Berlin: Springer) by permission from Springer Nature. Copyright 2011.

Table 13.1. Selected crosstalk signaling components in the human uterus.

Transmitter/modulator	Receptor type	$G_{(act)}$-protein	Pathway	Ion channel
ACh	μ_2	$G_{\alpha i}$	↓ AC*	
AD	α_1	$G_{\alpha q/11}$	↑ PLC	
	α_2	$G_{\alpha i}$	↓ AC*	
	β_1, β_3	$G_{\alpha s}$	↑ AC*	↑ BK_{Ca}
	β_2	$G_{\alpha s}$ and $G_{\alpha i}$	↑ AC*	↑ BK_{Ca}
$PrF_{2\alpha}$	FP	$G_{\alpha q/11}$	↑ PLC	↑ L-Ca_i^{2+}
PrE_2	$EP_{1,3D}$	—	—	↑ L-Ca_i^{2+}
	EP_{3A}	$G_{\alpha i}$	↓ AC*	
	EP_2	$G_{\alpha q/11}$	↑ PLC	
OT	OTR	$G_{\alpha q/11}$	↑ PLC	↑ T-Ca_i^{2+}
PR	mPR	$G_{\alpha i}$	↓ AC*	

terminal through voltage-gated Ca^{2+} channels. The concentration of cytosolic Ca_i^{2+} quickly rises reaching a maximum of 19.4 μM. Some of the ions are immediately absorbed by the buffer system, whereas others diffuse towards vesicles. These bind to the active centers to initiate the release of acetylcholine. During the whole cycle, about 10% of stored vesicular neurotransmitter is released (table 13.1).

Part of the postsynaptic acetylcholine undergoes degradation by acetylcholine esterase, max[ACh–E] = 0.47 μM being formed. The complex quickly dissociates into the enzyme and choline, S, which is reabsorbed and drawn into a new cycle of ACh synthesis.

The diffused fraction of ACh in the synaptic cleft equals 3.2 mM. The major part of the transmitter enters the postsynaptic membrane where it reacts with the surface receptors to form the ACh–R-complex: [ACh–R] = 0.123 μM. Their transformation to the active state triggers the generation of the excitatory postsynaptic potential, V_{syn}. It increases as a step function to reach 87 mV in 0.25 ms.

The myometrial fasciculus generates high amplitude, $V \simeq 30$ mV, and frequency, $\nu = 3.2$ Hz, action potentials on the crests of slow waves (figure 13.17). There is a concurrent increase in the level of intracellular calcium. A maximum concentration $[Ca_i^{2+}] = 0.49$ μM is recorded. As a result, the myofiber produces regular contractions of strength 15.8 mN cm^{-1} and duration 2.5 min.

The conjoint release of ACh and OT into the system causes a further rise in the amplitude of spikes, $V \simeq 38$ mV, and the concentration of intracellular calcium, $[Ca_i^{2+}] = 0.51$ μM. There is a slight increase in the intensity of contractions. The maximum active force, $T^a = 16.1$ mN cm^{-1}, is produced with an average duration of 2 min.

The washout of ACh abolishes high amplitude spiking activity. Oxytocin acting alone induces irregular action potentials of amplitude 7–10 mV. Remarkably, there are no significant changes in either the transient or the concentration of free cytosolic calcium. The fasciculus continues to contract with a strength of 16 mN cm^{-1}.

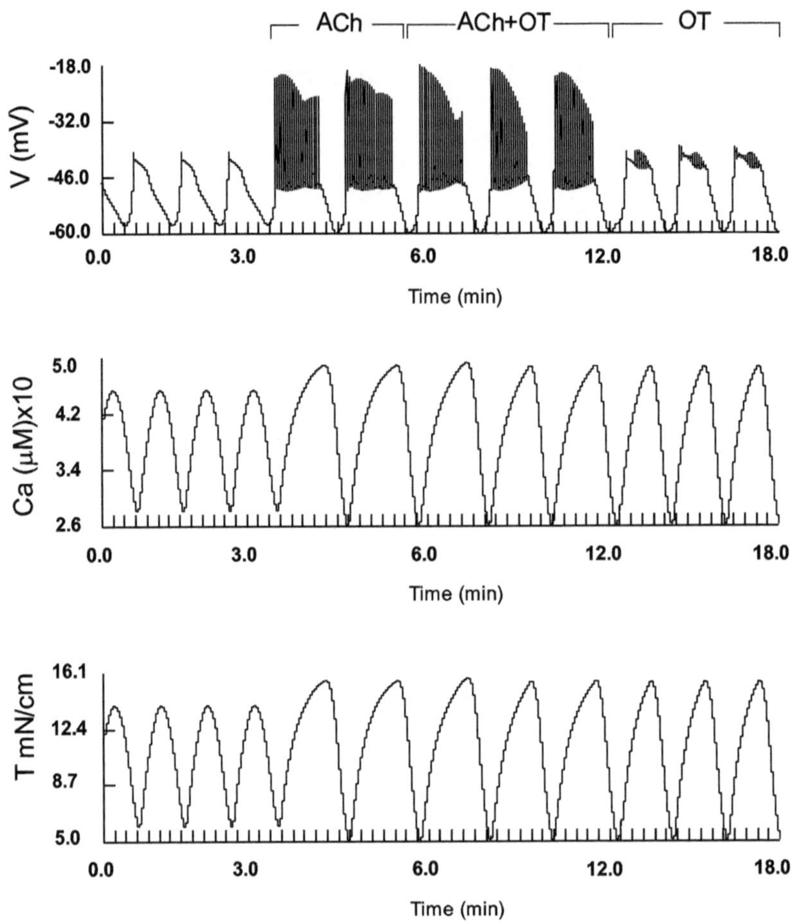

Figure 13.17. Selective and conjoint effects of ACh and OT on electromechanical activity of the fasciculus. Reprinted from Miftahof R M and Nam H G 2011 *Biomechanics of the Gravid Human Uterus* (Berlin: Springer) by permission from Springer Nature. Copyright 2011.

13.11.2 ACh and AD

In the case of co-transmission by ACh and adrenaline (AD) on the myoelectrical activity of the fasciculus, excitation of the nerve terminal triggers the release of vesicular AD. A maximum 86.3 μM of the free fraction of the neurotransmitter is released in the synaptic cleft. AD_c quickly diffuses towards the postsynaptic membrane where part of it, $[AD_c]$ = 35.2 μM, binds to $\beta_{2,3}$-adrenoceptors while another part is utilized by the re-uptake mechanisms. A total of 8.53 μM of the $AD_c{\cdot}R$ complex is formed causing a hyperpolarization of the myometrium to −78.8 mV.

The subsequent release of AD into the pre-excited ACh myometrial synapse has a detrimental effect on its electrical and mechanical activity (figure 13.18). The amplitude of slow wave oscillations reduces to 17 mV while their frequency increases two-fold. Their rate of spiking and amplitude decrease and the myometrium becomes hyperpolarized, V = −67 mV. These changes reflect the fall in the

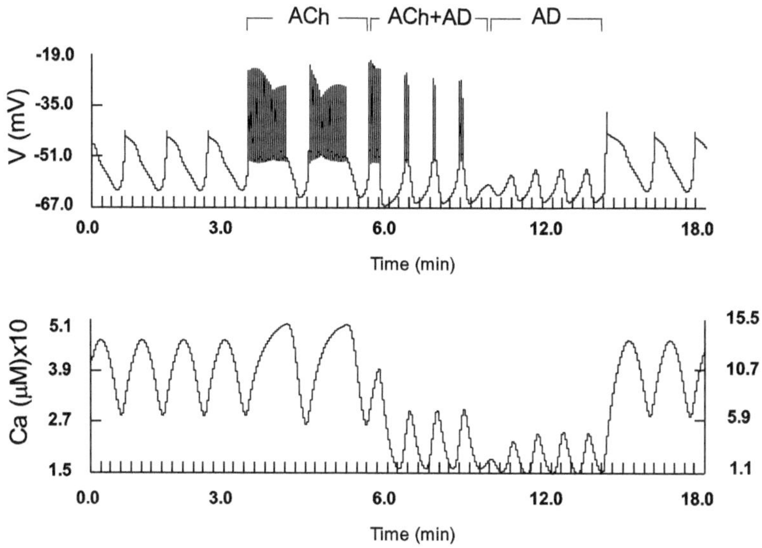

Figure 13.18. Selective and conjoint effects of ACh and AD on electromechanical activity of the fasciculus. Reprinted from Miftahof R M and Nam H G 2011 *Biomechanics of the Gravid Human Uterus* (Berlin: Springer) by permission from Springer Nature. Copyright 2011.

concentration of free cytosolic calcium, $[Ca_i^{2+}] = 0.27\ \mu M$, and contractility, max $T^a = 6.0$ mN cm^{-1}.

Adrenaline alone in low concentration reduces excitability of the fasciculus and suppresses the intensity of active forces. No action potentials are being generated and $T^a = 4.3$ mN cm^{-1} develops. A further increase in AD causes complete relaxation of the muscle.

13.11.3 OT and AD

The results of numerical simulations of the conjoint action of adrenaline and oxytocin on the myometrial fasciculus are shown in figure 13.19. Application of AD to a system already exposed to OT has a significant hyperpolarizing effect. The level of the resting membrane potential falls to −67 mV whilst the amplitude of slow waves decreases to 10 mV. These changes have a negative effect on the dynamics of Ca_i^{2+}. Only 0.17 μM of free cytosolic calcium ions are recorded, sustaining weak contractions of maximum strength 2.0 mN cm^{-1}. The washout of OT from the system abolishes spontaneous contractions and relaxes the myometrium.

13.11.4 OT and prostaglandins

The addition of prostaglandins to the myometrial fasciculus pre-treated with OT causes a short burst of high frequency spikes of various amplitudes. The intracellular calcium concentration reaches 0.53 μM and coincides with a maximum active force development $T^a = 17$ mN cm^{-1} of duration ~3 min (figure 13.20).

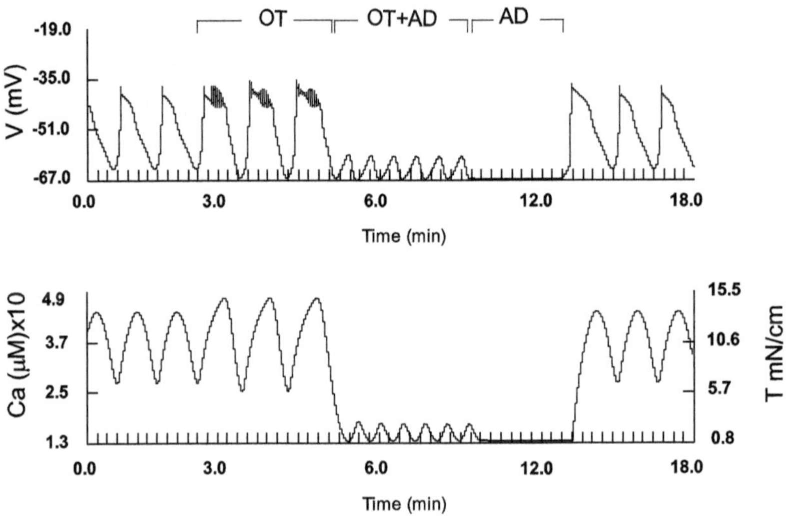

Figure 13.19. Selective and conjoint effects of OT and AD on electromechanical activity of the fasciculus. Reprinted from Miftahof R M and Nam H G 2011 *Biomechanics of the Gravid Human Uterus* (Berlin: Springer) by permission from Springer Nature. Copyright 2011.

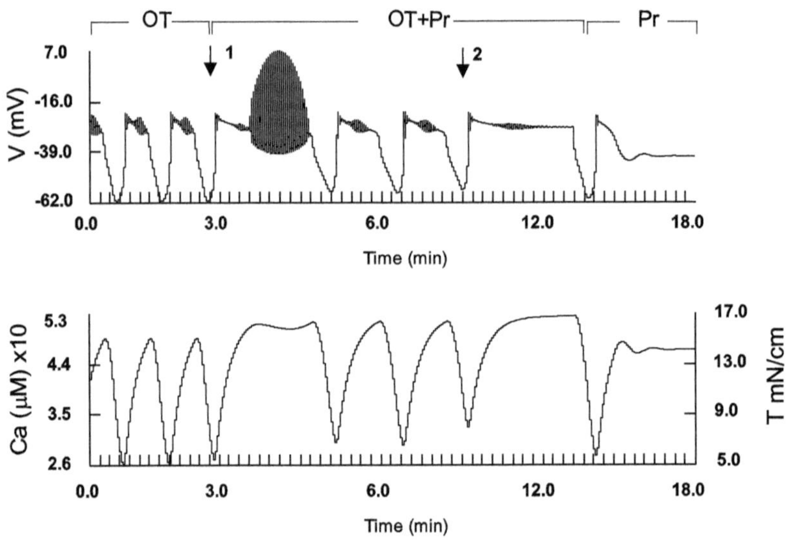

Figure 13.20. Selective and conjoint effects of OT and Pr on electromechanical activity of the fasciculus. Reprinted from Miftahof R M and Nam H G 2011 *Biomechanics of the Gravid Human Uterus* (Berlin: Springer) by permission from Springer Nature. Copyright 2011.

A further increase in the level of prostaglandins steadily depolarizes the membrane at −20 mV and causes a tonic-type contraction of the fasciculus, T^a = 17.2 mN cm^{-1}.

Prostaglandins acting alone abolish slow waves and depolarize the myometrium at V = −20 mV. The cytosolic calcium content falls to 44 μM along with the active force of contraction, T^a = 14.4 mN cm^{-1}.

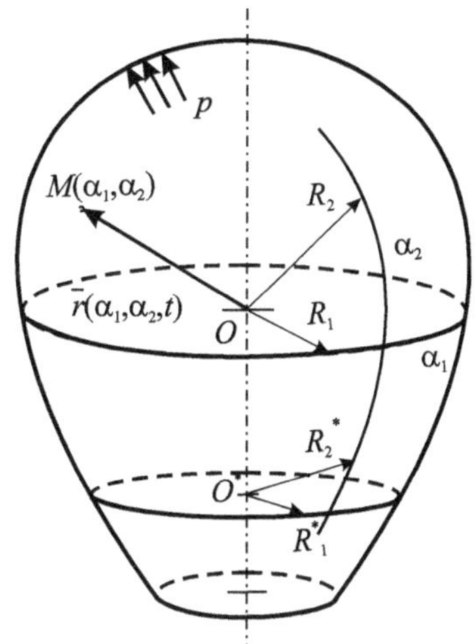

Figure 13.21. The gravid human uterus as a thin bioshell. Reprinted from Miftahof R M and Nam H G 2011 *Biomechanics of the Gravid Human Uterus* (Berlin: Springer) by permission from Springer Nature. Copyright 2011.

13.12 The gravid uterus as a soft biological shell

Let the middle surface of the pregnant uterus be associated with a cylindrical coordinate system $\{r, \varphi, z\}$ (figure 13.21). The first two—proliferative and synthetic phases in the organ are characterized by the extensive growth, remodeling, and homeomorphic change in shape without actual deformation. Therefore, it is reasonable to assume that during this stage the cut configuration coincides with the undeformed, $\overset{0}{S} = S$. Assume that stretch ratios $\lambda_{i,j} \equiv 1.0$, $(i, j = 1, 2)$, in-plane total forces and intrauterine pressure are zero throughout the bioshell, and intrauterine volume is $\breve{V} \simeq 450$–600 ml. The pregnant uterus attains the deformed $\overset{*}{S}$ state with $\lambda_{i,j} > 1.0$, $T_{ij} > 0$, $\breve{V} \simeq 800$ ml, and $p = 2$–12 mmHg only towards the end of the second synthetic phase to continue throughout the entire contractile phase.

The equations of motion of the bioshell satisfy equations (5.102), the dynamics of bursting and oscillatory myoelectrical activity, $V_{c,l}$, in the myometrial longitudinal and circumferential layers, respectively, are adequately described by the system of equations (10.5)–(10.9), the pacemaker activity in myometrial cells, V_{p}, yields equations (7.3)–(7.13), the propagation of the electrical wave of depolarization, $V_{c,l}^{s}$, along the myometrium in instances of generalized electrical anisotropy and isotropy is given by equations (10.10)–(10.18), and neurohormonal regulatory processes in the myometrium are described by equations (8.1)–(8.12), (8.24), (8.25).

The following anatomically and physiologically justifiable initial and boundary conditions assume that: (i) the organ is at rest, i.e. myoelectrically quiescent; (ii) an excitation of known intensity, $\overset{0}{V}_{\mathrm{p}}$, and duration, t_i^{d}, is provided by electrical discharges in the pacemaker regions; (iii) concentrations of the reacting substrates are known; (iv) the cervical end is electrically unexcitable and is either rigidly fixed or remains pliable throughout deformation; and (v) the condition of periodicity is imposed with respect to the angular coordinate, φ.

Thus, we have

$$\text{at } t = 0: \quad V_{\mathrm{p}} = \begin{cases} 0, & 0 < t < t_i^d \\ \overset{0}{V}_{\mathrm{p}}, & t \geqslant t_i^d \end{cases}, \quad V_{c,l} = V_{c,l}^r, \quad V_{c,l}^s = 0,$$
$$[\mathrm{Ca}_i^{2+}] = [\overset{0}{\mathrm{Ca}}{}_i^{2+}], \mathbf{X}(0) = \mathbf{X}_0, \mathbf{C}(0) = \mathbf{C}_0,$$
$$r(\alpha_1, \alpha_2) = r_0(\alpha_1, \alpha_2), \varphi(\alpha_1, \alpha_2) = \varphi_0(\alpha_1, \alpha_2), z(\alpha_1, \alpha_2) = z_0(\alpha_1, \alpha_2) \tag{13.36}$$

with the dynamic variables of ion channels involved defined as

$$\hat{m} = \hat{m}_\infty, \; \hat{h} = \hat{h}_\infty, \; \hat{n} = \hat{n}_\infty, \; z_{\mathrm{Ca}} = z_{\mathrm{Ca}\infty}, \; h_{\mathrm{Na}} = h_{\mathrm{Na}\infty}, \; n_{\mathrm{K}} = n_{\mathrm{K}\infty},$$
$$\tilde{h} = \tilde{h}_\infty, \; \tilde{n} = \tilde{n}_\infty, \; \tilde{x}_{\mathrm{Ca}} = \tilde{x}_{\mathrm{Ca}\infty}, \tag{13.37}$$

for $t > 0$:

$$r(\alpha_1, \alpha_2)_{\alpha_1=0,L} = r_0(0, \alpha_2) = r_0(L, \alpha_2),$$
$$\varphi(\alpha_1, \alpha_2)_{\alpha_1=0,L} = \varphi_0(0, \alpha_2) = \varphi_0(L, \alpha_2),$$
$$z(\alpha_1, \alpha_2)_{\alpha_1=0,L} = z_0(0, \alpha_2) = z_0(L, \alpha_2),$$
$$V_{c,l}^s(0, \alpha_2) = V_{c,l}^s(L, \alpha_2). \tag{13.38}$$

To close the problem constitutive relations for the tissue should be provided. Finally, the mathematical model as formulated above describes: (i) the pregnant uterus at term as a soft biological shell; (ii) pacemaker activity in the organ; (iii) the generation and propagation of electrical waves of excitation in the myometrial syncytia; and (iv) electromechanical coupling and neurohormonal regulation of contractile activity.

13.13 Investigations into the gravid human uterus

Labor is a series of continuous, progressive contractions of the uterus which help the cervix to open (dilate) and to thin (efface), allowing the fetus to move through the birth canal. It is divided into three stages. The first stage begins with the onset of true labor and ends when the cervix is completely dilated. Initial contractions are of low intensity, short in duration (30–45 s), and irregular (5–20 min apart), becoming stronger, longer in duration (60–90 s), regular, and more frequent, occurring every 0.5–1 min. At the end of the first stage the cervix dilates to 10 cm and the amniotic sac ruptures, releasing $\breve{V} \simeq 600$ ml of fluid. This leads to a fall in uterine pressure: $p =$ 2–4 mmHg. The womb changes its shape and size as a result of rising tonus in the myometrium.

The subsequent second stage is characterized by strong pushing contractions, which expel the baby through the birth canal to the outside world. The uterus contracts extensively during this stage and the intrauterine pressure rises to $p =$ 60–100 mmHg. Shortly after the baby is born and the placenta delivered—the third and final stage of labor—the uterus undergoes a significant reduction in size. The axial and transverse dimensions of the organ decrease by 20%–30%, a fact attributed to prevailing myometrial contractions. These mechanical and concomitant hormonal changes cause vasoconstriction and thus prevent postpartum bleeding.

13.13.1 The uterus close to term

The actual configuration and in-plane force–strain distribution in the pregnant womb depends on: (i) the fetal presentation—vertex (cephalic), oblique, or transverse; (ii) the fetal size; (iii) the amount of amniotic fluid; and (iv) the position and size of the placenta. Although the current mathematical formulation does not account explicitly for each of these factors, their joint contribution in the model, as a first approximation, can be attained through the variation of intrauterine pressure p.

The configuration of the electrically quiescent human uterus at 38 weeks, corresponding to the end of the proliferative phase of gestation, represents the initial undeformed state of the bioshell. It is the result of computer reconstruction of actual MRI data. Throughout simulations only a singleton pregnancy is considered.

A coronal view of the pear-like womb with the fetus in cephalic presentation at the beginning of the latent phase of the first stage of labor is shown in figure 13.22. Analysis of the static total force distribution in the bioshell indicates that the fundus and the body of the organ experience excessive longitudinal total forces, while the lower segment is predominantly circumferential. The cervix is closed with a min $T_{c,l} \simeq 0$ produced in the region.

The period from 38 to 40 weeks is associated with low intensity irregular contractions, known as Braxton Hicks. An increase in myometrial tonus leads to smoothing and shortening of the lower segment. The shape of the uterus becomes more rounded with a decrease in the fundal height. The redistribution and decrease in the spatial gradient of T_l along with a significant rise in T_c in the lower segment are observed. There is a simultaneous increase in the in-plane forces T_c and T_l in the cervical region.

In the case of oblique presentation, the initial configuration of the uterus is skewed and elongated in the direction of the crown–rump axis of the fetus (figure 13.23). Both the body and fundus undergo maximal tension in a longitudinal direction. The lower segment is unequally stretched with the presence of focal zones of excessive circumferential forces in that region. This pattern of $T_{c,l}$ distribution persists throughout the entire period of Braxton Hicks contractions. Compared to cephalic presentation, the cervical region is subjected to intense T_c forces and $T_l \approx 0$. These increase gradually with gestation to attain a maximum at the end of week 40.

Shapes and total force distributions in the uterus when the fetus is in transverse position are shown in figure 13.24. The results of simulations demonstrate that there is a constant increase in intensity of tension from 38 to 40 weeks in the longitudinal direction in the body and fundus of the organ. Small forces T_l are produced in the lower segment and cervical region. The lower segment is overstressed circumferentially with maximum T_c exceeding similar values for cephalic and oblique presentations. The circumferential force in the area of the cervix remains low, $T_c \approx 0$, throughout the progression of pregnancy. An increase in the intrauterine pressure above normal values, occurring in polyhydramnios, and changes in the mechanical

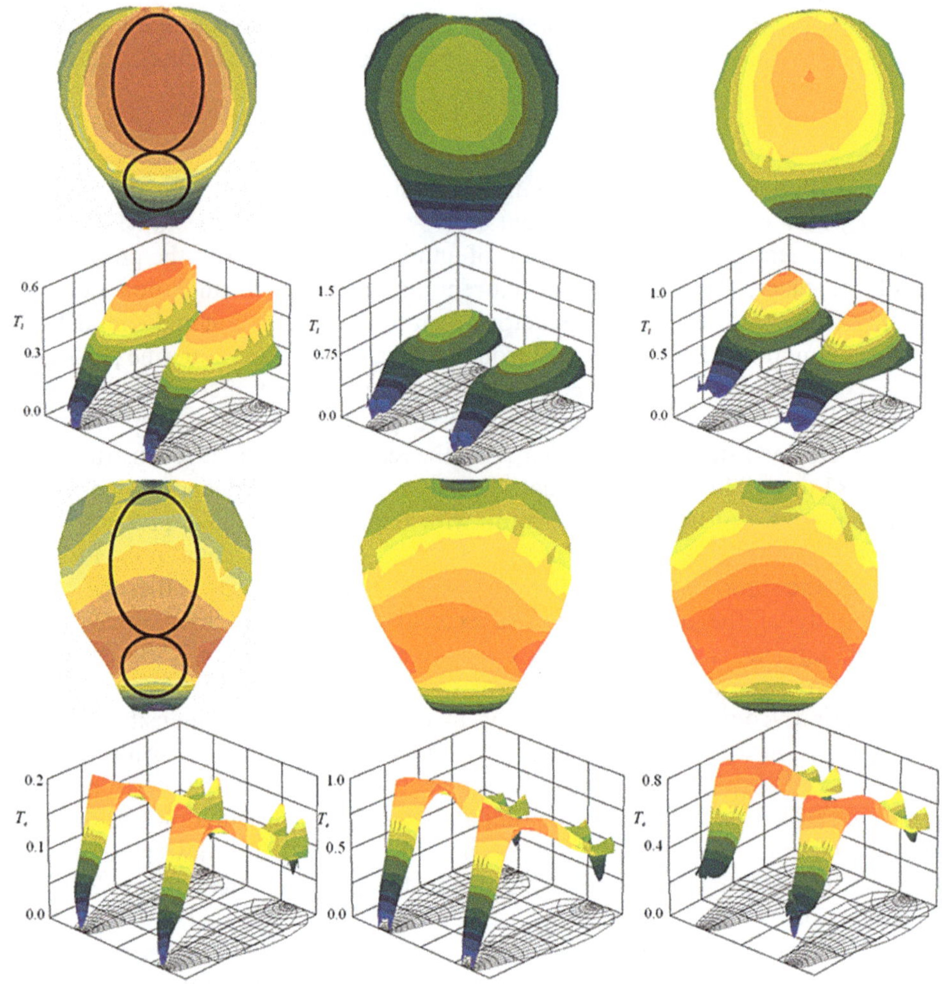

Figure 13.22. Coronal views and corresponding total in-plane force distributions in the longitudinal, T_l, and circumferential, T_c, myometrial striata in the pregnant gravid human uterus at term with the fetus in cephalic position. Henceforth, all forces are normalized to the maximum force generated by the uterus through the whole case of study. Reprinted from Miftahof R M and Nam H G 2011 *Biomechanics of the Gravid Human Uterus* (Berlin: Springer) by permission from Springer Nature. Copyright 2011.

characteristics of the myometrium do not affect the qualitative pattern of force–stretch ratio distribution in pregnant uteri.

A comparative analysis of forces at term in the cervical region, depending on fetal presentation and the assumption that the myometrium is physically and statistically homogeneous, is shown in figure 13.25. Results demonstrate that in the cephalic presentation, the cervix experiences pulling T_l and stretching T_c forces.

Surprisingly, with the fetus in oblique presentation, the cervical region undergoes intense circumferential stretching whilst in transverse presentation, relatively small and physiologically insignificant $T_{c,l}$ forces are produced. Such conditions play definite roles in the dynamics of cervical opening during labor as discussed below.

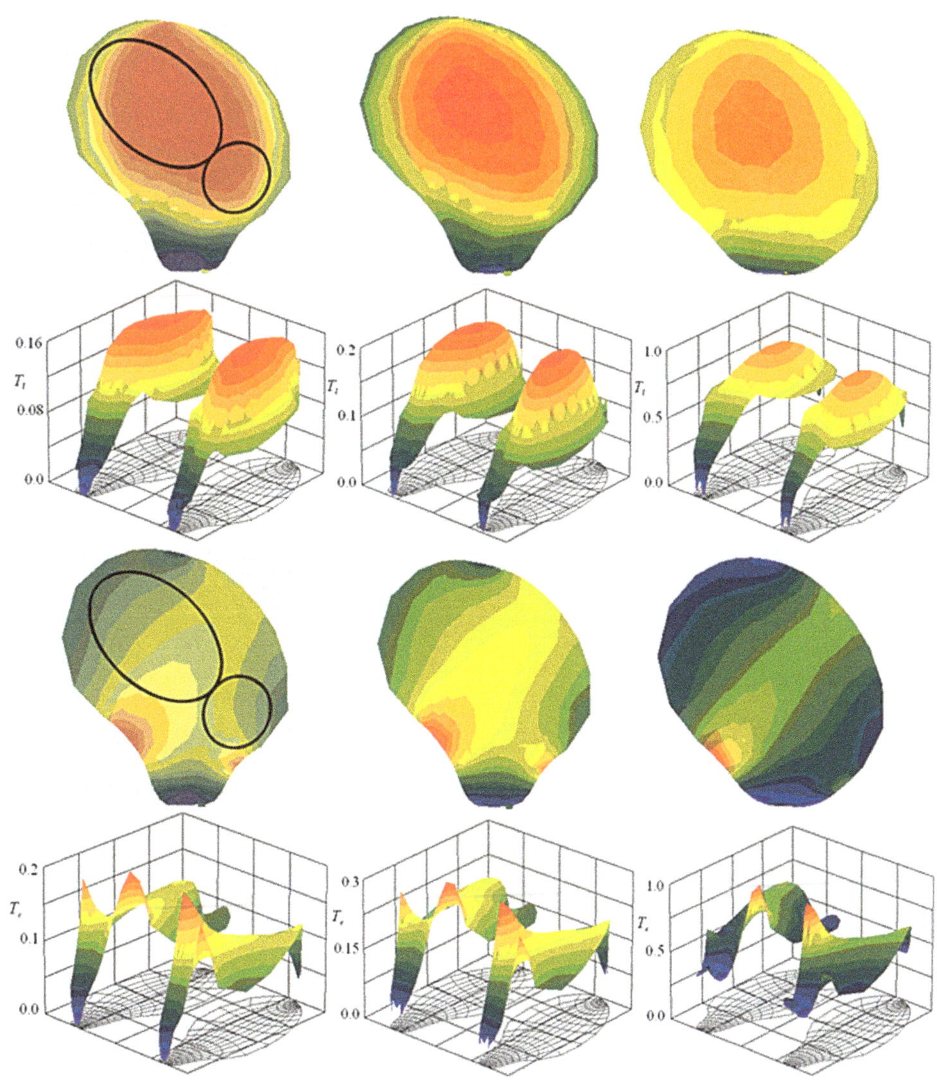

Figure 13.23. Same as in figure 13.22. The fetus is in oblique position. Reprinted from Miftahof R M and Nam H G 2011 *Biomechanics of the Gravid Human Uterus* (Berlin: Springer) by permission from Springer Nature. Copyright 2011.

13.13.2 The first stage of labor

At the end of the 40th week the uterus enters the first stage of labor marked by irregular contractions. Let two separate pacemaker zones in the longitudinal and circular layers be located in the uterotubal junctions. These discharge synchronously multiple impulses of constant amplitude $\overset{0}{V}_{\mathrm{p}} = 100$ mV and duration $t_i^d = 10$ ms to generate electrical waves of depolarization V_l and V_{c}, respectively. The wave V_l quickly spreads within the longitudinal fibers and encases a narrow zone along the

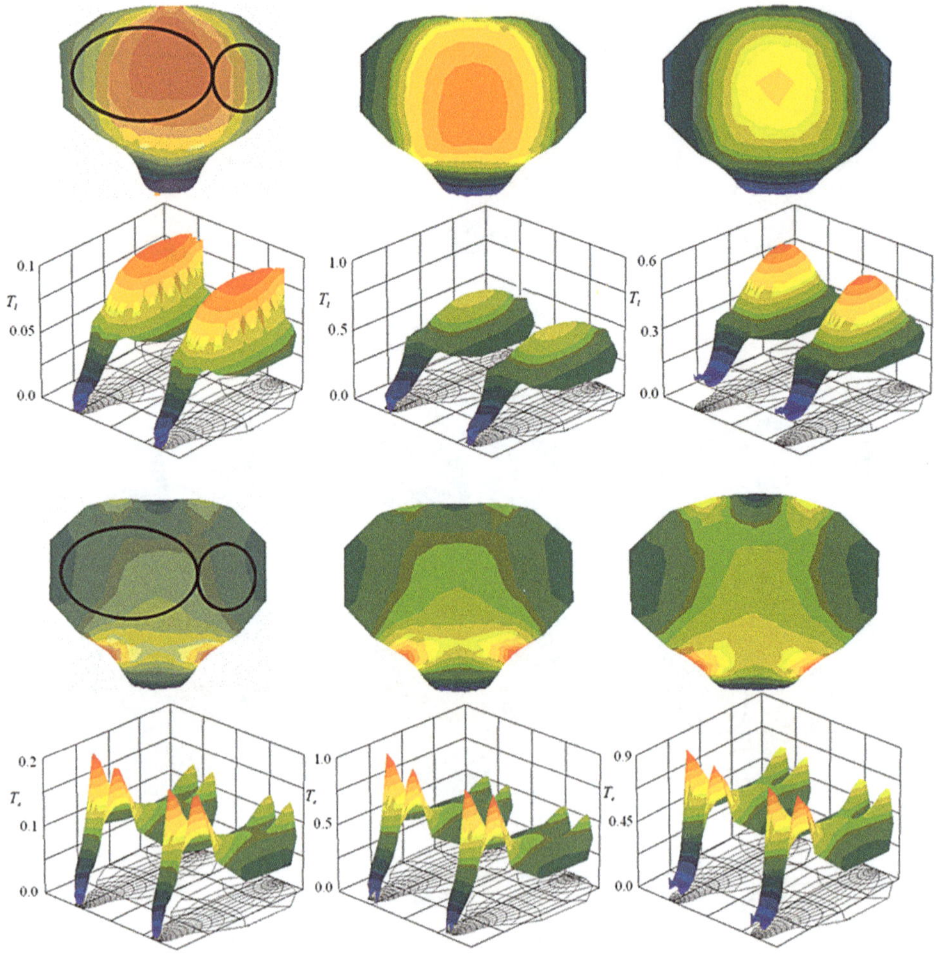

Figure 13.24. As in figure 13.22 with the fetus in transverse position. Reprinted from Miftahof R M and Nam H G 2011 *Biomechanics of the Gravid Human Uterus* (Berlin: Springer) by permission from Springer Nature. Copyright 2011.

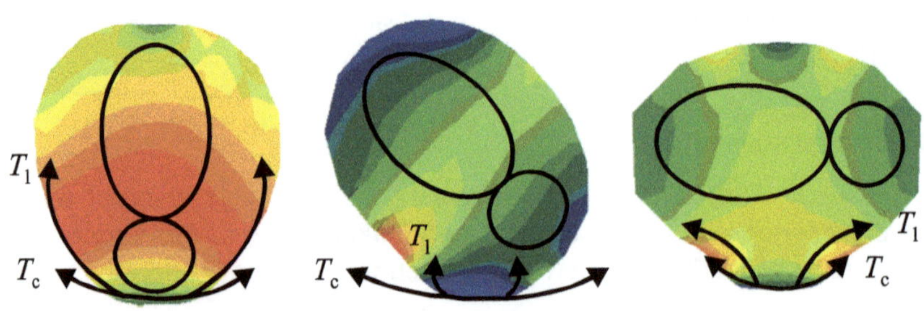

Figure 13.25. The intensity of total stretch forces, T_l and T_c, produced in the cervical region as a result of fetal presentation. Reprinted from Miftahof R M and Nam H G 2011 *Biomechanics of the Gravid Human Uterus* (Berlin: Springer) by permission from Springer Nature. Copyright 2011.

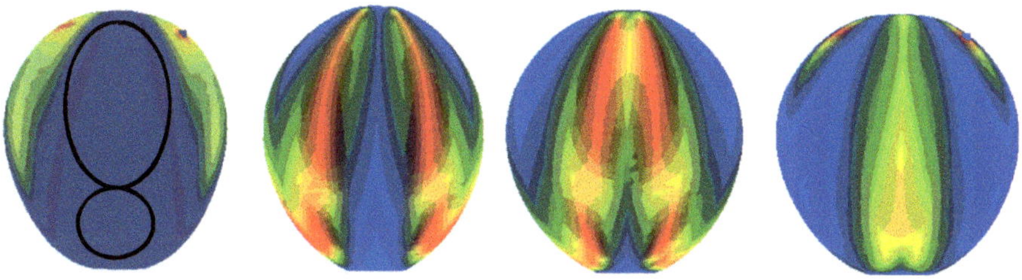

Figure 13.26. Dynamics of the first stage of labor. Propagation of the electrical waves of depolarization $V_{l,c}$ within the longitudinal and circular muscle layers of the uterus. Reprinted from Miftahof R M and Nam H G 2011 *Biomechanics of the Gravid Human Uterus* (Berlin: Springer) by permission from Springer Nature. Copyright 2011.

lateral sides of the womb (figure 13.26). As the two separate waves reach the lower segment, they begin to propagate circumferentially. The fronts of the waves of excitation collide in the region of the fundus and the body of the uterus with the generation of a single solitary wave V_l.

Within the circular syncytium the wave V_c extends circumferentially from the site of origin towards the lower segment. It provides uniform excitation to the organ. It may be noted that the fundus and body of the uterus experience strong depolarization if compared to the lower segment and cervical region.

The waves $V_{c,l}$ activate voltage-dependent calcium channels on the muscle membrane resulting in a rapid influx of extracellular Ca^{2+} inside cells. A rise in the free cytosolic calcium ion concentration leads to the activation of a cascade of mechanochemical reactions with production of the active forces of contraction (figure 13.27). Their pattern of propagation resembles the dynamics of spread of electrical waves. The most intense and lasting contractions are produced in the fundus and body of the uterus. The lower segment is subjected to strong circumferential forces that assist the dilation of the cervix.

The uterus undergoes biaxial stretching throughout the entire first stage. An analysis of passive force distribution in the wall of the bioshell shows that the stroma experiences the most intense tension in both directions in the body of the organ. It is related to the changes in shape of the region in the anterior–posterior dimension from rounded to flattened (figure 13.28).

The pattern of total force distribution in the womb demonstrates axial advancement, i.e. from the fundus to the body and lower segment, and a steady increase in the intensity of T_c. The dynamics are consistent with the generation of active forces of contraction by the myometrium (figure 13.29). A maximum T_c evenly encircling the body and lower segment of the uterus is observed close to the end of contraction. The force generated in the longitudinal striatum complements the process with a maximum T_l produced in the body along the anterior wall of the organ.

It is important to note that during the first stage of labor, the electromechanical wave processes sustain symmetry with respect to the axial dimension of the uterus and synchronicity of its pacemaker discharges. As a result, contractions cause the rupture of the amniotic sac with the release of 500–600 ml of fluid, the dilation of the cervix, and a change in shape, and decrease in the organ's fundal height.

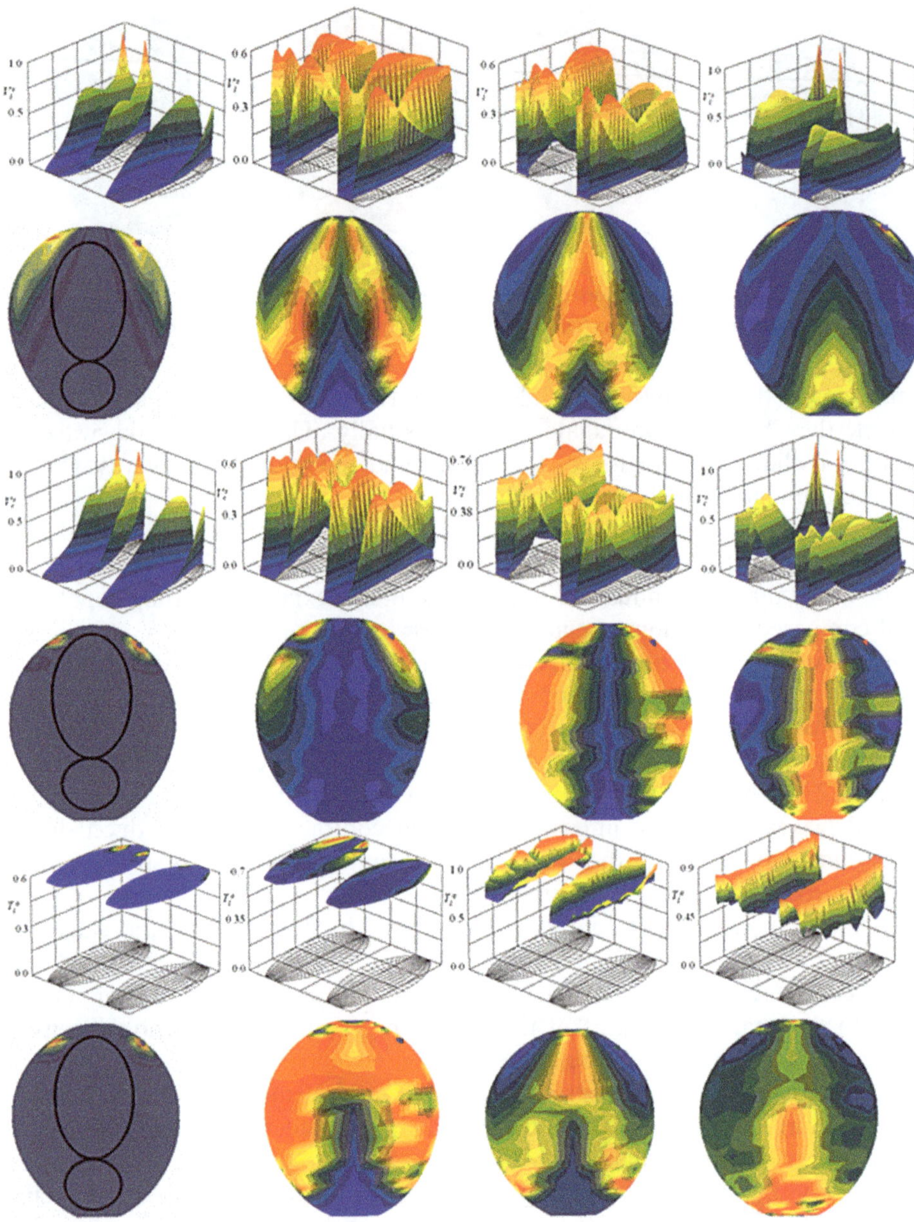

Figure 13.27. Dynamics of the first stage of labor. Active force, $T^{a}_{l,c}$, distribution in the pregnant uterus. Reprinted from Miftahof R M and Nam H G 2011 *Biomechanics of the Gravid Human Uterus* (Berlin: Springer) by permission from Springer Nature. Copyright 2011.

13.13.3 The second stage of labor

The subsequent second stage of labor is characterized by frequent strong uterine contractions aided by maternally controlled 'pushing down' efforts. They typically

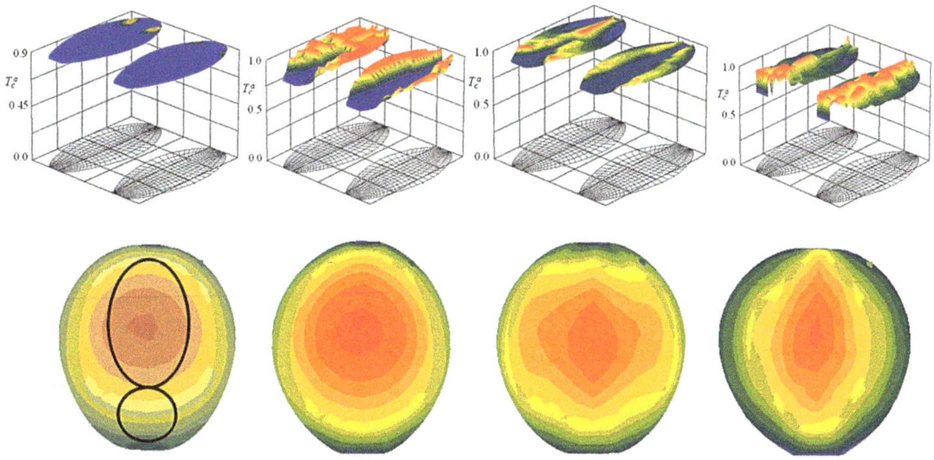

Figure 13.28. Dynamics of the first stage of labor. Passive force distribution in the pregnant uterus. Reprinted from Miftahof R M and Nam H G 2011 *Biomechanics of the Gravid Human Uterus* (Berlin: Springer) by permission from Springer Nature. Copyright 2011.

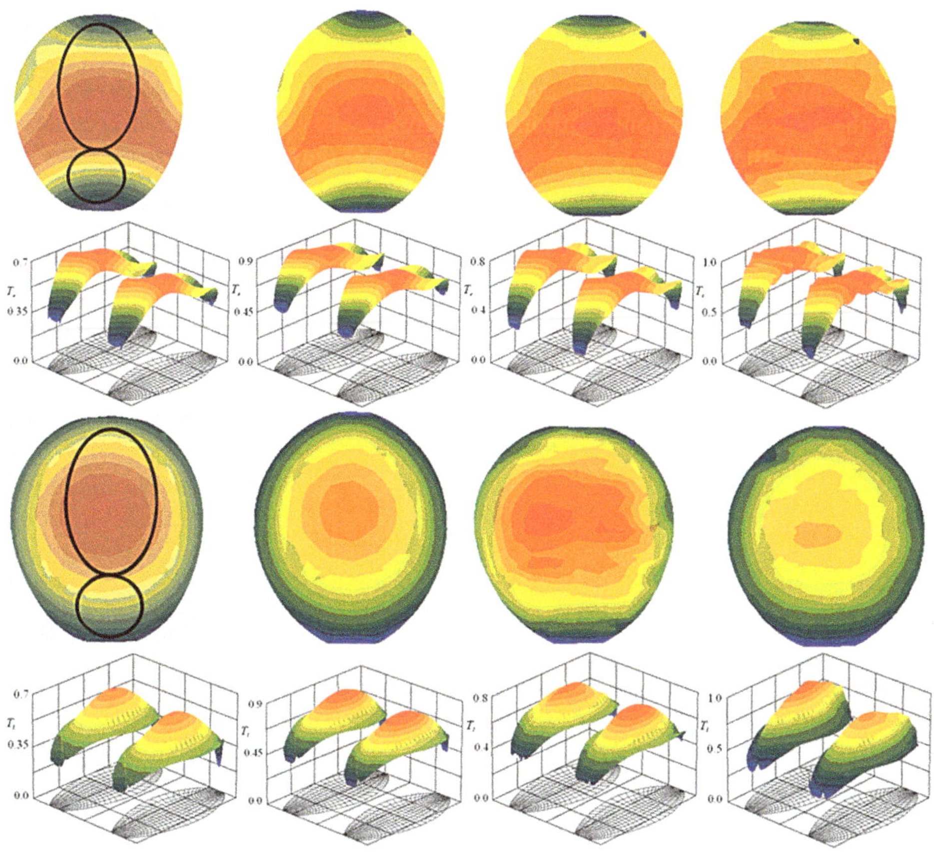

Figure 13.29. Dynamics of the first stage of labor. Total force distribution in the pregnant uterus. Reprinted from Miftahof R M and Nam H G 2011 *Biomechanics of the Gravid Human Uterus* (Berlin: Springer) by permission from Springer Nature. Copyright 2011.

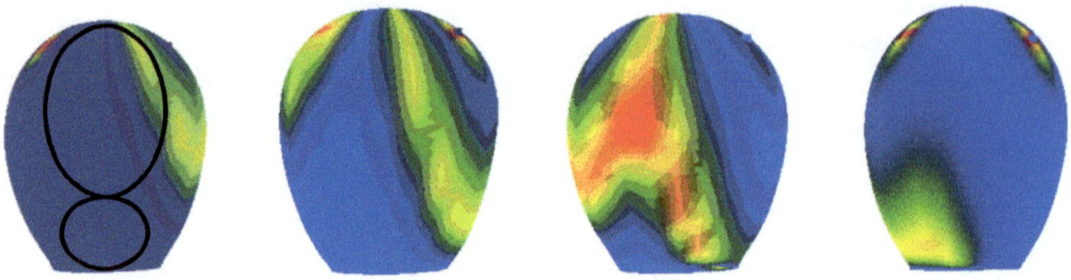

Figure 13.30. Dynamics of the second stage of labor. Propagation of the electrical waves of depolarization, V_c, within the circular myometrium. Reprinted from Miftahof R M and Nam H G 2011 *Biomechanics of the Gravid Human Uterus* (Berlin: Springer) by permission from Springer Nature. Copyright 2011.

occur before, during and after peak contraction force and are known as the 'triple' and 'peak' pushing styles. During this stage, the fetus is expelled from the womb. The process is associated with a series of internal deflections, translation and rotations of the head and body of the fetus, following a specific trajectory—the curve of Carus. (This is a curved twisted line representing the outlet of the pelvic canal with the end of the curve at a right angle to its beginning.)

Simulation results taken from the first stage of labor show that if the symmetry and synchronicity in electromechanical activity continue to prevail in to the second stage the fetus will undergo rapid translation only. No torque will be generated to initiate the necessary rotations. Although currently there is no experimental evidence to support the thought, it is reasonable to believe that the pattern of electrical activity changes. It can therefore be assumed that when the longitudinal syncytium is excited by synchronous discharges, there is a time delay between dischargers of the left and right pacemaker zones and the stimulation of the circular syncytium. During numerical experiments the intensity of impulses has been noticed to increase two-fold when compared to the first stage of labor.

The shape of the uterus with a fully dilated cervix supported by internal pressure $p = 19$ mmHg is given. The propagation of the wave of depolarization V_l, and passive T_l^{p}, active T_l^{a}, and total force T_l distribution in the organ are similar to those observed in the earlier stage.

The discharge of the left pacemaker zone precedes the firing of the pacemaker on the right. The anterior front of the wave V_{c} originating at the left uterotubal junction, envelops the uterus spirally before it collides with a similar wave propagating from the opposite right uterotubal junction (figure 13.30).

The formed single wave continues to spread towards the lower segment and down to the cervical region.

The myometrium produces intensive contractions of duration ~1.5 min, these being concomitant with oscillations of intracellular calcium, $\mathrm{Ca}_i^{2+}(t)$. Since the pattern of active force T_c^{a} distribution corresponds to the dynamics of the wave of depolarization V_{c}, it is reasonable to assume that the propagating mechanical wave of contraction produces a torque moment to rotate the fetus. Additionally, the total in-plane forces $T_{c,l}$ generated in the fundus and the body support its continual translation and later expulsion.

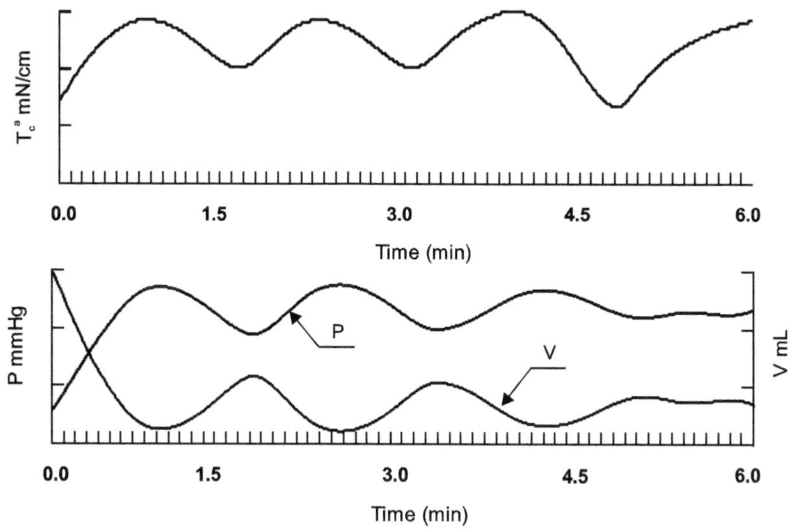

Figure 13.31. Typical trace of active force T_c^a progression in the circular myometrium layer of the pregnant uterus (top graph). Changes in intrauterine pressure and volume during the second stage of normal labor (bottom graph). The fetus is in cephalic presentation. Reprinted from Miftahof R M and Nam H G 2011 *Biomechanics of the Gravid Human Uterus* (Berlin: Springer) by permission from Springer Nature. Copyright 2011.

With each contraction, changes in volume of the uterus also reflect changes in intrauterine pressure (figure 13.31), increasing as much as five times from the resting value to peak at a maximum of $T_{c,l}^a$ and $T_{c,l}$. Interestingly, the rate dp/dt = const indicates that the myometrium at this stage behaves as pure elastic biomaterial.

13.13.4 The third stage of labor

The third stage of labor is characterized by a few strong regular contractions that separate the placenta from the wall and then deliver it through the birth canal. There is an associated increase in myometrial tonus, a thickening of the uterine wall (average $h \geqslant 2.4$ cm) with a significant reduction in size—the fundal height measures ~15–20 cm—and a flattening of the organ in the anterior–posterior dimension, ~8–12 cm. Detailed sonographic evaluation of *in vivo* changes in myometrial thickness after delivery have shown that the fundus measures 27.37 ± 3.5 mm, the anterior wall—40.94 ± 3.5 mm, and the posterior wall—42.34 ± 2.44 mm, respectively. The characteristic radii of the curvature of the middle surface of the uterus range within $15 \leqslant R_{1,2} \leqslant 20$ cm and $\max(h_i/R_i) \gg 1/20$. Thus, the organ at this stage does not satisfy the hypotheses of thin shells and needs to be treated as a thick shell of variable thickness.

Since the extension of the current thin shell approach to model the postpartum uterus is beyond the scope of this book, we shall only highlight a number of distinct features of thick shells that significantly influence the appropriateness of the model and give the results of stress–strain distribution in the organ. First, Kirchhoff–Love assumptions, i.e. that plane sections remain as a plane after deformation and are

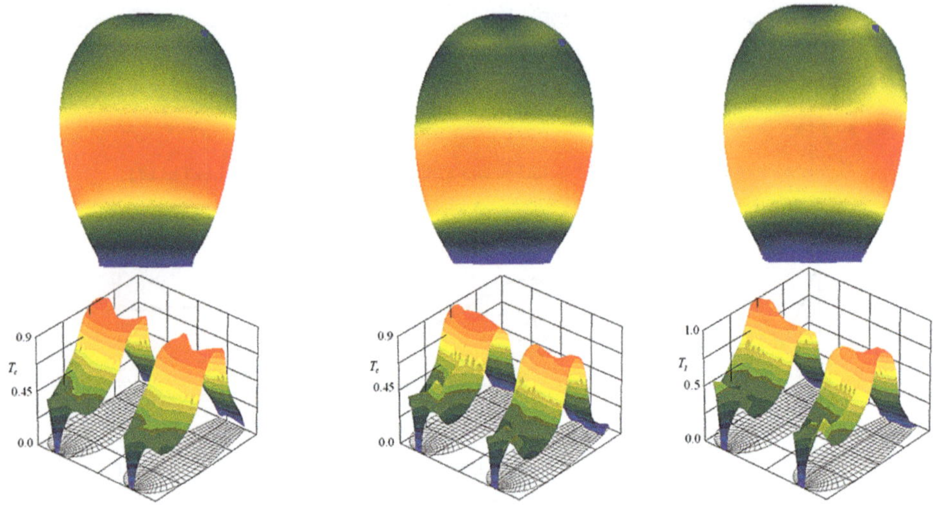

Figure 13.32. Dynamics of total force, T_c, development in the circular myometrium in the case of constriction ring. Reprinted from Miftahof R M and Nam H G 2011 *Biomechanics of the Gravid Human Uterus* (Berlin: Springer) by permission from Springer Nature. Copyright 2011.

perpendicular to the middle surface of the shell, are no longer valid. Therefore, the transverse shear strains cannot be neglected and the angle of rotation of the cross-section should be taken into consideration. Second, the initial curvatures of the thick shell contribute to the generated stress resultants and stress couples, causing a nonlinear distribution of in-plane stresses across the thickness of the shell. This happens because the length of the surface away from the middle surface has changed. Finally, in the case of the uterus it is imperative from a physiological point of view to consider the radial stress distribution over the thickness of the shell.

At the time of writing there has been no research to address the above questions with regard to the postpartum uterus.

13.13.5 Constriction ring

A constriction ring is a pathological condition that can occur at any stage of labor characterized by a persistent localized annular spasm of the circular myometrium. The exact pathophysiology of the phenomenon is not known. The predisposing factors, however, have been identified and include the malpositioning or malpresentation of the fetus and the improper stimulation of the uterus with oxytocin. The constriction can develop at any part of the uterus but most frequently it appears at the junction of the body and the lower segment. This is in concert with the oxytocin hypothesis and the pattern of OT receptor distribution in the womb. A critical analysis of relevant literature reveals that during labor, contractions are over expressed primarily in the fundus and body of the organ making them more susceptible to the hormone.

Consider the constriction ring—the constant active force T_c^{a} applied circumferentially—during the second stage of labor as shown in figure 13.32. The presence of a 'muscular band' does not affect the dynamics of spread of the waves of depolarization V_c and V_l. These freely pass the constricted zone to reach the cervical region. The intensity of T_c^a in the organ varies with each contraction, while T_c^a remains constant at the site of the ring. The region above the constriction experiences contractions, although the cervix remains lax: $T_{c,l}^a \approx 0$ and $T_{c,l} \approx 0$. At the zone of constriction, the passive force—the reaction of the fibrillar stroma to stretch—is less when compared to the values T_c^p observed during normal labor.

The addition of Atosiban™ to the system results in the relaxation of the constriction ring with a loss of productive contractions throughout the uterus.

Although the fetus *per se* is not included in the model, objective speculation can be made concerning the implications the constriction ring has on the dynamics of labor and delivery. Thus, ineffective mechanical activity and the resulting small forces generated during contractions may be associated with uterine dystocia, the delay in fetal descent or, if the ring occurs at the level of the internal cervix or around the fetal neck, retention of the placenta and postpartum hemorrhage.

13.13.6 Uterine dystocia

Uterine dystocia (dysfunctional labor) describes a difficult or prolonged labor and can be either cervical, i.e. the cervix does not efface and dilate, or uterine, e.g. constriction ring. Multiple causes have been implicated in the pathogenesis of this condition including an abnormal fetal size and position, fetopelvic disproportion, mineral and electrolyte imbalance, uncoordinated electromechanical myometrial activity, abnormal rigidity of the cervix, and cervical conglutination.

Consider the gravid uterus in the first stage of labor. Let numerous, in addition to ubiquitous, two uterotubal pacemaker zones be present and scattered across the organ. These fire at random impulses of constant amplitude $\overset{0}{V_p} = 100$ mV and duration $t_i^d = 10$ ms. Assume also that the tissue of the cervix is rigid and nonstretchable.

Under the conditions stated above, the induced waves of depolarization $V_{c,l}$ fail to propagate effectively along the longitudinal and circular myometrial syncytia (figure 13.33). Signals propagate over short distances only with multiple interferences and confluences preventing any powerful excitation of the organ.

The amplitude of both the active and total in-plane forces generated by the uterus is low. Contractions of the circular and longitudinal muscle layers are not synchronized. The anterior front of the electromechanical wave becomes irregular and there is a loss of directionality in its propagation from the fundus towards the lower segment. As a result, the cervix fails to efface and dilate, remaining closed throughout labor. This significantly affects the dynamics of expulsion of the fetus, noticeably impairing it.

13.13.7 Hyper- and hypotonic uterine inertia

Hypertonic uterine dysfunction describes the elevated tone of the uterus occurring most often in the latent phase during the first stage of labor. The uterus produces frequent strong and irregular contractions which are ineffective. The etiological

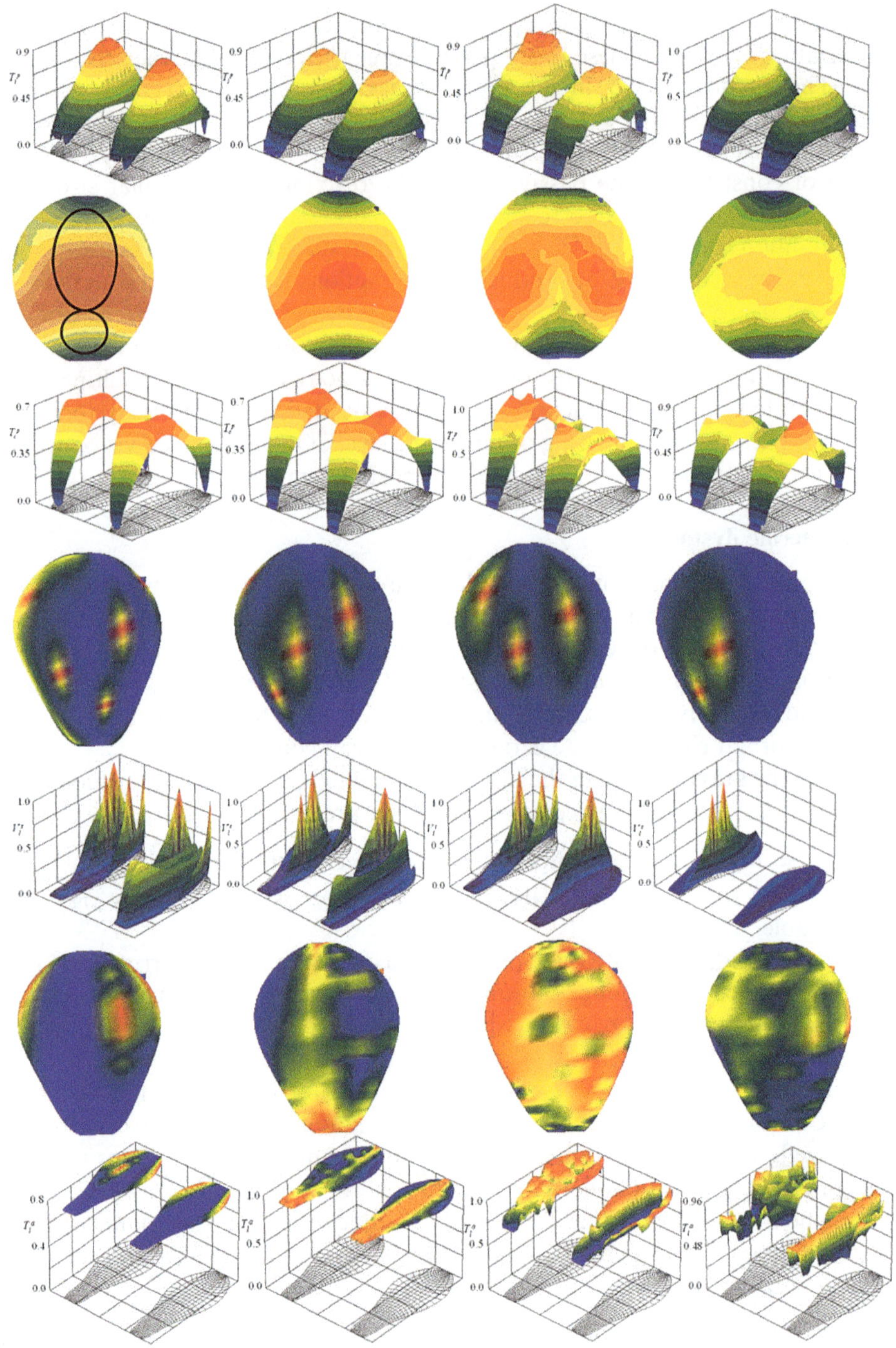

Figure 13.33. Uterine dystocia. Propagation of the electrical waves of depolarization, $V_{l,c}$, and active force, $T^{a}_{l,c}$, development within the longitudinal and circular muscle layers of the uterus. Reprinted from Miftahof R M and Nam H G 2011 *Biomechanics of the Gravid Human Uterus* (Berlin: Springer) by permission from Springer Nature. Copyright 2011.

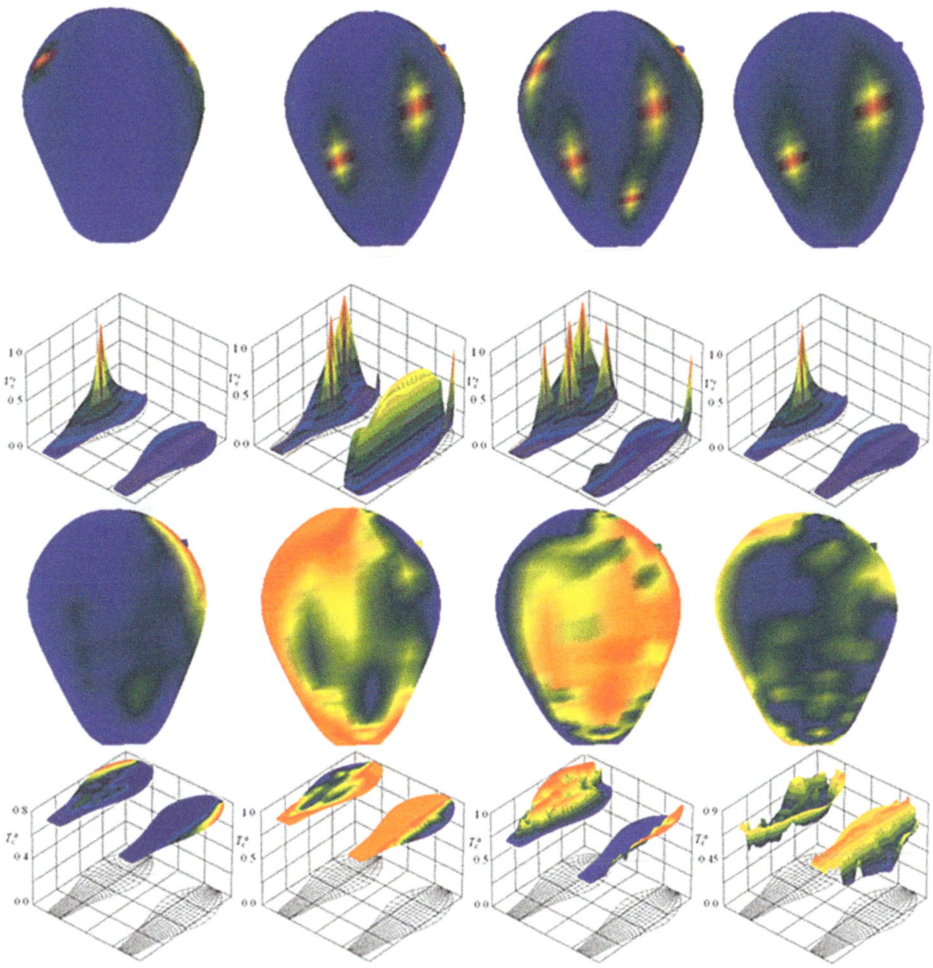

Figure 13.33. (Continued.)

factors concerned are not very clear but conditions including a state in which the body of the womb overreacts mechanically, and/or a lack of coordinated spread in the wave of depolarization and nerve pulse synchronization in the myometrium have been suggested. Resting intrauterine pressure between contractions is high (>12 mmHg). The cervix dilates slowly with the result that labor is prolonged.

To simulate the hypertonic uterine inertia, assume there is a time lag between discharges of the uterotubal pacemaker zones that triggers electrical waves of excitation in the longitudinal and circular myometrium. Let also the frequency and amplitudes of impulses produced by pacemakers exceed the normal values.

The results of calculations clearly demonstrate that initially the longitudinal myometrium of the fundus, body, and lower segment undergo uniform rigorous contractions. Their magnitude is higher than the values recorded during normal

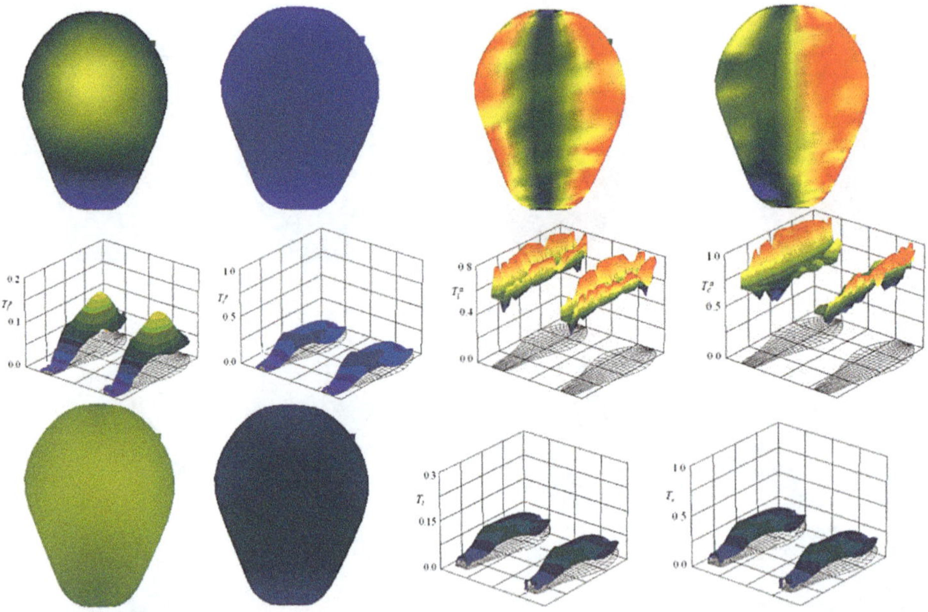

Figure 13.34. Hypertonic uterine inertia. Dynamics of passive, $T^{\mathrm{p}}_{l,c}$, active, $T^{\mathrm{a}}_{l,c}$, and total force, $T_{l,c}$, development in the longitudinal and circular myometria. Reprinted from Miftahof R M and Nam H G 2011 *Biomechanics of the Gravid Human Uterus* (Berlin: Springer) by permission from Springer Nature. Copyright 2011.

labor. In contrast, the circular myometrium generates intensive active forces mainly in the body and lower segment while both the strength and contractility of the fundal region remain low.

As the wave of depolarization quickly engulfs the uterus and the active and passive forces fully develop, the organ becomes stressed almost evenly throughout, with total in-plane forces $T_{c,l}$ attaining relatively constant values over the surface of the bioshell (figure 13.34). This effect is achieved by heterogeneous distribution of the forces $T^{\mathrm{p}}_{c,l}$ and $T^{\mathrm{a}}_{c,l}$ over different regions of the uterus. It is noteworthy here that the cervix fails to dilate and stays contracted throughout.

In clinics, pethidine, a drug with analgesic and antispasmodic properties, is being used to treat hypertonic uterine inertia. It exerts its pharmacological action through κ-opioid and μACh receptors and interactions with voltage-gated transmembrane Na^+ channels. Additionally, pethidine inhibits the dopamine and noradrenaline transporters and the uptake mechanisms.

The effect of the drug in the model has been achieved by simulating conjointly the following pharmacokinetic mechanisms—muscarinic antagonism, adrenergic agonism, and a decrease in the permeability of g_{Na}. The addition of pethidine into the system causes hyperpolarization with relaxation of the myometrium.

Infrequent contractions of small amplitude and of short duration during labor indicate hypotonic uterine inertia. Although the exact etiology of uterine inertia remains undetermined, the condition appears to be related to a combination of factors which include a deficiency of endogenous oxytocin and prostaglandins, an overdistension of the uterus, an acquired or inherited pathology of the myometrium, and uterine hypoplasia, but there may be others. Two types of hypotonic inertia, i.e. primary and secondary, are recognized. Weak and low frequency contractions occurring at the start of labor are characteristic of primary inertia while the substantial lessening of contractility after a period of good uterine electromechanical activity is suggestive of secondary hypotonic inertia.

A decrease in the firing strength and rate of pacemaker zones leads to a loss of synchronization in the depolarization of the myometrium and, as a result, the development of active forces. The intensity of total forces $T_{c,l}$ is lower when compared to normal labor. The shape of the organ stays unchanged whilst the cervix closes with each contraction.

The application of OT has a distinct excitatory effect. The resting tonus of the myometrium increases with the production of strong forceful contractions of normal amplitude and high frequency. Their dynamics are similar to those observed during normal labor.

Further reading

Åkerud A 2009 Uterine remodeling during pregnancy *PhD Thesis* (Sweden: Lund University)

Chkeir A, Moslem B, Rihana S G and Marque C 2011 *Phys. Procedia* **21** 85–92

Cochran A and Gao Y 2013 *Math. Mech. Solids* **20** 540–64

Manoogian S J, Bisplinghoff J A, Kemper A R and Duma S M 2012 *J. Biomech.* **45** 1724–7

Miftahof R N and Nam H G 2011 *Biomechanics of the Gravid Human Uterus* (Berlin: Springer)

Mizrahi J and Karni Z 1975 *Isr. J. Technol.* **13** 185–91

Mizrahi J, Karni Z and Polishuk W Z 1978 *J. Franklin Inst.* **306** 119–32

Testrow C P, Holden A V, Shmygol A and Zhang H 2018 *Nature: Sci. Rep.* **8** 9159

Vauge C, Carbonne B, Papiernik E and Ferré F 2000 *Acta Biotheor.* **48** 95–105

Wu X, Morgan K G, Jones C J, Tribe R M and Taggart M J 2008 *J. Cell Mol. Med.* **12** 1360–73

Young R C 2007 *Ann. N. Y. Acad. Sci.* **1101** 72–84

Zhang M, Tidwell V, La Rosa P S, Wilson J D, Eswaran H and Nehorai A 2016 *PLoS One* **11** e0152421

IOP Publishing

Soft Biological Shells in Bioengineering

Roustem N Miftahof and Nariman R Akhmadeev

Chapter 14

The urinary bladder

A one-dimensional mathematical model of the detrusor, a functional unit of the urinary bladder, is given followed by an analysis of its biomechanics, looking at the effects of changes in extracellular/intracellular ion environment and pharmacological interventions. These results are expanded to model the urinary bladder as a soft biological shell of revolution and to study the stress–strain distribution in the organ during both filling and voiding stages.

14.1 Anatomical considerations

The human urinary bladder is a musculomembranous hollow organ located deep in the pelvic cavity. Anatomically, the organ is divided into three major parts: the apex, body, and fundus (base), the latter consisting of the trigone and the neck (figure 14.1). The fundus is imbedded in the prostate in males and in the musculofibrous tissue in females being intimately attached to the internal urinary sphincter through the neck. The fibrous fascia endopelvina provides an additional connection between the base and pelvic wall and the rectum. The entire body of the organ is enclosed in loose fatty tissue of paravesicular fossa. The apex is covered by a thin stretchable peritoneum forming a series of folds—the false ligaments—which do not bear any biomechanical significance. The parts of the bladder are interconnected by the anterior, posterior, superior, right, and left lateral walls to form a smooth surface.

Histomorphologically the wall of the human urinary bladder consists of four layers: the mucous (urothelium), submucous, muscular, and serous layers. The details of their morphology can be found in many textbooks and research monographs with only a few aspects relevant to the biomechanics of the organ being discussed here. The innermost urothelium is made of polyhedral shaped cells of stratified transitional epithelium, including basal cells, intermediate cells, and umbrella cells. The outer umbrella cell layer interfaces with urine to form a primary barrier that includes a mucin/glycosaminoglycan layer, and an apical plasma membrane with low permeability to urea and water. In addition, umbrella cell tight

doi:10.1088/2053-2563/ab1a9ech14

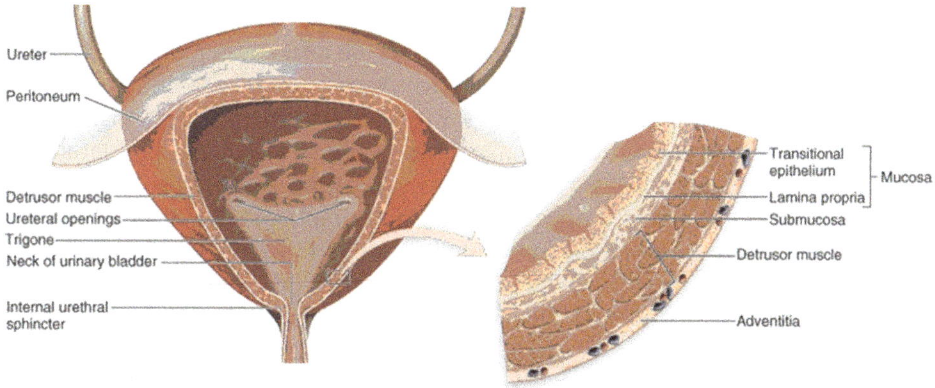

Figure 14.1. Anatomical divisions of the human urinary bladder. Reprinted from Miftahof R M and Nam H G 2013 *Biomechanics of the Human Urinary Bladder* (Berlin: Springer) by permission from Springer Nature. Copyright 2013.

junctions form a tight seal between adjacent cells being comprised of multiple claudin species to regulate paracellular transport. The uroepithelium maintains a barrier even as the bladder undergoes cycles of filling and voiding. The accommodation most likely reflects the ability of the highly wrinkled mucosal surface of the bladder to unfold, along with the increases in mucosal surface area that result from the fusion of a population of subapical discoidal/fusiform vesicles with the apical plasma membrane of the umbrella cell layer. On voiding, the mucosa refolds and the membrane plus the apical surface of the umbrella cells is thought to be recovered by endocytosis.

The submucous layer contains a large number of collagen and elastin fibers, myofibroblasts, and areolar tissue. Scanning electron microscopy studies have shown that fibrils are densely interwoven and make a loose network of three-dimensional stroma for both muscular and mucous layers. As a result of the fine arrangement of collagen and elastin fibers, the tunica mucosa possesses a high level of extensibility, i.e. when the bladder is empty it folds into rugae but stretches flat when the organ is filled with urine.

The muscular layer is the most prominent layer and is comprised of three layers: internal, middle, and external. Smooth muscle fibers of the inner and external layers run longitudinally from the fundus to the apex whereas the muscle elements of the middle layer have a predominantly circumferential orientation. Together, the three layers form the detrusor muscle with muscle fascicles and cells firmly covered with collagen sheaths. These not only provide a supporting connective tissue frame for the organ but also guarantee its deformability. Elastic fibers, on the other hand, are sparse throughout the bladder wall occurring only in denser networks around the blood vessels and muscle fascicles.

The serosa is partial as it only covers the superior and lateral walls, and is derived from the peritoneum. The latter contains wavy collagen bundles piled up in a sheet and intercalated by clusters of adipose cells. Ultrasonographic measurements of the wall thickness of the human urinary bladder have revealed that $h \approx 3.3 \pm 1.1$ mm. This figure remains relatively constant throughout the different regions of the organ.

The blood supply to the organ is through the superior, middle, and inferior vesical arteries derived from the anterior trunk of the hypogastric artery. Additionally, in the male the obturator and inferior gluteal arteries, and in the female the uterine and vaginal arteries, respectively, supply small visceral branches to the bladder. The venous drainage is through a complicated plexus that empties in the hypogastric veins.

The bladder receives autonomic innervation—sympathetic and parasympathetic—and somatic innervation mediated by pudendal nerves. The sympathetic nerves arise from within the thoracolumbar segments of the spinal cord, whereas the parasympathetic and somatic nerves originate in the sacrum. Along with their efferent function, each of these nerves conveys afferent signals concerning bladder distension. Light and electron microscopic studies have revealed the existence of intramural ganglia in the human urinary bladder. These intrinsic neurons are believed to be an extension of the pelvic plexus and may be involved in an integrative function of bladder activity.

The human urinary bladder, as described above, represents a dynamic multicomponent system. Optimal spatiotemporal arrangements among its anatomical and cellular/subcellular components guarantee normal function of the organ. It must be emphasized, however, that many of its behavioral patterns are determined by constant interactions among structural elements. Any instability in their integrated function results in the development of a variety of symptoms, e.g. urgency, frequency, incontinence, hesitancy, postmicturition dribble, all of which, if not corrected, may lead to serious pathological conditions. The key features of the main components giving rise to the physiological performance of the bladder are discussed below.

14.2 The detrusor

14.2.1 Morphological consideration

The morphostructural unit of the detrusor is the smooth muscle cell (myocyte) (chapter 6). Electron microscopy and freeze fracture studies have convincingly demonstrated that individual myocytes are interconnected by small and irregular gap junctions. Confocal immunofluorescence, Western blot techniques, transcriptase-PCR reaction, and *in situ* hybridization methods have shown that they are formed mainly of the subunit proteins connexin-43 and -45. They provide the structural basis for cytoplasmic continuity, mediate the movement of ions and small molecules, and support synchronization and long-range integration in the detrusor.

Immunohistochemical evidence has demonstrated the presence of mainly collagen (types I, III, and IV), elastin fibers, laminin, osteopontin, fibronectin, and integrins (α1–3, αvβ3, α5β1) in the lamina propria of the normal bladder. The three-dimensional hierarchy of the folding and coiling of the fine fibrillar matrix in concert with adhesive proteins ensures the property of the detrusor as a myogenic syncytium. It offers crucial mechanical characteristics such as high compliance, even stress–strain distribution, and coordinated phasic contractility during filling and emptying. In addition, continuous remodeling of the stromal network allows the organ to respond acutely and efficiently to prolonged periods of strain by adjusting its function and structure through dynamic myocyte–ECM interactions and by altering signaling pathways.

14.2.2 Electromechanical activity

Two types of contractions, tonic and phasic, are produced by the detrusor. Thus during the late stage of bladder filling the muscle generates tonic contractions but undergoes phasic contractions during bladder emptying.

The contractility of the detrusor is controlled by spontaneous and/or induced electrical processes. Their repertoire depends on the balanced function of plasmalemmal ion channels: L- and T-type Ca^{2+}, Ca^{2+}-activated K^+, voltage-dependent K^+, and Cl^- channels. The presence of L- and T-type Ca^{2+} channels in the human bladder has been confirmed by electrophysiological and pharmacological studies. Their morphology and function are similar to those present in the gastrointestinal tract and the uterus.

The resting membrane potential, V^r, of human bladder smooth muscle cells ranges between −55 mV and −38 mV. Both estimated and direct measurements of the input membrane resistance and capacitance of the detrusor myocytes have shown $R_m \simeq 125 \pm 49$ MΩ cm^2 and $C_m \simeq 1.0$ μF cm^{-2}, respectively. There is, however, controversy regarding the existence of spontaneous slow wave activity. Some authors claim that intracellular recording from isolated and intact strips of the detrusor do not show low-amplitude resting potential oscillations consistent with slow waves. In contrast, traces of simultaneous recordings of mechanical and intracellular electrical activity in human detrusor smooth muscle has convincingly demonstrated spontaneous fluctuations of the resting membrane potential of amplitude ~8–10 mV at a wide range of frequencies: $\nu = 0.33$–25 Hz. The detrusor muscle produces spontaneous action potentials (APs) or spikes of magnitude ≃34–46.5 mV and $\nu \simeq 0.07$–0.28 Hz. These occur as single clusters or bursts of 3–20 action potentials. Each spike has a relatively constant duration, ~1.3 s, a characteristic slow rising phase of depolarization, ~0.6 s, to be followed by a fast after-hyperpolarization phase, ~0.7 s. Spontaneous action potentials are resistant to tetrodotoxin (TTX), caffeine, ryanodine, thapsigargin, and cyclopiazonic acid, suggesting that extrinsic innervation and intracellular calcium stores do not contribute to their generation. However, spikes are abolished by L-type Ca^{2+} channels blockers, e.g. nifedipine, verapamil, or in calcium free solutions, indicating that they are of intrinsic (intramural) origin.

The conduction velocity, v_φ, of action potentials in mammals has been evaluated using the EMG mapping technique. The results have shown that a maximum v_φ in the rabbit detrusor is 3 cm s^{-1}, depending on the site and physiological status of the organ. Electrical coupling and passive cable properties of detrusor muscle cells from a pig bladder have been studied with the two-electrode method. Although the results are inconclusive, it is possible to assume that action potentials follow a preferred direction of propagation along the axis of the muscle cell over a short distance. The spread of excitation in the transverse direction is poor. Through observation it has been generally agreed that anatomical structure and distribution of gap junctions suggest that the detrusor syncytium possesses properties of electrical anisotropy. However, no direct attempts to measure preferential conductivity in the human bladder have been carried out.

14.2.3 Pacemaker activity

There is increasing experimental evidence that demonstrates that myofibroblasts—interstitial cells (ICs) (not to be confused with interstitial cells of Cajal)—modulate the spontaneous electrical activity of the bladder. Using methods of transmission, electron microscopy, immunostaining, and *c-kit* receptor labeling ICs have been found abundantly distributed immediately below the urothelium and between detrusor cells and smooth muscle bundles. According to their location, ICs are divided into three subpopulations: (i) boundary ICs—adjacent to the boundary of the bladder; (ii) intramuscular ICs—scattered among SMCs within muscle bundles; and (iii) interbundle ICs—distributed in connective tissues. They form close connections with intramural nerves and respond positively to various chemical mediators. Based mainly on their morphological similarities with those of ICC found in the gastrointestinal tract where their role as pacemakers is 'established', it has been hypothesized that myofibroblasts act themselves as pacemakers in the urinary bladder. This view is supported by evidence that the application of imatinib mesylate—a selective *c-kit* antagonist—disrupts spontaneous electrical activity in the organ. On the other hand, experiments on both single and groups of smooth muscle cells reveal that they are able to produce spontaneous discharges even without ICs. Moreover, it has been shown that Ca^{2+} transients in ICs occur independently of those of smooth muscles even when synchronous calcium waves sweep across muscle bundles. Therefore, there is reason to believe that ICs play a role in mediating the propagation of action potentials but not in providing a focus for their generation.

A comparative analysis of the behaviors of isolated cells and muscle strips from different regions of the bladder also suggests that the trigone myocytes may serve as the precursor for spontaneous electromechanical activity. However, the concept is based on speculative assumptions regarding their morpho-functional relationships and has not been fully tested experimentally.

The generation of strong regular electrical discharges is essential for the development of coordinated forceful contractions in the bladder during micturition. It is more likely to be achieved through the dense intramural parasympathetic innervation of the wall and network of intramural ganglia rather than through the syncytial cable properties guaranteed by existing adherens and gap junctions. Thus, sildenafil, a phosphodiesterase type 5 inhibitor, suppresses spontaneous contractions of the intact detrusor but does not affect spontaneous activity in single muscle bundles. Three types of spontaneous activity have been recorded: small amplitude membrane potentials, action potentials, and slow oscillatory conductance changes. However, no affirmative data on the dynamics of the propagation of excitation within the human detrusor to support or refute this view was available at the time of writing.

14.3 The neurohormonal regulatory system

14.3.1 Anatomical considerations

The storage and periodic elimination of urine by the bladder depend on the activity of smooth and striated muscles in the bladder and the urethral outlet. The coordination between these organs is mediated by a complex neural control system involving the brain, spinal cord, and major pelvic and intramural ganglia.

A meta-analysis of positron-emission tomography and fMRI studies of human and animal brains has demonstrated the existence of both non-specific—'level-setting'—and highly specific centers to regulate filling and voiding mechanisms. Non-specific centers are comprised of neuron populations located in the medullary raphe nuclei, locus coeruleus, and brainstem. Highly specific centers constitute the pontine micturition center (PMC), the periaqueductal gray (PAG), the preoptic and caudal hypothalamus, the thalamus, the insula, and cortical regions, the latter including the prefrontal cortex, anterior cingulated gyrus, and supplementary motor areas.

The neuronal tracts in the spinal cord include sympathetic, parasympathetic and somatic elements. Parasympathetic and sympathetic preganglionic neurons (PGNs) are found in the intermediate gray matter (laminae V–VII) sacral and lumbar segments, respectively, of the spinal cord. They project dendrites into the dorsal commissure, lateral funiculus, and the lateral dorsal horn to exhibit an extensive axon collateral branching that is distributed bilaterally. The somatic motor neurons that innervate the external urethral sphincter are located in the ventral horn (lamina IX) with a diverse arrangement of transverse dendrites.

The parasympathetic and sympathetic effector nerves of the bladder exit the sacral spinal cord in the anterior roots S2–S4 and T10–L2, respectively, and course through the pelvic and hypogastric nerves to the major pelvic ganglion. Pelvic ganglia are unique in that both preganglionic and postganglionic parasympathetic and sympathetic neurons are colocalized within the same ganglion capsule. Their postganglionic processes extend into the bladder wall where they contact intramural ganglia.

The ganglia are dispersed at random throughout the detrusor muscle bundles and adventitial connective tissue. The ganglia in the detrusor contain a variable number of cells ranging from one to six neurons although groups between 2 and 50 neurons have been described. The neurons possess typical multipolar characteristics and are interconnected via frequent axo-somatic and also less common axodendritic synapses to form an extensive neuronal network. The cells found in the adventitia have up to 20 nerve cells and are associated with large nerve trunks. These undoubtedly represent preganglionic inputs, either sympathetic or parasympathetic. Although there is little evidence for sympathetic (inhibitory) innervation of the human detrusor muscle, it has been proposed that an inhibitory effect is achieved through prejunctional inhibition via activation of possibly β_2-adrenoceptors and of nerve pulse conduction at the levels of intramural ganglia and/or the nerve terminal. It has also been suggested that excitatory presynaptic modulation of parasympathetic neurons is mediated by serotonin via 5-HT_4 receptors.

The sensory signals from the urinary bladder are conveyed to the spinal cord by the same pelvic, hypogastric, and pudendal nerves. They comprise thin myelinated Aδ-fibers that are present mainly in the detrusor, and unmyelinated C-fibers that originate largely from the uroepithelium and lamina propria. Both types of sensory fibers are diffusely and uniformly distributed throughout the organ. The Aδ-fiber endings are considered to be the primary mediators of the physiological sensation of organ fullness and are referred to as 'tension receptors'. In contrast, the C-fibers become active at a high level of bladder capacity. It has been proposed that their main roles are to provide a sensation of urgency and nociception. The cell bodies of the afferent nerve fibers are in the dorsal root ganglia (DRG) at the lower thoracolumbar and sacral spinal segments. Some of the afferent fibers synapse on intramural ganglia and it has been suggested that they complete integrative circuits capable of coordinating local autonomous activity of the organ.

Studies indicate that the urothelium functions as a transducer of some chemical and physical stimuli in the bladder. Multiple receptors for ACh, NA, ATP, neurotrophins, bradykinin, purines, etc, ion mechanosensitive Na^+ channels, myofibroblasts, and primary afferent and efferent neurons have been identified near to and within the sub- and urothelial layers. Through the channels and receptors, the urothelium is able to respond to various sensory inputs with the release of neurotransmitters—ACh, NA, ATP, prostaglandins, prostacyclin, NO, and cytokines, among others.

14.3.2 Neurotransmission

Acetylcholine is a ubiquitous excitatory neurotransmitter in the human urinary bladder. Recently, it has been established that there are two main sources of ACh release in the bladder: a neuronal source originating from intrinsic neurons, axons, and extrinsic neurons, and a non-neuronal source emanating from the urothelial cells. The main trigger for its release is cytosolic calcium, Ca_i^{2+}. Although all five types of muscarinic receptors (μ_1–μ_5) are found in the bladder, RT-PCR and Western blot analyses have demonstrated the dominance of type 2 (μ_2) and type 3 (μ_3), when compared to μ_1, μ_4, and μ_5 receptors. Quantitatively μ_2 type receptors outnumber the μ_3 type at a ratio of 3 to 1, although functional affinity is shown to be greater for μ_3 than it is for μ_2 receptors. The details of their distribution within the organ are still emerging, but existing experimental evidence suggests two main sites of location: the detrusor smooth muscle and interstitial cells of suburothelium. This evidence, along with clinical observations, supports the current hypothesis that μ_3 receptors are mainly responsible for the normal rhythmic electromechanical activity of the organ. Their regulatory effects are achieved through direct stimulation of smooth muscle and ICC cells. Non-neuronal cells of the urothelium, traditionally viewed as passive barriers, have been proposed as playing an essential part in bladder sensory mechanisms. They specifically respond to chemical and mechanical stretch stimuli and thus offer a reciprocal chemical communication with intramural nerves and the detrusor.

Acetylcholine along with ATP is commonly co-released from parasympathetic nerves. In the human bladder ATP acts at purinergic $P2X_1$ type receptors to function as non-specific cation channels. The hydrolysis of ATP ultimately yields adenosine which exerts its own effects on the detrusor through P1 type receptors. Four subtypes have been described so far: A_1, A_{2A}, A_{2B}, and A_3, coupled to G proteins either positively (A_2) or negatively ($A_{1/3}$). All types of receptors unequivocally regulate adenylyl cyclase activity. Despite its co-localization and co-release with ACh, the functional role of ATP in normal bladder mechanics is not significant.

Adrenaline acts via two main groups of G-protein coupled adrenoceptors. Low concentrations of α_{1A} and α_{1D}-mRNA adrenoceptors are present in the fundus, trigone, and base of the organ. They are linked to the $G\alpha_{q/11}$ protein system and PKA intracellular signaling pathways. Through cloning, *in situ* hybridization and pharmacological methods it has been demonstrated that the detrusor expresses three β subtypes of ARs, namely, β_1, β_2, and β_3. These are coupled to $G\alpha_s$, and $G_{i/0}$ proteins and are associated with the activation of the cAMP-dependent intracellular pathway. Selective $AR_{\beta 3}$ agonists cause effective inhibition of bladder contractions. This effect cannot be achieved through the use of specific β_1 and β_2 agonists indicating that it is mainly $AR_{\beta 3}$ that mediates relaxation. The results of recent *in vitro* investigations have suggested, however, that cAMP plays a minor role in β-adrenergic receptor-mediated relaxation. More specifically, it has been shown that a AR_β agonist can activate potassium channels, thus exerting an inhibitory effect.

Serotonin also has been suggested as playing a part in detrusor contractility. It has multiple sites of action, including the central nervous system, the dorsal and ventral horns in the lumbosacral spinal cord, and at presynaptical parasympathetic nerve terminals. In the human bladder, it acts at $5\text{-}HT_{2,3,4}$ type receptors. The stimulation of $5\text{-}HT_2$ receptors directly enhances contractility of the detrusor while activation of $5\text{-}HT_{3,4}$ receptors triggers contraction through the neuronal mechanism. Conversely, the inhibition of cholinergic neurotransmission at nerve terminals and relaxation of the bladder wall is controlled by $5\text{-}HT_{1A}$ receptors. Serotonin is metabolized in the liver by a two-step enzymatic oxidation to 5-hydroxyindoleacetic acid (5-HIAA). Monoamine oxidase and aldehyde dehydrogenase are essential enzymes that control this process.

Tachykinins, including SP and neurokinins A and B (NKA, NKB) are present in the human bladder. Radioligand binding, and autographic and pharmacological studies have helped identify three types of receptors—NK_1, NK_2, and NK_3—in the primary afferent nerves of intramural ganglia and the detrusor muscle. Tachykinins cause contractions of the organ via the excitation of NK_2 receptors. The effect is linked to activation of L-type Ca^{2+} channels.

In addition, many neuropeptides, e.g. endothelin 1, vasoactive intestinal polypeptide, somatostatin, angiotensin I, calcitonin-gene related peptide, nitric oxide, prostaglandins (PGI_2, E_2, $F_{2\alpha}$), thromboxane A_2, and neuropeptide Y among others, have been demonstrated as being synthesized, stored, and released in the organ. Their function has yet to be established but it has been hypothesized that their role as neuromodulators is small.

14.3.3 Electrophysiology of neurons

Studies of the electrical properties of pelvic ganglia neurons are limited to animal specimens only. *In vitro* preparations involving the enzymatic dissociation of cells, as well as *in vivo* intracellular recordings from intact ganglia, have provided a relatively concise description of electrophysiological characteristics and the patterns of neuron activity. The resting membrane potential for most neurons changes between −47.8 and −53.4 mV and the input resistance is 35–68 MΩ. The cells exhibit phasic and tonic types of discharges of amplitude 60–90 m followed by a short period of after-hyperpolarization (AHP). Furthermore, phasic neurons demonstrate both rapid ($\leqslant$4 APs) and slow adapting ($\geqslant$4 APs) responses to an injected depolarizing current. Tonic neurons fire with increasing frequency, $10 \leqslant \nu \leqslant 80$ Hz, which is proportional to the stimulus strength whilst the firing rate remains relatively stable for pulses applied at $\nu \leqslant 0.1$ Hz. However, discharge patterns change in both types of neurons if the frequency of excitation is increased. Thus, the tonic cells generate APs of a 'tonic bursting' characteristic, while the slowly adapting phasic cells produce spikes resembling an 'excitable' reaction in response to high frequency repetitive stimulation. In addition, the majority of phasic and tonic neurons in the major pelvic ganglion show rebound APs at the end of hyperpolarization.

Some tonic-type neurons also exhibit spontaneous activity with production of low $\simeq$5 mV, and high amplitude 60–90 mV APs. They can be blocked by the application of TTX, suggesting this activity is not intrinsic to their nature.

Data on the electrical characteristics and patterns of behavior of the urinary bladder intramural ganglia are even sparser. There are many similarities between the pelvic and intramural ganglia neurons. Intracellular recordings from neurons have shown that their resting membrane potential ranges between −40 and −60 mV, with an input resistance of $\simeq$58 MΩ. An injection of depolarizing currents into cells at frequencies $\geqslant$0.1 Hz causes the generation of either tonic or phasic spiking, similar to that observed in the major pelvic ganglion. Action potentials are usually followed by a period of fast AHP.

Intramural neurons are also capable of generating spontaneous low (1–3 mV) and high amplitude APs (50–60 mV) at a frequency of 60 Hz. Compared to the spontaneous activity recorded in pelvic ganglia, the spikes produced are not affected by hexamethonium, suggesting that they are intrinsic in origin.

14.4 Functional states in the bladder

14.4.1 Filling

The bladder functions, i.e. the storage and elimination of urine, are based on a coordinated interplay of the mechanical reactions of the detrusor and outflow region—the internal and external sphincters. Dynamic connections among intrinsic electrical, chemical (neurohormonal), and mechanical processes in the urinary bladder are required for the organ to function as a physiological entity. Existing ascending and descending pathways carry information between the brain, the spinal cord, and major pelvic and intramural ganglia to guarantee the effective regulation of bladder function. These forward-feedback interactions modulate the expression and activity of surface membrane and nuclear receptors, extra- and intracellular signaling pathways, ion channels, and contractile proteins, and define a variety of behavior patterns. Electro-chemo-mechanical coupling is a sequence of events resulting in the mechanical activity of the detrusor. It is preceded by a wave of depolarization of the cell membrane and/or ligand–receptor complex formation which triggers a sequence of intracellular processes leading to relaxation or contraction of the muscle.

Storage reflexes, known collectively as the 'guarding reflex', are organized primarily in the spinal cord and activated during bladder filling. Throughout this phase, the detrusor remains relaxed whilst the internal/external sphincters are contracted, thus preventing involuntary organ emptying. Such coordination is achieved by activation of the intramural stretch receptors whose distension produces low-amplitude afferent signals that are conveyed through the pelvic nerves to the spinal cord. Here they are organized by interneuronal circuitry to induce concurrent excitation to the sympathetic outflow in the hypogastric nerve and intramural ganglia of the organ. Some input from the lateral pons has been suggested as having a role in involuntary sphincter control. Additionally, the presumed connection between central and lateral PAG probably enables higher centers to control excitation to the PMC. During bladder filling PMC neurons and the parasympathetic pathway are turned off but at a critical level of distension the afferent signaling switches both to maximal activity.

The main neurotransmitter involved at this stage is noradrenalin. It binds positively to β_3-$G\alpha_s$, and $G_{i/0}$ coupled ARs located on the bodies of parasympathetic neurons and smooth muscle cells to activate the adenylyl cyclase enzyme. The latter catalyzes the conversion of ATP into cyclic adenosine monophosphate which subsequently activates the protein kinase A pathway. The binding of cAMP to the PKA enzyme causes the transfer of ATP terminal phosphates to myosin light chain kinase. As a result, there is a decrease in the affinity of myosin light chain kinase for the calcium–calmodulin complex with eventual detrusor relaxation. It has been hypothesized that PKA may augment the effect by inhibiting phospholipase C, intracellular Ca^{2+} turnover, and also by directly affecting the permeability of BK_{Ca} channels.

PKA activity is controlled entirely by cAMP. At low concentrations the enzyme remains catalytically inactive. The level of cAMP is regulated both by the activity of AC and by phosphodiesterases that degrade it to 5′-AMP. There is growing experimental evidence that phosphodiesterases 1, 4, and 5, play a role in the relaxation of the detrusor induced by parasympathetic stimulation. Another mechanism that decreases the production of cAMP is the activation of $G\alpha_{i-q/11}$ proteins which may directly inhibit AC through the MAPK signaling. However, no experiments have been conducted either to confirm or reject this theory of the mechanisms.

Another concomitant sequence of events related to the neurochemical processes described above is the electrical hyperpolarization of the detrusor. The generation of the inhibitory postsynaptic potential causes an increase in the BK_{Ca}, K_v, and Cl^-

channels' open state probability along with a reduction in permeability for voltage-gated L- and T-type Ca^{2+} channels with a resulting hyperpolarization of the cell. Deactivation of the L- and T-type Ca^{2+} channels affects the influx of extracellular calcium ions inside the cell. Non-selective cation channels, Ca^{2+} activated Cl^- channels, and Na^+/Ca^{2+} exchangers do not play a major role in Ca^{2+} influx. However, a basal level of free cytosolic calcium, 50–100 nM, and the release of Ca^{2+} from the SR through Ca^{2+}-induced calcium release, ryanodine, and inositol 1,4,5-trisphosphate receptor activation are insufficient to initiate or to sustain contractions. The detrusor muscle remains relaxed.

14.4.2 Voiding

The following micturition phase is mediated by reflexes starting in the brain which depend entirely on the neuromyogenic activity of the detrusor. Functional imaging studies of voiding have demonstrated that the process is associated with the generation of the activation signal in the prefrontal cortex, insula, hypothalamus, PAG, and PMC. The PAG receive inputs from sacral afferents and pass them to the PMC. The PMC and the paraventricular nucleus of the hypothalamus, in turn, connect non-specifically to the lumbosacral parasympathetic nuclei and autonomic preganglionic motor neurons in the spinal cord. From there the signal is transmitted to the parasympathetic neurons of intramural ganglia.

The excitation of the parasympathetic nerves, the release of acetylcholine (predominantly), and the depolarization of the smooth muscle membrane result in phasic mechanical contractions of the detrusor. Although the urinary bladder expresses different types of muscarinic receptors, contractions of the normal detrusor appear to occur largely via the stimulation of μ_3 muscarinic receptors. These receptors are coupled to a range of intracellular signaling pathways which involve $G_{i/0}$ and $G_{q/11}$ proteins. The activation of μ_3 receptors specifically triggers the cascade of $G_{q/11}$ protein reactions leading to a stimulation of PLC with a subsequent hydrolysis of phosphoinositide, formation of IP_3 and DAG, mobilization of intracellular Ca^{2+} ions from the sarcoplasmic reticulum, and ending in contraction. Various other signaling mechanisms have been demonstrated as linked to μ_3 receptor activation—Rho, tyrosine, and mitogen activated protein kinases and phospholipases D and A_2, among others. However, results of numerous *in vitro* and *in vivo* studies have suggested that these play a minor role in muscarinic receptor agonist induced contraction of the organ. Excitation of μ_2 receptors and the stimulation of the $G_{i/0}$ protein system causes downstream inhibition of the cAMP production. The latter is the main relay in the adrenergic pathway, causing the direct inactivation of membrane voltage-dependent Ca^{2+}–K^+ channels. The final result of the above cholinergic translations is the tight control of detrusor contractility.

Contractions of the bladder are comprised of localized 'micro-contractions' that occur in single or multiple discrete regions, electrical waves and micro-stretches. Tension, T = 1.0–2.0 g, is recorded in the organ at different locations, i.e. the detrusor and bladder base. Their intensity is small when compared to the contractions evoked through stimulation of the nervous system or those triggered by mechanical stretching. They cannot therefore significantly affect changes in the shape and intravesicular pressure, p, of the bladder. The evaluation of p as a function of volume, V, have shown that in a human with normal bladder compliance, $p(0) =$ 0–0.8 kPa and $p(300) =$ 1.46–3 kPa (numbers in brackets correspond to $V = 0$ and 300 ml, respectively). This phenomenon has been attributed partly to spontaneous contractility allowing the individual muscle bundles to adjust their length in response partly to filling and also partly to the viscoelastic properties of the tissue.

The average amount of urine that the bladder accommodates at one time is ~0.3–0.5 l. It varies from person to person and may be affected by underlying pathological conditions. In severe cases of fibrosis, the capacity is reduced to 0.2 liters whilst in the case of an obstruction, it may attain 2.5–3 l. The largest documented volume, 9.35 l, was recorded in a patient with severe obstruction caused by cancer of the bladder neck.

Despite its complex relationships with the rectum, uterus, pelvic bones, blood vessels, and ducts, the bladder expands during urinary filling without significant resistance from these surrounding structures. The actual size, position, and relationship of the bladder to other organs vary according to the amount of fluid the organ contains. Thus, an empty bladder is placed entirely within the pelvis, taking the form of a flattened tetrahedron with its vertex tilted forward. The configuration of the bladder during distension has been studied extensively using computed tomography and magnetic resonance imaging. However, since each imaging process takes several minutes, these traditional methods of data acquisition can only offer results which are qualitative in nature. Only recently, through the combination of high-resolution MRI technology with computer-based image rendering has it become possible to acquire a comprehensive insight into the dynamics of shape changes in the organ. It has been demonstrated clearly that during the filling stage, the bladder can assume diverse forms ranging from the most commonly observed ellipsoid to various irregular shapes. The radii of a fully distended bladder in the three principal directions, i.e. the anterior–posterior, R_l, superior–inferior, R_c, and left–right, R_v, measure $R_l \simeq 6$ cm, $R_c \simeq 4.3$ cm, and $R_v \simeq 4.3$ cm, respectively.

Voiding begins when a critical level of bladder distension is reached and strong afferent signals arising from stretch receptors switch the nervous system to maximal activity. In humans this process is voluntary. It involves multiple functional areas in the brain and rostral brainstem implying an interruption of the tonic suppression of input from periaqueductal gray cells to the pontine micturition center. Excitation passes from the PMC along intraspinal descending pathways to the sacral segment where it activates the parasympathetic outflow to the bladder. Stimulation of cholinergic pathways results in the contraction of the detrusor. During micturition, force generation and muscle shortening are initiated relatively quickly and are highly synchronized occurring over a large area. This efficiency is mainly achieved through the dense parasympathetic intramural network and intracellular mechanisms—IP_3 production and Ca^{2+} sensitization. A transient rise in $[Ca_i^{2+}]$ to 1 μM and the subsequent formation of an active Ca_4^{2+}–calmodulin–MLCK complex induce the myosin phosphorylation and contraction. Strong contractions with patent sphincters cause an increase in intravesicular pressure, p = 7.8 kPa, and a change in configuration of the bladder which becomes more rounded. With relaxation of the sphincter and urine outflow, the pressure falls to the resting level and the organ attains an undeformed configuration.

14.5 Biomechanics of the detrusor

A knowledge of the mechanical properties of the tissue of the bladder wall is crucial for the integration of motor functions into a biologically plausible biomechanical model. The combined study of urine flow in the bladder, the urinary sphincter, and the urethra is called urodynamics. A cystometric technique initially reported by Rose in 1927 has been extensively used from that time forward for both clinical and research purposes. Today, urodynamic investigations remain 'the golden standard' with the most definitive tests for the evaluation of the organ functioning objectively through a physiological micturition cycle. These constitute a series of tests to imply a real time monitoring of changes in bladder volume, intravesical p_{ves} and abdominal p_{abd}, pressures, uroflowmetry, surface electromyography and video-urodynamics during subsequent phases of artificial bladder filling and emptying. All recordings are made via a urethral catheter and a rectal balloon. The data acquired are used to calculate the cumulative bladder capacity V, detrusor pressure p_{det} ($p_{det} = p_{ves} - p_{abd}$) and contraction strength T, urine outflow rate Q, and urethral opening pressure and resistance. Although the method provides valuable quantitative information on the overall behavior of the bladder, it must be remembered that such studies are restricted solely to an assessment of micturition parameters dependent essentially on the theoretical concepts—physiological, mathematical, computational—employed in the evaluation of the organ's functionality.

As a part of urodynamic studies, detrusor electromyography (EMG) focuses primarily on recording electrical smooth muscle activity in living animals during active bladder emptying. It achieves this using either surface electrodes attached to the bladder wall or needle electrodes directly inserted into the detrusor muscle. This method is utilized for fundamental studies of bladder muscle physiology to test the integrity of neural circuits and intrinsic/extrinsic control mechanisms under normal and pathological conditions. EMG recordings offer higher spatial resolution and better dynamic estimates of bladder function than an assessment of pressure changes alone. Thus, spontaneous slow wave and repetitive spiking activities originating from the detrusor itself have been convincingly demonstrated through *in situ* experiments on rabbit bladders. A technique involving the positioning of multiple electrodes along the wall has put an estimate for the maximum conduction velocity of an arbitrary spike at ~3 cm s^{-1}. Both time domain and power spectrum analyses of recorded data clearly indicate a correlation between detrusor electromyogenic activity and an intravesical rise in pressure. Despite significant advancements in animal EMG studies, no electromyographic recordings have yet been obtained and verified from a human detrusor.

A large number of urodynamic studies to measure electromechanical activity in isolated and intact animal and human bladders have been conducted and a considerable number of publications on the topic are available in literature. These results, however, do not allow a reconstruction of active and passive uniaxial and biaxial force–stretch ratio relationships, an evaluation of structural changes in the detrusor and surrounding tissues, or an assessment of the spatiotemporal dynamics of variations in mechanical properties during the tension bearing process. Therefore, it comes as no surprise that credible models of the bladder tissue as a mechanical biologically active continuum have not as yet been constructed.

Most experiments on the bladder tissue under simple and complex loading protocols have been conducted on animals and only a few studies have been dedicated to the investigation of the human organ *per se*. Linear strips for uniaxial stretching were usually collected from different regions of the organ. Since the experiments have been performed on segments removed from the host, it has been assumed that muscle fibers are fully relaxed, the mechanical contribution being attributed to mechanochemically inert components of smooth muscle cells along with elastin and collagen fibers. *In vitro* quasi-static and dynamic tension tests have been performed along two structurally defined orthogonal directions of anisotropy—the longitudinal and circumferential. Their orientation coincides with the long and circumferential axes of the bladder, respectively. Assuming the homogeneity of both stress and strain fields and the tissue's incompressibility, passive force, and stretch ratios ($T^{\mathrm{p}}_{c,l} - \lambda_{c,l}$) have been calculated. The interpolation of data in the preferred axes of structural anisotropy yields

$$T^{\mathrm{p}}_{(c,l)} = c_1\left[\exp c_2(\lambda_{(c,l)} - 1) - 1\right], \quad \lambda_{(c,l)} > 1, \tag{14.1}$$

where c_1, c_2 are mechanical constants.

Experimental results have demonstrated that the tissue has nonlinear, pseudo-elastic properties and is similar to other biological materials. An analysis of the $T^{\mathrm{p}}_{c,l}(\lambda_{c,l})$ curves shows a characteristic 'triphasic' response with a nonlinear transition between the low and high elastic states. Histoarchitectural correlations with the dynamics of stress–strain development in the bladder wall have revealed that the uncoiling of ECM collagen fibers and small randomly oriented crack growth already begins at the early filling stages of the organ. These steadily increase in size as the distension of the bladder proceeds leading to a disrupture in the dense packaging of the fibrillary-collagen and elastin-matrix with an expansion and confluence of multiple small fractures. The distribution and orientation of elastin fibers in the bladder wall are both region and direction dependent. Most elastin is present in the ventral and lateral regions and appears to be oriented predominantly circumferentially. The detrusor muscle and collagen fibers, however, are most compact within the lower body with the trigone regions being the least affected by distension.

The viscoelastic properties of the bladder wall tissue have been studied extensively on uniaxially loaded strips *in vitro* and on the whole organ *in vivo* with ramp and quasi-static loading protocols employed in experimental settings. The quasi-linear viscoelastic model has been used to describe strain history dependence and hysteresis. This assumes that the relaxation function $K(\lambda, t)$ is the product of the pseudoelastic response $T(\lambda)$ and a reduced relaxation function $G(t)$

$$K(\lambda, t) = T_0(\lambda) + \int_0^t T[\lambda(t-\tau)]\frac{\partial G(\tau)}{\partial \tau}\partial\tau, \tag{14.2}$$

where

$$G(t) = \frac{1 + c_d[X(t/\tau_2) - X(t/\tau_1)]}{1 + c_d \ln(\tau_2/\tau_1)} \quad \text{for } \tau_1 \leqslant \tau \leqslant \tau_2, \tag{14.3}$$

and

$$X(t/\tau) = \int_0^\infty (e^{-t}/t)\mathrm{d}t, \quad \text{where } (t/\tau) \leqslant \pi. \tag{14.4}$$

In the above, c_d is the decay parameter, and τ_1, τ_2 are the fast and slow time constants, respectively.

The results of stress relaxation studies have revealed indifference in the biomaterial responses to quasi-static, ramp-and-hold, and oscillatory modes of loading along the structural axes of anisotropy. There is a shift in the stiffness and damping curves towards the smaller frequencies of the applied load. A decrease in the slope with higher stress levels indicates that larger stresses result in less relaxation with the damping more effective at smaller frequencies.

Biaxial tests to investigate *in vitro* pseudoelastic characteristics of the bladder wall tissue of different animals under quasi-static and dynamic loadings have been conducted on square-shaped specimens. These studies allow for the deduction of the full in-plane mechanical properties of the tissue. The edges of the specimens are aligned parallel and perpendicular to the orientation of the longitudinal and circular smooth muscle fibers. The experimental protocol to obtain force–stretch ratio curves $T^{\mathrm{p}}_{c,l}(\lambda_c, \lambda_l)$ uses constant stretch ratios of $\lambda_l : \lambda_c$.

The in-plane passive $T^{\mathrm{p}}_{c,l}$ forces under biaxial loading are calculated as

$$T^{\mathrm{p}}_{c,l} = \frac{\partial \rho W}{\partial(\lambda_{c,l} - 1)}. \tag{14.5}$$

The most general form of the pseudo-strain energy density function W is

$$\begin{aligned}\rho W = &\frac{1}{2}[c_3(\lambda_l - 1)^2 + 2c_4(\lambda_l - 1)(\lambda_c - 1) + c_4(\lambda_c - 1)^2 \\ &+ c_6 \exp(c_7(\lambda_l - 1)^2 + c_8(\lambda_c - 1)^2 + 2c_9(\lambda_l - 1)(\lambda_c - 1))],\end{aligned} \tag{14.6}$$

where ρ is the density of the undeformed tissue.

The bladders of pigs, rats, and dogs under biaxial loading exhibit a complex response including nonlinear pseudoelasticity, transverse anisotropy, and finite deformability with no dependence on the stretch rate. The curves $T^{\mathrm{p}}_{c,l}(\lambda_c, \lambda_l)$ show that as the stretch ratio in one direction gradually increases, the extensibility along the other decreases (figure 14.2). There is a concomitant increase in the stiffness of the biomaterial. The maximum force the tissue can bear during the biaxial tests depends on the ratio $\lambda_l : \lambda_c$. Experiments have shown that the shear force applied to

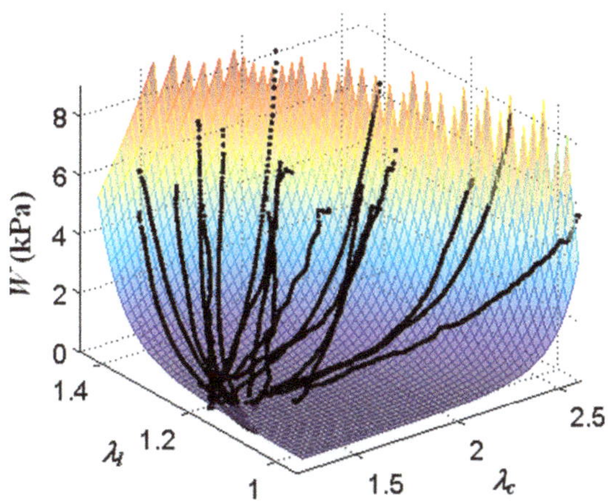

Figure 14.2. The strain energy function contour and fit of experimental biaxial data (black lines) for the rat bladder. Reprinted from Miftahof R M and Nam H G 2013 *Biomechanics of the Human Urinary Bladder* (Berlin: Springer) by permission from Springer Nature. Copyright 2013.

the tissue is significantly less $10^{-2}\ T^{\mathrm{p}}_{\max c,l}$ when compared with the stretch force. Unfortunately, no experimental results have been obtained from the human urinary bladder for any such analysis.

Investigations into the uniaxial and biaxial mechanical properties of actively contracting tissue remain the challenge in biomechanics. At the time of writing, no experimental data are available on the in-plane active behavior of the wall of the urinary bladder.

Over the years, surprisingly little attention has been given to the problem of constructing constitutive models of the bladder wall. The most common type of mathematical models used for soft tissues are phenomenological, these being usually of a polynomial or exponential form. Thus, earlier proposed descriptions of viscoelastic properties of the tissue employed a combination of Maxwell and Hooke elements. Here, elastic, time, and viscous parameters and constants of the models were evaluated from experimentally recorded cystometry curves. Despite their robustness and practicality, they do not capture the underlying mechanisms of biomaterial behavior and, therefore, have failed to integrate information about tissue composition and structure with its mechanical properties.

Under the assumptions that: (i) the soft tissue is an idealized network of muscle and undulated (in undeformed state) collagen fibers embedded into a compliant ground matrix; (ii) the mechanical net response is the sum of responses of individual fibers; (iii) the tissue is incompressible; and (iv) the strain energy density function W satisfies the decomposition

$$W = \phi_{\mathrm{ECM}} W_{\mathrm{ECM}}(\mathbf{E}) + \phi_{\mathrm{SM}} W_{\mathrm{SM}}(\mathbf{E}), \tag{14.7}$$

where ϕ_{ECM}, ϕ_{SM} are the extracellular matrix and smooth muscle volume fractions, respectively, and $\mathbf{E}$ is the Green–Lagrange strain tensor, the Piola–Kirchhoff stress $\mathbf{S}$ is obtained

$$\mathbf{S}(\mathbf{E}) = \frac{\partial W}{\partial \mathbf{E}} - l_{\mathrm{m}}\mathbf{C}^{-1} = \phi_{\mathrm{ECM}}\mathbf{S}_{\mathrm{ECM}}(\mathbf{E}_{\mathrm{ECM}}) + \phi_{\mathrm{SM}}\mathbf{S}_{\mathrm{SM}}(\mathbf{E}_{\mathrm{SM}}) - l_{\mathrm{m}}\mathbf{C}^{-1} \tag{14.8}$$

as a multiphase structural constitutive model of the mechanics of the urinary bladder wall. Here l_{m} is the Lagrange multiplier and $\mathbf{C}$ is the right Cauchy–Green strain tensor. The subsequent recruitment of fibers during loading in an ensemble of weight bearing elements suggests that the complete stress in the ECM and SM is

$$\mathbf{S}_{\mathrm{i}}(\mathbf{E}_{\mathrm{i}}) = \eta\phi_{\mathrm{f}}\int_{-\pi/2}^{\pi/2} R(\hat{\theta})\left\{\int_0^{E_{\mathrm{ens}}} D(x)E_{\mathrm{ens}}(\hat{\theta})dx\right\}\bar{\mathbf{r}} \otimes \bar{\mathbf{r}}d\hat{\theta} \quad i = \mathrm{ECM, SM}, \tag{14.9}$$

where the parameters and functions refer to the collagen/smooth muscle fiber: η is the modulus, ϕ_{f} is the volumetric fraction, $R(\hat{\theta})$ is the distribution function, $\hat{\theta}$ is the angle orientation in the undeformed configuration, E_{ens} is the fiber ensemble slack strain, $D(x)$ is the recruitment function, and $\bar{\mathbf{r}}$ is the orientation vector. The exact forms of $R(\hat{\theta})$ and $D(x)$ are assumed to be known *a priori*. For example, for collagen fibers their common representation is as a bimodal beta distribution whilst for smooth muscle, the two-parameter exponential model is widely adopted.

The general nature of this approach has the potential to explain the underlying remodeling mechanisms of individual constituents, i.e. the process of uncoiling, straightening, and reorientation of fibers along the direction of an applied force under normal physiological conditions along with an estimation of their role in various pathologies.

14.6 Models of the bladder

The earlier research into mathematical modeling of the biomechanics of the urinary bladder has been focused on modeling the organ as a reservoir with urinary bladder neuronal control mechanisms, and the simulation of urine-bladder–urethra interactions during filling and micturition. The bladder has been typically treated as a thin shell subjected to external and internal quasi-static loads. Initially, it was suggested that the organ could be approximated as a geometrically simple shape, namely a sphere. Assuming incompressibility, homogeneity, mechanical isotropy, and physical linearity of the wall, the dependence of the inflation pressure on the extension ratios λ_i ($i = 1, 2, 3$) was established:

$$p(\lambda) = \int_1^{\lambda} \frac{1}{\lambda^3 - 1}\frac{\mathrm{d}}{\mathrm{d}\lambda}W(\lambda, \lambda, \lambda^{-2})\mathrm{d}\lambda, \tag{14.10}$$

where the following form of strain energy function W was

$$W(\lambda, \lambda, \lambda^{-2}) = c(p_0, \dot{p}) + p_0\mathrm{P}(\dot{p}, \lambda)e^{\alpha(\lambda-1)}. \tag{14.11}$$

Here $p_0, \dot{p}$ are the initial intravesicular pressure and the rate of pressure change, respectively, $\mathrm{P}(\dot{p}, \lambda)$ is a third degree polynomial, $c(p_0, \dot{p})$ is a constant. The calculated Lagrangian stresses demonstrates a good correlation between both predicted and experimental stress–strain relations recorded from uniaxial loading tests of excised dog bladder strips, as well as slow and rapid cystometry studies performed on the whole organ.

The results of investigations into the role of more complex bladder shapes—the prolate and oblate spheroids—on the intravesicular pressure–volume $p(V)$ response during filling have shown that the $p(V)$ curves obtained for prolate and oblate spheroids for a wide range of eccentricities, $0.1 < \varepsilon < 0.9$, do not deviate significantly from the sphere.

The interaction of urine with the elastic urethra and bladder during filling and micturition has also been explored. In such experiments, the bladder–urethra system was modeled as an ellipsoid connected to a cylindrical tube. The wall of the bladder and urethra were considered to be isotropic and linear elastic whilst the urine was considered to be a Newtonian fluid with the flow non-stationary and turbulent. To reproduce dynamic (external body and volume related) forces, 'artificial' loading terms were included in the governing system of equations. Although the results have provided graphical outputs showing the urine velocity outflow, pressure distribution, and changes in the configuration of the urinary tract during voiding, the results of simulations are inconclusive, i.e. no detailed quantitative information can be derived from the data presented concerning the dynamics of micturition. A similar quasi-empirical analysis of variation in the intravesicular pressure, bladder volume, internal sphincter area, and urine outflow, including the parasympathetic signaling to the detrusor muscle and internal sphincter has been conducted recently. The parasympathetic signal has been chosen as a unit square function for $V_0 < V < V_{\mathrm{crit}}$, where V_{crit} is the critical volume when micturition starts. A sinusoidal oscillatory function has been employed to mimic intermittent voiding. Using experimental curves, e.g. cystograms, and adjusting a number of computational parameters during simulations, the authors achieved a satisfactory resemblance quantitatively and qualitatively to clinical observations.

In an inverse problem to determine the stress–strain relationships of the bladder based on the assumption that the organ is a thin spherical shell subjected to complex loading, the wall tension, σ, has been calculated from

$$\sigma = \frac{r}{2\delta}(p - p_{\mathrm{abd}}), \tag{14.12}$$

where p_{abd} is the intra-abdominal pressure, r is radius, and δ is the thickness of the sphere. Using actual cystometry and uroflowmetry readings as input data it is possible to reproduce the nonlinear profile of the $\sigma(\lambda)$ curve (λ–stretch ratio) either in a longitudinal or circumferential direction.

When the bladder is modeled as a thick-walled sphere, special emphasis is given to the evaluation of the effect of muscle fiber orientation and physical nonlinearity of the tissue on the dynamics of the organ's deformation. Three different geometries of fiber winding have been studied: the circumferential, longitudinal, and oblique. The total effective Cauchy stress, σ^{e}, is decomposed as

$$\sigma^{\mathrm{e}} = \sigma_{\mathrm{p}}^{\mathrm{e}} + \sigma_{\mathrm{a}}, \tag{14.13}$$

where σ_p^e is the passive stress—the result of stretch of the connective tissue elements, and σ_a is the active stress generated by muscle cells. The passive principal stress is obtained as

$$\sigma_p^e = \frac{\partial W(\mathbf{E})}{\partial \mathbf{E}}, \tag{14.14}$$

where the strain energy function, W, is chosen in the form

$$W(\mathbf{E}) = b_1 \mathrm{I}_E^2 + b_2 \mathrm{II}_E + c[\exp(a_1 \mathrm{I}_E^2 + a_2 \mathrm{II}_E) - 1].$$

Here I_E, II_E are the first and second invariants of $\mathbf{E}$, and a_1, a_2, b_1, b_2, c are empirical constants.

The classical Hill model composed of a parallel passive elastic, σ_p^e, and a series of passive elastic and contractile elements is used to simulate active stress. The activation, $A_r(t)$, deactivation, $A_d(t)$, and the length dependence, $A_l(l_c)$, functions are introduced to mimic the effect of regulatory mechanisms. They have been derived from experimental curves on single smooth muscle cells of a pig bladder,

$$\begin{aligned} A_r(t) &= 1 - \frac{1}{1 + (t/t_r)^4}, \\ A_d(t) &= \begin{cases} 1 - \dfrac{1}{1 + [(t_e - t)/t_d]^4}, & t \leqslant t_e \\ 0, & t > t_e \end{cases}, \\ A_l(l_c) &= \frac{(l_c - (l_{max} - l_w))(l_c - (l_{max} + l_w))}{l_w^2}. \end{aligned} \tag{14.15}$$

Here t_r, t_d are the time constants of contraction and relaxation, respectively, l_c is the actual length of a contractile element, and l_{max} is the length of a contractile element at maximal active force, l_w is the rate of curve width.

The cavity pressure during filling is calculated from

$$p = \int_{\lambda_i}^{\lambda_0} \frac{\partial W/\partial \lambda}{\lambda^3 - 1} d\lambda, \tag{14.16}$$

where the limits of integration refer to the stretch ratios of the outer and inner sphere radii. During micturition, however, it changes according to urine flow Q,

$$p = i\frac{\partial Q}{\partial t} + RQ, \tag{14.17}$$

where i and R are the inertia and urethral resistance.

The results of numerical simulations in cases of the circular winding of muscle fibers demonstrate a gradual change in the configuration of the shell (bladder) from spherical to that of a prolate spheroid during the collection phase. This reverses and resorts to the initial state at the end of the void. An analysis of stress distribution shows that the highest σ^e values are at the inner wall in the equator region whilst the lowest are at the poles. Having longitudinal fiber geometry, the bladder attains the shape of an oblate spheroid at the end of filling with the pattern of stress–strain distribution inverse to its circumferential geometry.

A conceptually analogous approach has been employed in a numerical modeling of the urinary bladder as an axisymmetric thin biologically active shell. The initial configuration of the organ closely resembles that observed clinically. In this approach, the wall tissue was assumed to be homogeneous and to possess nonlinear elastic properties. However, the supposition is valid for 'passive' biomaterials only and becomes invalid when any muscle activity is present or suspected. The results of these simulations for the passive relaxation and detrusor activation phases showed that maximum circumferential stress occurred at the lower part of the bladder and at the fundus. The body of the organ experienced a uniform axial and circumferential stress distribution throughout.

Although the mathematical models described above have provided useful insights into the investigation of clinical disorders related to bladder hypertony and urethral obstruction, they lack valid anatomical and physiological inputs, i.e. the neural regulatory elements, internal/external bladder and urethral sphincters, urine flow dynamics and neurotransmission mechanisms, among others. The first plausible attempt to address these issues was undertaken by Bastiaansen and colleagues (1996). Here the authors exercised a systems biology approach to simulate the bladder as a multi-hierarchical system that integrated neural networks with biomechanical and urodynamic components in one quantitative model. The dynamics of neural excitatory and inhibitory stimuli that trigger detrusor and urethral sphincter contraction and relaxation, respectively, are described in terms of normalized activity functions f_{aD}, f_{aS}:

$$\tau\frac{df_{aD}}{dt} = \omega_e^{D} - f_{aD}(1 - \omega_i^{D}) \quad f_{aD} \in [0, 1] \tag{14.18}$$

$$\tau\frac{df_{aS}}{dt} = \omega_s - f_{aS} \quad f_{aS} \in [0, 1], \tag{14.19}$$

where τ is a time constant, ω_e^{D}, ω_i^{D}, ω_s are the excitatory (subscript e), inhibitory (i), and excitatory somatic (s) inputs $((\omega_e^{D}, \omega_i^{D}, \omega_s) \in [0, 1])$.

Assuming quasi-static isometric contractions the detrusor was treated as a homogeneous incompressible viscoelastic continuum. The total actual tensile stresses in the smooth muscle and sphincter were decomposed into a sum of the active and passive stresses

$$\sigma_D = k_{area}(f_{aD}\sigma_{max}\sigma_v(v_D)\sigma_l(l_D) + \sigma_e(l_D) + \sigma_{ve}(v_D)), \tag{14.20}$$

$$\sigma_S = k_{thick}(f_{aS}\sigma_{max}\sigma_v(v_S)\sigma_l(l_S) + \sigma_e(l_S)). \tag{14.21}$$

Here, all functions are normalized on [0, 1], where σ_{max}, $\sigma_l(l_D)$, $\sigma_l(l_S)$ are the maximal and actual isometric stresses of the detrusor and urethral sphincter, respectively,

$\sigma_v(v_D)$, $\sigma_v(v_S)$ are velocity-dependent stresses obtained at an optimal length of muscle fibers to satisfy the Hill equation, $\sigma_e(l_D)$, $\sigma_e(l_S)$, $\sigma_{ve}(v_D)$ are the elastic and viscoelastic stresses, and k_{area}, k_{thick} are the ratio of the cross-sectional area of the detrusor taken at optimal muscle fiber length to the actual area and thickness of the sphincter, respectively.

The bladder was considered to be a thin spherical isotropic shell and the sphincter, a cylinder. Intravesicular and active sphincter pressures were calculated as $p_{D(S)} = \sigma_{D(S)} \ln (r^o_{D(S)}/r^i_{D(S)})$, where $r^o_{D(S)}$, $r^i_{D(S)}$ are the outer and internal radii of the shell and the sphincter, respectively. With regard to the passive elastic properties of the urethral sphincter, an exponential relationship between the radius of the urethra and urine pressure was selected.

An assumption of steady flow is made to describe the flow in different parts of the bladder–urethra system. The flow Q is obtained from

$$Q = \sqrt{\frac{p_u}{R_t(R_i, A_i)}} \qquad i = u_p, u_d, \tag{14.22}$$

where p_u ($p_u = p_S$) is the liquid pressure in the urethra, and $R_t(R_i, A_i)$ is the total resistance of the distal urethra, a function of the resistance and cross-sectional areas of the proximal and distal parts of the urethra.

In the above model, most parameters have both physiological and physical meanings. Therefore, it is possible for the authors to define a range of their variation and measure their actual values. Despite the mathematical and biological limitations, the results drawn from the model clearly resemble the traces obtained from urodynamic studies. Several other models of the lower urinary tract have been proposed which are, to a certain extent, variations of the Bastiaansen *et al* model. However, all of these models lack solid biological and mechanical foundations as a function in their design. Therefore, they cannot answer important questions related to the pathophysiological changes occurring in signal transduction mechanisms and biomechanical activity, or predict the effects of pharmacological interventions in various diseases.

More recently, a new class of models has emerged to study the dynamics of urinary flow in the bladder and urethra. These are a result of advancements in computational, software, and imaging technology, and in particular, in MRI with digital three-dimensional image processing and image reconstruction. The approach focuses primarily on the detailed description of geometry and an application of the principles of solid and fluid mechanics to simulate the anatomical structures of the lower urinary tract and their functions. Although existing models are still biologically and biomechanically deficient, i.e. no active forces and deformations are generated in the bladder and the urethra during micturition, with no regulatory (parasympathetic and sympathetic) inputs present, such models do provide an original insight into the dynamics of bladder–urethra–urine flow.

14.7 General model postulates

The basic anatomical and morphological data concerning the human urinary bladder are summarized as follows:

(i) The wall of the bladder is composed of two interspersed muscle layers, longitudinal and circumferential, with fasciculi running orthogonally within them.

(ii) The detrusor has the properties of an electrically isotropic syncytium. Multiple gap junctions provide low electrical resistance gating among smooth muscle cells.

(iii) The electrical activity represents the integrated function of ion channels: voltage-dependent Ca^{2+} channels of L- and T-types, large Ca^{2+}-activated K^+ channels (BK_{Ca}), potential sensitive K^+ channels, and Cl^- channels. The properties of the channels are neurohormonally modulated; this effect is assumed to be mainly chronotropic with an increase in the time of permeability for specific ions.

(iv) Although pacemaker cells *per se* have not been found in the organ, there are groups of cells that are responsible for the generation of electrical signals and coordinated rhythmic contractions of the bladder.

(v) Contractions are dependent on external and internal control. The coordination is provided by multiple neurotransmitters.

(vi) The key player in the process of electromechanical coupling is free cytosolic calcium. The active force T^{a}–Ca_{i}^{2+} relationship is characteristic for the smooth muscle.

(vii) The total force $T_{c,\mathrm{l}}$ generated by the muscle layers results from a deformation of its passive elements, $T^{\mathrm{p}}(\lambda_c, \lambda_{\mathrm{l}}, c_i)$, i.e. collagen and elastin fibers, and active contraction–relaxation of myofibrils, $T^{\mathrm{a}}(\lambda_{c,l}, Z_{\mathrm{mn}}^{(*)}, [Ca_{\mathrm{i}}^{2+}], c_i)$.

(viii) Electrochemical and chemoelectrical coupling in the system is guaranteed by separate and/or conjoint activation of multiple intracellular pathways as well as ligand-dependent transmembrane ion channels.

Assume that when the organ is empty of urine, its cut configuration coincides with the undeformed configuration ($S = \overset{0}{S}$) and stretch ratios $\lambda_{i,j} \equiv 1.0$, $(i,j = 1, 2)$, whilst in-plane total forces and intravesicular pressure equal zero throughout the bioshell. The bladder attains the deformed $\overset{*}{S}$ state with $\lambda_{i,j} > 1.0$, $T_{ij} > 0$, $\check{V} > 0$, and $p > 0$ during the filling phase.

14.8 Investigations into the detrusor

14.8.1 Mathematical model

Let a detrusor fasciculus of length L be referred to as a local Lagrange coordinate system α. Its equation of motion is given by equation (10.23) and the force–stretch ratio yields equation (10.2). Although the exact data pertaining to the sequence of mechanical events in the longitudinal and circular muscle syncytia during contractions of the detrusor are unavailable, it is reasonable to assume that both muscle syncytia contract simultaneously. Such coordination generates the strong active forces $T^{a}_{c,l}$ needed to expel urine from the bladder effectively. This assumption, together with the fine fibrillar structure of SM, suggests that $T^{a}_{c,l}$ are produced only in the preferred directions, longitudinal or circumferential, and as such can be characterized in full by uniaxial tests. The active force versus intracellular Ca_i^{2+} relationship for the detrusor yields equation (10.4). The system of equations for the oscillatory activity of the membrane potential V satisfies the system of equations (10.5)–(10.9). The evolution of L- and T-type Ca^{2+}-channels depends on the wave of depolarization, V^s, and is defined by equations (13.28). The propagation of the wave of excitation V^s is described by equations (13.29)–(13.32). At the initial moment of time the detrusor fasciculus is in an unexcitable state, described by equation (13.33), and is activated by a series of discharges of action potentials, equation (13.34). The ends of the detrusor fasciculus are clamped and are unexcitable, equation (13.35).

The mathematical formulation as above describes: (i) the self-oscillatory behavior and myoelectrical activity of the detrusor; (ii) the generation and propagation of the wave of depolarization along the detrusor; (iii) the generation of action potentials; (iv) the dynamics of the cytosolic Ca^{2+} transients; (v) the generation of both active and passive force; and (vi) the deformation of the detrusor followed by an excitation of the cell membrane with subsequent contractions.

14.8.2 Physiological responses

The resting membrane potential of the unexcited fasciculus is $V^{r} = -45$ mV. Continuous fluctuations at low rate and amplitudes of the T-type Ca^{2+} −0.006 and 0.01 nA, the BK_{Ca} −0.05 and 0.11 nA, and the small chloride −0.04 nA currents result in oscillations of the membrane potential V resembling slow waves. Their frequency, $\nu = 0.5$ Hz, and amplitude, $V = 6$–10 mV, vary in time. The maximum rate of depolarization is $dV/dt = 10$ mV s^{-1} and of repolarization is $dV/dt = -7.2$ mV s^{-1} (figure 14.3).

Slow waves induce the flux of Ca^{2+} ions inside the cell at an average rate of 0.04 μM s^{-1}. There is a short 0.65 s time delay in the intracellular calcium transients compared to the wave of depolarization. Free cytosolic calcium at max$[Ca_i^{2+}] =$ 0.42 μM activates the contractile protein system with the production of active contractions, max $T^{a} = 1.2$ mN cm^{-1}. These follow the dynamics of calcium oscillations in both phase and time being normally preceded by slow waves.

Electrical stimulation of the detrusor myofiber triggers the generation of high frequency and magnitude ion currents: $\tilde{I}^{s}_{Ca} = 1.1$, $\tilde{I}^{f}_{Ca} = 0.038$, $\tilde{I}_{K1} = 7.6$, $\tilde{I}_{Ca-K} = 1.5$, and $\tilde{I}_{Cl} = 0.4$ nA, respectively. Action potentials of amplitudes 35–40 mV at a frequency ranging from 4 to 6 Hz occur as single discharges or bursts of 4–10 spikes. Each spike consists of rapid depolarizing and repolarizing phases to be followed by after-hyperpolarizing phases. The rates of depolarization and repolarization are $dV/dt = 7.5-8$ mV ms^{-1} with the half-duration of a spike ~6 ms. The amplitudes of fast after-hyperpolarizing potentials vary between 8 and 12 mV. A concomitant rise

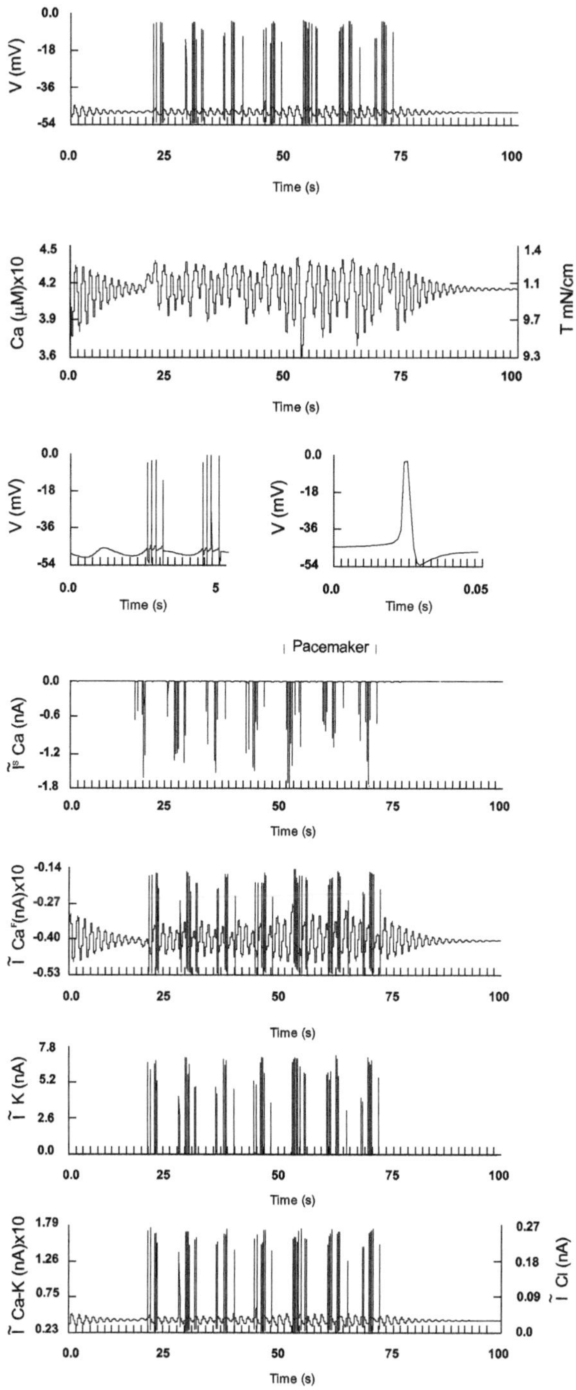

Figure 14.3. The dynamics of electrical pattern, intracellular Ca^{2+}, total force, and ion currents in the detrusor. Reprinted from Miftahof R M and Nam H G 2013 *Biomechanics of the Human Urinary Bladder* (Berlin: Springer) by permission from Springer Nature. Copyright 2013.

in intracellular calcium to 0.45 μM leads to the development of active force, max $T^a = 1.4$ mN cm^{-1}. Once the electrical charges are terminated, the myofiber returns to its unexcited state.

14.8.3 Effects of changes in K_0^+

A four-fold increase in the concentration of extracellular potassium depolarizes the detrusor cell membrane, $V^r = -17$ mV, and abolishes its oscillatory activity (figure 14.4) for a long period of time. The depolarization affects the transient dynamics of the fast Ca^{2+} as well as BK_{Ca} and K_v^+ channels which remain open and active throughout the period of depolarization. The strength of the T – Ca^{2+} current is $\tilde{I}_{Ca}^f =$ 0.028, $\tilde{I}_{Kv} = 0.03$, and $\tilde{I}_{Ca-K} = 0.06$ nA, respectively. There is a significant drop in the free intracellular calcium level, $[Ca_i^{2+}] = 0.35$ μM, with an associated reduction in the active force of the myofiber, $T^a = 0.9$ mN cm^{-1}.

The gradual decrease in $[K_0^+]$ that follows, hyperpolarizes the detrusor membrane: $V^r = -25, -36, -38$ mV. The intensity of the outward potassium current increases to 1.2 nA with a concomitant attenuation of both the T–Ca^{2+}, $\tilde{I}_{Ca}^f = 0.03$ nA, and calcium activated potassium, $\tilde{I}_{Ca-K} = 0.02$ nA, currents. The fast and slow Ca^{2+} channels regain their dynamics and the detrusor starts generating slow waves of small amplitude, $V = 3$ mV, and frequency, $\nu = 0.13$ Hz. There is a steady rise in $[Ca_i^{2+}]$ to $\simeq 5.0$ μM along with an intensity in contractions, max $T^a = 1.59$ mN cm^{-1}.

14.8.4 Effects of L- and T-type Ca^{2+} channel antagonists

The treatment of the fasciculus with the selective T-type Ca^{2+} channel blocker, mibefradil, produces a dose-dependent reduction not only of the fast inward Ca^{2+} current, but also in the frequency of spikes, calcium transients, and the intensity of contractions (figure 14.5). At low doses, the drug decreases the amplitude of the fast T-type Ca^{2+} current to 0.036 nA whilst the frequency of slow waves and action potentials diminish to 0.2 Hz and 1.5 Hz, respectively. The detrusor produces bursts of 2–4 action potentials at a time.

There is an influx and rise in the concentration of intracellular calcium, max $[Ca_i^{2+}] = 0.45$ μM, and the active force, $T^a = 1.41$ mN cm^{-1}. At 'high' concentrations mibefradil further reduces the frequency of spikes, although the pattern and strength of phasic contractions remain unaffected.

Nifedipine, a non-selective T- and L-type Ca^{2+} channels antagonist, hyperpolarizes the cell membrane and shifts the resting membrane potential to $V^r =$ -52 mV. There is an increase in both the amplitude, $V = 14$ mV, and frequency, $\nu =$ 0.7 Hz, of slow waves (figure 14.6). Electrical stimulation in the presence of nifedipine induces high amplitude action potentials, $V = 38$ mV, albeit at a lower frequency, $\nu = 3.5$ Hz, when compared to the physiological norm. No changes are seen in the dynamics of $\tilde{I}_{Ca}^s$. A decrease in the amplitude of the fast inward calcium current $\tilde{I}_{Ca}^f = 0.025$ nA also results in a decrease in the level of free cytosolic calcium,

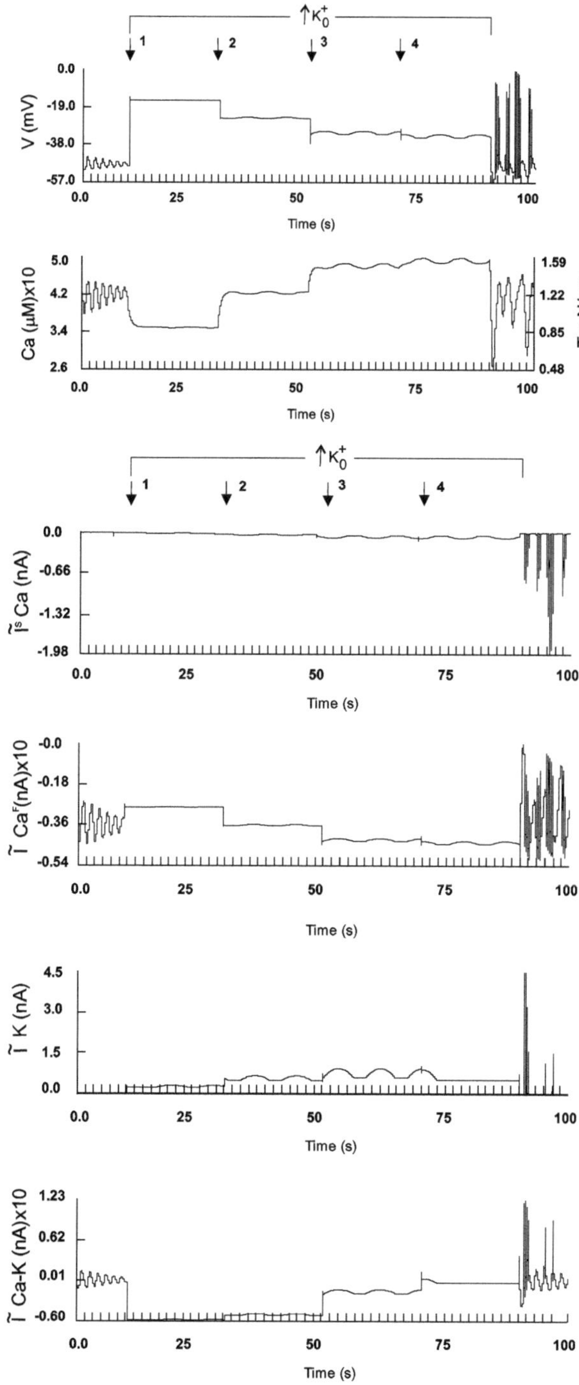

Figure 14.4. Electromechanical response of the detrusor to excess K_0^+. Reprinted from Miftahof R M and Nam H G 2013 *Biomechanics of the Human Urinary Bladder* (Berlin: Springer) by permission from Springer Nature. Copyright 2013.

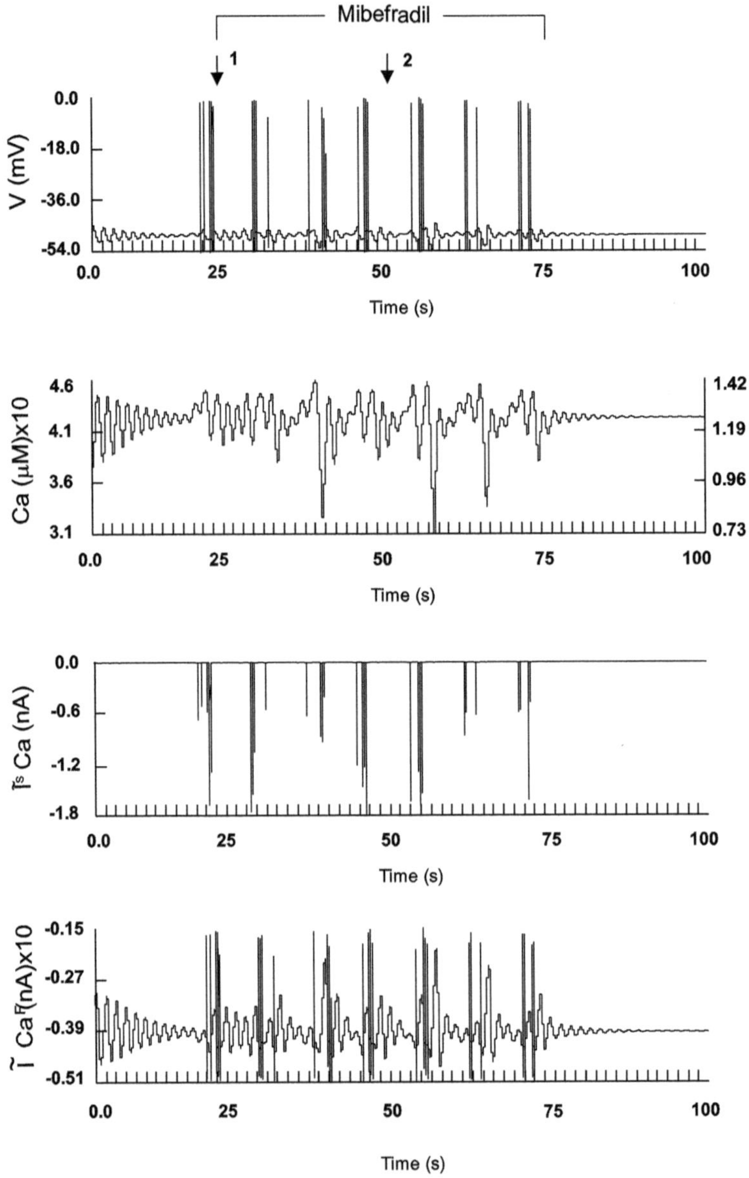

Figure 14.5. Dose-dependent effects of mifebradil on electromechanical activity and the dynamics of selective ion currents of the detrusor. Reprinted from Miftahof R M and Nam H G 2013 *Biomechanics of the Human Urinary Bladder* (Berlin: Springer) by permission from Springer Nature. Copyright 2013.

$[Ca_i^{2+}] = 0.16\ \mu M$. The myofiber continues to generate phasic contractions of $0.86\ mN\ cm^{-1}$.

The application of verapamil, a selective L-type Ca^{2+} channel blocker, inhibits spontaneous and induced myoelectrical activity in the detrusor. The intracellular calcium level decreases to $0.01\ \mu M$ and no contractions are produced.

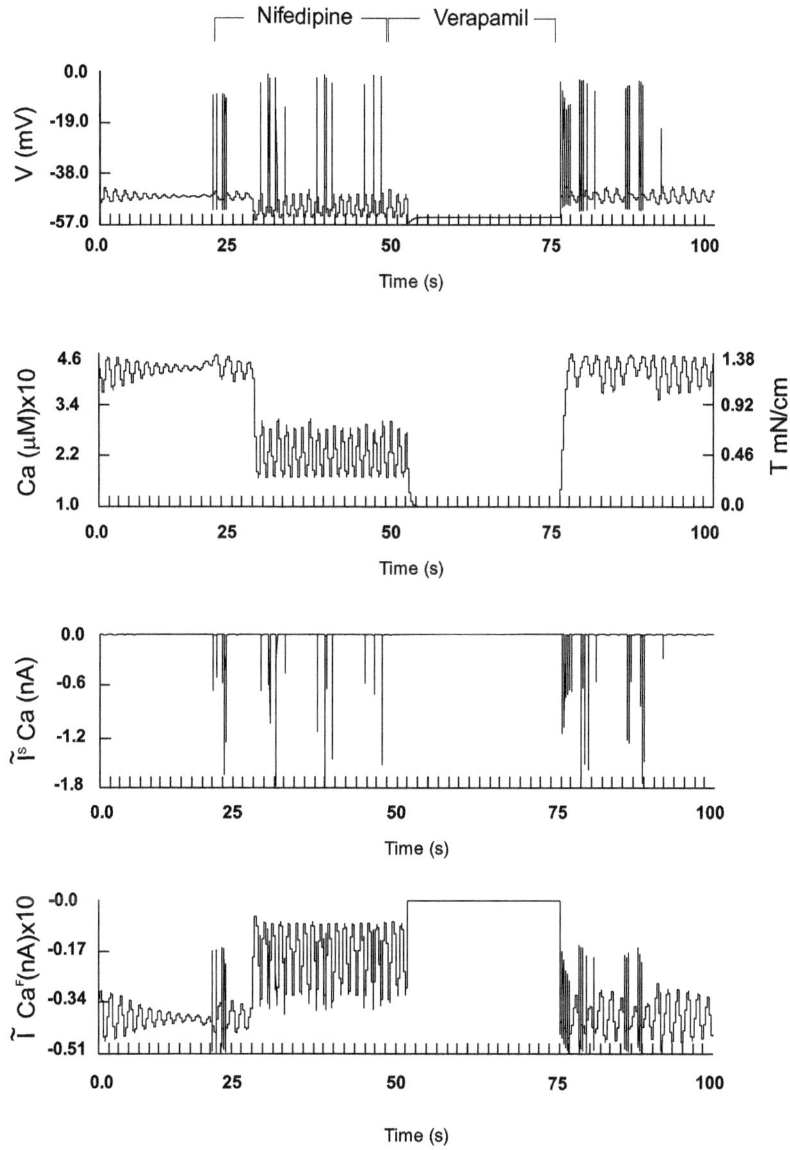

Figure 14.6. Effects of nifedipine and verapamil on electromechanical activity and the dynamics of selective ion currents of the detrusor. Reprinted from Miftahof R M and Nam H G 2013 *Biomechanics of the Human Urinary Bladder* (Berlin: Springer) by permission from Springer Nature. Copyright 2013.

14.8.5 Effects of BK_{Ca} channel agonists/antagonists

The application of forskolin (FSK), a Ca^{2+}-activated K^+ channel agonist, dose-dependently hyperpolarizes the detrusor, $V = -62, -68$ mV and abolishes slow wave oscillatory activity (figure 14.7). Although the conductivity of fast and slow Ca^{2+} channels remains unaltered, there is a fall in intracellular calcium concentration, $[Ca_i^{2+}] = 0.034\ \mu M$. As a result, the fasciculus remains relaxed throughout.

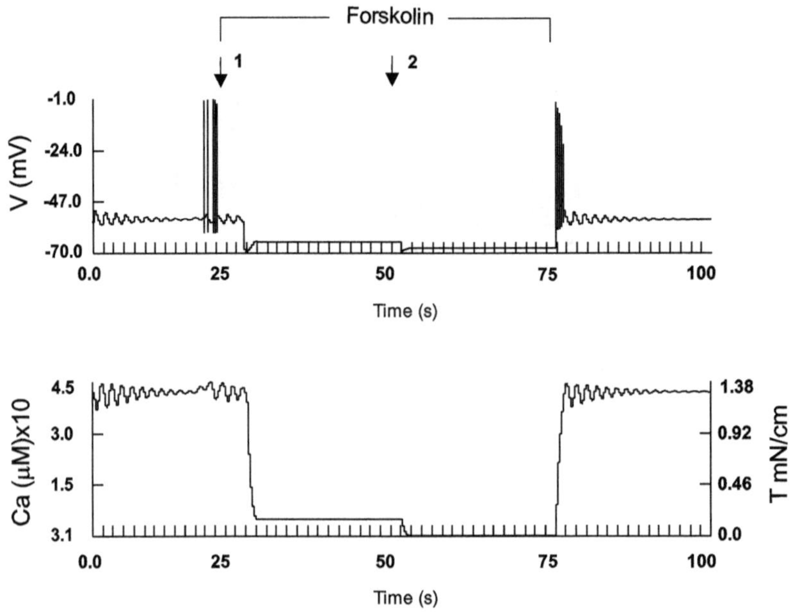

Figure 14.7. Dose-dependent effect of forskolin on electromechanical activity of the detrusor. Reprinted from Miftahof R M and Nam H G 2013 *Biomechanics of the Human Urinary Bladder* (Berlin: Springer) by permission from Springer Nature. Copyright 2013.

The treatment of the electrically stimulated detrusor with charybdotoxin (CTX), a selective max Ca^{2+}-activated K^+ channel blocker, exerts an excitatory effect on its myoelectrical activity. Charybdotoxin does not affect the resting membrane potential but abolishes slow waves and AHPs. There is an increase in the amplitude, $V =$ 50–55 mV and frequency, ν = 8 Hz, of action potentials. The level of free intracellular calcium rises to a maximum 0.48 μM and the myofiber generates tonic type contractions, max T^a = 1.5 mN cm^{-1} (figure 14.8). Similar electromechanical effects are observed after the application of iberiotoxin.

The concomitant addition of nifedipine disrupts high frequency bursting activity in the detrusor. The cell membrane becomes hyperpolarized $V^r = -52$ mV and the fasciculus generates steady slow waves of amplitude V = 20 mV and a constant frequency, ν = 0.85 Hz. Smooth muscle produces bursts of 7–9 action potentials, $V =$ 50–55 mV, at a frequency, ν = 2.5 Hz. Free intracellular calcium of 0.17 μM triggers an active force development with intensity max T^a = 0.9 mN cm^{-1}. The contractility pattern also changes from a tonic type to that of phasic.

14.8.6 Effects of K^+ channel agonists/antagonists

Lemakalim (LEM), a selective K^+-channel agonist, has a strong hyperpolarizing effect on the SMCs of the bladder reducing the resting membrane potential by 26 mV (V^r = −70 mV). LEM eliminates slow waves and action potentials. As the concentration of free intracellular calcium falls to zero, $[Ca_i^{2+}] \simeq 0$, the detrusor fails to contract (figure 14.9).

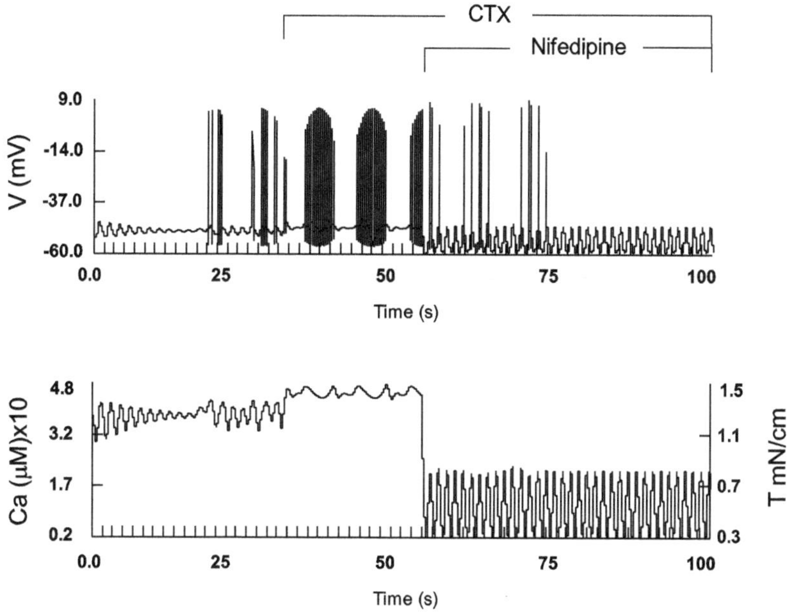

Figure 14.8. Selective and conjoint effects of charybdotoxin and nifedipine on electromechanical activity of the fasciculus. Reprinted from Miftahof R M and Nam H G 2013 *Biomechanics of the Human Urinary Bladder* (Berlin: Springer) by permission from Springer Nature. Copyright 2013.

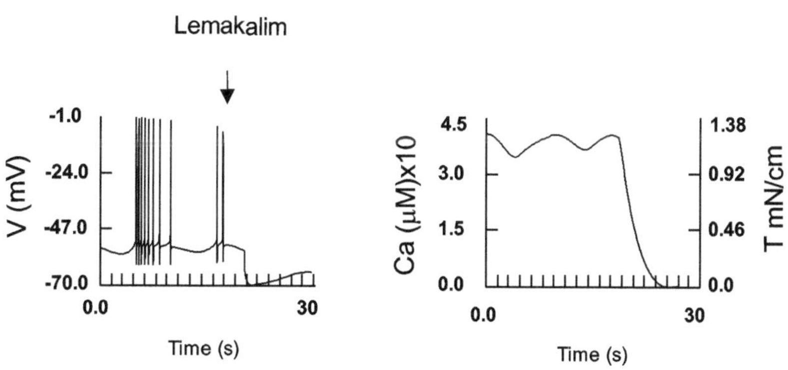

Figure 14.9. Electromechanical response of the detrusor to the application of LEM. Reprinted from Miftahof R M and Nam H G 2013 *Biomechanics of the Human Urinary Bladder* (Berlin: Springer) by permission from Springer Nature. Copyright 2013.

The treatment of the detrusor with tetraethylammonium chloride (TEA), a non-selective voltage-gated K^+-channel antagonist, increases the amplitude, $V = 55–60$ mV, and frequency, $\nu = 20$ Hz, of action potentials (figure 14.10). These effects are dose-dependent. There is an increase in the influx of calcium ions inside the cell, $[Ca_i^{2+}] = 0.47\ \mu$M, and a rise in the tension of contractions, $T^a = 1.46$ mN cm^{-1}.

The detrusor continues to generate spontaneously spikes of amplitude $V = 28–34$ mV and frequency, $\nu = 3.5$ Hz, in the presence of TEA even after external electrical stimuli

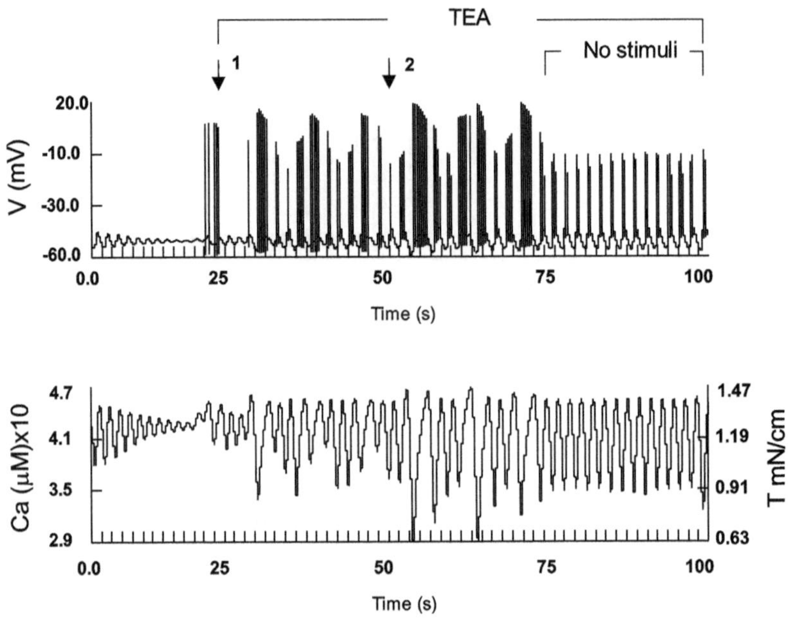

Figure 14.10. Electromechanical response of the detrusor to TEA. Reprinted from Miftahof R M and Nam H G 2013 *Biomechanics of the Human Urinary Bladder* (Berlin: Springer) by permission from Springer Nature. Copyright 2013.

are withdrawn. The smooth muscle fasciculus evokes long-lasting bursts of regular phasic contractions of a maximum 1.38 mN cm^{-1}.

4-aminopyridine (4-AP), a selective K^+-channel antagonist, depolarizes the membrane, $V^r = -42$ mV, but does not affect slow wave activity. There is an increase in the amplitude and frequency of spikes, $V = 47$ mV, $\nu = 7.1$ Hz, but without significant changes in the dynamics of their generation (figure 14.11). The intensity of $\tilde{I}_K$ is reduced by 25%, max $\tilde{I}_K = 5.6$ nA, although the effect is dose-dependent.

The maximum influx of extracellular calcium is not altered. Noticeable changes are seen in the amplitude of oscillations in free cytosolic Ca_i^{2+}. The detrusor smooth muscle contracts at a relatively constant strength of 1.44 mN cm^{-1}.

14.8.7 Effects of Ca^{2+}-ATPase inhibitors

Two agents have been described as selective inhibitors of Ca^{2+}-ATPase: cyclopiazonic acid (CPA), a mycotoxin from *Aspergillus* and *Penicillium*, and thapsigargin, a natural compound. CPA passes easily into the cytoplasm through the plasma membrane to reduce Ca^{2+}-ATPase activity. The effects of thapsigargin, however, are more complicated. At concentrations <1 μM, it prevents the filling of the Ca^{2+} stores, while at higher concentrations it interacts with voltage-dependent L-type Ca^{2+} channels in the plasma membrane.

The overall effect of CPA, with an increase in the magnitude of membrane ionic currents and the electromechanical activity of the detrusor, is time-dependent (figure 14.12). Thus, the inward slow and fast calcium currents reach $\tilde{I}_{Ca}^{s} = 2.0$ nA

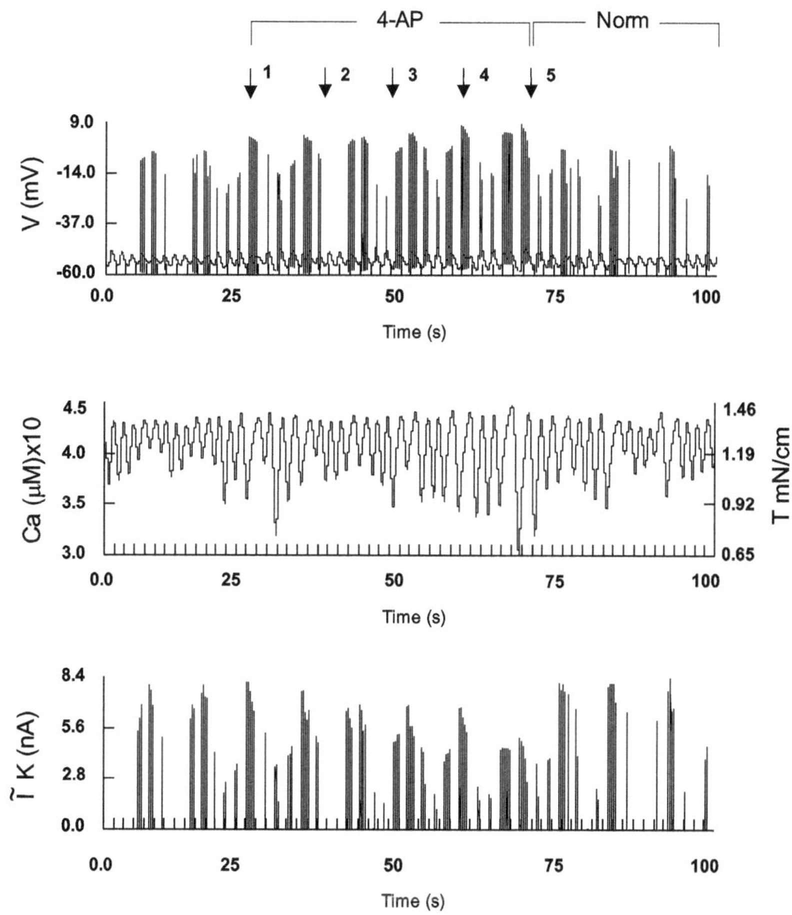

Figure 14.11. Dose-dependent effects of 4-aminopyridine on electromechanical activity of the detrusor. Reprinted from Miftahof R M and Nam H G 2013 *Biomechanics of the Human Urinary Bladder* (Berlin: Springer) by permission from Springer Nature. Copyright 2013.

and $\tilde{I}^{f}_{Ca} = 0.024$ nA, respectively, while the dynamics of the transient outward $\tilde{I}_{K}$ and $\tilde{I}_{Ca-K}$ currents are not affected.

CPA depolarizes the detrusor muscle membrane by 8 mV and abolishes slow waves. The detrusor muscle shifts to a new stable excitable state in which high amplitude, 52 mV, and high frequency, 30 Hz, action potentials are generated. The amount of free intracellular calcium is, however, slightly reduced, $\max[Ca^{2+}_{i}] =$ 0.51 μM with the result that the intensity of phasic contractions falls to $T^{a} =$ 1.2 mN cm^{-1}.

When compared with the norm, it is seen that thapsigargin causes an increase in the frequency of $\tilde{I}^{s}_{Ca}$ and $\tilde{I}^{f}_{Ca}$ currents and their amplitudes. The dynamics of the currents change to bursting. The amplitude of the influx of Ca^{2+} through the L-type Ca^{2+} channel is 0.18 nA whilst through the T-type Ca^{2+} channel it is 0.04 nA. In addition, there is an amplification of the outward $\tilde{I}_{K}$ and $\tilde{I}_{Ca-K}$ currents.

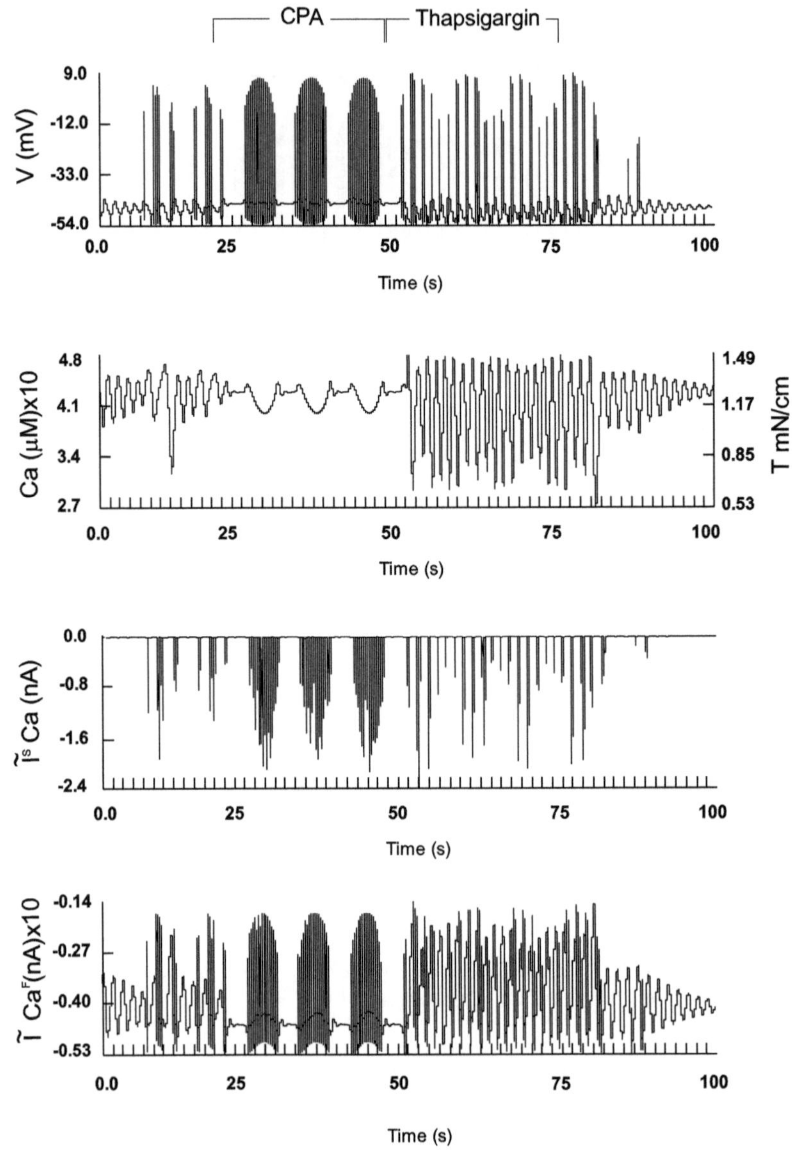

Figure 14.12. Effects of CPA and thapsigargin on electromechanical activity and the dynamics of selective ion currents in the detrusor. Reprinted from Miftahof R M and Nam H G 2013 *Biomechanics of the Human Urinary Bladder* (Berlin: Springer) by permission from Springer Nature. Copyright 2013.

Thapsigargin has little effect on muscle resting membrane potential but it does increase the frequency, $\nu = 0.57$ Hz, of self-oscillatory activity. Continuous bursts of action potentials, of amplitude 38–55 mV and frequency ~19 Hz, are generated. There is a rise in the concentration of intracellular calcium, $\max[\mathrm{Ca}_i^{2+}] = 0.48\ \mu\mathrm{M}$, with greater amplitude in its variation, 0.21 μM. The fasciculus produces high frequency phasic contractions, max $T^{\mathrm{a}} = 1.49\ \mathrm{mN\ cm}^{-1}$.

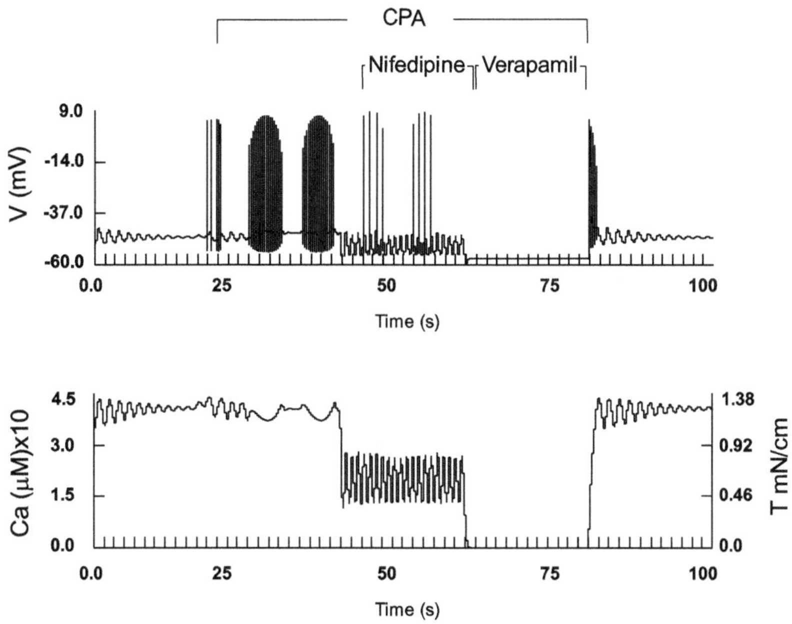

Figure 14.13. Selective and conjoint effects of CPA, nifedipine, and verapamil on electromechanical activity of the detrusor. Reprinted from Miftahof R M and Nam H G 2013 *Biomechanics of the Human Urinary Bladder* (Berlin: Springer) by permission from Springer Nature. Copyright 2013.

If pretreated with CPA, the response of the detrusor myofiber is sensitive to the concomitant addition of nifedipine and verapamil. Nifedipine has shown a detrimental effect on both $\tilde{I}^{s}_{Ca}$ and $\tilde{I}^{f}_{Ca}$ currents, and on the oscillatory and spiking activity of the urinary SM. The frequency of action potentials reduces significantly, $\nu = 0.03$ Hz, while their amplitude remains unchanged, $V = 52$ mV (figure 14.13). The drug has a positive effect on the amplitude and frequency of slow waves. A decrease in the amplitude of the inward calcium flux also results in a decrease in the level of free cytosolic calcium, $[Ca^{2+}_{i}] = 0.28$ μM. The myofiber sustains its phasic contractility to generate an active force of 0.9 mN cm^{-1}.

A subsequent washout of nifedipine and the application of verapamil abolishes electromechanical responses in the detrusor. The fasciculus becomes hyperpolarized, $V = 58$ mV, and remains relaxed, $T^{a} = 0$.

In an environment free of extracellular calcium, $[Ca^{2+}_{0}] = 0$, the detrusor smooth muscle cell fails to respond to CPA. Instead it becomes hyperpolarized, $V = 52$ mV, with no active forces being produced (figure 14.14). An increase in the concentration of Ca^{2+}_{0} has an excitatory effect on the fasciculus with the development of strong slow calcium $\tilde{I}^{s}_{Ca} = -1.1$ and -3.2 nA and fast calcium $\tilde{I}^{f}_{Ca} = -0.014$ and -0.045 nA ion currents. High frequency and amplitude spikes, max $V = 60$ mV, are generated. The amount of free intracellular calcium also rises, max $[Ca^{2+}_{i}] = 0.37$ μM, and, as a result, an active force of contraction develops of intensity 1.3 mN cm^{-1}.

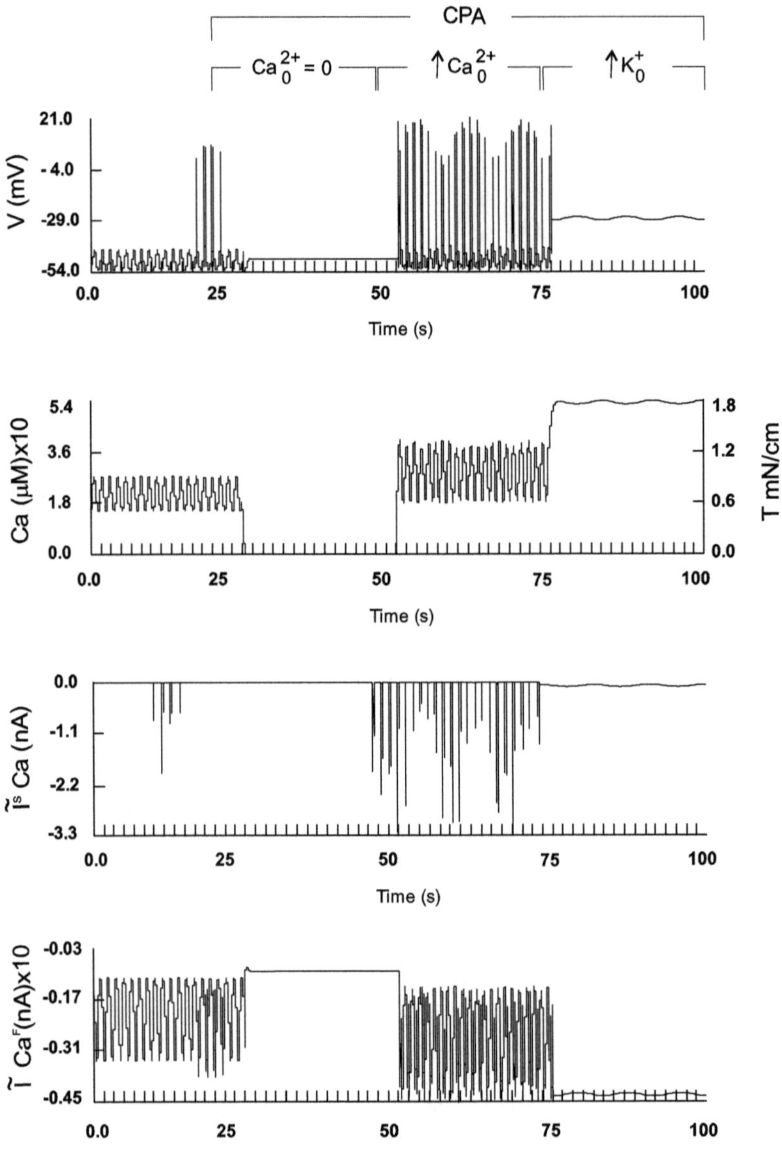

Figure 14.14. Conjoint effects of cyclopiazonic acid and excess extracellular Ca^{2+} and K^+ ions on electromechanical activity and the dynamics of selective ion currents in the detrusor. Reprinted from Miftahof R M and Nam H G 2013 *Biomechanics of the Human Urinary Bladder* (Berlin: Springer) by permission from Springer Nature. Copyright 2013.

The concomitant application of CPA with the elevation in concentration of extracellular potassium ions leads to a stable depolarization of the detrusor by ~21 mV ($V = -29$ mV) and development of a long-lasting tonic-type contraction, $T^a = 1.8$ mN cm^{-1}.

14.9 Pharmacology of detrusor

14.9.1 Therapies of bladder dysfunction

The control of detrusor excitability has important therapeutic implications since its malfunction may lead to bladder overactivity and either urinary incontinence or urinary retention. These syndromes can be the result of pathological changes in: the anatomical structure of the bladder and surrounding organs, e.g. benign prostatic hyperplasia, bladder calculus, or developmental abnormality; the central and peripheral nervous system involved in bladder control, e.g. brain and spinal cord lesions, or sacral nerve damage; the detrusor, e.g. hyperreflexia, instability or areflexia, intramuscular fibrosis, or ischemia; the coordinated function of the external sphincter and detrusor muscle; and/or urethral sphincter bradykinesia. Such syndromes may also be a complication of multiple sclerosis, Parkinson's disease, dementia, spinal cord injury, and myelomeningocele, among others. These conditions are of health, hygiene, and social concern to the patient. Patients with neurogenic bladders are highly susceptible to urinary tract infections, whilst those with spinal cord injury are susceptible to stone formation in the bladder and kidneys and also bladder cancer. Unfortunately, no adequate pharmacological modalities are available at the moment to treat these conditions.

Approximately 17% of both men and women over the age 40 experience the symptoms of an overactive bladder, a figure which increases to 33% as the years progress. The mainstay therapy for an overactive bladder depends on the use of μ_2 and μ_3 receptor antagonists—oxybutynin, darifenacin, fesoterodine, propiverine, solifenacin, tolterodine, and trospium. Although the drugs offer a significant improvement in the management of symptoms, their overall efficacy, tolerability, and toxicity are still less than optimal. Potential novel formulations such as selective α_{1D}-adrenoceptor, serotonin 5-HT_{1A} and 5-HT_7, neurokinin NK_1 and NK_2 receptor antagonists (SP-saponin, aprepirant), β_3-adrenoceptors (terbutaline, clenbuterol), potassium channel agonists (retigabine, forskolin), vanilloids (capsaicin, resiniferatoxin), and botulinum toxin are currently under investigation. Despite many new biological insights, very few drugs with a mechanism of action other than antimuscarinics pass the proof-of-concept stage.

14.9.2 Cholinergic antagonists/agonists

The addition of ACh-antagonists causes a deactivation of chemical processes on the postsynaptic membrane with the effects being dose-dependent. According to numerical results, the compound at concentrations of 0.13–0.26 mM causes a complete blockade in excitation transmission, $V_{syn} = 0$ while at lower concentrations of 0.026 mM, the number of choline receptors available for interaction decreases, $[R] = 17\ \mu M$. Consequently, the concentration of the (ACh–R)-complex is reduced to 0.016 mM, which, however, is enough to produce a depolarization of the postsynaptic membrane with the generation of EPSP, $V_{syn} = 69.6$ mV.

In the case of partial chemical equilibrium, the compounds in a concentration of 0.26 mM, do not cause a blockade of synaptic transmission. This figure represents

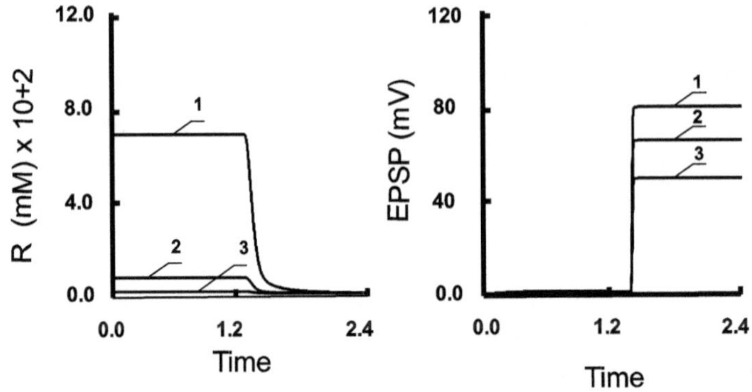

Figure 14.15. Receptor availability on the postsynaptic membrane and excitatory postsynaptic potential development in the case of the physiological norm (1), in the presence of a cholinergic antagonist (2), and in the case of chemical equilibrium (3). Reprinted from Miftahof R M and Nam H G 2013 *Biomechanics of the Human Urinary Bladder* (Berlin: Springer) by permission from Springer Nature. Copyright 2013.

twice the number of ACh receptors found on the postsynaptic membrane. A maximum of [ACh–R] = 1.87 μM is formed leading to the generation of EPSP with an amplitude of 53.2 mV (figure 14.15).

In addition to the drugs that completely or partially block synaptic transmission, there is also a large group of chemical agents that facilitate cholinergic transmission. Their primary mechanism of action is to inhibit the activity of acetylcholinesterase enzyme in the synaptic cleft, and to increase the effectiveness of ACh release from the nerve terminals.

Strictly reversible anticholinesterase agents, such as galantamine, ambenonium, endorphonium, and aceclidine, are not hydrolyzed by cholinesterase and relatively quickly dissociate intact from the enzyme. Others, such as neostigmine and its derivatives, remain bound to the esteric site of the enzyme for a long time, undergoing a reaction of hydrolysis in the same manner as ACh, but at a very slow rate.

The treatment of the nerve terminal by cholinesterase inhibitors at a concentration 0.1 mM causes a significant decrease in the active enzyme content in the synaptic cleft [E] = 3.5 μM. The presence of the inhibitor leads to an expected accumulation free fraction of ACh in perfusate: max[ACh_c] = 5.42 mM. The amount in the neurotransmitter left inactivated in the cleft is [AChE] = 0.22 mM (figure 14.16). Consequently, 0.124 mM of (ACh–R)-complex is developed on the postsynaptic membrane to induce a generation of EPSP of an amplitude 89.08 mV. In the case of 0.05 mM, being added V_{syn} = 88 mV is registered.

Interestingly, when a partial chemical equilibrium between the inhibitor and the enzyme is achieved, an application of 0.15 mM of the drug does not abolish the enzyme's activity. The level being applied here is three times higher than the concentration of acetylcholinesterase. The concentration of the free enzyme falls to 1.3 μM. A slight increase in ACh content in the cleft, max[ACh_c] = 5.44 mM, with a significant decrease in inactivated acetylcholine, [AChE] = 1.22 μM, are observed. The amplitude of EPSP attains 89.1 mV.

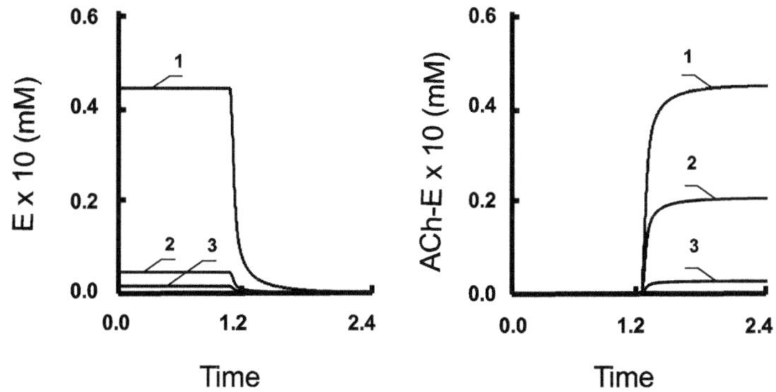

Figure 14.16. Changes in acetylcholinesterase enzyme and inactivated ACh in the synaptic cleft as a result of the application of cholinesterase inhibitors in concentrations 0.1 mM (2) and 0.15 mM (3). The curve (1) corresponds to the case of physiological norm. Reprinted from Miftahof R M and Nam H G 2013 *Biomechanics of the Human Urinary Bladder* (Berlin: Springer) by permission from Springer Nature. Copyright 2013.

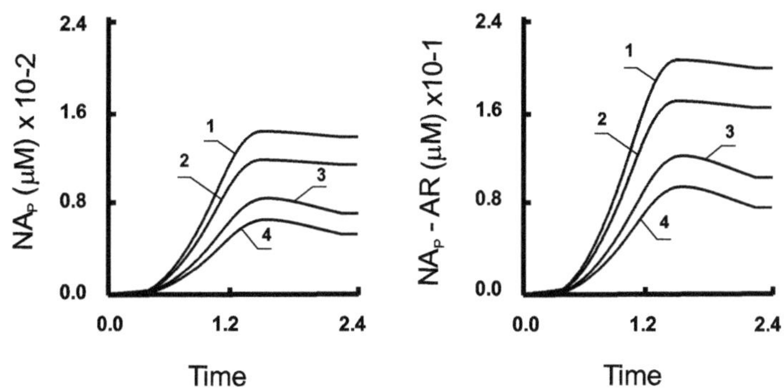

Figure 14.17. Changes in NA and noradrenaline-receptor complex on the postsynaptic membrane in the presence of COMT inhibitors. The curves (1), (2) refer to the concentrations of 0.13 mM and 0.2 mM of the inhibitor present in a state of chemical equilibrium, and the curves (3), (4) correspond to the addition of 0.15 mM and 0.2 mM of the inhibitor. Reprinted from Miftahof R M and Nam H G 2013 *Biomechanics of the Human Urinary Bladder* (Berlin: Springer) by permission from Springer Nature. Copyright 2013.

14.9.3 Inhibitors of catechol-*O*-methyltransferase

Catechol, pyrogallol, quercin, and rutin substances described as flavenoids of the vitamin P group, along with tropolones and a group of benzoic acid derivatives, are potent COMT inhibitors. Their addition causes a significant increase in the concentration of NA_f on the postsynaptic membrane. The response is nonlinear depending on the concentration of compound added. Thus, if the adrenergic neuron is treated with 0.15 mM of the drug, $[NA_p] = 58.2\ \mu M$ is formed. After the application of 0.2 mM of the inhibitor, $\max[NA_p] = 80.5\ \mu M$ is produced (figure 14.17). As a result $[NA_p - AR_\beta] = 15.5$ and $19.8\ \mu M$ are formed and $18.8\ \mu M$ versus $13.8\ \mu M$ of the β_3-adrenoceptors are bound, respectively. The amount of NA utilized by COMT also decreases to $25.2\ \mu M$. However, following treatment with a 'high' dose of the inhibitor, 0.2 mM, only $20.04\ \mu M$ are produced.

This affects the level of hyperpolarization of the postsynaptic membrane: $V_{syn} = -83.3$ mV (-78.7 mV) is recorded.

In a state of partial chemical equilibrium between the inhibitor and the enzyme the addition of IK in concentrations of 0.13 mM and 0.2 mM causes an increase in $[NA_p]$ to 119.3 and 135.5 μM, respectively. Consequently, the concentration of bound NA_p to adrenoceptors on the postsynaptic membrane increases: $\max[NA_p - AR_\beta] = 24.5$ and 26.98 μM. The blockage of 81%–87% of COMT leads to a decrease in the intensity of degradation of NA_p. Only 9.59 μM and 13.0 μM of the $(NA_p - COMT)$ complex is formed. As a result, the amplitude of IPSP increases: $V_{syn} = -85.6$ and -86.1 mV.

14.9.4 β-adrenoceptor antagonists

Drugs that block the adrenoceptors for sympathomimetic amines are classified on the basis of their chemical structure: haloalkylamines (phenozybenzamine), imidazolines (phentolamine, tolazoline), and phenoxyalkylamines (thymoxamine). The mechanism of their action is rather complex and not completely understood. It is supposed that the antagonism is competitive and slowly reversible due to the high strength of the covalent bond formed with the receptor. As well as acting on postsynaptic receptors, the drugs can affect adrenergic transmission to prevent the uptake of released NA into neuronal and extraneuronal sites, and inhibit the action of adrenoceptors on the presynaptic membrane. The latter mechanism is more important since the compounds that inhibit NA uptake cause only a slight increase in NA release.

In rising concentrations, the addition of antagonist blocks 55.4%–67.5% of the receptors on the postsynaptic membrane. The concentration of free β_3-adrenoceptors also decreases to 44.6–33.51 μM with the result that the rate and maximum concentration of $(NA_p - AR_\beta)$-complex development falls. Thus, $\max[NA_p - AR_\beta] = 4.81$ μM is formed (figure 14.18). At a 'high' dose, the inhibitor dose causes a further

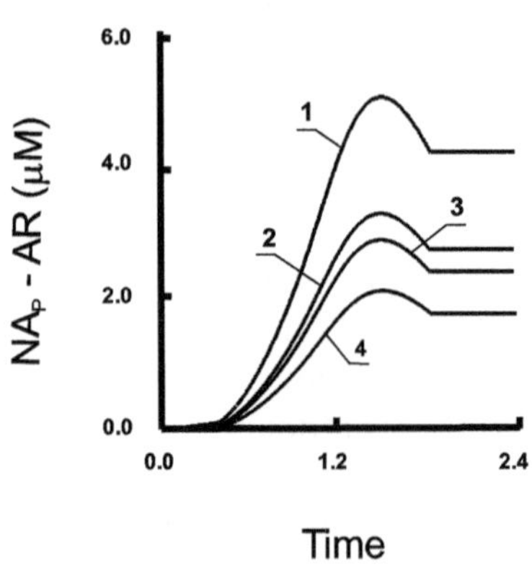

Figure 14.18. Dose-dependent changes of the noradrenaline-receptor complex after application of adrenoceptor antagonist at concentrations of 0.15 mM and 0.25 mM (1), (2), and in the case of partial chemical equilibrium (3), (4) in the presence of 0.2 mM and 0.3 mM of a drug. Reprinted from Miftahof R M and Nam H G 2013 *Biomechanics of the Human Urinary Bladder* (Berlin: Springer) by permission from Springer Nature. Copyright 2013.

decrease in the amount of active complex, 3.49 μM. The above changes affect the postsynaptic response to produce IPSPs of amplitude $V_{syn} = -71.42$ and -66.24 mV.

After achieving a partial chemical equilibrium, the added drug in concentrations of 0.2 and 0.3 mM blocks 69.2%–75% of β_3-receptors. This is associated with a decrease in the formation of $[NA_p - AR_\beta]$—3.12 μM and 2.36 μM. As a result, a higher level of hyperpolarization is attained: $V_{syn} = -64.3$ and -58.86 mV.

14.10 The urinary bladder as a soft biological shell

Let the middle surface of the human urinary bladder be associated with a cylindrical coordinate system. Consider that the equations of motion of the bioshell satisfy equations (5.102); the dynamics of bursting and oscillatory myoelectrical activity, $V_{c,l}$, in the muscle longitudinal (subscript l) and circumferential (c) layers, respectively, are adequately described by the system of equations (10.5)–(10.9); the pacemaker activity in cells, V_p, yields equations (7.3)–(7.13); and the propagation of the electrical wave of depolarization, $V_{c,l}^s$, along the smooth muscle syncytia in cases of generalized electrical anisotropy and isotropy is given by equations (10.10)–(10.18).

The following are anatomically and physiologically justifiable initial and boundary conditions. They assume that: (i) the initial undeformed configuration of the bladder is defined by the intrauterine pressure, p, and that the organ is at rest, i.e. myoelectrically quiescent; (ii) an excitation of known intensity, $\overset{0}{V}_p$, and duration, t_i^d, is provided by electrical discharges in the 'pacemaker regions'; and (iii) the urethral end is either rigidly fixed or remains pliable throughout deformation. To close the problem, the above equations should be complemented by constitutive relations.

The results of numerical experiments to study the statics and dynamics of changes in shapes, force–stretch ratio distributions, electromechanical activity, and pharmacological modulation of the urinary bladder are presented below. It must be recognized that the model contains numerous parameters and constants that have not yet been evaluated experimentally. For example, no information is currently available on mechanical constants c_i of the human bladder under biaxial loading, chemical reactions k_i, and electrical properties of the detrusor as an electro-conductive medium. To overcome the problem of missing data during simulations, the wall of the organ is regarded as a curvilinear anisotropic nonlinear viscoelastic material with constitutive parameters derived to resemble similar soft human tissues. Thus, the uniaxial passive force–stretch ratio $T^p(\lambda, c_i)$ relationship is assumed to show 'pseudoelastic' behavior, the active force function exhibits nonlinear dependence on the intracellular calcium concentration, and the biaxial in-plane $T^{ij}(\lambda_i, \lambda_j)$ function is a generalized form of the uniaxial constitutive relationship. Other parameters and constants are adjusted to resemble the physiological and diseased states of the organ.

14.11 Investigations into the urinary bladder

14.11.1 Filling state

Anatomical shapes of the human urinary bladder are highly variable. The fundus is located in the lower pelvis and is significantly restricted in its movements, while the body and the apex undergo extensive deformations and changes in configuration.

The cut shape of the bioshell corresponds to the electrically quiescent organ when empty of urine. It can attain many forms simultaneously which depend on the status of the tissue *per se* and surrounding organs. The initial undeformed configuration of the bladder, however, is determined by the amount of urine it contains at any given moment in time and the intravesicular pressure, p. In simulations it has been assumed that at $t = 0$ the bioshell is loaded by $p = 1.0$ kPa. Coronal, sagittal, and transverse views of the three commonly observed anatomical shapes of the organ for $p = 1.0$ kPa are shown in figure 14.19. Although urine, as a second phase, is not present in a mathematical formulation of the problem, its mechanical effect has been reproduced numerically by a gradual increase (in the case of filling) or decrease (in the case of voiding) in p. Such an approach through modeling has allowed the dynamics of changes to be followed in both shapes and stress–strain fields in the organ during different stages of its function.

During the filling stage, it is assumed that the detrusor remains actively relaxed, i.e. no excitatory or inhibitory signals are generated in the tissue. Analysis of the total force distribution during this stage indicates that initially, $p = 1.2$ kPa, with excessive tensions developing along a longitudinal direction in the body and apex of

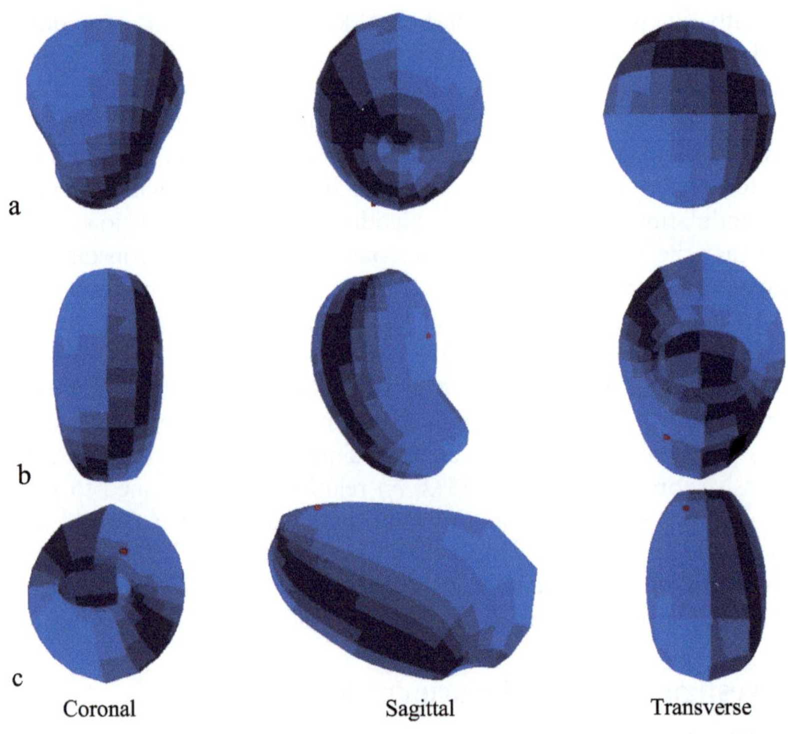

Figure 14.19. Coronal, sagittal, and transverse views of actual configurations of different anatomical shapes of the human urinary bladder at $p = 1$ kPa. Reprinted from Miftahof R M and Nam H G 2013 *Biomechanics of the Human Urinary Bladder* (Berlin: Springer) by permission from Springer Nature. Copyright 2013.

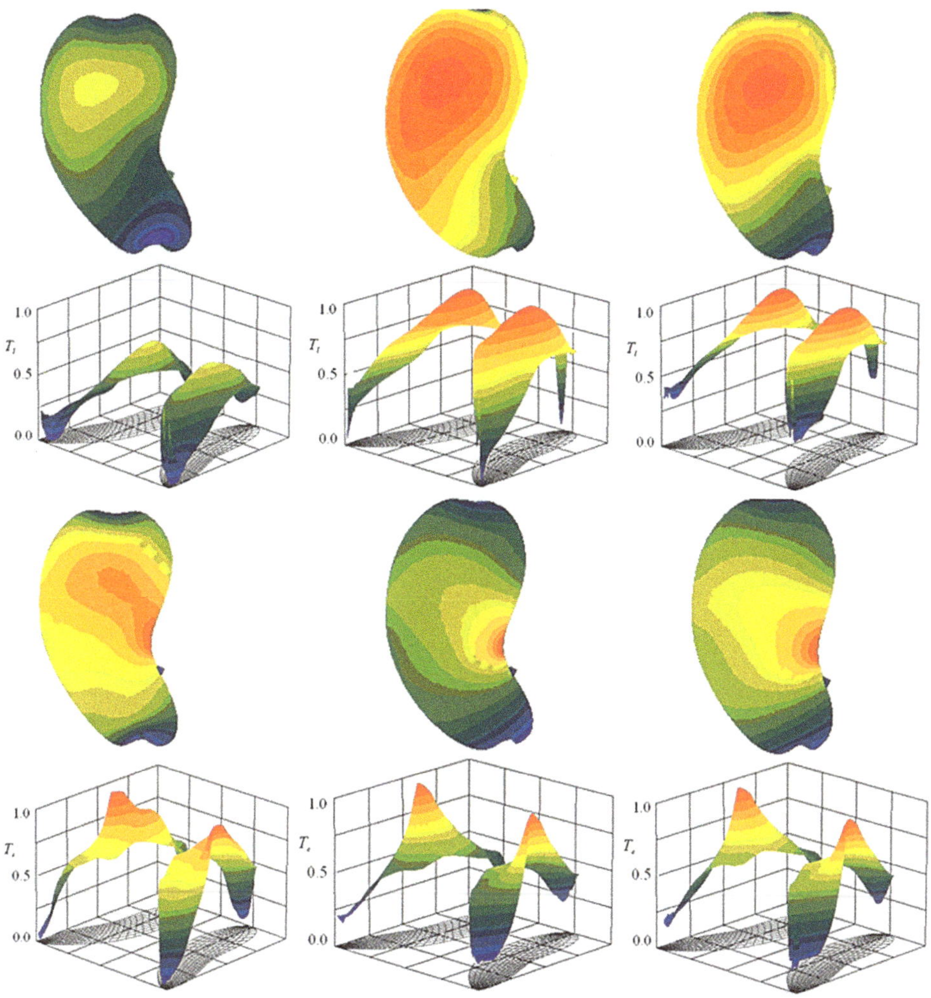

Figure 14.20. Dynamics of changes in the longitudinal, T_l, and circumferential, T_c, tension fields in the bladder during filling. Reprinted from Miftahof R M and Nam H G 2013 *Biomechanics of the Human Urinary Bladder* (Berlin: Springer) by permission from Springer Nature. Copyright 2013.

the organ (figure 14.20). A high level of circumferential force is observed in the region of the flexure appearing along the posterior wall of the bladder. It extends bilaterally and upwards to the body of the organ. Low intensity longitudinal and circumferential stretch forces are seen in the fundus. With a gradual increase in p to 2.7 and 6.5 kPa, respectively, maximum T_l and T_c values are produced in the body and apex of the bioshell which undergo even biaxial tension. A persistent zone of high degree T_c, is recorded at the flexure. Throughout the process of filling, all regions of the organ experience biaxial stretching with $\lambda_{l,c} \gg 1.0$.

The pattern of total force and strain distribution differ significantly depending on the initial configuration of the bladder. Thus in the bladder of the given shape (c) (figure 14.19), the excessive in-plane forces T_l, T_c develop along the posterior wall of

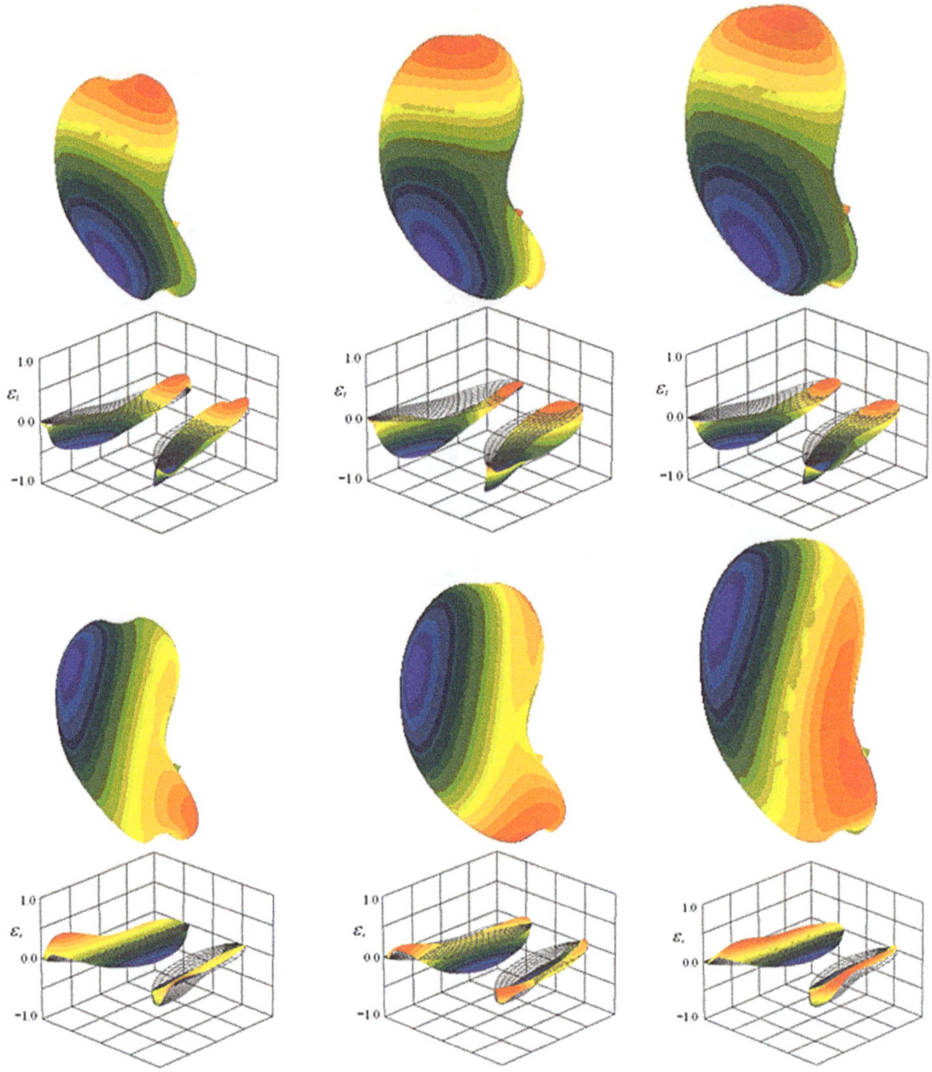

Figure 14.21. Dynamics of changes in axial, ε_l, and circumferential, ε_c, deformation fields in the bladder during filling. Reprinted from Miftahof R M and Nam H G 2013 *Biomechanics of the Human Urinary Bladder* (Berlin: Springer) by permission from Springer Nature. Copyright 2013.

the body and apex of the organ whereas the fundal region remains almost free of tension. The smooth gradient in $T_{c,l}$, should also be noted, i.e. the change in intensity extends from the fundus to the apex of the bioshell (figures 14.21 and 14.22).

14.11.2 Voiding state

The distension of the bladder caused by urine along with the activation of intramurally located mechanoreceptors leads to 'micro-contractions' of the organ.

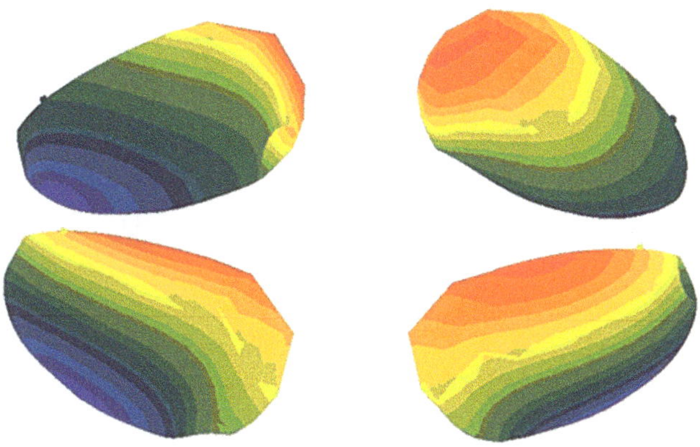

Figure 14.22. Circumferential, λ_c, (top) and axial, λ_l, (bottom) stretch ratio fields in the fully filled bladder. Oblique views of the bladder are shown. Reprinted from Miftahof R M and Nam H G 2013 *Biomechanics of the Human Urinary Bladder* (Berlin: Springer) by permission from Springer Nature. Copyright 2013.

This mechanism is attributed to self-excitatory, pacemaker type reactions detectable throughout the entire detrusor.

Let multiple 'pacemakers' be randomly distributed over the surface of the bioshell. They discharge impulses of average amplitude, $\overset{0}{V}_p$ = 70–80 mV, and duration, t_i^d = 10 ms, to incite waves of depolarization V_l and V_c, in the longitudinal and circular smooth muscle layers of the detrusor. These quickly spread over a long distance in a longitudinal direction but only over a short distance circumferentially (figure 14.23). The fronts of the waves may collide with a generation of a single solitary wave, V_l. However, both the strength of excitation and poor electrical connectivity within the muscle tissue prevent the propagation of $V_{c,l}$ throughout the organ. Only an area that includes the posterior wall of the body, the fundus. and the apex appears to be depolarized.

The activation of L- and T-type Ca^{2+} channels, along with the influx and rise in intracellular calcium concentration leads to contractions of the detrusor. Extremely localized, patchy areas mainly encircling the 'pacemaker' zones are subjected to weak active forces $T^a_{c,l}$, which are consistent with experimental observations described as 'micro-contractions'.

A chain of signal transduction events involving the pontine micturition center, the lumbosacral nuclei, and parasympathetic ganglionic motor neurons is marked by widespread long-lasting, intense, tonic type contractions of the detrusor. The general topology of intercellular arrangements, electrochemical coupling, and mechanical processes, along with the mathematical aspects of model formulation, have been discussed earlier. Throughout these numerical experiments the aim has been to reproduce and analyze the following sequence of physiological and mechanical events that occur during voiding: deformation of free nerve endings of mechanoreceptors; generation of action potentials and their propagation along the unmyelinated fibers; action potential generation at the soma of neurons; electrochemical

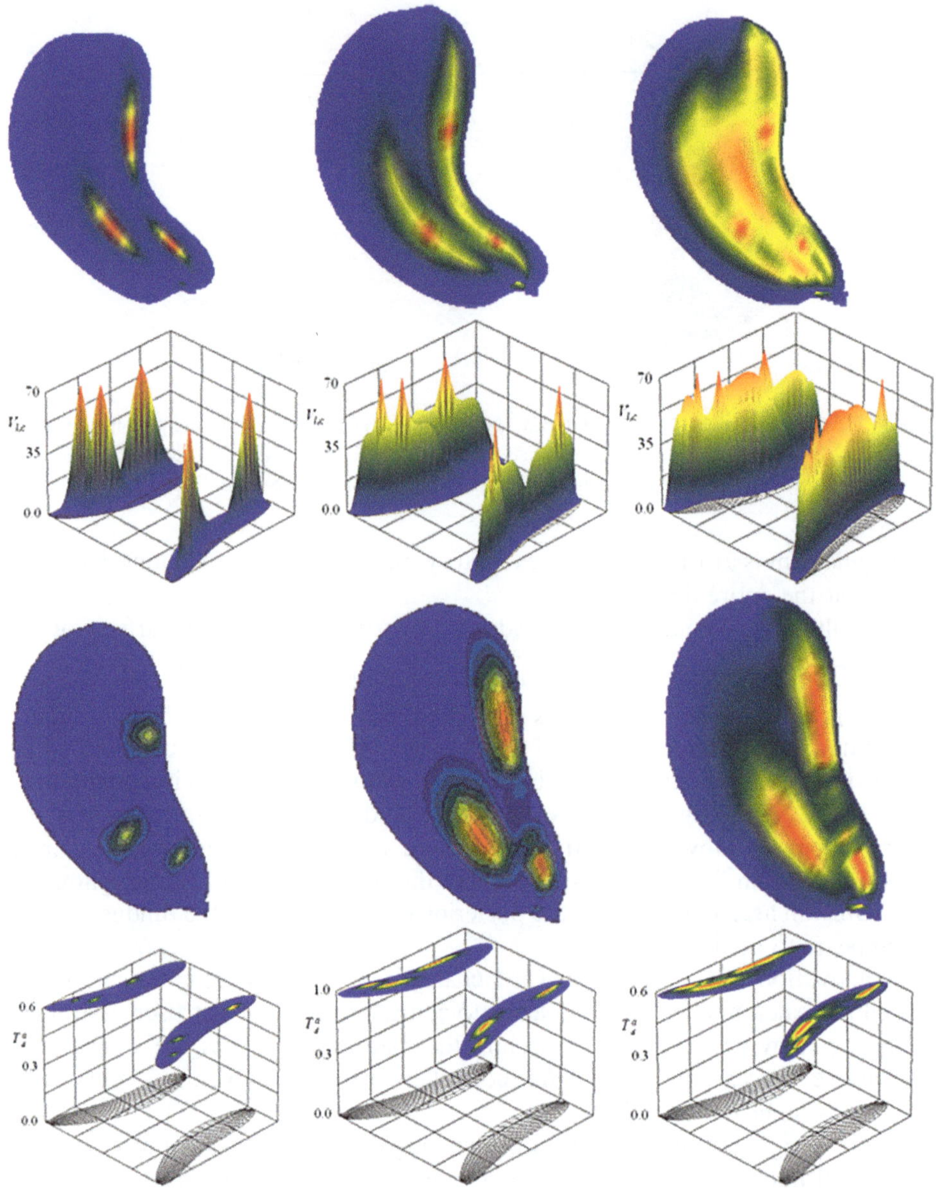

Figure 14.23. Dynamics of micro-contractions in the fully distended urinary bladder. Reprinted from Miftahof R M and Nam H G 2013 *Biomechanics of the Human Urinary Bladder* (Berlin: Springer) by permission from Springer Nature. Copyright 2013.

coupling at synapses with the production of fast excitatory and inhibitory post-synaptic potentials; ion channel dynamics and the spread of a wave of depolarization within the detrusor; and active force generation and configuration changes of the bladder—bioshell.

A mechanical stretch of the bladder with urine, $\varepsilon = 0.75$, evokes single receptor potentials of maximum amplitude 82.5 mV and duration ~2.3 ms at the mechanosensitive afferents of the pelvic nerve. These trigger the development of action potentials of amplitude 69 mV in the unmyelinated nerve fibers that propagate towards the somas of neurons in the lumbosacral nuclei. Here they initiate high frequency, 8–10 Hz, APs of amplitude 81.3 mV. The further efferent spread of the electrical excitation with a subsequent activation of the ganglionic motor neurons and muscarinic cholinergic synapses on smooth muscle results in the generation of fEPSPs and waves of depolarization, V_l, V_c.

The waves $V_{c,l}$ extend rapidly along the muscular syncytium throughout the organ. The bladder undergoes a uniform electrical excitation with average intensity, 80 mV. This level of depolarization is strong enough to produce a rapid influx of Ca^{2+} inside cells.

A rise in the free cytosolic calcium ion concentration leads to the activation of a cascade of mechanical reactions with the production of active forces of contraction, $T_{c,l}$ (figure 14.24). Their pattern of propagation resembles the dynamics of spread of electrical waves. Weak in strength, localized contractions quickly proliferate throughout different areas of the bladder. The intensity increases over time so that the whole organ becomes uniformly contracted—a condition essential for its effective emptying. Note that there are no changes in the actual configuration of the bioshell despite the presence of strong active forces. The intravesicular pressure rises to ~10 kPa.

The relaxation of the internal urinary sphincter and emptying of the bladder, achieved in the model by decreasing p values, results in gradual changes in shape and a reduction in the organ's dimensions (figure 14.25). During this process, the bioshell attains homeomorphic configurations.

14.11.3 Pharmacology of voiding

Currently there are but a limited number of therapeutics available to treat bladder dysmotility. The leading edge of therapy relies on selective and non-selective muscarinic μ_{1-3} receptor antagonists, e.g. oxybutynin, darifenacin, fesoterodine, etc, and, to a lesser extent, $\beta_{2,3}$ adrenergic receptor agonists, e.g. terbutaline and clenbuterol. Their effects on the fully distended urinary organ have been studied.

The application of cholinergic antagonists has a negative effect on the dynamics of signal transduction processes both at the neuro-neuronal synapses and at the detrusor, by significantly reducing the amplitude of fEPSPs and APs, respectively, and inhibiting depolarization of the muscle membrane. Adrenergic receptor agonists facilitate the generation of fIPSPs postsynaptically, thus inhibiting the spread of excitation along the parasympathetic pathways and depolarization of the detrusor. As a result, the wall of the bladder either remains relaxed or produces low intensity active forces of contraction $T^a_{l,c} \simeq 0$. Remarkably, the strength of total in-plane forces, T_l and T_c, increase throughout the bioshell while its shape remains unchanged.

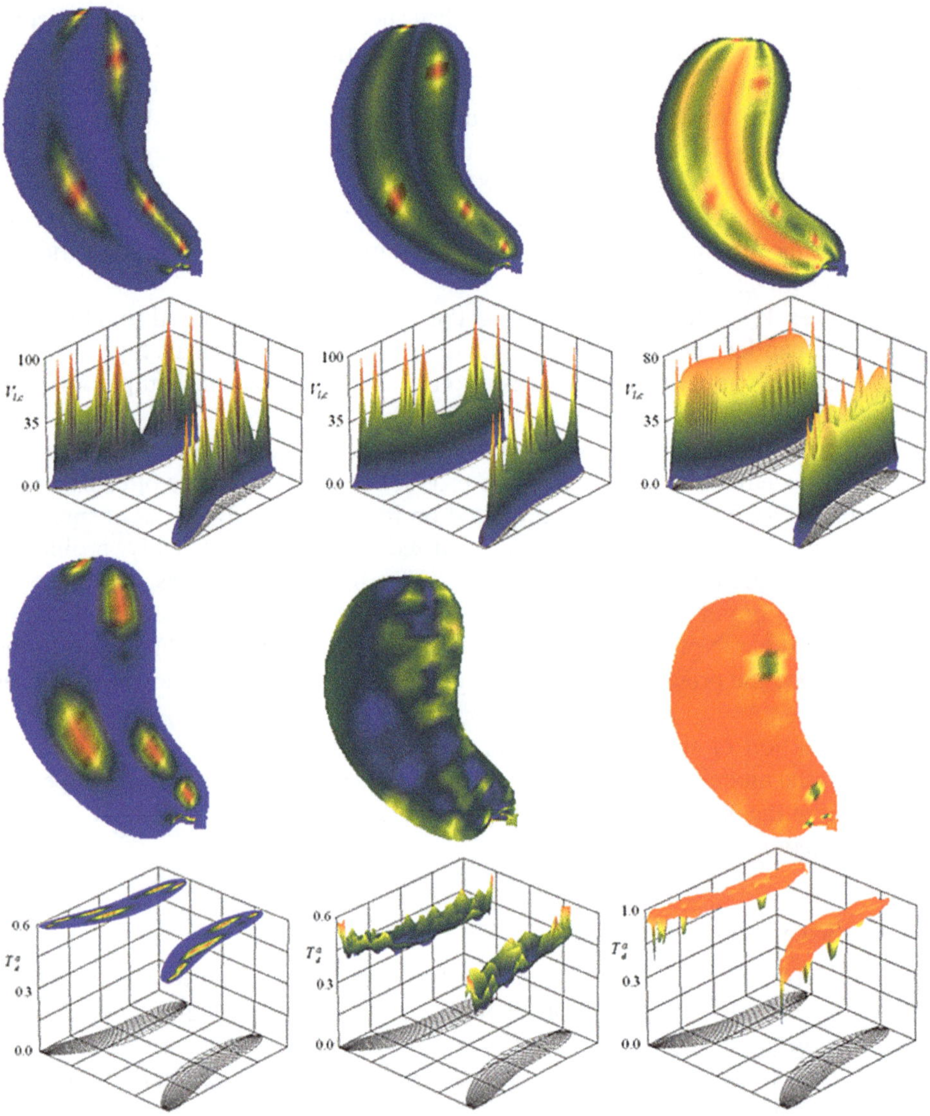

Figure 14.24. Dynamics of contractions of the detrusor as a result of activation of the micturition regulatory mechanisms. Reprinted from Miftahof R M and Nam H G 2013 *Biomechanics of the Human Urinary Bladder* (Berlin: Springer) by permission from Springer Nature. Copyright 2013.

These results are not unexpected and are easy to predict from the reductionist analysis of the neuronal arrangements and detrusor conducted separately. The mysteries of bladder function are concealed in the multifunctional integration of its morphostructural elements. Although the extension of the current model to simulate (i) co-localization and co-transmission by multiple neurotransmitters, (ii) receptor polymodality, (iii) receptor distribution, (iv) mechanical heterogeneity, and (v)

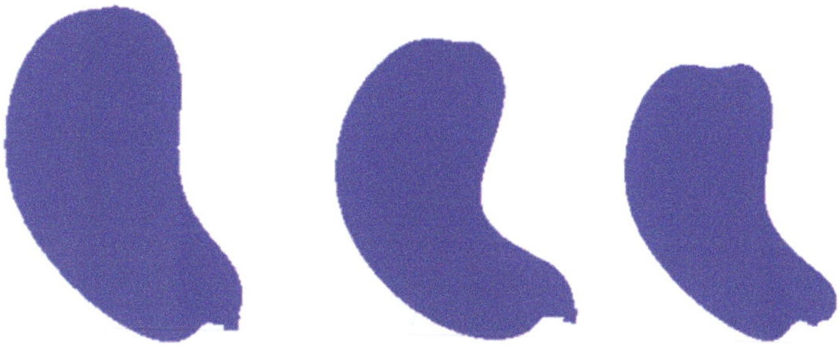

Figure 14.25. Changes in the configuration of the bladder during voiding. Reprinted from Miftahof R M and Nam H G 2013 *Biomechanics of the Human Urinary Bladder* (Berlin: Springer) by permission from Springer Nature. Copyright 2013.

detailed neuromorphological (intraganglionic) ensembles, is beyond the scope of the current book, it is important to recognize their implications on the functionality of the bladder.

Further reading

Bastiaanssen E H C, van Leeuwen J L, Vanderschoot J and Redert P A 1996 *J. Theor. Biol.* **178** 113–33

Fry C H, Sadananda P, Wood D N, Thiruchelvam N, Jabr R I and Clayton R 2011 *Neurourol. Urodyn.* **309** 692–9

Kim J, Lee M K and Choi B 2011 *Int. J. Precis. Eng. Manuf.* **12** 679–85

Mandge D and Manchanda R 2018 *PLoS Comput. Biol.* **14** e1006293

Miftahof R N and Nam H G 2013 *Biomechanics of the Human Urinary Bladder* (Berlin: Springer)

Parekh A, Cigan A D, Wognum S, Heise R L and Chancellor M B 2010 *J. Biomech.* **43** 1708–16

Pérez F M, Chamizo J M G, Payá A S and Fernández D R 2008 *Neurocomput.* **71** 743–54

Wognum S 2010 A multi-phase structural constitutive model for insights into soft tissue remodeling mechanisms *PhD Thesis* University of Pittsburgh, PA, USA

IOP Publishing

Chapter 15

Conclusion

Modeling and models in biomedicine

Recent technological advancements in various fields of applied science have radically transformed the strategies and vision of biomedical research. While only a few decades ago scientists were largely restricted to studying parts of biological systems in isolation, mathematical and computational modeling now enable a holistic approach to the analysis of data spanning multiple biological levels and combining traditionally disconnected fields.

Mathematics is a powerful tool to explore, understand, and predict reality. The mode of operation of mathematics is a model. This constitutes a theoretical projection based on a comprehension of the event, the accuracy of application of physical laws and principles, and the precision of the mathematical formulations and algorithms employed. In addition to summarizing a given set of hypothetical concepts, it also places them in the mind of the user, demanding that he/she conceptualizes a relationship between the object of study and the model. This can bring the system in line with the concepts but it can equally well bring the concepts in line with the system.

The recent explosion in the quantity of experimental data available at the molecular, sub-cellular, and cellular levels has presented difficulties in interpretation when related to the physiological behavior of tissues and organs. This has demanded the development of effective new tools to integrate intricate physiological processes at multiscale levels. Systems biology modeling refers to the application of a systems theory used to study biological functions at various spatiotemporal scales through a common representation. The complexity in this comes from a combination of different factors: (i) a limited knowledge of the underlying mechanisms, (ii) the diversity of spatial and temporal scales, (iii) the range of physicochemical reactions, (iv) the high level of interdependence among functions, and (v) the intrinsic dynamic nonlinearity of processes. To take some examples, the spatial scales span from the gene ($\sim 10^{-10}$ m) to the whole body (~ 1 m) while the temporal scales range from the

doi:10.1088/2053-2563/ab1a9ech15

dynamics of ion channels ($\sim 10^{-6}$ s) to a whole life ($\sim 10^{9}$ s); the level of interdependence emerges from gene and protein interactions with intra- and extracellular structures; nonlinear physicochemical phenomena arise from signal transduction cascades, metabolic pathways, coupled electromechanical processes, etc.

Conventional *in vivo* and *in vitro* approaches have proved inept at unraveling the elaborate pathways of hierarchical interactions. Modern physiological methodologies, including cerebral evoked responses, positron emission tomography scanning, and fMRI, can be employed to study communications among organs in the body. However, none of the existing technologies and clinical protocols offer the desired depth of accessibility to a combined analysis of the underlying functional mechanisms. Most conclusions are drawn from 'technically deficient' experiments providing only an implicit and partial insight into pathological mechanisms and, as a result, can only offer poor prediction and management of many diseases.

To build a biologically feasible mathematical model demands a continuous balanced iteration, i.e. inclusion versus elimination, reduction versus integration, and selection versus rejection, between experimental datasets and theoretical concepts. Promising attempts have been made in developing plausible models of the human heart, the lung, the kidney, and the digestive tract. It is a considerable challenge for the coming years to construct unified biologically realistic mathematical models of all the various organs in the human body incorporating their genes, proteins, and both cellular and tissue diversity.

Before a model can be applied to study a particular system, it has to be evaluated for its accuracy of working hypotheses and for the robustness of its algorithm. This is achieved through a series of test simulations spanning a wide range of empirical conditions, with a subsequent qualitative and quantitative comparison of both theoretical and experimental results. This process is highly dependent on the, at times variable, quality of data input, a condition which has always been a problem with any model. Finally, each model should be transparent with regard to its working hypotheses, its mathematical description, and its method of solution. Unless all requirements are met, any model bears a certain ambiguity and can be accepted only with reservations.

Without the help of mathematical modeling and computer simulation, any understanding of the physiology of the human body will remain inadequate. In this book, only the problems involved in developing and integrating models of a few visceral organs have been touched upon. It is hoped that the ideas put forward will provide both motivation and encouragement for interested readers to undertake new research in the fascinating and rapidly expanding field of computational systems biology.

Lightning Source UK Ltd.
Milton Keynes UK
UKHW051639070120
356513UK00003B/37/P

9 780750 321938